Hepatology: A Handbook of Liver Disease

Hepatology: A Handbook of Liver Disease

Editor: Tiffany Brown

FOSTER ACADEMICS
www.fosteracademics.com

www.fosteracademics.com

FOSTER ACADEMICS

Cataloging-in-Publication Data

Hepatology : a handbook of liver disease / edited by Tiffany Brown.
p. cm.
Includes bibliographical references and index.
ISBN 978-1-63242-955-1
1. Hepatology. 2. Liver--Diseases. 3. Liver--Diseases--Diagnosis. 4. Gastroenterology. I. Brown, Tiffany.
RC845 .H47 2020
616.362--dc23

Foster Academics,
118-35 Queens Blvd., Suite 400,
Forest Hills, NY 11375, USA

ISBN 978-1-63242-955-1 (Hardback)

Contents

Preface

The field of hepatology encompasses the study of the liver, pancreas, gallbladder and biliary tree, as well as their disorders and management. The scope of hepatology is wide, from investigating conditions as varied as drug overdose, fever with features suggestive of a hepatological anomaly, the management of jaundice/ hepatitis, advanced liver disease, systemic diseases of the liver and biliary tree, and cancer. The most common conditions dealt with are viral hepatitis and alcohol related liver pathologies. Hepatitis B virus infects nearly two billion people across the globe and up to 350 million people are persistent carriers. Nearly 80% of all cases of liver cancers may be attributed to hepatitis B or C virus. Excessive alcohol consumption has been linked with the high incidence of cirrhosis. Endoscopic retrograde cholangiopancreatography (ERCP) and transhepatic pancreato-cholangiography (TPC) are two important diagnostic tools for the diagnosis of hepatic diseases. This book discusses the fundamentals as well as modern approaches of hepatologic studies. Also included in this book is a detailed explanation of the various diagnostic tools and treatment procedures in hepatology. The extensive content of this book provides the readers with a thorough understanding of the subject.

After months of intensive research and writing, this book is the end result of all who devoted their time and efforts in the initiation and progress of this book. It will surely be a source of reference in enhancing the required knowledge of the new developments in the area. During the course of developing this book, certain measures such as accuracy, authenticity and research focused analytical studies were given preference in order to produce a comprehensive book in the area of study.

This book would not have been possible without the efforts of the authors and the publisher. I extend my sincere thanks to them. Secondly, I express my gratitude to my family and well-wishers. And most importantly, I thank my students for constantly expressing their willingness and curiosity in enhancing their knowledge in the field, which encourages me to take up further research projects for the advancement of the area.

Editor

Liver Stiffness Value-Based Risk Estimation of Late Recurrence after Curative Resection of Hepatocellular Carcinoma: Development and Validation of a Predictive Model

Kyu Sik Jung[1,§], Ji Hong Kim[1,§], Seung Up Kim[1,2,6,7*], Kijun Song[3], Beom Kyung Kim[1,2,6,7], Jun Yong Park[1,2,6,7], Do Young Kim[1,2,6,7], Sang Hoon Ahn[1,2,6,7], Do Chang Moon[1], In Ji Song[1], Gi Hong Choi[4], Young Nyun Park[5], Kwang-Hyub Han[1,2,6,7]

1 Department of Internal Medicine, Yonsei University College of Medicine, Seoul, Korea, **2** Institute of Gastroenterology, Yonsei University College of Medicine, Seoul, Korea, **3** Department of Biostatistics, Yonsei University College of Medicine, Seoul, Korea, **4** Department of Surgery, Yonsei University College of Medicine, Seoul, Korea, **5** Department of Pathology, Yonsei University College of Medicine, Seoul, Korea, **6** Liver Cancer Special Clinic, Yonsei University College of Medicine, Seoul, Korea, **7** Liver Cirrhosis Clinical Research Center, Seoul, Korea

Abstract

Background: Preoperative liver stiffness (LS) measurement using transient elastography (TE) is useful for predicting late recurrence after curative resection of hepatocellular carcinoma (HCC). We developed and validated a novel LS value-based predictive model for late recurrence of HCC.

Methods: Patients who were due to undergo curative resection of HCC between August 2006 and January 2010 were prospectively enrolled and TE was performed prior to operations by study protocol. The predictive model of late recurrence was constructed based on a multiple logistic regression model. Discrimination and calibration were used to validate the model.

Results: Among a total of 139 patients who were finally analyzed, late recurrence occurred in 44 patients, with a median follow-up of 24.5 months (range, 12.4–68.1). We developed a predictive model for late recurrence of HCC using LS value, activity grade II-III, presence of multiple tumors, and indocyanine green retention rate at 15 min (ICG R15), which showed fairly good discrimination capability with an area under the receiver operating characteristic curve (AUROC) of 0.724 (95% confidence intervals [CIs], 0.632–0.816). In the validation, using a bootstrap method to assess discrimination, the AUROC remained largely unchanged between iterations, with an average AUROC of 0.722 (95% CIs, 0.718–0.724). When we plotted a calibration chart for predicted and observed risk of late recurrence, the predicted risk of late recurrence correlated well with observed risk, with a correlation coefficient of 0.873 ($P<0.001$).

Conclusion: A simple LS value-based predictive model could estimate the risk of late recurrence in patients who underwent curative resection of HCC.

Editor: William Alazawi, Queen Mary University of London, United Kingdom

Funding: This study was supported by the Liver Cirrhosis Clinical Research Center, in part by a grant from the Korea Healthcare technology R & D project, Ministry of Health and Welfare, Republic of Korea (no. HI10C2020), and by the Yonsei Liver Blood Bank (YLBB), in part by a grant from sanofi-aventis Korea. The funders had no role in study design, data collection and analysis, decision to publish, or preparation of the manuscript.

Competing Interests: This study was supported by the Liver Cirrhosis Clinical Research Center, in part by a grant from the Korea Healthcare technology R & D project, Ministry of Health and Welfare, Republic of Korea (no. HI10C2020), and by the Yonsei Liver Blood Bank (YLBB), in part by a grant from sanofi-aventis Korea.

* E-mail: ksukorea@yuhs.ac

§ These authors contributed equally to this work.

Introduction

Hepatic resection is the treatment of choice for hepatocellular carcinoma (HCC) in non-cirrhotic patients and remains the mainstay of treatment in cirrhotic patient with well-preserved liver function.[1] Although adequate patient selection, optimized surgical technique and postoperative management increased treatment efficacy, recurrence remains the main cause of a unsatisfactory long-term prognosis rate after resection of HCC.[2] Thus, identifying risk factors for recurrence after curative resection is important when selecting optimal candidates for resection and predicting a postoperative prognosis.

As recent study revealed that the prognosis and underlying mechanism are different for early and late recurrence, independent risk factors for each type of recurrence have been investigated respectively.[2–5] Among these, advanced liver fibrosis or cirrhosis is a known risk factor for late recurrence, as it contributes to multicentric recurrence at the remnant liver.[2,3,6] Furthermore, advanced liver fibrosis or cirrhosis is closely correlated with the development of postoperative mortality or complications, such as liver failure, worsening encephalopathy, or ascites.[7–9] Thus, a preoperative assessment of liver fibrosis severity is essential for prediction of postoperative outcomes.

Recently, liver stiffness (LS) measurement using transient elastography (TE, FibroScan) has been used to assess the degree of liver fibrosis noninvasively with high reproducibility and reliability.[10,11] After much research into the role of LS value in predicting future development of clinical endpoints such as hepatic decompensation or HCC[12–14], several studies revealed that preoperative LS value could be used in the preoperative setting to predict postoperative outcomes such as hepatic insufficiency or operative blood loss.[7,15] Furthermore, a recent study demonstrated that preoperative LS value was significantly correlated with intrahepatic recurrence after curative resection of HCC, particularly with late recurrence, suggesting that LS value could be used to stratify the risk of recurrence in patients with a remnant fibrotic liver.[16]

Thus, this prospective study was designed to investigate the correlation of LS value with the risk of late recurrence of HCC, and if such a correlation was identified, to construct and validate a LS value-based predictive model for late recurrence in patients who underwent curative resection of HCC.

Materials and Methods

Predictive model derivation

Between August 2006 and January 2010, patients with HCC, who were due to undergo curative resection of HCC at Severance Hospital, Yonsei University College of Medicine, Seoul, Korea, were prospectively enrolled in this study. Inclusion criteria were as follows; (1) age >20 years, (2) volunteered to participate in the study, (3) no previous diagnosis or treatment for HCC. TE was performed after enrollment to obtain preoperative LS value within 1 month prior to the operation by study protocol.

The database of our cohort included information on patient demographics, preoperative laboratory results, preoperative LS values, and pathological results of extracted liver and HCC specimens. The study protocol was consistent with the ethical guidelines of the 1975 Declaration of Helsinki. Written informed consent was obtained from each participant. This study was approved by the Ethics Committee/Independent Institutional Review Board of Severance Hospital, Yonsei University College of Medicine, Seoul, Korea.

Diagnosis of HCC

The preoperative diagnosis of HCC was made based on dynamic imaging studies, biopsy, and alpha-fetoprotein (AFP) serology according to the AASLD guideline.[17] Before surgery, the size, number, and location of HCC, and the presence of extrahepatic metastatic lesions were confirmed by imaging studies including computed tomography (CT), magnetic resonance imaging (MRI), positron emission tomography, and angiography.

Preoperative LS measurement

The principles of LS measurement have been described previously.[10] Briefly, TE generates an elastic wave using a vibrator ultrasound transducer applied to the intercostal spaces at the level of the right lobe of the liver and measures the propagation velocity of the shear wave, which is directly related to LS. LS values were obtained according to the instructions provided by the manufacturer. Immediately after ultrasonographic evaluation of the right hepatic lobe to avoid interference by HCC, LS measurement was performed on the right lobe of the liver through the intercostal spaces on patients lying in the dorsal decubitus position with the right arm in maximal abduction. A single experienced technician (more than 10,000 examinations), who was blind to the patients' clinical data, performed TE. The results were expressed as kilopascals (kPa).

Before surgery, TE was performed once at a single visit and LS values were measured more than 10 times during a single performance of TE. The interquartile range (IQR) was defined as an index of intrinsic variability of LS values corresponding to the interval of LS value containing 50% of the valid measurements between the 25th and 75th percentiles. The median value of successful measurements was selected as representative of the LS values in a given patient. Only LS values with at least 10 validated measurements, an IQR to median value ratio (IQR/M) of <0.3, and a success rate of at least 60% were considered reliable. LS value that did not satisfy these conditions was considered unreliable and excluded from further analysis.

Surgery and follow-up

The time of surgery was determined after diagnostic work up of HCC considering the status of the patient and the operation schedule. All resections were performed by three experienced surgeons (GH Choi, KS Kim, and JS Choi). The type and extent of resection were determined according to tumor size, location, and liver reserve function estimated by the Child-Pugh score and indocyanine green retention rate at 15 min (ICG R15).[18] Intraoperative ultrasonography was performed routinely to determine tumor location and extent and to exclude the presence of additional lesions in the residual liver. Curative resection was defined as a negative histopathological surgical margin and the absence of residual tumor, as demonstrated by abdominal CT scans 1 month after hepatectomy.

Patients were followed up 1 month after surgery and every 3 months thereafter with tumor markers (AFP and des-gamma carboxy prothrombin) and imaging studies including abdominal CT or MRI. Recurrence was diagnosed based on the combined findings of these clinical examinations, and sub-classified as early (<1 year) and late (≥1 year) recurrence [3,19].

Histological evaluation of extracted liver specimens

A histological evaluation of the extracted liver specimens was performed by one experienced hepatopathologist (YN Park) who was blind to the patients' clinical information. Gross tumor classification, tumor size and number, tumor capsule formation and invasion, macroscopic or microscopic vascular invasion, satellite nodule, and the Edmondson-Steiner grade were determined.[20,21] All HCCs were histologically confirmed in 139 patients and tumor stage was determined using the tumor, node, metastasis (TNM) staging system of the American Joint Commission on Cancer (7th edition).[22] _ENREF_20_ENREF_20Liver fibrosis and necroinflammatory activity were evaluated semi-quantitatively in non-cancerous tissues according to the Metavir system.[23] Fibrosis was staged on a 0–4 scale: F0, no fibrosis; F1, portal fibrosis without septa; F2, portal fibrosis and a few septa; F3, numerous septa without cirrhosis and F4, cirrhosis. Histological activity grade (degree of necroinflammatory activity in the lobules and periportal area) was scored as follows: A0, no activity; A1, mild activity; A2, moderate activity and A3, severe activity. Activity grade was defined as lobule or periportal activity (whichever was higher) [23].

Statistical analyses

Data are expressed as means ± standard deviation (SD), medians (range), or n (%), as appropriate. Comparisons between patients with late recurrence and those without were performed using Student's t-test or the Mann-Whitney test for continuous variables and the chi-square or Fisher's exact tests for categorical variables. In a univariate analysis, patient demographics including background liver etiology, preoperative laboratory results including ICG R15, preoperative LS values, surgical factors (types and extent of resections, resection margin, intraoperative blood loss, and perioperative transfusion) and pathological results of the extracted liver (fibrosis and necroinflammatory activity) and HCC (gross tumor classification, tumor size and number, tumor capsule formation and invasion, macroscopic or microscopic vascular invasion, satellite nodule, and the Edmondson-Steiner grade) were evaluated in terms of their relationship with late recurrence. Based on variables with clinical relevance and a univariate statistical significance, multivariate predictive model was constructed using a logistic regression model. The output of the model was expressed as regression coefficients, odd ratios (ORs), and 95% confidence intervals (CIs), which were used to predict late recurrence of HCC.

The model was validated by discrimination and calibration. Discrimination was assessed with the receiver operating characteristic curve, area under the receiver operating characteristic curve (AUROC), sensitivity, and specificity. We calculated the predicted risk of late recurrence based on our predictive model and then estimated the observed risk of late recurrence to assess calibration. Observed risk estimates were plotted against the predicted risk in the group to create a calibration chart. All statistical analyses were conducted using the SAS software, ver. 9.2 (SAS Institute, Cary, NC, USA).

Results

Baseline characteristics

A total of 164 patients with HCC who underwent curative resection of HCC were enrolled. Five patients were excluded due to LS measurement failure (no valid shot) or an unreliable LS value. Thereafter, since the purpose of our study was to investigate the risk factor and construct a model to predict late recurrence of HCC, two patients with perioperative mortality (death within 1 month of the operation) and 18 with early recurrence (<1 year) were also excluded from the analysis (**Fig. 1**). Finally, the study cohort consisted of 139 patients, who were used to develop the predictive model for late recurrence after curative resection. With exception of 16 patients who died during study period due to recurrence, the patients were followed-up until October 2012, and the median follow-up period was 42.9 months (range, 20.4–72.7 months).

The baseline characteristics of the study population are summarized in **Table 1**. Median age (119 males and 20 females) was 59 years. The most common etiology of underlying liver disease was chronic hepatitis B (n = 113, 81.3%). Liver cirrhosis was histologically confirmed in 56 (40.3%) patients. Median tumor size was 3.0 cm, and most tumors (n = 118, 84.9%) were single. According to the TNM staging system, 84 (60.5%) patients were classified as stage I, 7 (5.0%) stage II, and 48 (34.5%) stage IIIA.

Late recurrence was observed in 44 (31.7%) patients at a median of 24.5 months (range, 12.4–68.1 months). Intrahepatic recurrence was identified in all patients with late recurrence. Among these patients, simultaneous extrahepatic metastasis with intrahepatic recurrence were identified in seven patients at the time of recurrence (lung, n = 4; bone, n = 3).

LS values and the performance to predict liver fibrosis

LS value using TE was obtained for all patients within 1 month before surgery (median 5 days; range 1–30 days). The median LS value was 10.5 kPa (range, 4.0–45.0 kPa). LS values according to fibrosis stage were 5.1 kPa for F0-1 (range, 4.1–5.5 kPa), 8.5 kPa for F2 (range, 4.0–35.3 kPa), 9.2 kPa for F3 (range, 4.1–38.0 kPa), and 13.4 kPa for F4 (range, 5.8–45.0 kPa) (**Fig. 2**). The median LS value increased significantly with fibrosis stage (all $P<0.05$). The AUROCs of LS values to predict ≥F2, ≥F3, and F4 were 0.951 (95% CI, 0.913–0.988), 0.796 (95% CI, 0.702–0.889), and 0.837 (95% CI, 0.755–0.919), respectively.

Multivariate logistic regression model

The influence of each variable was tested in a univariate analysis (**Table S1**). In our cohort, ICG R15, the presence of multiple tumors, activity grade II-III, and LS value were significantly related with late recurrence in the univariate analysis (all $P<0.05$), whereas other variables were not statistically significant. A multivariate analysis was performed using the variables that exhibited statistical significance in the univariate analysis. **Table 2** shows the β-regression coefficient estimates in the multivariate logistic regression model. In the multivariate analysis, activity grade II-III, and LS value were identified as independent predictors of late recurrence (all $P<0.05$), whereas ICG R-15 and the presence of multiple tumors did not achieve statistical significance ($P>0.05$).

Development of a predictive model of late HCC recurrence

In addition to the two independent variables (activity grade II-III, and LS value), ICG R-15 and the presence of multiple tumors were also incorporated as constituent variables to develop a predictive model for late HCC recurrence, which is a known significant risk factor for late recurrence.[24,25] This predictive model showed a fairly good discrimination capability, with an AUROC of 0.724 (95% CIs, 0.632–0.816).

$$\text{Probability of recurrence} = \exp(-2.9733 + 0.0616 \times A + 1.2470 \times B + 0.3750 \times C + 0.0213 \times D) \div (1 + \exp(-2.9733 + 0.0616 \times A + 1.2470 \times B + 0.3750 \times C + 0.0213 \times D))$$

Where A = LS value (kPa); B = activity grade II-III (0: no, 1: yes); C = multiple tumors (0: no, 1: yes); D = ICGR15 (%)

Discrimination and calibration

We used a bootstrap method to assess discrimination, in which 1,000 random samples were drawn with replacement from the original dataset, and AUROCs were recalculated in each sample. The AUROCs remained largely unchanged between iterations, with an average AUROC of 0.722 (95% CIs, 0.718–0.724). We plotted a calibration chart that compared the predicted and observed risks of late HCC recurrence (**Fig. 3**). The predicted risk of late recurrence calibrated well with the observed risk, with a correlation coefficient of 0.873($P<0.001$).

Discussion

Although the risk factors for postoperative recurrence have been investigated extensively, few mathematical models are available to

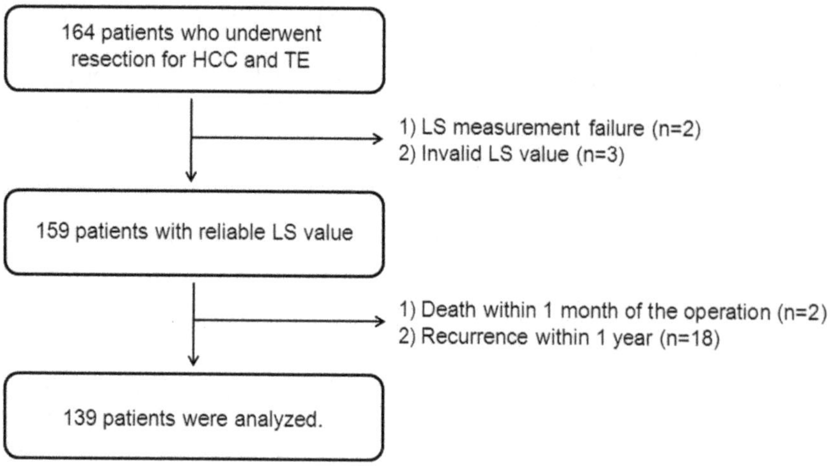

Figure 1. Flow chart of patient selection. A total of 164 patients with HCC undergoing curative resection were recruited. Five patients were excluded due to LS measurement failure or an unreliable LS measurement. Of the 159 patients with a reliable LS value, 20 were excluded due to postoperative death within 1 month, or early recurrence within 1 year. Thus, a total of 139 patients were selected for statistical analysis. HCC, hepatocellular carcinoma; LS, liver stiffness measurement.

Table 1. Baseline characteristics (n = 139).

Variable	
Host factors	
Age (years)	59 (32–80)
Male	119 (85.6)
Body mass index (kg/m^2)	23.3 (15.9–32.5)
Etiology, HBV/HCV/non-B non-C	113 (81.3)/11 (7.9)/15 (10.8)
Total bilirubin (mg/dL)	0.7±0.2
Albumin (g/dL)	4.3±0.4
Prothrombin time (%)	93.1±7.6
Aspartate aminotransferase (IU/L)	35.5±17.9
Alanine aminotransferase (IU/L)	40.0±30.1
Alpha-fetoprotein (ng/mL)	24.4 (1–83,000)
Des-gamma carboxy prothrombin (mAU/mL)	56.0 (5–2,000)
Indocyanine green retention rate at 15 min (%)	8.5 (1.0–31.2)
Tumor factors	
Tumor size (cm)	3.0 (1.0–9.5)
Tumor number, single/multiple	118 (84.9)/21 (15.1)
Tumor stage, I/II/IIIA	84 (60.4)/7 (5.0)/48 (34.5)
Portal vein invasion	9 (6.5)
Satellite nodule	3 (2.2)
Edmonson-Steiner grade, I-II, III-IV	97 (69.8)/42 (30.2)
Non-tumor liver pathology	
F0-1/F2/F3/F4	5 (3.6)/44 (31.7)/34 (24.5)/56 (40.3)
A1/A2/A3	47 (33.8)/89 (64.0)/3 (2.2)
Liver stiffness measurement	
Liver stiffness value (kPa)	10.5 (4.0–45.0)
Interquartile range (kPa)	1.6 (0.3–9.8)
Success rate (%)	97.0 (63–100)

Variables are expressed as median (range) or n (%).
HBV, hepatitis B virus; HCV, hepatitis C virus; kPa, kilopascal.

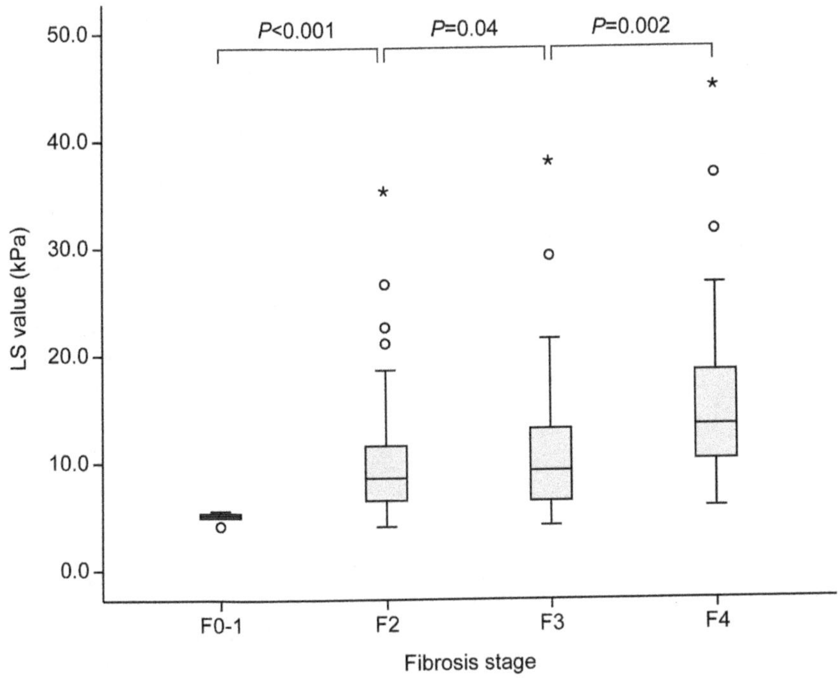

Figure 2. Distribution of LS values according to fibrosis stage. The median LS value increased significantly with fibrosis stage (P<0.001). LS, liver stiffness.

predict recurrence after resection of HCC. [26–29] As none of the previous models included the effect of fibrosis in the formula, this is the first study to validate a specified prediction model for late recurrence of HCC based on LS value, which accurately reflects the burden of liver fibrosis. Finally, this study demonstrated that LS value-based predictive model could estimate the risk of late recurrence in patients who have undergone curative resection of HCC with considerable accuracy.

Compared to other risk factors, for a long time, the impact of liver fibrosis on recurrence has generally been underestimated. In previous studies, the influence of liver fibrosis was attenuated by other risk factors such as pathological factors, because recurrence was not classified into early and late one.[2,28,30] However, when types of recurrence were considered in the analysis, advanced liver fibrosis was selected as one of the independent risk factors for late recurrence.[3,16,24,31] Additionally, as advances in surgical technique and proper patient selection have reduced early recurrence, which has a poorer prognosis than late recurrence, the effect of underlying fibrosis on long-term prognosis has gained greater importance. Despite its clinical importance, in most cases, it is difficult to assess histological staging of liver fibrosis prior to surgical resection. This suggests the need for a preoperative and non-invasive method of estimating liver fibrosis for selecting optimal candidates for resection or making individualized treatment and follow-up plans.

Recently, it has been proposed that preoperative LS value assessed using TE is significantly associated with recurrence, suggesting that clinicians can estimate fibrosis status noninvasively and accurately before surgery.[16] Consistently, preoperative LS value was selected as independent risk factor for late recurrence in this study, whereas histological fibrosis stage was not significant even in a univariate analysis.[16] These results might suggest that risk stratification using preoperative LS value could add more prognostic information for patients undergoing resection regardless of the histological findings, as LS might enable more precise quantification of liver fibrosis, expressed as continuous values, than simple stepwise histological grading. These findings also support a theoretical concept that the main mechanism of late recurrence is *de novo* development of HCC from a remnant fibrotic liver, rather than from dissemination of primary tumor cells [2].

Because the mechanism of late recurrence could not be explained solely by liver fibrosis, we developed a prediction model that included other important clinical factors and that could be validated internally. At first, as necroinflammatory activity was

Table 2. Multivariate analysis to identify independent predictors ofHCC occurrence.

Factor	Beta	*P* value	Odd ratios (95% CIs)
ICG R15	0.0213	0.5715	1.022 (0.949–1.100)
Multiple tumors	0.3750	0.4565	1.455 (0.542–3.904)
Activity grade II-III	1.2470	0.0121	3.480 (1.313–9.221)
Liver stiffness value	0.0616	0.0172	1.063 (1.011–1.119)

HCC, hepatocellular carcinoma; CIs, confidence intervals; ICG R15, Indocyanine green retention rate at 15 min (%).

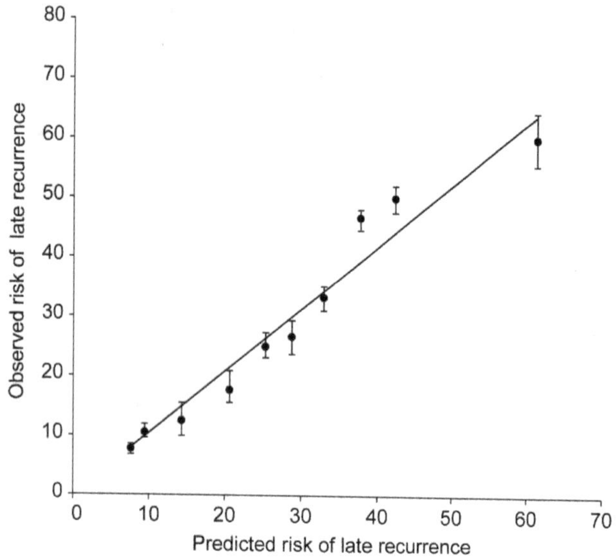

Figure 3. Calibration chart for predicted versus observed risk of late recurrence after curative resection of HCC. The predicted risk of recurrence calibrated well with the observed risk, with a correlation coefficient of 0.873 (P<0.001).HCC, hepatocellular carcinoma.

significantly associated with late recurrence in the multivariate analysis, consistent with previous studies, it was included in our predicting model.[24,32,33] Because liver fibrosis and necroinflammation are associated with a risk of carcinogenesis, it may enhance the performance to assess the risk of HCC development by incorporating simultaneously LS value and necroinflammatory activity into our prediction model.[4,17] _ENREF_17Nevertheless, there can be a concern regarding potential overestimation of the influence of necroinflammation on LS values, which affected the overall performance of our prediction model.[34,35] However, because we did not detect a correlation between LS and necroinflammatory activity in our patient cohort in a univariate analysis (P>0.05 by Spearman's correlation analysis), it was possible to use these two variables which reflect the degree of fibrosis and activity for our prediction model.

In addition, ICG R15, which had significant correlation with late recurrence in a univariate analysis, was included in our prediction model. Indeed, ICG R15 was significantly correlated with late recurrence in previous studies.[4,24] _ENREF_24Although ICG R15 has been used to estimate remnant liver function after hepatectomy[18], the value of ICG R15 for predicting late recurrence was attenuated in our cohort. However, because ICG R15 could reflect the degree of functional liver status by estimating hepatic metabolic capacity whereas LS values could reflect the degree of physical status of liver fibrosis, we incorporated ICG R15 in our prediction model based on the hypothesis that the combination of these two parameters would strengthen the accuracy of our prediction model. Lastly, the presence of multiple tumors was included in our prediction models. Previous studies have demonstrated that the presence of multiple tumors was significantly related to late recurrence, suggesting that tumor multiplicity reflects increased carcinogenicity of the background liver.[2,4] In this study, the presence of multiple tumors, which was confirmed histologically, was successfully diagnosed by radiological methods in all patients prior to resection. This result suggests that an advanced imaging modality can detect multiple tumors sensitively, thus the presence of multiple tumors, which was assessed by preoperative imaging, could be incorporated in the model.

Our new prediction model consisted of four variables: LS value, activity grade, presence of multiple tumors, and ICG R15, but other risk factors such as vascular invasion, tumor differentiation, and preoperative AFP level were not included in our model. Although these factors were identified as significant risk factors of recurrence in previous studies[36,37], they did not achieve significance, even in the univariate analysis in this study. Additionally, because these factors did not enhance accuracy of our model, they were excluded from our final prediction model.

Although our study proposed a LS values-based HCC prediction model after curative resection, several issues remain unresolved in our study. First, this prediction model was developed using a relatively small sized cohort with various liver disease etiologies and validated internally and its accuracy seemed modest (AUROC = 0.724). Although, the etiology of liver disease was not significantly related to late recurrence in this study, consistently with the results of previous studies (P>0.05), further research with a larger and more homogenous study population should be followed by external validation.[2] Second, cross-sectional methods of identifying the risk factors for late recurrence in a cohort with variable follow-up time and exclusion of patients with early recurrence might lead to a selection bias. However, because the aim of our study was to develop a model to predict the risk of late recurrence itself, not the increasing risk of late recurrence over time, we used logistic regression instead of longitudinal statistical methods. Additionally, a short follow-up time less than 3 years was identified in 10 patients who died after recurrence and the remaining patients (n = 129) were followed up more than 3 years, suggesting that the current cross-sectional approach might be adequate for our cohort to compensate for the wide range of follow-up durations. Similar to our work, previous studies used cross-sectional methods to identify the risk factors for the late recurrence after resection of HCC.[3,38] However, additional studies of a prediction model based on a survival analysis, such as Cox-regression or standardization of follow-up time, are required in the future. Third, as histological necroinflammatory activity grade was included, our model cannot be used prior to resection. Consequently, it does not seem feasible to use this model for stratification of an appropriate treatment modality such as liver transplantation, instead of surgical resection, especially for patients at high risk of recurrence after resection. Thus, it will be important to determine whether other noninvasive surrogate markers of the degree of necroinflammatory activity grade may be used as a preoperative risk calculator. Serum aminotransferase or apolipoprotein A1 are possible candidates as they revealed a significant correlation with necroinflammatory activity in a previous study.[39] Lastly, this model did not include gene expression profiles of surrounding non-cancerous liver tissue, which has been emphasized in recent studies as a significant risk factor for late recurrence after curative resection for HCC.[40,41] However, from a different point of view, our results might suggest the importance of the characteristics of the remnant liver, such as LS values, ICG R15, and necroinflammation in predicting late recurrence in patients who have undergone curative resection of HCC.

In conclusion, this study constructed and validated a novel LS value-based model for predicting late HCC recurrence. This model, which involved tumor and non-tumor characteristics, demonstrated acceptable accuracy in patients who underwent curative resection of HCC. However, further studies with a larger sample size are warranted for external validation of our prediction model.

Acknowledgments

The authors are grateful to Dong-Su Jang, (Medical Illustrator, Medical Research Support Section, Yonsei University College of Medicine, Seoul, Korea) for his help with the figures.

Author Contributions

Conceived and designed the experiments: SUK KJS. Analyzed the data: SUK KJS KSJ. Contributed reagents/materials/analysis tools: JHK BKK JYP DYK SHA GHC YNP KHH IJS DCM. Wrote the paper: KSJ JHK SUK.

References

1. Llovet JM, Schwartz M, Mazzaferro V (2005) Resection and liver transplantation for hepatocellular carcinoma. Semin Liver Dis. 25: 181–200.
2. Tung-Ping Poon R, Fan ST, Wong J (2000) Risk factors, prevention, and management of postoperative recurrence after resection of hepatocellular carcinoma. Ann Surg 232: 10–24.
3. Poon RT, Fan ST, Ng IO, Lo CM, Liu CL, et al. (2000) Different risk factors and prognosis for early and late intrahepatic recurrence after resection of hepatocellular carcinoma. Cancer. 89: 500–507.
4. Imamura H, Matsuyama Y, Tanaka E, Ohkubo T, Hasegawa K, et al. (2003) Risk factors contributing to early and late phase intrahepatic recurrence of hepatocellular carcinoma after hepatectomy. J Hepatol. 38: 200–207.
5. Qu LS, Jin F, Huang XW, Shen XZ (2010) High hepatitis B viral load predicts recurrence of small hepatocellular carcinoma after curative resection. J Gastrointest Surg. 14: 1111–1120. Epub 2010 Apr 1127.
6. Sasaki Y, Imaoka S, Masutani S, Ohashi I, Ishikawa O, et al. (1992) Influence of coexisting cirrhosis on long-term prognosis after surgery in patients with hepatocellular carcinoma. Surgery 112: 515–521.
7. Kim SU, Ahn SH, Park JY, Kim do Y, Chon CY, et al. (2008) Prediction of postoperative hepatic insufficiency by liver stiffness measurement (FibroScan((R))) before curative resection of hepatocellular carcinoma: a pilot study. Hepatol Int. 2: 471–477. Epub 2008 Sep 2009.
8. van den Broek MA, Olde Damink SW, Dejong CH, Lang H, Malago M, et al. (2008) Liver failure after partial hepatic resection: definition, pathophysiology, risk factors and treatment. Liver Int. 28: 767–780.
9. Friedman LS (2010) Surgery in the patient with liver disease. Trans Am Clin Climatol Assoc. 121: 192–204; discussion 205.
10. Sandrin L, Fourquet B, Hasquenoph JM, Yon S, Fournier C, et al. (2003) Transient elastography: a new noninvasive method for assessment of hepatic fibrosis. Ultrasound Med Biol. 29: 1705–1713.
11. Jung KS, Kim SU (2012) Clinical applications of transient elastography. Clin Mol Hepatol. 18: 163–173. doi: 110.3350/cmh.2012.3318.3352.3163. Epub 2012 Jun 3326.
12. Jung KS, Kim SU, Ahn SH, Park YN, Kim do Y, et al. (2011) Risk assessment of hepatitis B virus-related hepatocellular carcinoma development using liver stiffness measurement (FibroScan). Hepatology. 53: 885–894. doi: 810.1002/hep.24121. Epub 22011 Feb 24111.
13. Chon YE, Jung ES, Park JY, Kim do Y, Ahn SH, et al. (2012) The accuracy of noninvasive methods in predicting the development of hepatocellular carcinoma and hepatic decompensation in patients with chronic hepatitis B. J Clin Gastroenterol. 46: 518–525. doi: 510.1097/MCG.1090b1013e31825079f31825071
14. Kim SU, Lee JH, Kim do Y, Ahn SH, Jung KS, et al. (2012) Prediction of liver-related events using fibroscan in chronic hepatitis B patients showing advanced liver fibrosis. PLoS One. 7: e36676. doi: 36610.31371/journal.pone.0036676. Epub 0032012 May 0036674.
15. Wong JS, Wong GL, Chan AW, Wong VW, Cheung YS, et al. (2013) Liver stiffness measurement by transient elastography as a predictor on posthepatectomy outcomes. Ann Surg. 257: 922–928. doi: 910.1097/SLA.1090-b1013e318269d318262ec
16. Jung KS, Kim SU, Choi GH, Park JY, Park YN, et al. (2012) Prediction of recurrence after curative resection of hepatocellular carcinoma using liver stiffness measurement (FibroScan(R)). Ann Surg Oncol. 19: 4278–4286. doi: 4210.1245/s10434-10012-12422-10433. Epub 12012 Jul 10433.
17. Bruix J, Sherman M (2011) Management of hepatocellular carcinoma: an update. Hepatology. 53: 1020–1022. doi: 1010.1002/hep.24199
18. Makuuchi M, Sano K (2004) The surgical approach to HCC: our progress and results in Japan. Liver Transpl. 10: S46–52.
19. Shimada M, Takenaka K, Gion T, Fujiwara Y, Kajiyama K, et al. (1996) Prognosis of recurrent hepatocellular carcinoma: a 10-year surgical experience in Japan. Gastroenterology. 111: 720–726.
20. Edmondson HA, Steiner PE (1954) Primary carcinoma of the liver: a study of 100 cases among 48,900 necropsies. Cancer 7: 462–503.
21. Kanai T, Hirohashi S, Upton MP, Noguchi M, Kishi K, et al. (1987) Pathology of small hepatocellular carcinoma. A proposal for a new gross classification. Cancer 60: 810–819.
22. Edge S, Byrd DR, Compton CC, Fritz AG, Greene FL, et al. (2010) AJCC cancer staging handbook. New York: Springer-Verlag. 237–245 p.
23. Bedossa P, Poynard T (1996) An algorithm for the grading of activity in chronic hepatitis C. The METAVIR Cooperative Study Group. Hepatology. 24: 289–293.
24. Wu JC, Huang YH, Chau GY, Su CW, Lai CR, et al. (2009) Risk factors for early and late recurrence in hepatitis B-related hepatocellular carcinoma. J Hepatol. 51: 890–897. doi: 810.1016/j.jhep.2009.1007.1009. Epub 2009 Jul 1023.
25. Mazzaferro V, Romito R, Schiavo M, Mariani L, Camerini T, et al. (2006) Prevention of hepatocellular carcinoma recurrence with alpha-interferon after liver resection in HCV cirrhosis. Hepatology. 44: 1543–1554.
26. Huang X, Wei W, Ya N, Zeng J, Zeng Y, et al. (2013) A mathematical model to predict short-term recurrence and metastasis of primary hepatocellular carcinoma larger than 10 cm in diameter. Hepatogastroenterology. 60: 225–230. doi: 210.5754/hge
27. Zhao WH, Ma ZM, Zhou XR, Feng YZ, Fang BS (2002) Prediction of recurrence and prognosis in patients with hepatocellular carcinoma after resection by use of CLIP score. World J Gastroenterol. 8: 237–242.
28. Okada S, Shimada K, Yamamoto J, Takayama T, Kosuge T, et al. (1994) Predictive factors for postoperative recurrence of hepatocellular carcinoma. Gastroenterology. 106: 1618–1624.
29. Woo HG, Park ES, Cheon JH, Kim JH, Lee JS, et al. (2008) Gene expression-based recurrence prediction of hepatitis B virus-related human hepatocellular carcinoma. Clin Cancer Res. 14: 2056–2064. doi: 2010.1158/1078-0432.CCR-2007-1473
30. Ng IO, Lai EC, Fan ST, Ng MM, So MK (1995) Prognostic significance of pathologic features of hepatocellular carcinoma. A multivariate analysis of 278 patients. Cancer. 76: 2443–2448.
31. Ko S, Kanehiro H, Hisanaga M, Nagao M, Ikeda N, et al. (2002) Liver fibrosis increases the risk of intrahepatic recurrence after hepatectomy for hepatocellular carcinoma. Br J Surg. 89: 57–62.
32. Hanazaki K, Matsushita A, Nakagawa K, Misawa R, Amano J (2005) Risk factors of intrahepatic recurrence after curative resection of hepatocellular carcinoma. Hepatogastroenterology. 52: 580–586.
33. Ko S, Nakajima Y, Kanehiro H, Hisanaga M, Aomatsu Y, et al. (1996) Significant influence of accompanying chronic hepatitis status on recurrence of hepatocellular carcinoma after hepatectomy. Result of multivariate analysis. Ann Surg. 224: 591–595.
34. Oliveri F, Coco B, Ciccorossi P, Colombatto P, Romagnoli V, et al. (2008) Liver stiffness in the hepatitis B virus carrier: a non-invasive marker of liver disease influenced by the pattern of transaminases. World J Gastroenterol. 14: 6154–6162.
35. Kim SU, Kim JK, Park YN, Han KH (2012) Discordance between liver biopsy and Fibroscan(R) in assessing liver fibrosis in chronic hepatitis b: risk factors and influence of necroinflammation. PLoS One. 7: e32233. doi: 32210.31371/journal.pone.0032233. Epub 0032012 Feb 0032223.
36. Yamamoto J, Kosuge T, Takayama T, Shimada K, Yamasaki S, et al. (1996) Recurrence of hepatocellular carcinoma after surgery. Br J Surg. 83: 1219–1222.
37. Li T, Qin LX, Gong X, Zhou J, Sun HC, et al. (2013) Hepatitis B virus surface antigen-negative and hepatitis C virus antibody-negative hepatocellular carcinoma: clinical characteristics, outcome, and risk factors for early and late intrahepatic recurrence after resection. Cancer. 119: 126–135. doi: 110.1002/cncr.27697. Epub 22012 Jun 27626.
38. Portolani N, Coniglio A, Ghidoni S, Giovanelli M, Benetti A, et al. (2006) Early and late recurrence after liver resection for hepatocellular carcinoma: prognostic and therapeutic implications. Ann Surg 243: 229–235.
39. Cheong JY, Kim DJ, Hwang SG, Yang JM, Kim YB, et al. (2011) Serum markers for necroinflammatory activity in patients with chronic viral hepatitis and normal or mildly elevated aminotransferase levels. Liver Int. 31: 1352–1358. doi: 1310.1111/j.1478-3231.2011.02570.x. Epub 02011 Jun 02523.
40. Sato F, Hatano E, Kitamura K, Myomoto A, Fujiwara T, et al. (2011) MicroRNA profile predicts recurrence after resection in patients with hepatocellular carcinoma within the Milan Criteria. PLoS One. 6: e16435. doi: 16410.11371/journal.pone.0016435
41. Hoshida Y, Villanueva A, Kobayashi M, Peix J, Chiang DY, et al. (2008) Gene expression in fixed tissues and outcome in hepatocellular carcinoma. N Engl J Med. 359: 1995–2004. doi: 1910.1056/NEJMoa0804525. Epub 0802008 Oct 0804515.

2

The Osteopontin Level in Liver, Adipose Tissue and Serum is Correlated with Fibrosis in Patients with Alcoholic Liver Disease

Stéphanie Patouraux[1,2,3], Stéphanie Bonnafous[1,4], Cosmin S. Voican[5,6,10], Rodolphe Anty[1,2,4], Marie-Christine Saint-Paul[1,2,3], Maria-Alessandra Rosenthal-Allieri[8], Hélène Agostini[5,6,7], Micheline Njike[5,6,7], Nadége Barri-Ova[5,6,7], Sylvie Naveau[5,6,7], Yannick Le Marchand-Brustel[1,2,4], Pascal Veillon[9], Paul Calès[9], Gabriel Perlemuter[5,6,7], Albert Tran[1,2,4], Philippe Gual[1,2,4]*

1 INSERM, U1065, Equipe 8 «Complications hépatiques de l'obésité», Nice, France, **2** Université de Nice-Sophia Antipolis, Faculté de Médecine, Nice, France, **3** Centre Hospitalier Universitaire de Nice, Hôpital de l'Archet, Département de Biologie, Nice, France, **4** Centre Hospitalier Universitaire de Nice, Hôpital de l'Archet, Département Digestif, Nice, France, **5** INSERM, U996, IPSIT, Clamart, France, **6** Univ. Paris-Sud, Faculté de Médecine Paris-Sud, Kremlin-Bicêtre, France, **7** AP-HP, Hôpital Antoine Béclère, Service d'hépato-gastroentérologie, Clamart, France, **8** Centre Hospitalier Universitaire de Nice, Hôpital de l'Archet, Département d'Immunologie, Nice, France, **9** Centre Hospitalier Universitaire d'Angers, Service d'Hépatologie, Angers, France, **10** Universitatea de Medicina si Farmacie Craiova, Craiova, Romania

Abstract

Background: Osteopontin (OPN) plays an important role in the progression of chronic liver diseases. We aimed to quantify the liver, adipose tissue and serum levels of OPN in heavy alcohol drinkers and to compare them with the histological severity of hepatic inflammation and fibrosis.

Methodology/Principal Findings: OPN was evaluated in the serum of a retrospective and prospective group of 109 and 95 heavy alcohol drinkers, respectively, in the liver of 34 patients from the retrospective group, and in the liver and adipose tissue from an additional group of 38 heavy alcohol drinkers. Serum levels of OPN increased slightly with hepatic inflammation and progressively with the severity of hepatic fibrosis. Hepatic OPN expression correlated with hepatic inflammation, fibrosis, TGFβ expression, neutrophils accumulation and with the serum OPN level. Interestingly, adipose tissue OPN expression also correlated with hepatic fibrosis even after 7 days of alcohol abstinence. The elevated serum OPN level was an independent risk factor in estimating significant ($F \geq 2$) fibrosis in a model combining alkaline phosphatase, albumin, hemoglobin, OPN and FibroMeter® levels. OPN had an area under the receiving operator curve that estimated significant fibrosis of 0.89 and 0.88 in the retrospective and prospective groups, respectively. OPN, Hyaluronate (AUROC: 0.88), total Cytokeratin 18 (AUROC: 0.83) and FibroMeter® (AUROC: 0.90) estimated significance to the same extent in the retrospective group. Finally, the serum OPN levels also correlated with hepatic fibrosis and estimated significant ($F \geq 2$) fibrosis in 86 patients with chronic hepatitis C, which suggested that its elevated level could be a general response to chronic liver injury.

Conclusion/Significance: OPN increased in the liver, adipose tissue and serum with liver fibrosis in alcoholic patients. Further, OPN is a new relevant biomarker for significant liver fibrosis. OPN could thus be an important actor in the pathogenesis of this chronic liver disease.

Editor: Wing-Kin Syn, Institute of Hepatology London, United Kingdom

Funding: This work was supported by grants from the Institut National de la Santé et de la Recherche Médicale (France), the University of Nice, the Programme Hospitalier de Recherche Clinique (Centre Hospitalier Universitaire de Nice), and charities (AFEF/Schering-Plough and AFEF/ROCHE to PG and AT). SP was supported by the Fondation Recherche Médicale. PG is the recipient of an Interface Grant from Centre Hospitalier Universitaire de Nice. The funders had no role in the study design, data collection and analysis, decision to publish, or preparation of the manuscript.

Competing Interests: The authors have read the journal's policy and have the following conflicts: PC has mentioned potential conflict of interest due to stock ownership in a company (BioLiveScale) that owns the license for FibroMeters, which is patented by the University of Angers. PC has consultancy and stock ownership with BioLiveScale.

* E-mail: gual@unice.fr

These authors contributed equally to this work.

Introduction

Excessive alcohol consumption is the third leading preventable cause of death in the United States [1]. Regular alcohol use can result in hepatic steatosis, which eventually progresses to steatohepatitis, fibrosis and cirrhosis. Up to 40% of patients with severe acute alcoholic hepatitis die within six months [1]. A better understanding of the molecular mechanisms leading to the progression of liver disease and the identification of new potential actors of the pathogenesis of alcoholic liver diseases (ALD) are thus important challenges. Modification of gut permeability, production of acetaldehyde, NADH and ROS, activation of Endoplasmic

Reticulum stress, recruitment of immune cells into the liver and hepatocyte apoptosis may be key mechanisms of alcohol-induced liver injury [1,2]. In line with the involvement of death of hepatocytes, we recently showed that serum markers of hepatocyte death and apoptosis are non invasive biomarkers of advanced fibrosis in patients with alcoholic liver disease [3]. Others factors involved in the pathogenesis of ALD can originate from extra-hepatic sites, particularly adipose tissue. The pioneers in this field have reported excess weight to be an independent risk factor for steatosis, acute alcoholic hepatitis (AAH) and cirrhosis in patients with ALD [4]; body mass index (BMI) is an independent risk factor for fibrosis in non-obese alcoholic patients [5] and high blood pressure, apolipoprotein A-1 concentration and BMI are predictive of steatosis [6]. More recently, Naveau *et al.* demonstrated that adipose tissue inflammation correlated with the severity of pathological features in the liver of alcoholic patients [7].

Recently, altered hepatic expression of osteopontin (OPN), a Th1 cytokine, chemokine and profibrogenic extracellular matrix protein, has been reported in an animal model of alcohol-induced liver injury [8,9,10] and in the liver of patients with alcoholic hepatitis and fibrosis [11,12]. In female rats fed an ethanol containing Lieber-DeCarli liquid diet for 6 weeks and then challenged with LPS, the elevated circulating and hepatic levels of OPN play an important role in neutrophil accumulation and liver injury [8,10,13,14]. OPN could also be involved in fibrogenesis. Indeed, OPN was upregulated in rodent liver fibrosis models [15,16,17] and in activated hepatic stellate cells [17,18,19]. OPN was required for myofibroblast differentiation [20] and upregulation of OPN expression in the liver of patients with ALD-cirrhosis was recently reported [12].

Similarly, OPN appears to play an important role in the occurrence of liver complications in a mouse model of non alcoholic fatty liver disease (NAFLD) [15,21,22,23]. We also reported recently that the elevated expression of OPN was associated with adipose tissue macrophage accumulation and liver steatosis in humans [24] and evidence of OPN overexpression with progressive NAFLD has been confirmed recently [12].

Based on the evidence that OPN can be considered as a potential actor in alcohol-induced hepatic complications in rodents, we focused our study on serum, liver and adipose tissue OPN levels in patients with ALD and searched for a correlation with the disease severity. The evaluation of this marker in estimating significant fibrosis was also examined

Materials and Methods

Study population

1) Alcoholic patients. Estimation group: From October 1997 to June 1998, 109 consecutive heavy alcohol drinkers (82 males, 27 females, 47±1 years old) admitted to our Liver unit for detoxification and/or inpatient rehabilitation were entered into this study as previously described [3,25,26]. **Validation group:** 95 additional consecutive heavy alcohol drinkers (73 males, 22 females, 48±9 years old) were entered into this study from November 2006 to December 2009. All patients had consumed over 80 g ethanol per day for more than 5 years. All patients were negative for circulating hepatitis B surface antigen, hepatitis C virus, and human immunodeficiency virus. No patient had osteoarthritis or rheumatoid arthritis. Fasting blood samples were obtained and used to measure alanine amino transferase (ALT), aspartate aminotransferase (AST), gamma glutamyl transferase (γGT). A needle liver biopsy was performed in all patients by the transparietal approach. Biopsies were processed routinely and stained with hematoxylin-eosin-saffron and Sirius Red. The quality of biopsies was sufficient for interpretation [27]. The length of the liver biopsy was over 15 mm. Histopathological features were semi-quantitatively evaluated (**Table 1**): the grade of steatosis (0, <5%; 1, 5%–30%; 2, >30%–60%; 3, >60%) and stage of fibrosis (from 0, none, to 4, cirrhosis). The grading of hepatic inflammation was done according to the Activity score of Orrego et al. [28]. Briefly, hepatic inflammation was determined by the presence (I1) or absence (I0) of hepatocellular necrosis and ballooning degeneration, alcoholic Mallory's hyaline bodies, associated with an inflammatory reaction. Sera and liver tissues were stored at −80°C until use. **Second gene group:** 38 consecutive heavy alcohol drinkers admitted to the Hepatogastroenterology Department of Antoine Béclère University Hospital, Clamart, France, due to alcoholism and ALD, were prospectively included into this study. All patients underwent ultrasound-guided liver biopsy at admission. One specimen of liver tissue was used for histological analysis and another was immediately frozen in liquid nitrogen and stored at −80°C for subsequent RNA extraction. Specimens were stained with hematoxylin-eosin-saffron, Masson's trichrome and picrosirius red. All biopsy samples were evaluated by a pathologist blind to the patient's clinical and biological data and to the duration of alcoholism and daily alcohol intake. Histopathological features were evaluated semi-quantitatively as described above (**Table 1**). Subcutaneous adipose tissue biopsies were performed at admission and after 7 days of abstinence from ethanol consumption. Adipose tissue samples were removed by needle aspiration as previously described [7]. **2) Patients with chronic viral hepatitis C.** 86 patients with chronic viral hepatitis C were included from June 1999 to May 2009. Anti-HCV antibodies and HCV RNA were detected in their serum. Selected patients had an available liver biopsy and some blood markers. Fasting blood samples were collected immediately before or no more than 12 months after liver biopsy. Exclusion criteria comprised additional causes of liver disease, particularly HBV and HIV infections, complicated cirrhosis, anti-fibrotic treatment in the previous 6 months, alcohol consumption of more than 30 g/day in the five years prior to inclusion. Liver biopsies were performed using Menghini's technique with a 1.4–1.6 mm diameter needle. Biopsy specimens were fixed in a formalin–alcohol–acetic solution and embedded in paraffin; 5-µm thick sections were then cut and stained with hematoxylin–eosin–saffron. Liver fibrosis was staged from F0 to F4 according to the Metavir staging system [29]. The diagnostic target, significant fibrosis, was defined as follows: F2+F3+F4. Readings were performed by independent, senior pathologists specialized in hepatology. These pathologists were blinded to blood tests. **3) Obese patients.** Obese patients were recruited through the Department of Digestive Surgery and Liver Transplantation, where they underwent bariatric surgery for morbid obesity (Nice and Paris hospitals). Bariatric surgery was indicated for these patients in accordance with the French Guidelines for surgery for obesity. Briefly, they had a BMI of 40 or 35 kg/m^2 with at least one complication. Exclusion criteria were as follows: presence of a hepatitis B or hepatitis C virus infection, excessive alcohol consumption (>20 g/day), or another cause of chronic liver diseases (primary biliary cirrhosis, autoimmune hepatitis, Wilson disease, genetic hemochromatosis, or biliary disease). Fasting blood samples were obtained before surgery. Surgical liver biopsies were obtained at the time of bariatric surgery. Liver bridging fibrosis was assessed by sirius red staining and was classified into five stages as follows: absent, mild, significant (incomplete septa), advanced (with complete septa) and cirrhotic.

All subjects gave their informed written consent to participate in this research study according to French legislation regarding Ethics and Human Research (Huriet-Serusclat law, the "Comité

Table 1. Characteristics of the Estimation, Second Gene and Validation groups.

	Estimation group		Second gene group	Validation group
	Serum	Liver	Adipose tissue and liver	Serum
N (female/male)	109 (27/82)	34 (5/29)	38 (7/31)	95 (22/73)
Age (years)	47±1	47±1	47±1	49±1
Alcohol (g/day)	163±10	169±16	148±17	159±9
AST (IU/L)	95±10	98±13	152±31	98±8
ALT (IU/L)	70±15	61±9	98±15	76±7
AST/ALT	1.8±0.1	1.8±0.2	1.5±0.1	2±0.1
γGT (IU/L)	361±38	429±73	472±65	379±43
Fibrosis n(%)				
F0	16(15)	6(17.6)	9(23.7)	9(9.5)
F1	49(45)	14(41.2)	13(34.2)	38(40)
F3	15(14)	6(17.6)	7(18.4)	8(8.4)
F3	23(21)	3(8.8)	5(13.2)	39(41.1)
F4	6(6)	5(14.7)	4(10.5)	1(1.1)
Inflammation n(%)	26(24)	6(17.6)	12(31.6)	
Steatosis n(%)				
<5%	8(7)	1(2.9)	4(10.5)	
5–30%	62(57)	18(52.9)	10(26.3)	
>30–60%	27(25)	9(26.5)	12(31.6)	
>60%	12(11)	6(17.6)	12(31.6)	

Data are expressed as Means ± SEM or N (%). AST: aspartate amino-tranferase; ALT: alanine amino-transferase; γGT: Gamma Glutamyl Transpeptidase.

Consultatif de Protection des Personnes dans la Recherche Biomédicale de Nice" (N°03.613)(DGS 2003/0395), the "Ethics committee of Bicêtre Hospital" and "Ethics committee of Centre Hospitalier Universitaire of Angers Hospital" (N°2010-01) approved this study).

Circulating levels of OPN, Leptin and FibroMeter®

Circulating OPN levels were evaluated with an ELISA (R&D Systems, Lille, France), as described in the manufacturer's instructions. All samples were analyzed in duplicate, in random order and blinded to the clinical/pathological data. The CV (%) of intra-assay precision and inter assay precision ranged from 2.6 to 4 and 5.4 to 6.6, respectively. The minimum detectable dose of OPN ranged from 0.006 to 0.024 ng/mL. Serum was validated for use in this assay as indicated by the manufacturer. However, serum values are approximately 50% of the plasma values because of proteolytic cleavage by thrombin during the clotting process. Leptin was assessed in the serum by MILLIPLEX MAP Human Adipokine Panel A kit (HADK1-61K-A, Millipore) using a Luminex instrument (Luminex) according to manufacturer's recommendations. The FibroMeter® index of fibrosis was calculated using an algorithm including hyaluronate, the prothrombin index, α2-macroglobulin and platelets [30].

Immunostaining

Liver biopsies were fixed in 4% buffered formol, paraffin embedded and sectioned at a thickness of 2 micron Slides were then dewaxed at pH = 6 using PT link (cycle :start at 65°C ,20′ at 95°C, back to 65°C), and washed for 5 minutes in Envision Flex Wash Buffer. Immunohistochemical staining was done using Autostainer Link, with anti-CD15 antibodies (347420 BD Biosciences) as the primary antibody, and diaminobenzidine (DAB) as activated chromogen. Nuclear counterstaining was done with Hematoxylin. CD15+ cells were counted in 2 or 3 portal spaces for each patient at 400× magnification. Counting was performed blindly by one observer.

Real-time quantitative PCR analysis

Total RNA was extracted from human tissues using a RNeasy Mini Kit (Qiagen, Courtaboeuf, France). The samples were treated with Turbo DNA-free™ (Applied Biosystems, Courtaboeuf, France) or RNAse-free DNAse kit (Qiagen) following the manufacturer's protocols. The quality of the isolated RNA was determined using the Agilent 2100 Bioanalyser with RNA 6000 Nano Kit (Agilent Technologies, Massy, France). Total RNA (0.5 or 0.35 µg) was reverse-transcribed with the High Capacity cDNA Reverse Transcription Kit (Applied Biosystems, Courtaboeuf, France) or with the RT^2 First Strand kit (SABiosciences) for the "estimation" and "second gene" groups, respectively. For the estimation group, real-time quantitative PCR was performed using the ABI PRISM 7500 Fast Real Time PCR System and FAM™ dyes (Applied Biosystems, Courtaboeuf, France) following the manufacturer's protocols in C3M Genomics facilities. The TaqMan® gene expression assays were purchased from Applied Biosystems: OPN, (Hs00167093_m1); TGFβ (Hs00171257_m1), RPLP0 (Hs99999902_m1) and 18S (Hs99999901_s1). For the second gene group, real-time quantitative PCR was performed using a custom-made PCR array (SABiosciences) in the LightCycler® 480 instrument (Roche) with the RT^2 SYBR® Green qPCR Master Mix (SABiosciences) according to the manufacturer's instructions. Gene expression values were normalized to the value of the housekeeping gene *RPLP0* (Ribosomal Phosphoprotein Large P0) or *18S* and calculated based on the comparative cycle threshold Ct method ($2^{-\Delta\Delta C_t}$) as previously described [24,31].

Statistical analysis

Statistical significance of the differential gene expression or circulating levels between the two study groups was determined using the non-parametric Mann-Whitney test with the ΔCt or amount for each group, respectively. The non-parametric Kruskal-Wallis test was used for the comparison of more than two study groups. $P<0.05$ was considered as significant. As a post-hoc correction for Kruskal-Wallis test, the Scheffe's test has been performed (data not shown). Correlations were analyzed using the Spearman's rank correlation test. Comparisons were done using the Chi^2 test or Fischer's exact tests for nominal data and by two-sample *t* tests for continuous data. Multivariate analyses were performed using binary logistic regression with estimation of odds ratios (OR) and 95% confidence intervals (95%CI). Diagnostic performance was determined by constructing a "receiver-operating characteristic" (ROC) curve and calculating the area under the ROC (AUROC) curve for determination of patients with significant fibrosis (F≥2) for serum OPN. From these curves, the best cut-off values were established for OPN, which were the values that maximized the sum of the sensitivity and specificity to identify patient status. Statistical analyses were performed using NCSS 2007 software.

Results

Clinical Characteristics of Patients

Two cohorts of heavy alcohol drinkers were included in this study, which examines retrospective (estimation cohort) and prospective (validation cohort) data. In the estimation cohort (109 patients), 36% of the patients had moderate or severe steatosis (S≥2), 24% presented with hepatic inflammation, 14% with moderate fibrosis (F = 2) and 27% with advanced fibrosis (F≥3) (**Table 1**). The estimation (**Table 1**) and validation (95 patients) cohorts were similar in terms of age, gender, alcohol consumption, AST, AST/ALT, γGT and hepatic fibrosis. The serum OPN level was evaluated in all patients, while OPN gene expression was evaluated in the liver of 34 patients from the estimation group (**Table 1: Liver**) and in the liver and adipose tissue in 38 patients from the second group (**Table 1: Second gene group**).

The serum and hepatic OPN level increased with liver fibrosis in patients with alcoholic liver diseases

We first evaluated the serum OPN levels in the estimation cohort of 109 alcoholic patients. While hepatic steatosis had no effect on the serum OPN level (**Figure 1A**), the level was increased in patients with hepatic inflammation (I1) compared with patients without liver inflammation (I0) (**Figure 1B**) and was progressively increased in association with the stage of fibrosis (**Figure 1C**). The serum OPN concentrations of F0/F1 alcoholic patients (14 F0 and 51 F1) were comparable to those found in 16 lean subjects without diagnosed liver complications (BMI = 21±1 kg/m^2) and in 14 morbidly obese patients (BMI = 43±1 kg/m^2) with a minimal stage of fibrosis (4 F0 and 10 F1) and without hepatic steatosis, inflammation and ballooning (**Figure S1**). The serum OPN level further correlated strongly with fibrosis ($r_s = 0.681$, $P<0.001$) and, to a lesser extent with the hepatic inflammation ($r_s = 0.193$, $P = 0.047$). We then evaluated the hepatic expression level of OPN and TGFβ, a pro-fibrogenic factor [32], in 34 alcoholic patients from the estimation group (**Table 1**). Gene expression of OPN was increased in patients with moderate (F2) and advanced fibrosis (F3/F4) compared with patients with no fibrosis (F0) (**Figure 2A**). The liver OPN and TGFβ expression correlated with each other and with the grade of fibrosis (**Figures 2A and 2B**). The serum OPN level also

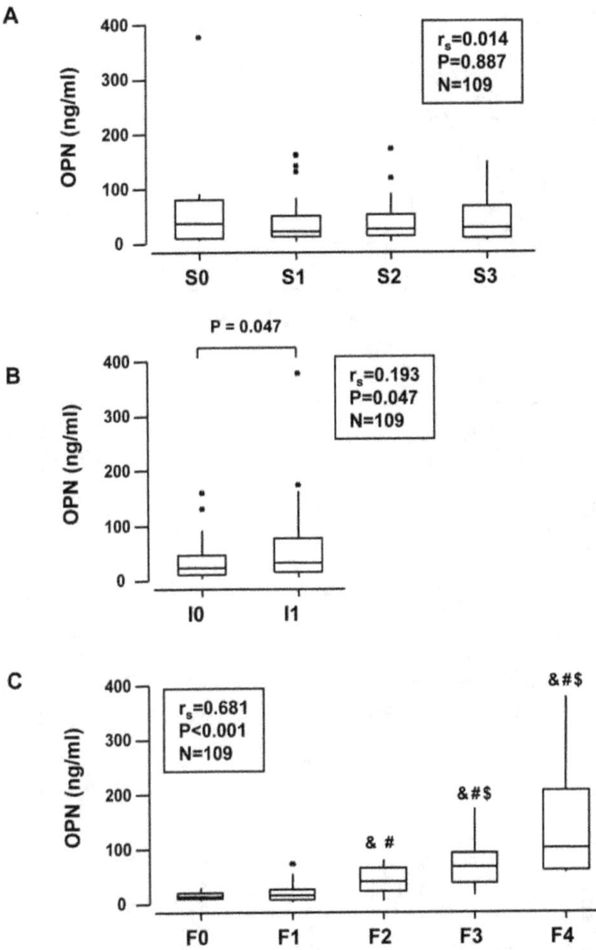

Figure 1. The serum OPN level correlated with fibrosis and steatohepatitis in 109 alcoholic patients (estimation cohort). The circulating levels of OPN were measured in the serum of 109 alcoholic patients (Table 1) and analyzed according to the grade of steatosis (S0, S1, S2, S3)(**A**), the presence of hepatic inflammation (I0, I1) (Hepatic inflammation was determined by the presence (I1) or absence (I0) of hepatocellular necrosis and ballooning degeneration, alcoholic Mallory's hyaline bodies, associated with an inflammatory reaction) (**B**) and the stage of fibrosis (F0, F1, F2, F3, F4)(**C**) (as described in Materials and Methods). Results were expressed as the median (25th, 75th percentile). The Kruskal-Wallis test was used to compare the 4 groups S0, S1, S2 and S3, $P = 0.900$ and the 5 groups F0, F1, F2, F3 and F4, $P<0.001$. The Mann Whitney test compared A0 A1: $P = 0.047$. The Mann Whitney test compared the two groups (C): &, $P<0.015$, compared with F0; #, $P<0.028$, compared with F1; $, $P = 0.007$, compared with F2. Correlations between the serum OPN level with hepatic steatosis, hepatitis or fibrosis were analyzed using the Spearman's rank correlation test.

correlated with its hepatic expression. Since OPN plays an important role in neutrophil accumulation and liver injury in the rat model of ASH [8,10,13,14], we then evaluated OPN expression compared to the accumulation of neutrophil in the liver of patients with different grades of hepatic fibrosis (N = 11). The number of neutrophils in the portal space correlated with the circulating and hepatic OPN level ($r_s = 0.917$, $P<0.001$; $r_s = 0.907$, $P<0.001$; respectively) (**Figure 2C**). These results indicate that the circulating OPN level could reflect its hepatic expression and that there is a strong link between hepatic OPN expression and fibrogenesis.

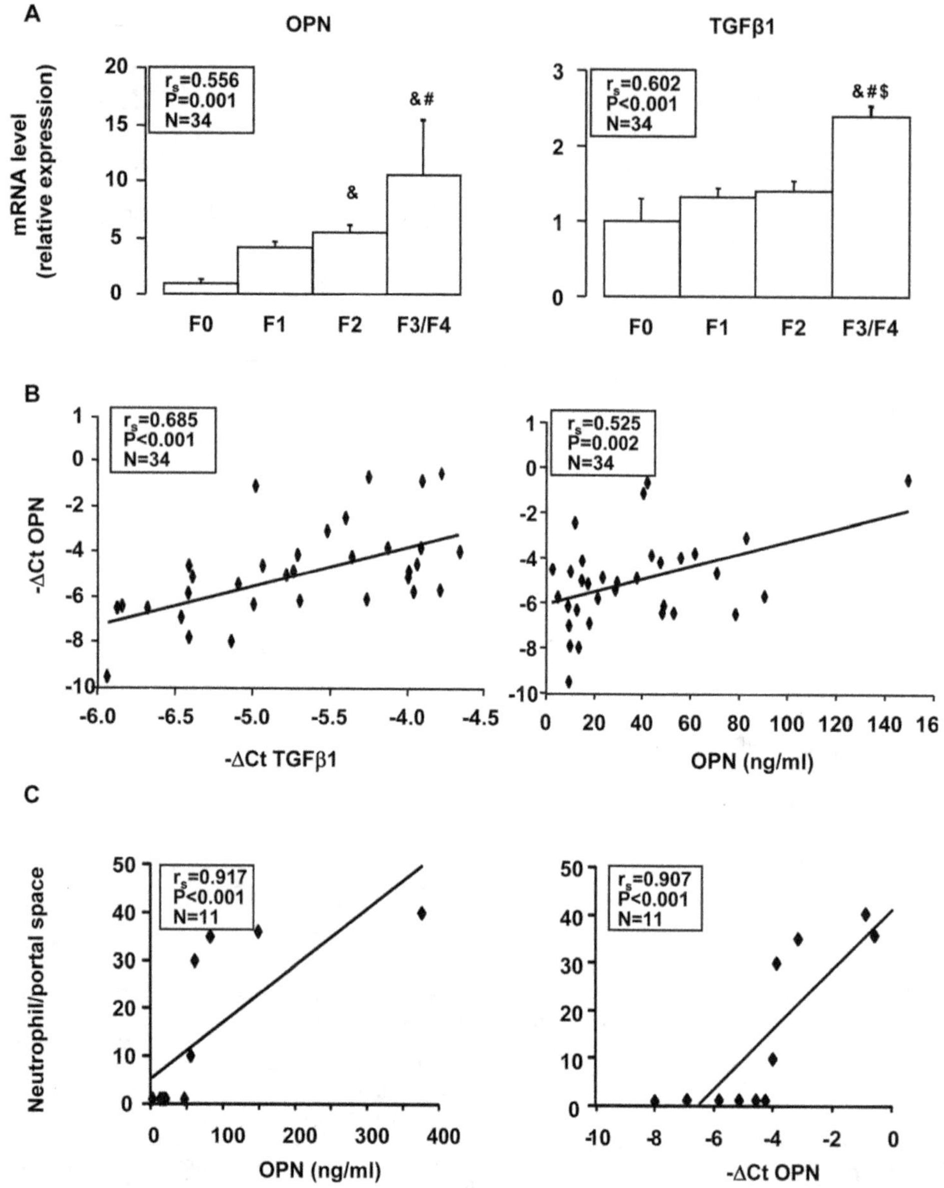

Figure 2. Hepatic OPN expression correlated with hepatic TGFβ expression, portal space neutrophils and the serum OPN level. A) Hepatic OPN and TGFβ1 expression levels were analyzed by real-time quantitative PCR in 34 alcoholic patients from the estimation group without (**F0**) (N = 6) or with mild (**F1**) (N = 14), moderate (**F2**) (N = 6) or advanced (**F3/4**) (N = 8) fibrosis. The mRNA levels were normalized to the mRNA levels of RPLP0. Results are expressed relative to the expression levels in F0 patients and expressed as means ± SEM. The Kruskal-Wallis test compared the 4 groups F0, F1, F2 and F3/F4: OPN, $P = 0.037$; TGFβ1, $P = 0.002$. Mann Whitney test compared the two groups: &, $P \leq 0.011$, compared with F0; #, $P \leq 0.029$, compared with F1; $, $P = 0.008$, compared with F2. **B)** Correlation between hepatic OPN gene expression (ΔCt) and either the hepatic TGFβ1 expression level (ΔCt) or the serum OPN level were analyzed using the Spearman's rank correlation test. **C)** Correlation between the number of portal space neutophils (Cf. Materials and methods) and serum OPN level or hepatic OPN gene expression (ΔCt) in 11 alcoholic patients (2F0/3F1/1F2/5F4) were analyzed using the Spearman's rank correlation test.

The adipose tissue OPN level increased with liver fibrosis in patients with alcoholic liver diseases

Since adipose tissue inflammation correlated with the severity of pathological features in the liver [7], we evaluated OPN expression in 38 ongoing alcoholic patients in both liver and adipose tissue biopsies (BMI = 24±4 kg/m^2) (**Table 1: Second gene group**). In adipose tissue, the OPN level was already increased in patients with mild fibrosis (F1) compared with patients without liver fibrosis (3.10±0.51 fold increase, $P = 0.0082$) and correlated with hepatic fibrosis but not with liver steatosis and inflammation (**Table 2**). OPN level in adipose tissue did not correlate with BMI ($r_s = 0.073$, $P = 0.689$, N = 37) and the leptin level in adipose tissue ($r_s = 0.138$, $P = 0.415$, N = 37) or serum ($r_s = 0.099$, $P = 0.577$, N = 34). Expression in the liver correlated with fibrosis, as found in the estimation group (**Figure 1**), and with steatosis and inflammation (**Table 2**). Because recent alcohol intake could influence these results, the adipose tissue OPN expression was evaluated after 7 days of alcohol abstinence. Its expression still correlated with liver fibrosis (**Table 2**). Since OPN is mainly expressed by the inflammatory and immune cells in adipose tissue [22,24], the

Table 2. Correlation between hepatic and adipose tissue OPN expression and hepatic steatosis, inflammation and fibrosis in alcoholic patients (the second gene group).

OPN expression in	Steatosis			Inflammation			Fibrosis		
	r_s	P	N	r_s	P	N	r_s	P	N
Liver	0.432	0.007	38	0.712	<0.001	38	0.766	<0.001	38
Adipose tissue	0.077	0.652	37	0.117	0.492	37	0.361	0.028	37
Adipose tissue after 7 days of alcohol abstinence	0.063	0.722	34	0.170	0.337	34	0.342	0.048	34

Spearman's rank correlation test.

adipose tissue of alcoholic patients could be inflamed at the early stage of liver fibrogenesis.

The serum OPN level was an independent risk factor in estimating significant (F≥2) liver fibrosis in patients with alcoholic liver diseases

Since the circulating level of OPN was higher in patients with moderate fibrosis (F2) compared with patients with no or mild fibrosis (F0/F1) (**Figure 1C**), we investigated the pertinence of the serum OPN level for the estimation of significant fibrosis (F≥2). Using the univariate analysis (**Table 3**), patients with significant fibrosis (F≥2) were older and had a higher levels of OPN, γGT, alkaline phosphatase, bilirubin, hyaluronate and of the FibroMeter® index of fibrosis and lower levels of platelets, albumin, red blood cells, hemoglobin and of the prothrombin index compared to patients with mild fibrosis (F<2) (**Table 3**). In contrast, the gender, AST and ALT were not associated with F≥2. In a multivariate analysis including the OPN, alkaline phosphatase, albumin, hemoglobin and FibroMeter® level, OPN and FibroMeter® were the only independent variables when F≥2 was the judgment criterion (**Table 4**). Since FibroMeter® is a test that combines analysis for hyaluronate, the prothrombin index, α2-macroglobulin and platelets, we did not include these items in this analysis. The serum OPN level could thus be considered as an independent factor in estimating significant liver fibrosis in patients with alcoholic liver disease.

Table 3. Univariate analysis of the Estimation group according to the severity of the liver disease.

Data	F<2 (N = 65)	F≥2 (N = 44)	P
Age (years)	45.4±8.2	49.8±8.2	0.008279
Gender (female/male)	14/51	13/31	0,342053
Platelets (10^9/L)	208.5±82.4	161.4±72.5	0.002715
AST (IU/L)	79.7±57.4	116.3±139.6	0.060470
ALT (IU/L)	62.0±45.1	82.1±240.2	0.512052
γGT (IU/L)	247.1±301.8	527.9±464.9	0.000221
Bilirubin (μmol/L)	9.8±5.97	56.2±94.6	0.000142
Alkaline phosphatase (IU/L)	85.2±37.7	142.7±68.2	<0.000001
Red blood cells (10^{12}/L)	4.2±0.4	3.5±0.5	<0.000001
Albumin (g/L)	48.4±4.2	37.9±8.3	<0.000001
Prothrombin index (%)	98.4±3.9	75.9±22.4	<0.000001
Hemoglobin (g/dL)	13.8±1.6	11.9±1.7	<0.000001
OPN (ng/mL)	18.6±14.1	73.0±65.5	<0.000001
Hyaluronate (μg/L)	40.7±30.4	293.6±309.9	<0.000001
FibroMeter®	0.18±0.15	0.72±0.33	<0.000001

Patients were classified according to Fibrosis (F) <2 or ≥2.. Quantitative results are expressed as means ± standard deviations. AST: aspartate amino-tranferase; ALT: alanine amino-transferase; γGT: Gamma Glutamyl Transpeptidase; OPN: Osteopontin.

The serum OPN levels estimated significant fibrosis in alcoholic patients

As shown in **Figure 3**, the area under the ROC curve in the estimation and validation cohorts for discrimination between F<2 and significant (F≥2) fibrosis with the serum OPN level was 0.89 (95% CI: 0.81–0.94) and 0.88 (95% CI: 0.79–0.93), respectively. Thus, the retrospective (estimation cohort) and prospective (validation cohort) studies led to the same result. Several cut-off values were calculated for the serum OPN level for the prediction of F≥2 in the estimation group (**Table S1**). For example, the cut-off point at 29 ng/mL estimated F≥2 with a sensitivity of 84%, a specificity of 81%, a Positive and Negative Predictive Value of 75.5% and 88.3%, respectively. To validate the performance of OPN in estimating significant fibrosis, we compared the OPN to the FibroMeter® level, a specific blood test using four biomarkers to predict fibrosis in ALD [30], and hyaluronate, serum cell death (Cytokeratin 18 total) and apoptotic markers (caspases generated cytokeratin 18 fragment), single biomarkers reflecting increased fibrogenesis [3,33]. The area under the ROC curve in the estimation cohort for discriminating F<2 from significant (F≥2) fibrosis with the FibroMeter®, hyaluronate, cell death marker and apoptotic marker was 0.90 (95% CI: 0.82–0.95), 0.88 (95% CI: 0.79–0.94), 0.83 (95% CI: 0.73–0.89) and 0.74 (95% CI: 0.63–0.82), respectively. While OPN was more efficient than the apoptotic marker in estimating significant fibrosis (OPN AUROC

Table 4. Multivariate analysis of the Estimation group for the assessment of significant hepatic fibrosis.

Data	F≥2 (N = 44) versus F<2 (N = 65)		
	P	OR	95% CI
Alkaline phosphatase	0.925	0.999	0.9842–1.0143
Albumin	0.684	0.962	0.8018–1.1559
Hemoglobin	0.269	0.778	0.4987–1.2143
OPN	0.033	1.044	1.0033–1.0865
FibroMeter®	0.001	59.405	4.7129–748.7968

Patients were classified according to Fibrosis (F)<2 or ≥2. Multivariate analysis was realized using logistic regression.

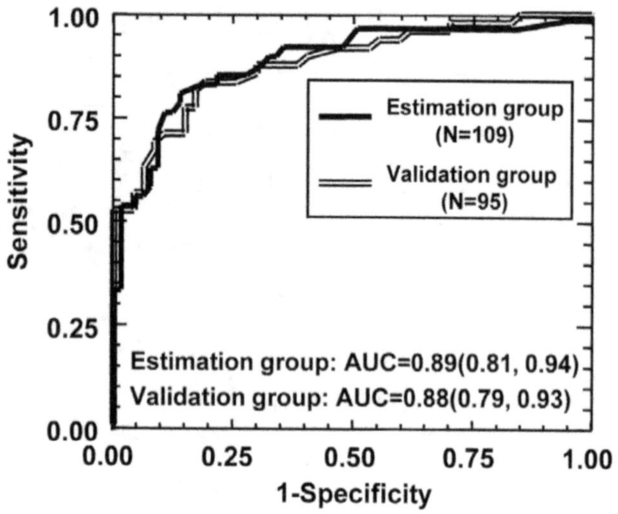

Figure 3. Levels of serum OPN for diagnosis of significant fibrosis (F≥2) in cohorts of alcoholic patients. The area under the ROC curves are shown for the performance of serum OPN levels in evaluating significant fibrosis (F≥2) in estimation (109 patients) and validation (95 patients) cohorts.

versus serum apoptotic marker AUROC: $P=0.0011$), OPN, FibroMeter®, hyaluronate and cell death marker levels estimated significant fibrosis with the same accuracy (OPN AUROC versus FibroMeter® AUROC: $P=0.752$; versus hyaluronate AUROC: $P=0.791$, versus cell death marker AUROC: $P=0.100$) indicating that OPN should be an important actor or manifestation of liver fibrosis induced by chronic alcohol consumption.

The serum OPN levels correlated with hepatic fibrosis and estimated significant (F≥2) fibrosis in patients with chronic viral hepatitis C

To explore whether the previous findings were specific to ALD, we evaluated the serum OPN levels in 86 patients with chronic viral hepatitis C including 25 patients with mild fibrosis (F1), 34 patients with moderate fibrosis (F2), 19 patients with severe fibrosis (F3) and 8 patients with cirrhosis (F4). The OPN level was increased in patients with moderate, severe fibrosis or cirrhosis compared with patients with mild fibrosis (F1) (**Figure 4A**). The serum OPN level further correlated strongly with fibrosis ($r_s=0.617$, $P<0.001$) (**Figure 4A**) and, to a lower extent with hepatic inflammation ($r_s=0.360$, $P=0.047$). However, the serum OPN level in patients with chronic viral hepatitis C and significant fibrosis (F≥2) was lower than in alcoholic patients with significant fibrosis (F≥2) (HCV group: OPN median = 43.2 ng/mL, N = 61; Alcoholic group (estimation cohort): OPN median = 59.5 ng/mL, N = 44; Mann-Whitney test: $P=0.005$). As shown in **Figure 4B**, the area under the ROC curve in patients with chronic viral hepatitis C to estimate significant (F≥2) and advanced (F≥3) fibrosis with the serum OPN level were 0.75 (95% CI: 0.62–0.84) and 0.81 (95% CI: 0.68–0.89), respectively. This indicated that circulating OPN could be a conserved response to chronic liver injury induced, *per se*, by alcohol and HCV.

Discussion

We report here for the first time that the serum OPN level correlated with hepatic inflammation and fibrosis in heavy alcohol drinkers. The hepatic OPN expression level strongly correlated

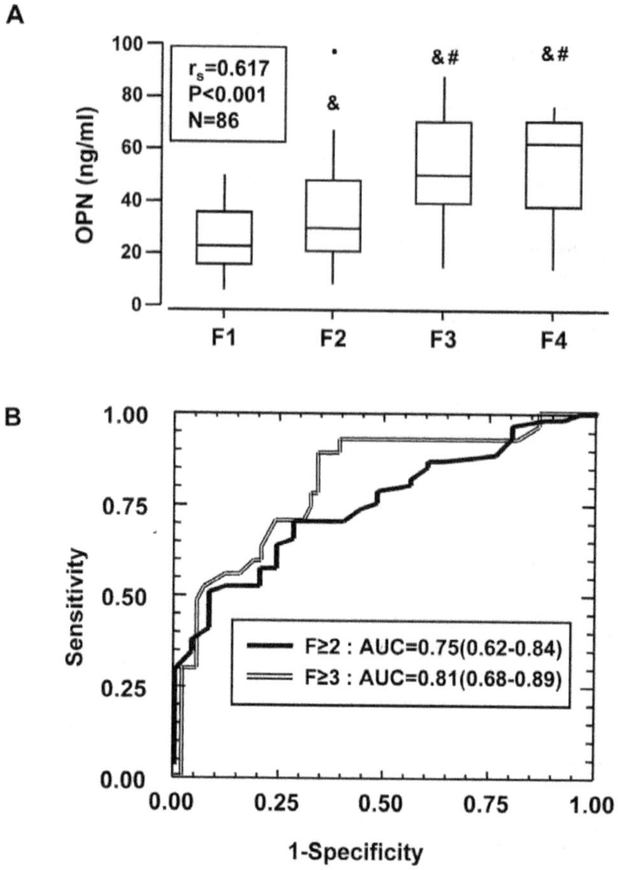

Figure 4. Levels of serum OPN in patients with chronic viral hepatitis C. (**A**) The circulating levels of OPN were measured in the serum of 86 patients with chronic hepatitis C (25 F1, 34 F2, 19 F3, 8 F4) and analyzed according to the stage of fibrosis. Results were expressed as the median (25th, 75th percentile). The Kruskal-Wallis test was used to compare the 4 groups F1, F2, F3 and F4: $P<0.001$. The Mann-Whitney test compared the two groups: &, $P\leq0.048$, compared with F1; #, $P\leq0.026$, compared with F2. Correlation between the serum OPN level with hepatic fibrosis was analyzed using the Spearman's rank correlation test. (**B**) The areas under the ROC curves are shown for the performance of serum OPN levels in estimating significant fibrosis (F≥2) or advanced fibrosis (F≥3) in this cohort.

with hepatic neutrophils accumulation, the pro-fibrogenic factor TGFβ and hepatic fibrosis. Expression of OPN in adipose tissue correlated with hepatic fibrosis reinforcing the concept that adipose tissue was also inflamed in ALD. The serum level of OPN was an accurate independent factor in estimating significant liver fibrosis in both the estimation and validation cohort.

OPN expression detected in adipose tissue and in the liver of alcoholic patients was enhanced by the presence of hepatic fibrosis. The relative contribution of these two tissues in circulating OPN is difficult to estimate. While hepatic OPN expression correlated with the serum OPN level in our patients, further studies will be required to determine the relative role of these two tissues in modulating circulating OPN concentrations. Although the cellular origin of the increased hepatic OPN expression has not been precisely determined, increased OPN gene expression has been reported in macrophages, Kupffer cells, stellate cells, biliary epithelial cells and in inflammatory cells of the necrotic areas in rodent liver fibrosis models [15,16,18]. The observation that hepatic inflammation was associated with elevated serum OPN levels is in favor of a role for OPN in liver inflammation. Recent studies have highlighted the role of OPN in inflammatory liver diseases such as alcoholic and non alcoholic liver diseases and T cell-mediated hepatitis [8,10,13,15,23,34,35,36,37]. In rodent models of alcoholic liver diseases, neutrophils accumulation in the liver was mediated by OPN [8,10,13]. In agreement with these reports, we showed in a small number of patients that hepatic and systemic OPN expression correlated with neutophil infiltration in the portal space. OPN also facilitated the infiltration and accumulation of macrophages at sites of injury during the initial steps after carbon tetrachloride intoxication [16]. The recruitment and activation of the inflammatory and immune cells by OPN could enhance hepatic inflammation, which in turn may activate hepatic stellate cells and fibrogenesis. In agreement with this mechanism, the invalidation of the OPN gene decreased hepatic inflammation and consequently fibrosis in mice fed a choline-methione-deficient diet [12,15]. Furthermore, it has been suggested that OPN could have fibrogenic properties. OPN expression was increased in activated hepatic stellate cells [17,18,19] and was required for myofibroblast differentiation [20]. OPN was regulated by the hedgehog pathway and directly promoted pro-fibrogenic responses [12]. The upregulation of OPN has been reported in the liver of patients with ALD-cirrhosis but also with NASH-cirrhosis, primary biliary cirrhosis, autoimmune hepatitis and primary sclerosing cholangitis, which suggested that OPN induction is a conserved response to chronic liver injury [12]. Excess weight was as an independent risk factor for fibrosis and cirrhosis in patients with ALD [4,5]. More recently, Naveau *et al.* demonstrated that adipose tissue inflammation correlated with the severity of pathological features in the liver [7]. The increase in the production of OPN in adipose tissue could result from the activation of adipose tissue macrophages by LPS and cytokines such as TNFα and IL6. The latter were strongly increased in serum and adipose tissue of heavy alcohol drinkers [1,7]. OPN plays an important role in the infiltration and accumulation of macrophages in the early stages of obesity. Indeed, we recently reported that elevated OPN expression in adipose tissue paralleled with adipose tissue macrophage infiltration and both phenomena were reversed after weight loss in obese patients [24]. While further investigation is necessary to determine the molecular mechanism of adipose tissue inflammation, adipose tissue OPN expression could lead to enrichment of adipose tissue in macrophages and to increased adipose tissue inflammation. The OPN level in adipose tissue could be related more to inflammation than adipose tissue gain. Indeed, OPN expression in adipose tissue did not correlate with BMI, leptin expression and leptinemia.

We have shown for the first time that the serum OPN level was an independent factor that estimates significant fibrosis in two independent cohorts of patients with ALD. A larger group of alcoholic patients with all the data allowing to repeat the univariate and multiple regression modeling will be done in the future. Since circulating OPN could increase in obese individuals and that obesity is also associated with a higher propensity to fibrosis and progression of chronic liver diseases, we analyzed 60 alcoholic patients with available BMI to determine an independent association between OPN and fibrosis. In these patients (39% with a significant fibrosis (F≥2)), serum OPN correlated with hepatic fibrosis ($r_s = 0.497$, $P<0.001$, N = 60) but not with BMI ($r_s = 0.128$, $P = 0.328$, N = 60). Using the univariate analysis, OPN but not BMI was associated with F≥2 (**Table S2**). In a multivariate analysis including the OPN, γGT and BMI, OPN was the only independent variable when F≥2 was the judgment criterion (**Table S3**). The serum OPN level could thus be considered as an independent factor estimating significant liver fibrosis. However, additional validations on a large number of alcoholic patients, controls subjects and morbidly obese group included patients with the full range of liver fibrosis with available BMI will be required. Liver biopsy remains the gold standard for assessment of liver fibrosis. However, problems with liver biopsy include sampling error and inter-observer variability. Fibroscan and the currently available blood-algorithm tests (Fibrotest®, FibroMeter®) or direct biomarker (Hyaluronate) can differentiate between mild and advanced disease [2,33,38,39]. In the case of borderline results two or more methods can be combined. However, identification of novel markers is needed to improve blood-algorithm tests leading to quantification of fibrosis and to monitor the dynamic nature of fibrosis.

Interestingly, the OPN and FibroMeter® levels were the only independent variables when the F≥2 was the judgment criterion in a multivariate analysis including OPN, alkaline phosphatase, albumin, hemoglobin and FibroMeter® levels. Furthermore, OPN, FibroMeter® and hyaluronate estimated significant fibrosis with the same accuracy. OPN was a good marker in both retrospective (AUROC = 0.89 (0.81, 0.94)) and prospective (AUROC = 0.88 (0.79, 0.93)) studies. Moreover, the serum OPN levels accurately estimated advanced fibrosis (F≥3: AUROC = 0.91 (0.83, 0.95)) and cirrhosis (F = 4: AUROC = 0.91 (0.80, 0.96)) in alcoholic patients (from the estimation group).

Circulating levels of OPN were also modified in patients with liver complications related to the hepatitis C and B viruses. An elevated circulating OPN level was an excellent predictor of cirrhosis in patients with a hepatitis B infection [40]. The circulating levels of OPN were also modified in patients with liver complications induced by a hepatitis C infection. Indeed, we report here that the serum OPN in patients with chronic viral hepatitis C correlates with hepatic fibrosis, as previously reported for plasma of hepatitis C virus infected subjects [41]. OPN enhanced tumor development and metastases, since OPN was highly expressed in hepatocellular carcinoma (HCC) and correlated with worse prognosis [42]. However, the role of OPN in these diseases is still poorly understood. It was recently proposed that OPN could be a potential target for the control of HCC [43,44].

In summary, circulating levels of OPN estimate, with good accuracy, significant fibrosis in heavy alcohol drinkers. Hepatic OPN also correlated with serum OPN and with hepatic inflammation, neutrophils infiltration, fibrosis and TGFβ expression. Infiltration of liver by parenchymal neutrophils is a prominent feature of Alcoholic Hepatitis [45]. Up-regulation of OPN in liver could contribute to this infiltration and the severity of Alcoholic Hepatitis. Multiple factors stimulate parenchymal and nonparenchymal cells to produce this chemokine including LPS, IL6 and TNFα. Adipose tissue of alcoholic patients was further inflamed, as evaluated by OPN expression. OPN adipose tissue level also correlated with hepatic fibrosis. Since TNFα and IL6 were strongly increased in adipose tissue and serum of heavy alcohol drinkers [1,7], cytokines secreted by adipose tissue could enhance the inflammation and up-regulation of OPN in liver. The recruitment and activation of the inflammatory and immune cells by OPN could also enhance hepatic inflammation, which in turn may activate hepatic stellate cells and fibrogenesis. Furthermore, it has been suggested that OPN could have fibrogenic properties [12,15,16,17,18,19,20]. Studies focusing on the role of OPN in liver and adipose tissue function will be appropriate approaches to acquire more insight into the pathogenesis of human ALD.

Supporting Information

Figure S1 The serum OPN level in lean, obese and alcoholic patients with minimal stage (F0–F1) of fibrosis.

The circulating levels of OPN were measured in the serum of 16 lean subjects (**Lean**) without diagnosed liver complications (BMI = 21±1 kg/m^2); of 14 morbidly obese patients (**Obese**) (BMI = 43±1 kg/m^2) with a minimal stage of fibrosis (4 F0 and 10 F1) and without hepatic steatosis, inflammation and ballooning; and of 61 alcoholic patients (**Alcoholic**) with a minimal stage of fibrosis (14 F0 and 51 F1). Results were expressed as the median (25th, 75th percentile). The Kruskal-Wallis test was used to compare the 3 groups $P = 0.55$.

Table S1 Osteopontin levels forsignificant fibrosis (F≥2) assessment in the Estimation group.

Table S2 Univariate analysis of 60 patients from Validation group according to the severity of liver disease.

Table S3 Multivariate analysis in 60 patients from Validation group for the estimation of significant hepatic fibrosis.

Acknowledgments

We thank Dr. M.C. Brahimi-Horn for editorial correction and Z. Neffati for statistical assistance.

Author Contributions

Conceived and designed the experiments: SP SB PG. Performed the experiments: SP SB CSV MCSP PC. Analyzed the data: SP SB PG MCSP. Contributed reagents/materials/analysis tools: RA MARA HA MN NBO SN AT GP PC PV. Wrote the paper: SP PG CSV GP. Critical reading: YLMB AT.

References

1. Lucey MR, Mathurin P, Morgan TR (2009) Alcoholic hepatitis. N Engl J Med 360: 2758–2769.
2. Bataller R, Rombouts K, Altamirano J, Marra F (2011) Fibrosis in alcoholic and nonalcoholic steatohepatitis. Best Pract Res Clin Gastroenterol 25: 231–244.
3. Lavallard VJ, Bonnafous S, Patouraux S, Saint-Paul MC, Rousseau D, et al. (2011) Serum markers of hepatocyte death and apoptosis are non invasive biomarkers of severe fibrosis in patients with alcoholic liver disease. PLoS One 6: e17599.
4. Naveau S, Giraud V, Borotto E, Aubert A, Capron F, et al. (1997) Excess weight risk factor for alcoholic liver disease. Hepatology 25: 108–111.
5. Raynard B, Balian A, Fallik D, Capron F, Bedossa P, et al. (2002) Risk factors of fibrosis in alcohol-induced liver disease. Hepatology 35: 635–638.
6. Naveau S, Thaury J, Barri-Ova N, Balian A, Dauvois B, et al. (2009) Predictive factors for pure steatosis in alcoholic patients. Alcohol Clin Exp Res 33: 1104–1110.
7. Naveau S, Cassard-Doulcier AM, Njike-Nakseu M, Bouchet-Delbos L, Barri-Ova N, et al. (2010) Harmful effect of adipose tissue on liver lesions in patients with alcoholic liver disease. J Hepatol 52: 895–902.
8. Apte UM, Banerjee A, McRee R, Wellberg E, Ramaiah SK (2005) Role of osteopontin in hepatic neutrophil infiltration during alcoholic steatohepatitis. Toxicol Appl Pharmacol 207: 25–38.
9. Banerjee A, Burghardt RC, Johnson GA, White FJ, Ramaiah SK (2006) The temporal expression of osteopontin (SPP-1) in the rodent model of alcoholic steatohepatitis: a potential biomarker. Toxicol Pathol 34: 373–384.
10. Banerjee A, Apte UM, Smith R, Ramaiah SK (2006) Higher neutrophil infiltration mediated by osteopontin is a likely contributing factor to the increased susceptibility of females to alcoholic liver disease. J Pathol 208: 473–485.
11. Seth D, Gorrell MD, Cordoba S, McCaughan GW, Haber PS (2006) Intrahepatic gene expression in human alcoholic hepatitis. J Hepatol 45: 306–320.
12. Syn WK, Choi SS, Liaskou E, Karaca GF, Agboola KM, et al. (2011) Osteopontin is induced by hedgehog pathway activation and promotes fibrosis progression in nonalcoholic steatohepatitis. Hepatology 53: 106–115.
13. Banerjee A, Lee JH, Ramaiah SK (2008) Interaction of osteopontin with neutrophil alpha(4)beta(1) and alpha(9)beta(1) integrins in a rodent model of alcoholic liver disease. Toxicol Appl Pharmacol 233: 238–246.
14. Koh A, da Silva AP, Bansal AK, Bansal M, Sun C, et al. (2007) Role of osteopontin in neutrophil function. Immunology 122: 466–475.
15. Sahai A, Malladi P, Melin-Aldana H, Green RM, Whitington PF (2004) Upregulation of osteopontin expression is involved in the development of nonalcoholic steatohepatitis in a dietary murine model. Am J Physiol Gastrointest Liver Physiol 287: G264–273.
16. Lorena D, Darby IA, Gadeau AP, Leen LL, Rittling S, et al. (2006) Osteopontin expression in normal and fibrotic liver. altered liver healing in osteopontin-deficient mice. J Hepatol 44: 383–390.
17. De Minicis S, Seki E, Uchinami H, Kluwe J, Zhang Y, et al. (2007) Gene expression profiles during hepatic stellate cell activation in culture and in vivo. Gastroenterology 132: 1937–1946.
18. Kawashima R, Mochida S, Matsui A, YouLuTu ZY, Ishikawa K, et al. (1999) Expression of osteopontin in Kupffer cells and hepatic macrophages and Stellate cells in rat liver after carbon tetrachloride intoxication: a possible factor for macrophage migration into hepatic necrotic areas. Biochem Biophys Res Commun 256: 527–531.
19. Lee SH, Seo GS, Park YN, Yoo TM, Sohn DH (2004) Effects and regulation of osteopontin in rat hepatic stellate cells. Biochem Pharmacol 68: 2367–2378.
20. Lenga Y, Koh A, Perera AS, McCulloch CA, Sodek J, et al. (2008) Osteopontin expression is required for myofibroblast differentiation. Circ Res 102: 319–327.
21. Sahai A, Malladi P, Pan X, Paul R, Melin-Aldana H, et al. (2004) Obese and diabetic db/db mice develop marked liver fibrosis in a model of nonalcoholic steatohepatitis: role of short-form leptin receptors and osteopontin. Am J Physiol Gastrointest Liver Physiol 287: G1035–1043.
22. Nomiyama T, Perez-Tilve D, Ogawa D, Gizard F, Zhao Y, et al. (2007) Osteopontin mediates obesity-induced adipose tissue macrophage infiltration and insulin resistance in mice. J Clin Invest 117: 2877–2888.
23. Kiefer FW, Neschen S, Pfau B, Legerer B, Neuhofer A, et al. (2011) Osteopontin deficiency protects against obesity-induced hepatic steatosis and attenuates glucose production in mice. Diabetologia 54: 2132–2142.
24. Bertola A, Deveaux V, Bonnafous S, Rousseau D, Anty R, et al. (2009) Elevated expression of osteopontin may be related to adipose tissue macrophage accumulation and liver steatosis in morbid obesity. Diabetes 58: 125–133.
25. Tran A, Benzaken S, Saint-Paul MC, Guzman-Granier E, Hastier P, et al. (2000) Chondrex (YKL-40), a potential new serum fibrosis marker in patients with alcoholic liver disease. Eur J Gastroenterol Hepatol 12: 989–993.
26. Tran A, Hastier P, Barjoan EM, Demuth N, Pradier C, et al. (2000) Non invasive prediction of severe fibrosis in patients with alcoholic liver disease. Gastroenterol Clin Biol 24: 626–630.
27. Rockey DC, Caldwell SH, Goodman ZD, Nelson RC, Smith AD (2009) Liver biopsy. Hepatology 49: 1017–1044.
28. Orrego H, Blake JE, Blendis LM, Medline A (1987) Prognosis of alcoholic cirrhosis in the presence and absence of alcoholic hepatitis. Gastroenterology 92: 208–214.
29. (1994) Intraobserver and interobserver variations in liver biopsy interpretation in patients with chronic hepatitis C. The French METAVIR Cooperative Study Group. Hepatology 20: 15–20.
30. Cales P, Oberti F, Michalak S, Hubert-Fouchard I, Rousselet MC, et al. (2005) A novel panel of blood markers to assess the degree of liver fibrosis. Hepatology 42: 1373–1381.
31. Bertola A, Bonnafous S, Anty R, Patouraux S, Saint-Paul MC, et al. (2010) Hepatic expression patterns of inflammatory and immune response genes associated with obesity and NASH in morbidly obese patients. PLoS One 5: e13577.
32. Friedman SL (2008) Mechanisms of hepatic fibrogenesis. Gastroenterology 134: 1655–1669.
33. Manning DS, Afdhal NH (2008) Diagnosis and quantitation of fibrosis. Gastroenterology 134: 1670–1681.
34. Kiefer FW, Zeyda M, Gollinger K, Pfau B, Neuhofer A, et al. (2010) Neutralization of osteopontin inhibits obesity-induced inflammation and insulin resistance. Diabetes 59: 935–946.
35. Diao H, Kon S, Iwabuchi K, Kimura C, Morimoto J, et al. (2004) Osteopontin as a mediator of NKT cell function in T cell-mediated liver diseases. Immunity 21: 539–550.
36. Mimura S, Mochida S, Inao M, Matsui A, Nagoshi S, et al. (2004) Massive liver necrosis after provocation of imbalance between Th1 and Th2 immune reactions in osteopontin transgenic mice. J Gastroenterol 39: 867–872.
37. Kon S, Ikesue M, Kimura C, Aoki M, Nakayama Y, et al. (2008) Syndecan-4 protects against osteopontin-mediated acute hepatic injury by masking functional domains of osteopontin. J Exp Med 205: 25–33.
38. Naveau S, Gaude G, Asnacios A, Agostini H, Abella A, et al. (2009) Diagnostic and prognostic values of noninvasive biomarkers of fibrosis in patients with alcoholic liver disease. Hepatology 49: 97–105.
39. Nguyen-Khac E, Chatelain D, Tramier B, Decrombecque C, Robert B, et al. (2008) Assessment of asymptomatic liver fibrosis in alcoholic patients using

fibroscan: prospective comparison with seven non-invasive laboratory tests. Aliment Pharmacol Ther 28: 1188–1198.
40. Zhao L, Li T, Wang Y, Pan Y, Ning H, et al. (2008) Elevated plasma osteopontin level is predictive of cirrhosis in patients with hepatitis B infection. Int J Clin Pract 62: 1056–1062.
41. Huang W, Zhu G, Huang M, Lou G, Liu Y, et al. (2010) Plasma osteopontin concentration correlates with the severity of hepatic fibrosis and inflammation in HCV-infected subjects. Clin Chim Acta 411: 675–678.
42. Ramaiah SK, Rittling S (2008) Pathophysiological role of osteopontin in hepatic inflammation, toxicity, and cancer. Toxicol Sci 103: 4–13.
43. Zhao J, Dong L, Lu B, Wu G, Xu D, et al. (2008) Down-regulation of osteopontin suppresses growth and metastasis of hepatocellular carcinoma via induction of apoptosis. Gastroenterology 135: 956–968.
44. Sun BS, Dong QZ, Ye QH, Sun HJ, Jia HL, et al. (2008) Lentiviral-mediated miRNA against osteopontin suppresses tumor growth and metastasis of human hepatocellular carcinoma. Hepatology 48: 1834–1842.
45. Gao B, Bataller R (2011) Alcoholic liver disease: pathogenesis and new therapeutic targets. Gastroenterology 141: 1572–1585.

3

New Insight into the Antifibrotic Effects of Praziquantel on Mice in Infection with *Schistosoma japonicum*

Yue-Jin Liang[1], Jie Luo[1], Quan Yuan[1], Dan Zheng[1], Ya-Ping Liu[1], Lei Shi[1], Ying Zhou[1], Ai-Ling Chen[1], Yong-Ya Ren[2], Ke-Yi Sun[3], Yan Sun[1], Yong Wang[1]*, Zhao-Song Zhang[1]

1 Department of Pathogen Biology, Key Laboratory of Pathogen Biology of Jiangsu Province, Nanjing Medical University, Nanjing, Jiangsu, China, **2** Department of Pathology, Nanjing Medical University, Nanjing, Jiangsu, China, **3** Department of Microbiology and Immunology, Nanjing Medical University, Nanjing, Jiangsu, China

Abstract

Background: Schistosomiasis is a parasitic disease infecting more than 200 million people in the world. Although chemotherapy targeting on killing schistosomes is one of the main strategies in the disease control, there are few effective ways of dealing with liver fibrosis caused by the parasite infection in the chronic and advanced stages of schistosomiasis. For this reason, new strategies and prospective drugs, which exert antifibrotic effects, are urgently required.

Methods and Findings: The antifibrotic effects of praziquantel were assessed in the murine models of schistosomiasis japonica. Murine fibrosis models were established by cutaneous infection with 14±2 *Schistosoma japonicum* cercariae. Then, the mice of both chronic (8 weeks post-infection) and advanced (15 weeks post-infection) schistosomiasis were treated by gavage of praziquantel (250 mg/kg, once daily for 3 days) to eliminate worms, and followed by praziquantel anti-fibrosis treatment (300 mg/kg, twice daily for 30 days). The fibrosis-related parameters assessed were areas of collagen deposition, content of hydroxyproline and mRNA expressions of Col1α1, Col3α1, α-SMA, TGF-β, MMP9, TIMP1, IL-4, IL-10, IL-13 and IFN-γ of liver. Spleen weight index, alanine aminotransferase activity and liver portal venous pressure were also measured. The results showed that anti-fibrosis treatment improved liver fibrosis, splenomegaly, hepatic function, as well as liver portal hypertension. In order to confirm the anti-fibrotic properties of praziquantel, we established a CCL_4-induced model and revealed that CCL_4-induced liver fibrosis was inhibited by PZQ treatment for 30 days. Furthermore, we analyzed the effects of praziquantel on mouse primary hepatic stellate cells (HSCs). It is indicated that mRNA expressions of Col1α1, Col3α1, α-SMA, TGF-β, MMP9 and TIMP1 of HSCs were all inhibited after praziquantel anti-parasite treatments.

Conclusions: The significant amelioration of hepatic fibrosis by praziquantel treatment validates it as a promising drug of anti-fibrosis and offers potential of a new chemotherapy for hepatic fibrosis resulting from schistosomiasis.

Editor: David Joseph Diemert, The George Washington University Medical Center, United States of America

Funding: This work was supported by National Basic Research Program of China (973 Program) (No. 2007CB513102). The funders had no role in study design, data collection and analysis, decision to publish, or preparation of the manuscript.

Competing Interests: The authors have declared that no competing interests exist.

* E-mail: yongwsh@njmu.edu.cn

Introduction

Schistosomiasis is a tropical parasitic disease caused by blood-dwelling fluke, schistosome. According to WHO, 200 million people are infected by the parasite worldwide, leading to the loss of 1.53 million disability-adjusted life years [1]. The main pathologic lesions of hepatic schistosomiasis are the granuloma formation around schistosome eggs at acute stage of the infection, followed by the liver fibrosis at chronic and advanced stages [2]. Hepatic fibrosis of schistosomiasis results from a massive deposition of extracellular matrix (ECM) in the periportal spaces, leading to blockage of the portal veins, portal hypertension, splenomegaly, portocaval shunting, and gastrointestinal varices [1]. The persistent fibrosis of chronic schistosomiasis may cause hepatic cirrhosis and high mortality rate for liver cancer [3]. Although chemotherapy eliminates matured worms effectively and prevents the accumulation of schistosome eggs, less effective durgs are direct to reverse the existing hepatic fibrosis, especially at chronic and advanced stages of schistosomiasis. Therefore, treatment targeting hepatic fibrosis of schistosomiasis remains a challenging proposition [4].

Hepatic stellate cells(HSCs) are considered as an important liver resident cells, which are the major cellular sources of extracellular matrix (ECM) and play a key role in the process of hepatic fibrosis [5,6]. Deposition of collagen, imbalance of matrix metalloproteinase (MMP)/tissue inhibitor of metalloproteinase(TIMP) and secretion of profibrotic cytokines caused by activated HSCs are described previously in schistosomiasis and other infectious diseases [7,8]. According to their pivotal role, HSCs have been recognized as the therapeutic targets of hepatic fibrosis caused by permanent alcohol abuse [9], nonalcoholic steatohepatitis [10], Hepatitis C [11] and schistosomiasis [12].

Praziquantel (PZQ), as a safe anti-schistosome drug, has been used for more than 30 years [13]. It has been documented that PZQ has only mild side-effect and very low toxicity in animals [14]. No important long term safety problems have been observed in people and the safety is also considered in both children and pregnant women [15]. Reversal of schistosome-induced pathology after treatment of PZQ has been described. Parasitological cure of murine *Schistosoma monsoni* infection was followed by eventual partial reversal of liver fibrosis [16]. Researchers showed that patients in Ethiopia and Uganda had improvement or resolution

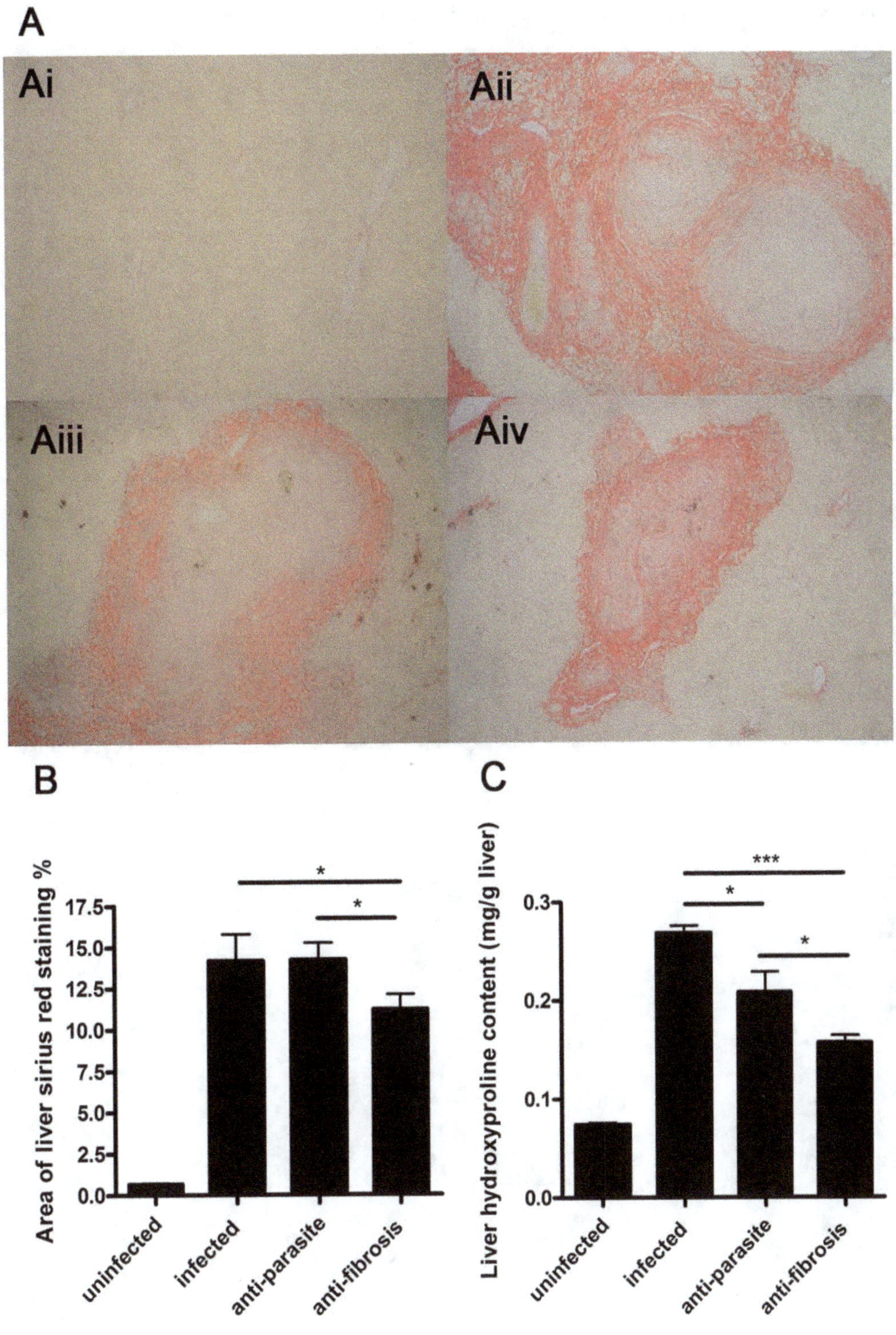

Figure 1. Anti-fibrosis treatment with prizaquantel reduced areas of liver Sirius Red staining and liver hydroxyproline contents of mice 8 weeks post infection with *Schistosoma japonicum*. (A) Representative images of Sirius Red staining by light microscope (×100). Ai, uninfected; Aii, infected; Aiii, anti-parasite; Aiv, anti-fibrosis. (B) Statistical analysis of scanned images in Sirius Red staining by software IPP6.0. (C) Measurement of liver hydroxyproline content. (* $p<0.05$, ** $p<0.01$, *** $p<0.001$).

of schistosomal periportal thickening/fibrosis after parasitologic cure of PZQ [17,18]. The main explanations of these results are presumed to be probably a removal of schistosomal worms and subsequent reduction of egg deposition. However, the exact mechanism is not clear.

Recent years, in addition to anti-helminth effect, anti-inflammation of PZQ has been reported [19]. Report also showed that eight- weeks- continuing treatment with PZQ could inhibit the development of pulmonary granulomas caused by vein injection of *Schistosoma japonicum* (*S. japonicum*) eggs, suggesting that PZQ may have the effect on fibrosis [20]. It seems that PZQ may not only eliminate the parasites, but also influence the immune response of the host, and consequently exerts dual effects on the infection. The aim of our study is to investigate whether PZQ has

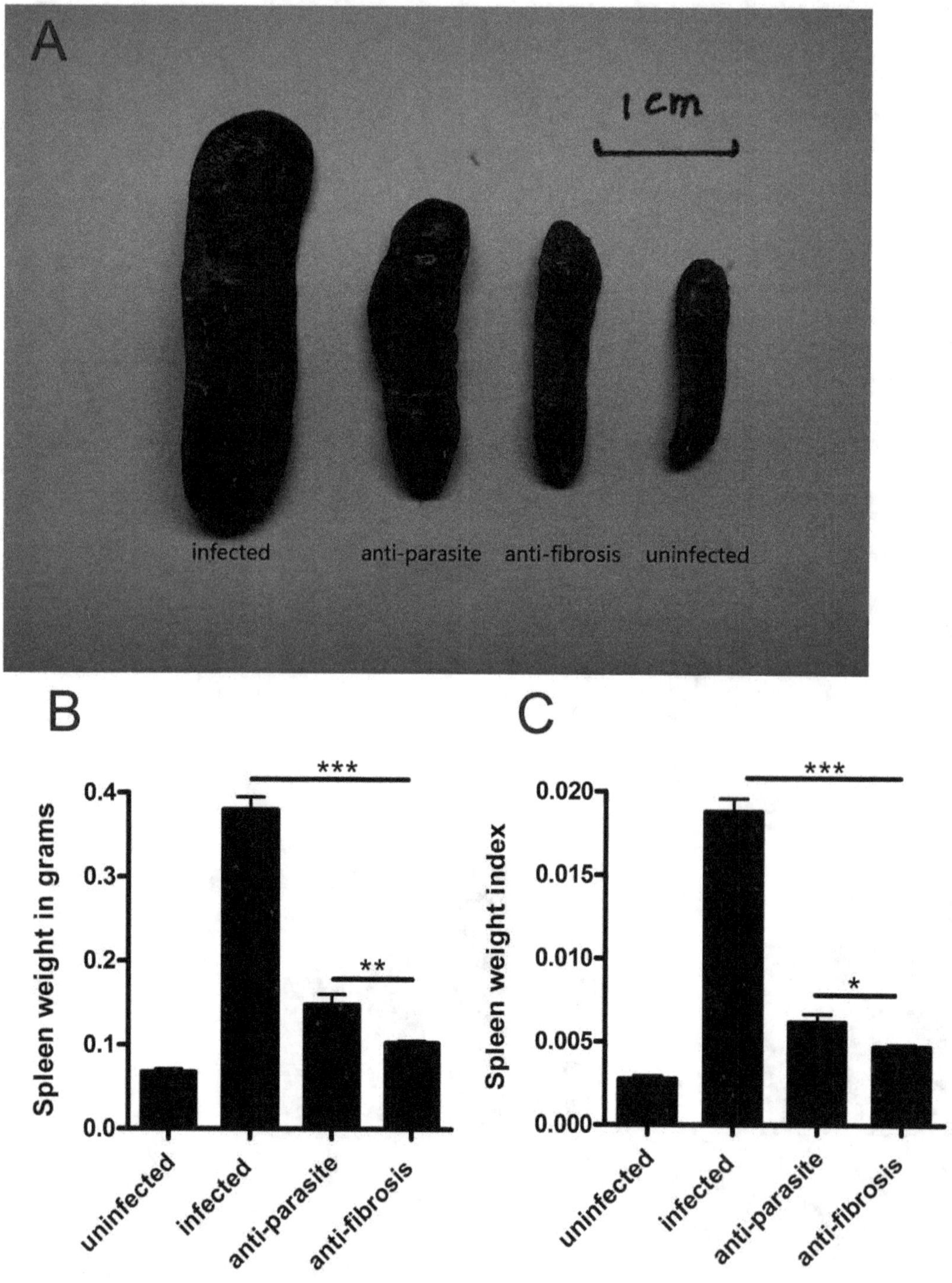

Figure 2. Anti-fibrosis treatment with prizaquantel reduced spleen weights in mice 8 weeks post infection with *Schistosoma japonicum*. (A) images of representative spleens in different groups. The bar is 1 cm. (B) Statistical analysis of spleen weights. (C) Spleen weight index (spleen weight/body weight). (* $p<0.05$, ** $p<0.01$, *** $p<0.001$).

the direct therapeutic action on liver fibrosis of schistosomiasis japonica and prospect it as a well tolerated, easily administered and inexpensive drug for new treatment strategy of hepatic schistosomiasis.

Materials and Methods

Animals and drug

Female BABL/c mice (Comparative Medicine Center of Yangzhou University, Yangzhou, China), 6–8 weeks old, were used throughout the study and maintained according to guidelines approved by the Nanjing Medical University Animal Experiment and Care Committee. *S. japonicum* cercariae of chinese mainland strain were obtained from the infected *Oncomelania hupensis* (Jiangsu Institute for Schistosomiasis Control, Wuxi, China). PZQ was purchased from Sigma and resuspanded in 1% carboxymethyl cellulose carrier for use.

Establishment of infection model and strategy of PZQ treatment

The BABL/c mice were infected cutaneously with 14±2 *S. japonicum* cercariae [21].The liver fibrosis models were established after the mice being infected for 8 weeks and 15 weeks, respectively. Intragastric administrations of PZQ (250 mg/kg/24 hours) for 3 days and continuing 1% carboxymethyl cellulose carrier up to 30 days were carried out as an anti-parasite intervention [16]. Intragastric administrations of PZQ (300 mg/kg/12 hours) for one month were carried out as an anti-fibrosis intervention. Both interventions were carried out for the mice of eight- weeks-infection and fifteen- weeks-infection, respectively (n = 10 in each group). A low dose administration of PZQ (75 mg/kg/12 hours) for one month was also used for the mice of fifteen-weeks-infection (n = 10). Concurrent control of untreated mice (n = 10) with liver fibrosis and uninfected mice (n = 8) were intragastric administrations of equal value of carboxymethyl cellulose carrier. When animals were sacrificed at the last time of treatment, liver portal venous pressures were measured, and tissues (livers and spleens) and serum were collected. Perfusions of hepatic portal system were performed to detect the number of adult worms as described [22]. For *in vivo* experiments on primary mouse HSCs, the mice getting the infection for 12 weeks and then administrating 250 mg/kg PZQ for 3 days were employed (n = 6 in each group).

Sirius Red staining and measure of liver hydroxyproline content

Mice livers were fixed in 10% neutralized formaldehyde and embedded in paraffin, and tissue sections (4-µm thick) were stained with aqueous saturated solution of picric acid containing 0.1% Sirius Red (Sigma-Aldrich, St. Louis, MO). Images of six random microscopic fields of red- stained collagen fibers in the liver section of each mouse were recorded using an inverted microscope (ZEISS, Goettingen, Germany) and then digitized and analyzed on Image-Pro Plus software 6.0 as previously described [21]. The content of liver hydroxyproline was determined according to the protocol of the Hydroxyproline Testing Kit (Jiancheng, Nanjing, China) as described [23].

Immunohistochemistry assay for α-SMA of liver

Smooth muscle actin alpha (α-SMA) (Sigma-Aldrich, St. Louis, MO), a marker of activated HSCs, was detected on formaldehyde-fixed paraffin-embedded sections by immunohisto- chemistry method. Images of six random microscopic fields in the sections of each mouse were recorded using an inverted microscope (ZEISS, Goettingen, Germany) and the α-SMA positive area of each image was analyzed by Image-Pro Plus software 6.0 software [21].

Measurement of mice serum alanine aminotransferase (ALT) and aspartate aminotransferase(AST)

Mice blood were collected in 1.5 ml Eppendorf tubes and standing in room temperature for 4 hours. The serums were separated by centrifugation at 3500 r/min for 15 minutes and serum ALT/AST was detected by Olympus AU5400 automatic biochemistry analyzer.

Measurement of liver portal venous pressure

Mouse was anesthetized with 2% Pentobarbital Sodium, then peritoneal cavity was opened and hepatic portal vein was canulated. Strain gauge transducer was used to get the signal from liver portal vein and the signal was recorded by Power-Lab8SP (ADInstruments, Castle Hill, Australia). Data acquisition was performed using Chart software v5.4 [24].

Isolation and culture of mice primary HSCs

HSCs were isolated from mice by the modified mothed as described [25]. Mice were anesthetized with 2% Pentobarbital Sodium. Peritoneal cavity was opened and hepatic portal vein was canulated. In situ perfusion of the livers was initiated with 40 mL DMEM (Hyclone, Thermo Fisher Scientific, Beijing, China) and at the same time the suprahepatic inferior vena cava was cut. The liver was removed, placed in a dish and perfused continually with DMED containing 0.04% collagenase type IV and 0.2% pronase (Gibco Life Technologies, Grand Island, NY, USA) at 37°C for 10 minutes. Then, the liver was further digested with DMEM containing 0.08% collagenase type IV, 0.08% pronase and 10 U/ml DNase I (Sigma-Aldrich, St. Louis, MO) at 37°C bath shaking for 30 minutes. The resulting cell suspension was filtered through

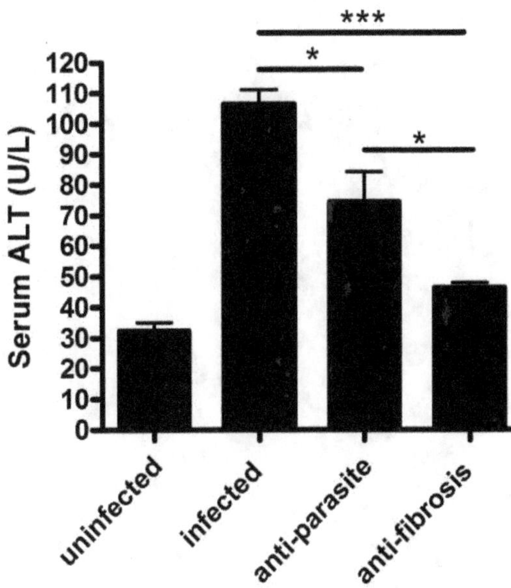

Figure 3. Anti-fibrosis treatment with prizaquantel reduced serum alanine aminotransferase (ALT) levels in mice 8 weeks post infection with *Schistosoma japonicum*. Serum ALT was assessed by Olympus AU5400 automatic biochemistry analyzer. (* $p<0.05$, ** $p<0.01$, *** $p<0.001$).

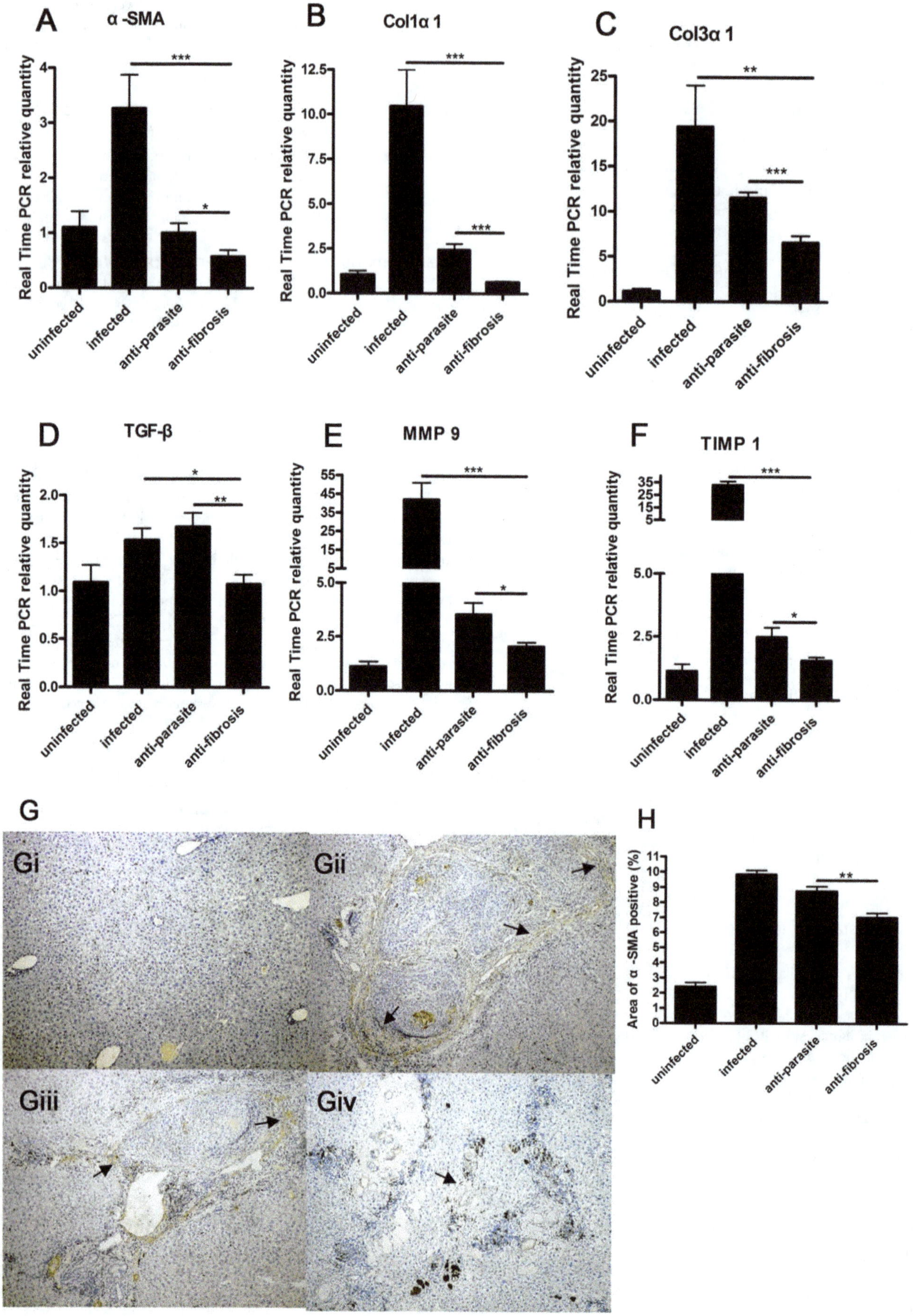

A
α -SMA
B
Col1α 1
C
Col3α 1
D
TGF-β
E
MMP 9
F
TIMP 1
Real Time PCR relative quantity
uninfected
infected
anti-parasite
anti-fibrosis
G
Gi
Gii
Giii
Giv
H
Area of α -SMA positive (%)

Figure 4. Anti-fibrosis treatment with prizaquantel inhibited expressions of liver profibrotic genes and α-SMA protein expression in mice 8 weeks post infection with *Schistosoma japonicum*. The expressions of mRNA were detected by Real Time PCR. (A) Expression of α-SMA. (B) Expression of Col1α1. (C) Expression of Col3α1. (D) Expression of TGF-β. (E) Expression of MMP9. (F) Expression of TIMP1. α-SMA protein expression was assessed by immunohistochemistry (G) Representative images of immunohistochemistry by light microscope (×100). Gi, uninfected; Gii, infected; Giii, anti-parasite; Giv, anti-fibrosis. Arrows showed the positive staining. (H) α-SMA positive areas were measured by software IPP6.0. (* $p<0.05$, ** $p<0.01$, *** $p<0.001$).

a nylon mesh and washed with cold DMEM for three times. Ten percent Optiprep(Axis-Shield PoC AS, Oslo, Norway) was used for density gradient centrifugation to isolate HSCs [26,27] and purity of HSCs was estimated based on the autofluorescence of the cells by ultraviolet-excited fluorescence microscopy. Cell viability was examined by Trypan blue exclusion. Both cell purity and viability were in excess of 90% [28].

RNA isolation and Real Time PCR

Tissues or cells were homogenized in Trizol (Invitrogen, Carlsbad, CA) and their RNAs were extracted according to the manufacturer's protocol. The RNA purity was assessed by spectrophotometry and 2% (w/v) agarose gel electrophoresis. Reverse transcriptase (RT) reactions for cDNA synthesis were carried out using RevertAid^{TM} First Strand cDNA Synthesis Kit with oligo-dT primer (Fermentas,EU). Relative expression of mRNA species was determined by Real Time PCR with Faststart Universal SYBR Green PCR Master(Roche Diagnostics, Indianapolis, IN, USA) using ABI7300. The primers formouse GAPDH (Forward 5′-TGGAAAGCTGTGGCGTGAT-3′, Reverse 5′-TGCTTCACCACCTTCTTGAT-3′) [29], mouse TGF-β (Forward 5′-CACCGGAGAGCCCTGGATA-3′, Reverse 5′-TGTACAGCTGCCGCACACA-3′) [30],mouse α-SMA(Forward 5′-TCAGCGCCTCCAGTTCCT-3′, Reverse 5′-AAAAAAAACCACGAGTAACAAATCAA-3′) [30],mouse Coll α1(Forward 5′-ACGTCCTGGTGAAGTTGGTC-3′, Reverse 5′-CAGGGAAGCCTCTTTCTCCT-3′) [31],mouse Col3α1(Forward 5′-TGGTCCTCAGGGTGTAAAGG-3′, Reverse 5′-GTCCAGCATCACCTTTTGGT-3′) [32],mouse MMP9(Forward 5′-GCTCATGTACCCGCTGTATAGCT-3′, Reverse 5′-CAGATACTGGATGCCGTCTATGTC-3′) [33], mouse TIMP1(Forward 5′-TGGGAAATGCCGCAGATATC-3′, Reverse 5′-TGGGACTTGTGGGCATATCC-3′) [33], mouse IL-4(Forward 5′-GGTCTCAACCCCCAGCTAGT-3′, Reverse 5′-GCCGATGATCTCTCTCAAGTGAT-3′), mouse IL-10(Forward 5′-GCTCTTACTGACTGGCATGAG-3′, Reverse 5′-CGCAGCTCTAGGAGCATGTG-3′), mouse IL-13(Forward 5′-CCTGGCTCTTGCTTGCCTT-3′, Reverse 5′-GGTCTTGTGTGATGTTGCTCA-3′) and mouse IFN-γ(Forward 5′-ATGAACGCTACACACTGCATC-3′, Reverse 5′-CCATCCTTTTGCCAGTTCCTC-3′) were gained from articles orPrimerBank (http://pga.mgh.harvard.edu/primerbank/), and used for PCR. Cycling conditions were 2 min at 50°C, then 10 min at 95°C and followed by 40 cycles of 95°C for 15 s and 60°C for 1 min. Melt curve analysis and 2% agarose gel electrophoresis of the amplicon were used to determine the specificity of the amplicon. Data were normalized with GAPDH and results were expressed as fold amplification using the method described by Pfaffl [34]. Each experiment was repeated three times.

Statistics

The data were analyzed using two-tailed Student's *t*-test when compared between two groups. A p-value<0.05 was considered statistically significant. All statistical analyses were operated by GraphPad Prism software 5.0.

Results

PZQ Treatment Decreases Liver Fibrosis and Its Related Gene Expressions in the Mice with Chronic Schistosomiasis

PZQ was administrated to the mice infected with *S. japonicum* at week 8 post-infection for either 3 days (anti-parasite group, 250 mg/kg/day) or 30 days (anti-fibrosis group,300 mg/kg/12 hours). Homochronous normal mice (uninfected group) and untreated mice (infected group) were also used in the experiments. The perfusion of hepatic portal system showed that no adult worm was detected in anti-parasite group at the end of the treatment (data not shown), which demonstrated that the administration of PZQ for anti-parasite treatment resulted in parasitologic cure. As shown in figures 1A and 1B, the areas of Sirius Red- stained liver were significantly decreased in anti-fibrosis group in comparison to both infected group and anti-parasite group. The accordant results were observed in measurement of liver hydroxyproline contents (Figure 1C). In addition, the spleen weight and the spleen index (spleen weight/body weight) of the mice were also reduced in anti-fibrosis group in comparison to both infected group and anti-parasite group (Figure 2). Serum ALT which was dramatically increased after the infection was decreased by anti-fibrosis therapy of PZQ (Figure 3).

Hepatic mRNA expressions of the genes associated with liver fibrosis were detected by Real Time PCR. Results showed that the levels of Coll α1, Col3α1, α-SMA, MMP9 and TIMP1 were decreased while TGF-β was increased in anti-parasite group in comparison to infected group and all of them were decreased in anti-fibrosis group in comparison to both infected group and anti-parasite group (Figure 4A–F). Immunohistochemistry assay showed that α-SMA positive cells around the hepatic egg granulomas were dramatically decreased in anti-fibrosis group in comparison to both infected group and anti-parasite group (Figure 4G–H).

Besides, CCL_4-induced early and established liver fibrosis mice [35] was brought into our experiment (Text S1). PZQ treatment significantly reduced the collagen areas in CCL_4-induced fibrotic liver assessed by Sirius Red staining (Figure S1A–D). Content of hepatic hydroxyproline (Figure S1E) as well as serum ALT and AST (Figure S1F) was also decreased significantly in PZQ treated mice.

PZQ Treatment Decreases Liver Fibrosis and Enhances MMP9 gene Expression of Mice with Advanced Schistosomiasis

In this study, PZQ was administrated to the mice infected with *S.japonicum* at week 15 post-infection for either 3 days (anti-parasite group, 250 mg/kg/day) or 30 days (anti-fibrosis low dose group, 75 mg/kg/12 hours; anti-fibrosis high dose group, 300 mg/kg/12 hours). Homochronous normal mice (uninfected group) and untreated infected mice (infected group) were also used in the experiments. As expected, the areas of Sirius Red staining on the liver sections were significantly decreased in high dose group in comparison to both infected group and anti-

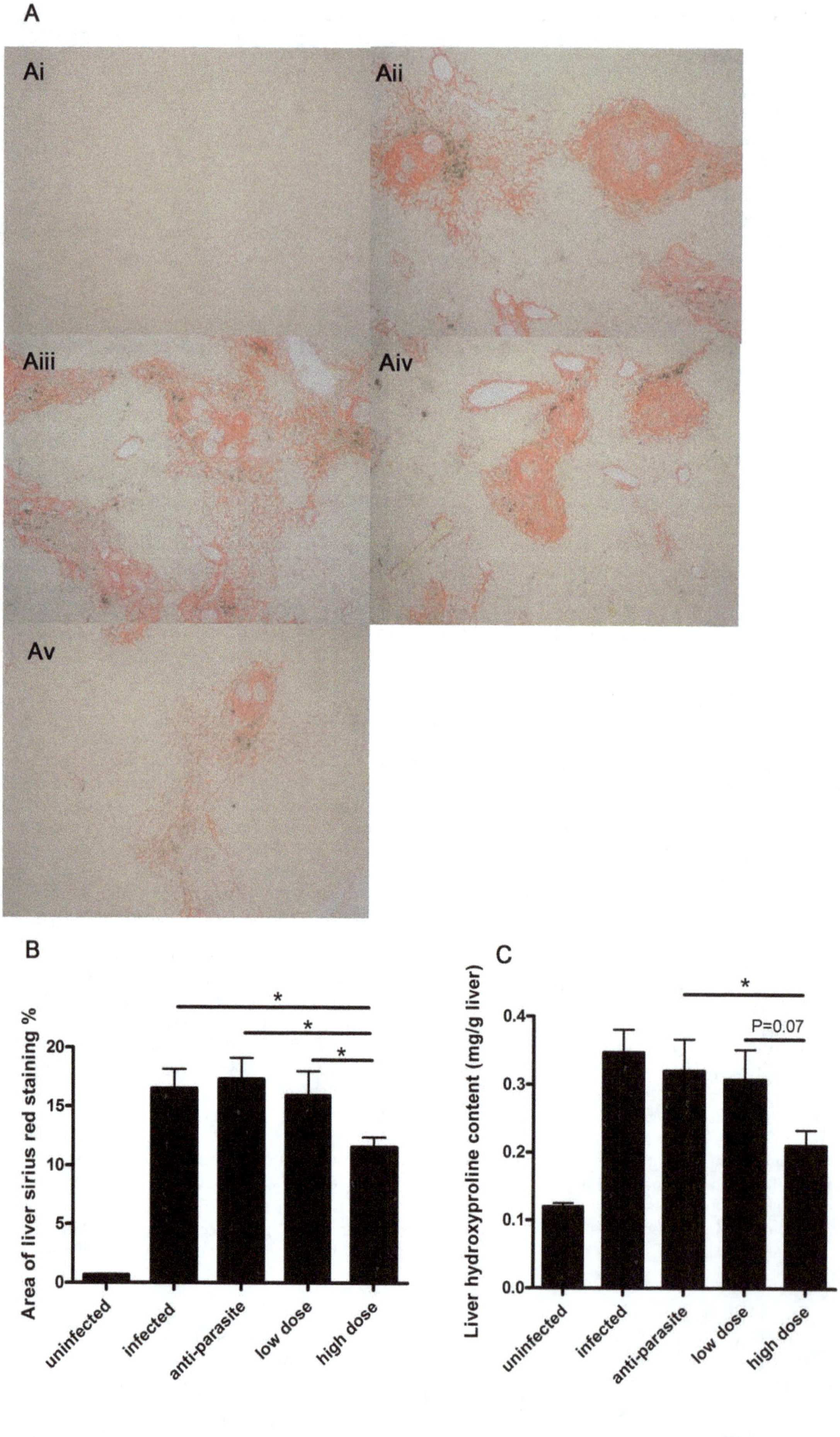
A
Ai
Aii
Aiii
Aiv
Av
B
Area of liver sirius red staining %
0
5
10
15
20
*
*
*
uninfected
infected
anti-parasite
low dose
high dose
C
Liver hydroxyproline content (mg/g liver)
0.0
0.1
0.2
0.3
0.4
*
P=0.07
uninfected
infected
anti-parasite
low dose
high dose

Figure 5. Anti-fibrosis treatment with prizaquantel reduced areas of liver Sirius Red staining and liver hydroxyproline content in mice 15 weeks post infection with *Schistosoma japonicum.* (A) Representative images of Sirius Red staining by light microscope (×100). Ai, uninfected; Aii, infected; Aiii, anti-parasite; Aiv, low dose; Av, high dose. (B) Statistical analysis of scanned images in Sirius Red staining by software IPP6.0. (C) Measurement of Liver hydroxyproline content. (* $p<0.05$).

parasite group. In low dose group, the Sirius Red stained-areas decreased without statistical significance in comparison to anti-parasite group. Also, the change profiles of the liver hydroxyproline contents were in accordance with those of Sirius Red staining (Figure 5). The spleen weights of mice in anti-parasite group and anti-fibrosis groups (both low dose and high dose) were decreased in comparison to infected group, but no significant differences between them (Figure 6). Portal hypertension is a characteristic manifestation of advanced schistosomiasis japonica and resulted mainly from severe hepatic fibrosis. To evaluate the anti-fibrosis effects of PZQ on the mice with advanced schistosomiasis, we measured liver portal venous pressure. The results showed that the pressure of the mice were significantly decreased after anti-parasite treatment and further decreased to nearly normal levels after both low dose and high dose treatment of PZQ (Figure 7). Serum ALT levels were significantly decreased only in high dose group, which were nearly back to normal baselines (Figure 8).

We also detected the expressions of fibrosis-related genes. Col1α1, Col3α1, α-SMA and TGF-β mRNAs of liver were all markedly decreased in high dose group in comparison to both infected group and anti-parasite group (Figure 9A–D), which were similar to those changes in the mice with chronic schistosomiasis. Liver TIMP1 mRNA was reduced in low dose group, but more significantly decreased in high dose group in comparison to anti-parasite group. However, the expression of liver MMP9 mRNA was increased nearly five-fold in high dose group in comparison to both anti-parasite group and low dose group (Figure 10E–F). Hence, PZQ did not inhibit all kinds of fibrosis-related genes in liver. The immunohistochemistry change of liver α-SMA in each group was accordant with its α-SMA mRNA expression (Figure 9G–H). Gene Expressions of Th1/Th2 cytokines of IL4, IL10, IL13 and IFN-γ were all reduced in high dose group in comparison to infected, anti-parasite and low dose group, respectively (Figure 9I–L). Normal mice treated with high dose PZQ for 30 days (Text S2) showed reduced mRNA expression of Col1α1, TGF-β and TIMP1 in liver in comparison to untreated control mice (Figure S2A, D and F). Col3α1 and α-SMA (Figure S2B and C) showed a tendency to decrease, while MMP9 (Figure S2E) showed a tendency to increase, but the changes were not significant statistically. We also demonstrated that PZQ did not inhibit the proliferation of splenic mononuclear cells stimulated by schistosomal egg antigens detected by incorporation of ^{3}H-thymidine (TDR) (Text S3 and Figure S3).

PZQ Treatment Inhibits Activation or Fibrosis-related gene expressions of Primary HSCs in Mice with Chronic Schistosomiasis

PZQ was administrated to the mice infected with *S.japonicum* at week 12 post-infection for 3 days (250 mg/kg/day) and primary HSCs were isolated for detection of mRNA expression. Consistent with anti-fibrosis treatment experiment of the mice with chronic schistosomiasis, the expressions of activation or fibrosis-related genes such as Col1α1, Col3α1, α-SMA, TGF-β, MMP9 and TIMP1 were all decreased significantly after the anti-parasite treatment with PZQ (Figure 10).

Discussion

Although it remain a neglected transmissible disease, affecting people mainly in developing countries, schistosomiasis are second only to malaria as a major parasitic disease [36]. So far, although chemotherapy makes a great success in against all schistosome species, few admitted and widely used interventions of anti-fibrosis can be accepted to improve the hepatic fibrosis and treatment of hepatic fibrosis for the patients with schistosomiasis is neglected all the while. The patients with severe diseases have no choice but surgery for enlarged spleens or fibrotic liver to avoid the risk of death [37,38]. Consequently, radical therapy of hepatic fibrosis remains an imperative requirement and new effective drugs of anti-fibrosis are eager to be applied in clinical.

PZQ, as an antihelminthic drug, is widely used now. After PZQ anti-parasite therapy, hepatic fibrosis is reversal in murine schistosomiasis model and the reversal is considered due to pathogenic cure [39]. Other effects have been reported too in recent years [19,20], suggesting that PZQ may have direct effect on host. However, there is no report about the direct anti-fibrosis effect and mechanism of PZQ on liver. In our experiments, we adopted continuous and therapeutic dose (600 mg/kg/day for murine approximately converts to 60 mg/kg/day for human [40]) of PZQ for anti-fibrosis treatment and investigated whether it has

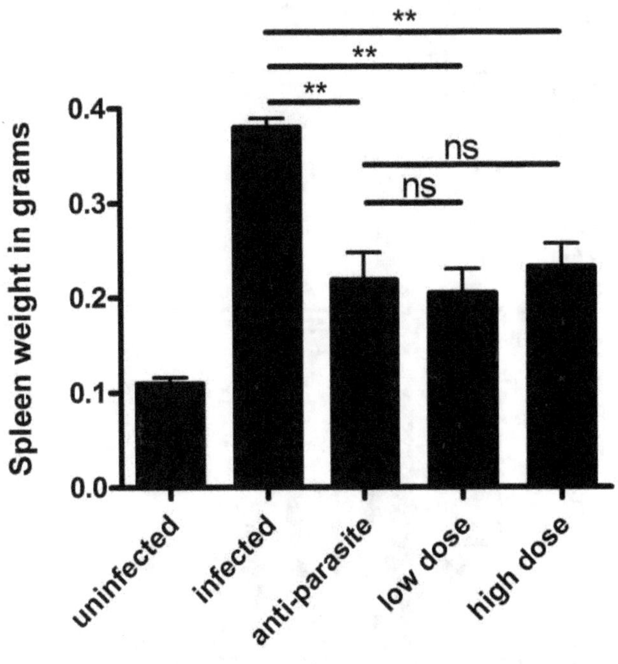

Figure 6. Spleen weights were not changed after Anti-fibrosis treatment with low dose or high dose prizaquantel compared with anti-parasite treatment in mice 15 weeks post infection with *Schistosoma japonicum.* Spleen weights were reduced in anti-parasite, anti-fibrosis low dose and high dose groups compared with infected group, but no significant changes were found between treated groups. (** $p<0.01$).

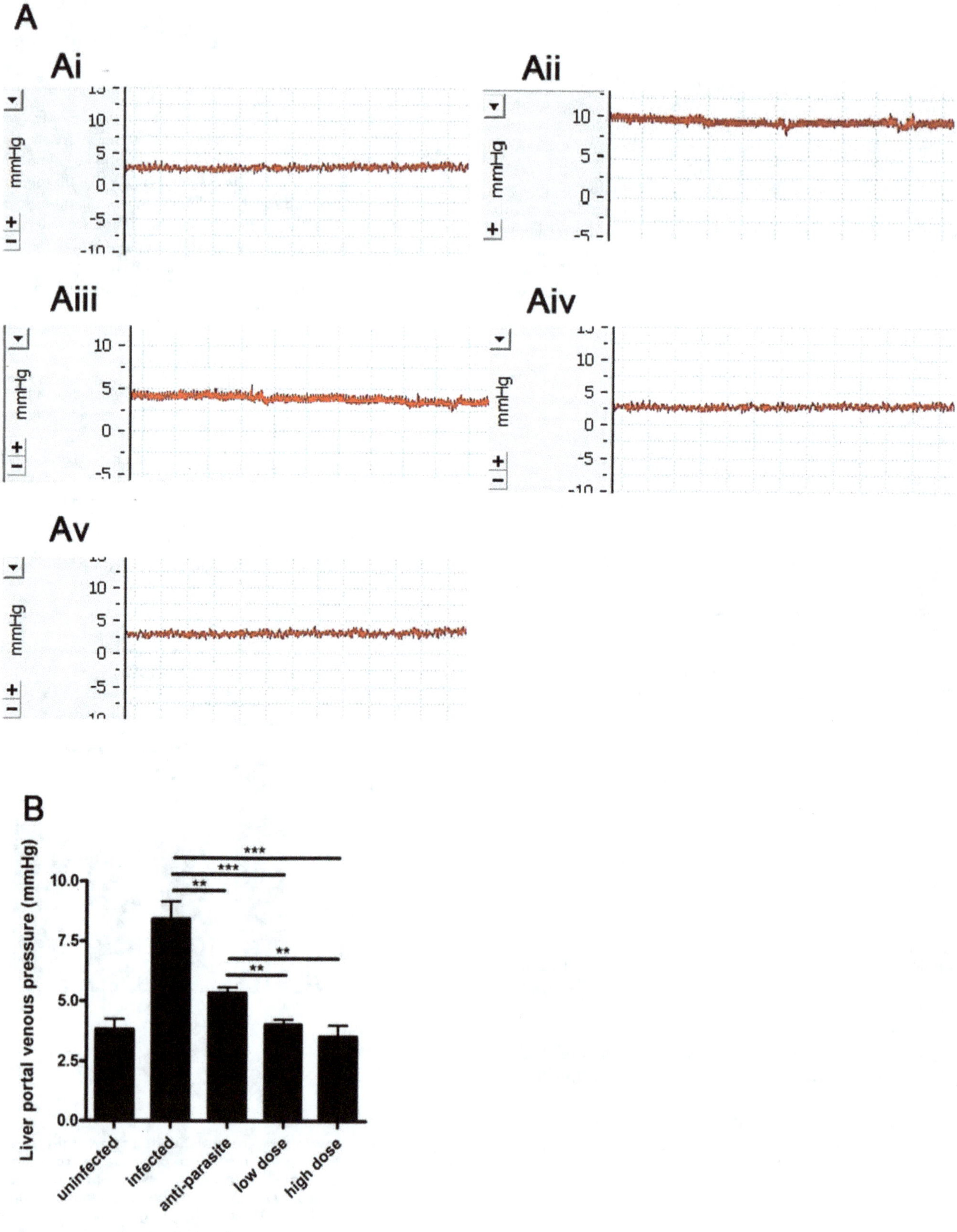
A
Ai
Aii
Aiii
Aiv
Av
mmHg
10
5
0
-5
B
Liver portal venous pressure (mmHg)
10.0
7.5
5.0
2.5
0.0
***
**
uninfected
infected
anti-parasite
low dose
high dose

Figure 7. Anti-fibrosis treatment with prizaquantel reduced hepatic portal venous pressure. Hepatic portal venous pressure was measured by PowerLab8SP and analyzed by chart5 software. (A) Representative recording images were showed: Ai, uninfected; Aii, infected; Aiii anti-parasite; Aiv, low dose; Av, high dose. (B) Statistical analysis of each group hepatic portal venous pressure. Although anti-parasite treatment reduced portal venous pressure compared with infected group, anti-fibrosis treatment (both low dose and high dose group) further reduced the pressure to nearly uninfected level. (** $p<0.01$, *** $p<0.001$).

the effect of anti-fibrosis and contributes to the strategy of schistosomiasis hepatic fibrosis treatment.

Because mouse model is of high homologization and has similar course with human schistosomiasis, we thus established the mouse schistosomiasis model [41]. In the study, we demonstrated that anti-fibrosis treatment with PZQ significantly improved the hepatic fibrosis of schistosomiasis japonica at both 8 weeks and 15 weeks post-infection, as measured by Sirius Red staining areas and hydroxyproline content. We also detected the clinical parameters, such as spleen weight, portal venous pressure and serum ALT. The results showed that clinical symptoms, such as splenomegaly [42,43], portal hypertension [44,45] and dysregulated liver function [46,47] were ameliorated by anti-fibrosis treatment with PZQ. Low dose treatment with PZQ did not show significant effects on hepatic fibrosis, which may be due to the quick metabolism of this drug in liver [48]. Because of the probable formation of fibrotic spleens [47], the enlarged spleens were not reversed by treatment of PZQ in advanced schistosomiasis mice. Meanwhile, hepatic fibrosis was more serious in 15 weeks- post-infected mice than in 8 weeks- post-infected mice before and after treatment. Herein, we suggest that anti-fibrosis treatment with PZQ should be used as early as possible and delayed treatment will be difficult to reverse the splenomegaly and hepatic fibrosis.

To further confirm the reversal of hepatic fibrosis, we detected the transcriptional level of some profibrotic genes in liver, such as Col1α1 and Col1α3 which are predominant collagens in the liver of schistosomiasis mice [49,50]. TGF-β is considered as typical profibrotic gene in the progress of hepatic fibrosis [51,52], and also plays an important role in hepatic fibrosis of schistosomiasis [53,54]. The expressions of TGF-β, as well as α-SMA which is the activated marker of HSCs [7,55], were detected between each group. All of them were decreased after anti-fibrosis treatment of PZQ, suggesting that anti-fibrosis treatment of PZQ inhibits transcriptional levels of profibrotic gene expressions in schistosomiasis mouse liver.

Besides, gene expressions of Th1/Th2 cytokines such as IL-4, IL-10, IL-13 and IFN-γ, which were important in schistosomiasis liver fibrosis [21,56,57], were also detected in our experiment. Studies in schistosomiasis demonstrated that the development of fibrosis requires the production of the profibrotic cytokines IL-4 and IL-13 [58,59,60]. Oppositely, IL-10 and IFN-γ showed antifibrotic effects [57]. Our results demonstrated that anti-fibrosis treatment with PZQ significantly inhibited the gene expression of both Th1 and Th2 cytokines, which suggested that the alteration of Th1/Th2 cytokines in hepatic microenvironment after PZQ treatment might finally influence the resolution of hepatic fibrosis. Furthermore, although expressions of fibrosis associated genes in liver of normal mice were low, PZQ treatment could also inhibit the expression of them such as Col1α1, TGF-β and TIMP1 in our experiment. Therefore, PZQ treatment could regulate the expression of fibrosis associated genes not only on schistosomiasis mice but also on normal mice.

The balance of the activities between matrix metalloproteinases (MMPs) and TIMPs(tissue inhibitors of metalloproteinases) plays an important role in extracellular matrix(ECM) production and degradation in hepatic fibrosis [61,62]. MMP9 with the activity of collagen degradation [21,63] has multi-source and is produced by Kupffer cells [64], hepatocytes [65] and HSCs [66]. Meanwhile, HSCs is also the main source of TIMP1 [8]. In our chronic fibrosis model, we showed that treatment of anti-fibrosis with PZQ reduced transcriptional levels of MMP9 and TIMP1. Meanwhile, TIMP1 was more close to the normal level than MMP-9. Unexpectedly, we observed a high transcriptional level of MMP9 by anti-fibrosis treatment with PZQ in liver of advanced infected mice, whereas TIMP1 was significantly reduced. Thus, the imbalance that favors MMP9 by PZQ treatment is helpful to reverse hepatic fibrosis.

Unlike schistosome egg induced hepatic granuloma and fibrosis, CCL_4-induced liver fibrosis is mainly due to the damage of hepatocyte [35]. However, the mechanism of resulting liver fibrosis is the same that is the activation of HSCs and subsequent ECM deposition [5]. In order to confirm the anti-fibrotic properties of PZQ, we established mice model of CCL_4-induced liver fibrosis. As expected, PZQ treatment significantly reduced liver collagen areas and hydroxyproline content in mice of CCL_4-induced liver fibrosis. Level of serum ALT and AST were also significantly reduced after PZQ treatment. These results further confirmed the anti-fibrosis effects of PZQ.

To further investigate cellular mechanism of anti-fibrosis with PZQ, we focused on HSCs, which is one of liver resident cells and plays the key role in liver fibrosis [5,7]. In recent researches,

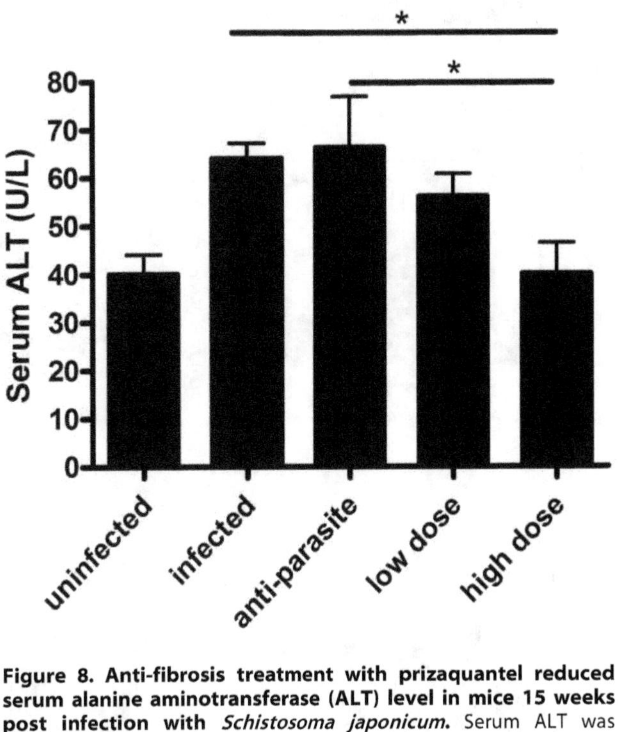

Figure 8. Anti-fibrosis treatment with prizaquantel reduced serum alanine aminotransferase (ALT) level in mice 15 weeks post infection with *Schistosoma japonicum*. Serum ALT was assessed by Olympus AU5400 automatic biochemistry analyzer. Levels of serum ALT were significantly decreased nearly to the normal level after anti-fibrosis treatment with high dose prizaquantel. (* $p<0.05$).

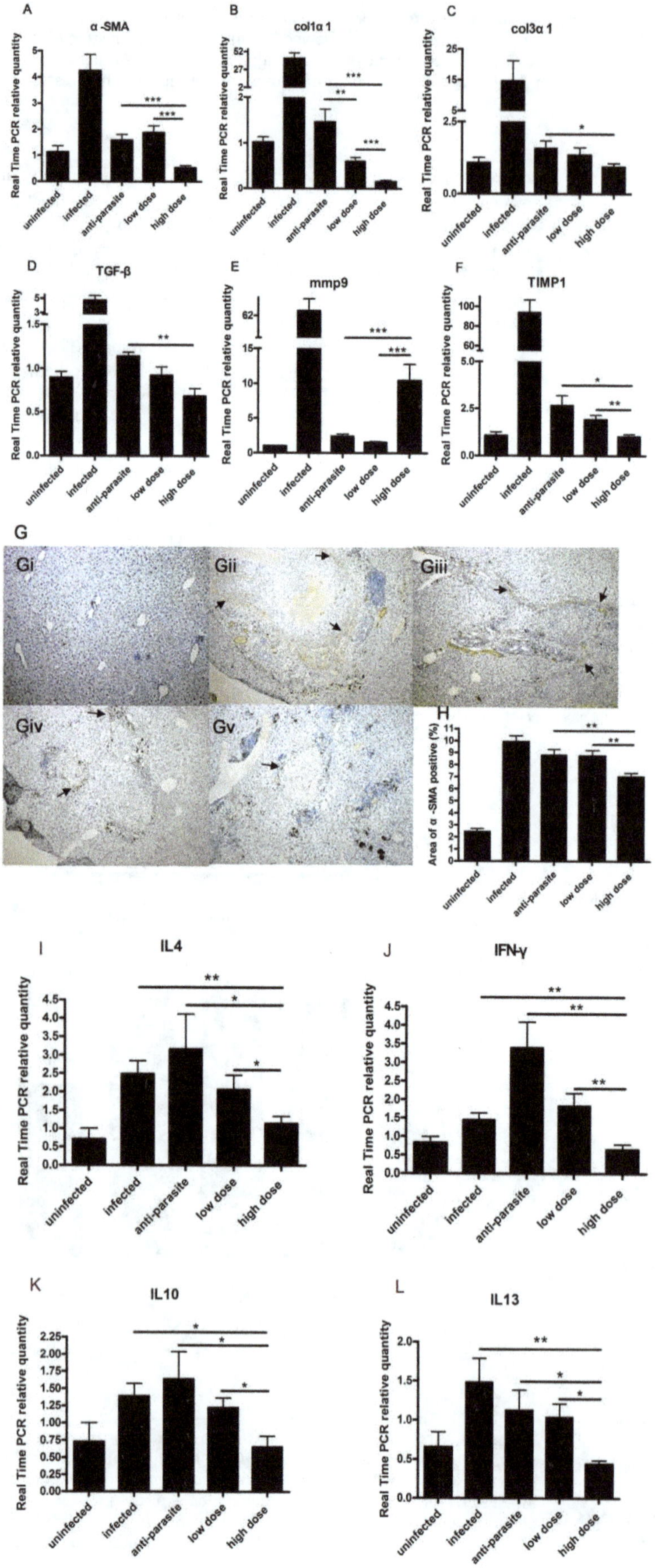
A
α -SMA
B
col1α 1
C
col3α 1
D
TGF-β
E
mmp9
F
TIMP1
G
Gi
Gii
Giii
Giv
Gv
H
Area of α -SMA positive (%)
I
IL4
J
IFN-γ
K
IL10
L
IL13
Real Time PCR relative quantity
uninfected
infected
anti-parasite
low dose
high dose

Figure 9. Anti-fibrosis treatment with prizaquantel inhibited expressions of profibrotic genes and α-SMA protein expression in liver, but increased MMP9 mRNA expressions of mice 15 weeks post infection with *Schistosoma japonicum.* (A)α-SMA; (B)Col1α1; (C)Col3α1; (D)TGF-β were reduced by anti-fibrosis treatment with high dose prizaquantel. (E)MMP9 levels in high dose group were increased about 10 fold compared with uninfected group, whereas (F) TIMP1 levels were decreased nearly to uninfected level. α-SMA protein expressions was assessed by immunohistochemistry. (G) Representative images of immunohistochemistry by light microscope (×100). Gi, uninfected; Gii, infected; Giii, anti-parasite; Giv, low dose; Gv, high dose. Arrows showed the positive staining. (H) α-SMA positive areas were measured by software IPP6.0. Expression of IL-4 (I), IL-10 (J), IL-13(K) and IFN-γ (L) were significantly reduced in high dose group compared respectively with infected, anti-parasite or low dose group. (* $p<0.05$, ** $p<0.01$, *** $p<0.001$).

HSCs is the promising target of anti-fibrosis drugs [67]. In our experiments with mouse models, we found the reduced transcriptional levels of the fibrosis-related genes Col1α1, Col3α1, α-SMA, TGF-β, MMP9 and TIMP1 in primary HSCs by PZQ treatment for 3 days. This result was consistent with anti-fibrosis treatment experiment of mice with chronic schistosomiasis, indicating that inhibition of HSCs activation by PZQ occured rapidly after the treatment. More importantly, the inhibition was persistence and no rebounding of this effect was observed at the end of anti-parasite treatment. Therefore, PZQ might exhibit the anti-fibrosis property by affecting activation of HSCs. Although the appropriate dose-course of anti-fibrosis treatment by PZQ is not determined and the exact pathway is not clear, our results suggest that PZQ is a promising drug for the treatment of hepatic fibrosis.

In conclusion, although the pathways about anti-fibrosis property of PZQ are enigmatic, we demonstrated the effects of anti-fibrosis of PZQ in mice with both chronic and advanced schistosomiasis as well as in CCL_4-induced liver fibrosis mice. Our study also provided clues that based on the changes following PZQ treatment, the levels of TGF-β and TIMP-1 were potential biomarkers for regression of liver fibrosis. It is suggested that new treatment strategy in clinical is that treatment of pathogenic intervention could be adopted at first and followed by anti-fibrosis treatment with PZQ for several times. The inhibition of transcriptional levels of profibrotic genes in HSCs by treatment

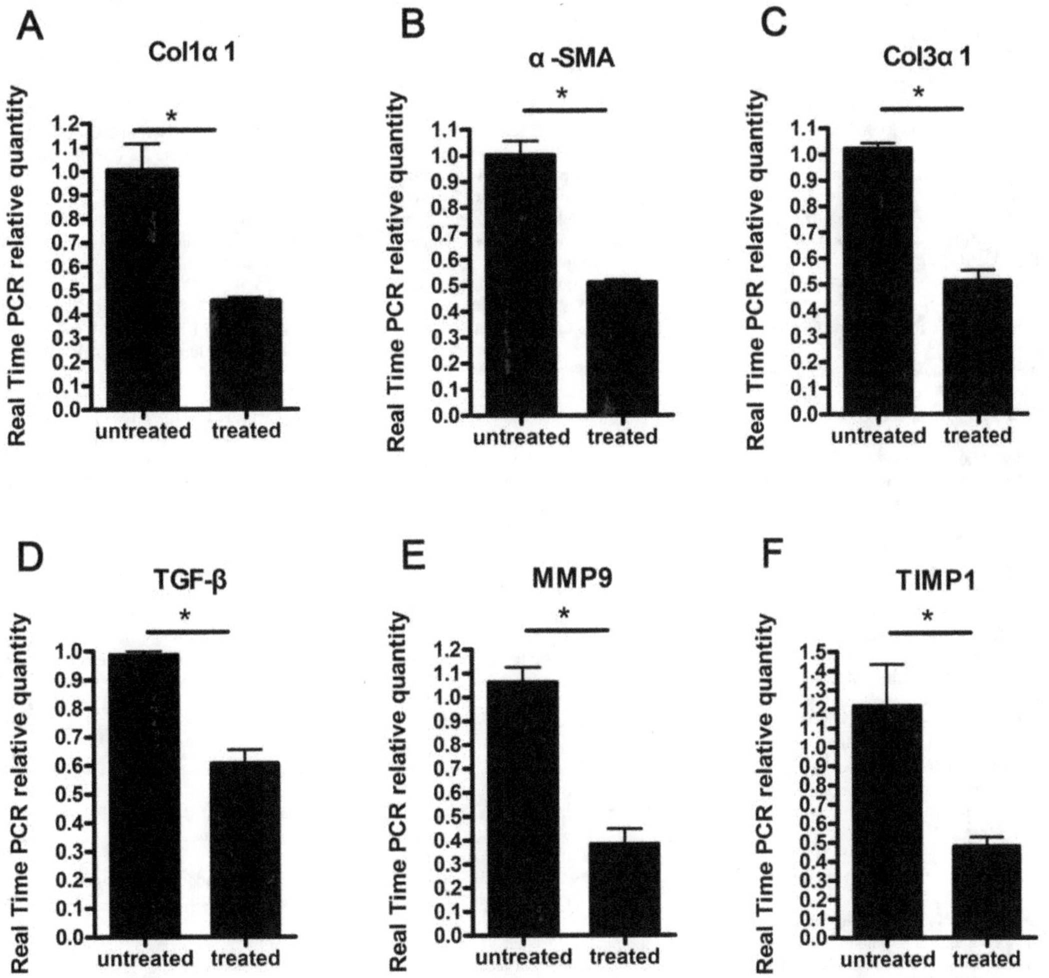

Figure 10. Treatment of prizaquantel for 3 days inhibited expressions of HSC profibrotic genes of mice 12 weeks post infection with *Schistosoma japonicum.* Prizaquantel (250 mg/kg/day) was administrated to mice for 3 days. Primary HSCs were isolated and transcriptional levels were assessed by Real Time PCR. Transcriptional level of (A) Col1α1, (B) α-SMA,(C) Col3α1, (D) TGF-β, (E) MMP9 and (F) TIMP1 in HSC of treated mice were significantly reduced compared with untreated mice. (* $p<0.05$).

with PZQ is probably part mechanism of its anti-fibrosis property. Further molecular mechanism and clinical application of PZQ are deserved to be investigated.

Supporting Information

Figure S1 PZQ treatment improved CCL_4 -induced liver fibrosis and serum transaminase. Liver sections of mice from normal (A), CCL_4 -induced liver fibrosis (B), and PZQ treatment (C) groups were stained with Sirius Red, respectively. Statistical analysis showed that PZQ treatment significantly decreased collagen areas (D). PZQ treatment also decreased the liver hydroxyproline content (E) and serum ALT/AST (F). (*, $p<0.05$;**, $p<0.01$; ***, $p<0.001$).

Figure S2 PZQ treatment inhibited the expressions of liver fibrosis associated genes in normal mice detected by Real Time PCR. Results showed that PZQ treatment significantly decreased the expression of Col1α1 (A), TGF-β (D) and TIMP1 (F) ($p<0.001$), and the changes of Col3α1(B), α-SMA(C), and MMP9(E) were not significant. ($p>0.05$).

Figure S3 Proliferation of spleen mononuclearcells were not significantly changed by stimulation of SEA. 12 weeks post-infected schistosomiasis mice were first treated by prizaquantel or control solution. Then spleen mononuclearcells were isolated and stimulated by SEA or anti-CD3. The method of incorporation of ^{3}H-thymidine (TDR) was used to assess the proliferation. (ns, no significance).

Text S1

Text S2

Text S3

Acknowledgments

We thank Ming-Juan Tan at the Department of Laboratory Medicine, Nanjing First Hospital for ALT analysis and Yu-Hua Li at the Department of Pathology, Nanjing Medical University for help with the Immunohistochemistry assay.

Author Contributions

Conceived and designed the experiments: YW Z-SZ Y-JL. Performed the experiments: Y-JL JL QY DZ Y-PL LS YZ A-LC Y-YR K-YS YS. Analyzed the data: Y-JL JL YW. Wrote the paper: Y-JL YW JL.

References

1. Gryseels B, Polman K, Clerinx J, Kestens L (2006) Human schistosomiasis. Lancet 368: 1106–1118.
2. Cheever AW (1997) Differential regulation of granuloma size and hepatic fibrosis in schistosome infections. Mem Inst Oswaldo Cruz 92: 689–692.
3. Takemura Y, Kikuchi S, Inaba Y (1998) Epidemiologic study of the relationship between schistosomiasis due to Schistosoma japonicum and liver cancer/cirrhosis. Am J Trop Med Hyg 59: 551–556.
4. Andrade ZA (2008) Schistosomiasis and hepatic fibrosis regression. Acta Trop 108: 79–82.
5. Friedman SL (2008) Mechanisms of hepatic fibrogenesis. Gastroenterology 134: 1655–1669.
6. Friedman SL (2008) Hepatic stellate cells: protean, multifunctional, and enigmatic cells of the liver. Physiol Rev 88: 125–172.
7. Bartley PB, Ramm GA, Jones MK, Ruddell RG, Li Y, et al. (2006) A contributory role for activated hepatic stellate cells in the dynamics of Schistosoma japonicum egg-induced fibrosis. Int J Parasitol 36: 993–1001.
8. Arthur MJ, Mann DA, Iredale JP (1998) Tissue inhibitors of metalloproteinases, hepatic stellate cells and liver fibrosis. J Gastroenterol Hepatol 13 Suppl: S33–38.
9. Breitkopf K, Haas S, Wiercinska E, Singer MV, Dooley S (2005) Anti-TGF-beta strategies for the treatment of chronic liver disease. Alcohol Clin Exp Res 29: 121S–131S.
10. Cortez-Pinto H, Baptista A, Camilo ME, de Moura MC (2001) Hepatic stellate cell activation occurs in nonalcoholic steatohepatitis. Hepatogastroenterology 48: 87–90.
11. Tomanovic NR, Boricic IV, Brasanac DC, Stojsic ZM, Delic DS, et al. (2009) Activated liver stellate cells in chronic viral C hepatitis: histopathological and immunohistochemical study. J Gastrointestin Liver Dis 18: 163–167.
12. Burke ML, Jones MK, Gobert GN, Li YS, Ellis MK, et al. (2009) Immunopathogenesis of human schistosomiasis. Parasite Immunol 31: 163–176.
13. Fenwick A, Savioli L, Engels D, Robert Bergquist N, Todd MH (2003) Drugs for the control of parasitic diseases: current status and development in schistosomiasis. Trends Parasitol 19: 509–515.
14. Stelma FF, Talla I, Sow S, Kongs A, Niang M, et al. (1995) Efficacy and side effects of praziquantel in an epidemic focus of Schistosoma mansoni. Am J Trop Med Hyg 53: 167–170.
15. WHO (2002) Report of the WHO informal consultation on the use of praziquantel during pregnancy/lactation and albendazole/mebendazole in children under 24 months (WHO/CDS/CPE/PVC/2002.4). Geneva: World Health Organization.
16. Morcos SH, Khayyal MT, Mansour MM, Saleh S, Ishak EA, et al. (1985) Reversal of hepatic fibrosis after praziquantel therapy of murine schistosomiasis. Am J Trop Med Hyg 34: 314–321.
17. Berhe N, Myrvang B, Gundersen SG (2008) Reversibility of schistosomal periportal thickening/fibrosis after praziquantel therapy: a twenty-six month follow-up study in Ethiopia. Am J Trop Med Hyg 78: 228–234.
18. Frenzel K, Grigull L, Odongo-Aginya E, Ndugwa CM, Loroni-Lakwo T, et al. (1999) Evidence for a long-term effect of a single dose of praziquantel on Schistosoma mansoni-induced hepatosplenic lesions in northern Uganda. Am J Trop Med Hyg 60: 927–931.
19. Pinlaor S, Hiraku Y, Yongvanit P, Tada-Oikawa S, Ma N, et al. (2006) iNOS-dependent DNA damage via NF-kappaB expression in hamsters infected with Opisthorchis viverrini and its suppression by the antihelminthic drug praziquantel. Int J Cancer 119: 1067–1072.
20. Xu YL, Huang YX, Yu CX, Liang YS, Wu YY, et al. (2007) Effect of praziquantel on schistosomal ovum granuloma and hepatic fibrosis I Effect of praziquantel on schistosomal ovum granuloma in the lung of mice. Chin J Schisto Control 19: 357–359.
21. Tao FF, Yang YF, Wang H, Sun XJ, Luo J, et al. (2009) Th1-type epitopes-based cocktail PDDV attenuates hepatic fibrosis in C57BL/6 mice with chronic Schistosoma japonicum infection. Vaccine 27: 4110–4117.
22. Zhang L, Yang Y, Yang X, Zhao J, Yang J, et al. (2008) T cell epitope-based peptide-DNA dual vaccine induces protective immunity against Schistosoma japonicum infection in C57BL/6J mice. Microbes Infect 10: 251–259.
23. Yue HY, Yin C, Hou JL, Zeng X, Chen YX, et al. (2010) Hepatocyte nuclear factor 4alpha attenuates hepatic fibrosis in rats. Gut 59: 236–246.
24. Gonzalez-Forero D, Portillo F, Sunico CR, Moreno-Lopez B (2004) Nerve injury reduces responses of hypoglossal motoneurones to baseline and chemoreceptor-modulated inspiratory drive in the adult rat. J Physiol 557: 991–1011.
25. Weiskirchen R, Gressner AM (2005) Isolation and culture of hepatic stellate cells. Methods Mol Med 117: 99–113.
26. Bachem MG, Schneider E, Gross H, Weidenbach H, Schmid RM, et al. (1998) Identification, culture, and characterization of pancreatic stellate cells in rats and humans. Gastroenterology 115: 421–432.
27. Peterson TC, Rowden G (1998) Drug-metabolizing enzymes in rat liver myofibroblasts. Biochem Pharmacol 55: 703–708.
28. Shimizu I, Mizobuchi Y, Yasuda M, Shiba M, Ma YR, et al. (1999) Inhibitory effect of oestradiol on activation of rat hepatic stellate cells in vivo and in vitro. Gut 44: 127–136.
29. Mendias CL, Bakhurin KI, Faulkner JA (2008) Tendons of myostatin-deficient mice are small, brittle, and hypocellular. Proc Natl Acad Sci U S A 105: 388–393.
30. Henderson NC, Mackinnon AC, Farnworth SL, Poirier F, Russo FP, et al. (2006) Galectin-3 regulates myofibroblast activation and hepatic fibrosis. Proc Natl Acad Sci U S A 103: 5060–5065.
31. Nagase Y, Iwasawa M, Akiyama T, Kadono Y, Nakamura M, et al. (2009) Anti-apoptotic molecule Bcl-2 regulates the differentiation, activation, and survival of both osteoblasts and osteoclasts. J Biol Chem 284: 36659–36669.
32. Huang XR, Chung AC, Wang XJ, Lai KN, Lan HY (2008) Mice overexpressing latent TGF-beta1 are protected against renal fibrosis in obstructive kidney disease. Am J Physiol Renal Physiol 295: F118–127.

33. Wu J, Liu J, Waalkes MP, Cheng ML, Li L, et al. (2008) High dietary fat exacerbates arsenic-induced liver fibrosis in mice. Exp Biol Med (Maywood) 233: 377–384.
34. Pfaffl MW (2001) A new mathematical model for relative quantification in real-time RT-PCR. Nucleic Acids Res 29: e45.
35. Constandinou C, Henderson N, Iredale JP (2005) Modeling liver fibrosis in rodents. Methods Mol Med 117: 237–250.
36. Ross AG, Li YS, Sleigh AC, McManus DP (1997) Schistosomiasis control in the People's Republic of China. Parasitol Today 13: 152–155.
37. Andersson KL, Chung RT (2007) Hepatic schistosomiasis Current Treatment Options in Gastroenterology 10: 504–512.
38. Parsons CJ, Takashima M, Rippe RA (2007) Molecular mechanisms of hepatic fibrogenesis. J Gastroenterol Hepatol 22 Suppl 1: S79–84.
39. Homeida MA, el Tom I, Nash T, Bennett JL (1991) Association of the therapeutic activity of praziquantel with the reversal of Symmers' fibrosis induced by Schistosoma mansoni. Am J Trop Med Hyg 45: 360–365.
40. Reagan-Shaw S, Nihal M, Ahmad N (2008) Dose translation from animal to human studies revisited. Faseb J 22: 659–661.
41. Abdul-Ghani RA, Hassan AA (2010) Murine schistosomiasis as a model for human schistosomiasis mansoni: similarities and discrepancies. Parasitol Res 107: 1–8.
42. Maia MD, Lopes EP, Ferraz AA, Barros FM, Domingues AL, et al. (2007) Evaluation of splenomegaly in the hepatosplenic form of mansonic schistosomiasis. Acta Trop 101: 183–186.
43. Rakotonirina E, Andrianjaka P, Rakotoarivelo R, Ramanampamonjy R, Randria M, et al. (2010) Relation between Shistosoma mansoni and hepatosplenomegalies. Sante 20: 15–19.
44. Christian J, Steib MH, Frigga Beitinger (2010) Amiloride reduces portal hypertension in rat liver cirrhosis. Gut. pp 827–836.
45. Reynaert H, Thompson MG, Thomas T, Geerts A (2002) Hepatic stellate cells: role in microcirculation and pathophysiology of portal hypertension. Gut 50: 571–581.
46. Olds GR, Dasarathy S (2001) Recent Advances in Schistosomiasis. Curr Infect Dis Rep 3: 59–67.
47. Freitas CR, Barbosa AA, Jr., Fernandes AL, Andrade ZA (1999) Pathology of the spleen in hepatosplenic schistosomiasis. Morphometric evaluation and extracellular matrix changes. Mem Inst Oswaldo Cruz 94: 815–822.
48. Watson M (2009) Praziquantel Journal of Exotic Pet Medicine 18: 229–231.
49. Biempica L, Dunn MA, Kamel IA, Kamel R, Hait PK, et al. (1983) Liver collagen-type characterization in human schistosomiasis. A histological, ultrastructural, and immunocytochemical correlation. Am J Trop Med Hyg 32: 316–325.
50. Dunn MA, Rojkind M, Warren KS, Hait PK, Rifas L, et al. (1977) Liver collagen synthesis in murine schistosomiasis. J Clin Invest 59: 666–674.
51. Fichtner-Feigl S, Strober W, Kawakami K, Puri RK, Kitani A (2006) IL-13 signaling through the IL-13alpha2 receptor is involved in induction of TGF-beta1 production and fibrosis. Nat Med 12: 99–106.
52. Seki E, De Minicis S, Osterreicher CH, Kluwe J, Osawa Y, et al. (2007) TLR4 enhances TGF-beta signaling and hepatic fibrosis. Nat Med 13: 1324–1332.
53. Jacobs W, Kumar-Singh S, Bogers J, Van de Vijver K, Deelder A, et al. (1998) Transforming growth factor-beta, basement membrane components and heparan sulphate proteoglycans in experimental hepatic schistosomiasis mansoni. Cell Tissue Res 292: 101–106.
54. Chu D, Luo Q, Li C, Gao Y, Yu L, et al. (2007) Paeoniflorin inhibits TGF-beta1-mediated collagen production by Schistosoma japonicum soluble egg antigen in vitro. Parasitology 134: 1611–1621.
55. Carpino G, Morini S, Ginanni Corradini S, Franchitto A, Merli M, et al. (2005) Alpha-SMA expression in hepatic stellate cells and quantitative analysis of hepatic fibrosis in cirrhosis and in recurrent chronic hepatitis after liver transplantation. Dig Liver Dis 37: 349–356.
56. Coutinho HM, Acosta LP, Wu HW, McGarvey ST, Su L, et al. (2007) Th2 cytokines are associated with persistent hepatic fibrosis in human Schistosoma japonicum infection. J Infect Dis 195: 288–295.
57. Arnaud V, Li J, Wang Y, Fu X, Mengzhi S, et al. (2008) Regulatory role of interleukin-10 and interferon-gamma in severe hepatic central and peripheral fibrosis in humans infected with Schistosoma japonicum. J Infect Dis 198: 418–426.
58. Cheever AW, Williams ME, Wynn TA, Finkelman FD, Seder RA, et al. (1994) Anti-IL-4 treatment of Schistosoma mansoni-infected mice inhibits development of T cells and non-B, non-T cells expressing Th2 cytokines while decreasing egg-induced hepatic fibrosis. J Immunol 153: 753–759.
59. Kaplan MH, Whitfield JR, Boros DL, Grusby MJ (1998) Th2 cells are required for the Schistosoma mansoni egg-induced granulomatous response. J Immunol 160: 1850–1856.
60. Kaviratne M, Hesse M, Leusink M, Cheever AW, Davies SJ, et al. (2004) IL-13 activates a mechanism of tissue fibrosis that is completely TGF-beta independent. J Immunol 173: 4020–4029.
61. Gomez DE, De Lorenzo MS, Alonso DF, Andrade ZA (1999) Expression of metalloproteinases (MMP-1, MMP-2, and MMP-9) and their inhibitors (TIMP-1 and TIMP-2) in schistosomal portal fibrosis. Am J Trop Med Hyg 61: 9–13.
62. Hemmann S, Graf J, Roderfeld M, Roeb E (2007) Expression of MMPs and TIMPs in liver fibrosis - a systematic review with special emphasis on anti-fibrotic strategies. J Hepatol 46: 955–975.
63. Roderfeld M, Weiskirchen R, Wagner S, Berres ML, Henkel C, et al. (2006) Inhibition of hepatic fibrogenesis by matrix metalloproteinase-9 mutants in mice. Faseb J 20: 444–454.
64. Knittel T, Mehde M, Kobold D, Saile B, Dinter C, et al. (1999) Expression patterns of matrix metalloproteinases and their inhibitors in parenchymal and non-parenchymal cells of rat liver: regulation by TNF-alpha and TGF-beta1. J Hepatol 30: 48–60.
65. Giannelli G, Bergamini C, Marinosci F, Fransvea E, Napoli N, et al. (2006) Antifibrogenic effect of IFN-alpha2b on hepatic stellate cell activation by human hepatocytes. J Interferon Cytokine Res 26: 301–308.
66. Han YP, Zhou L, Wang J, Xiong S, Garner WL, et al. (2004) Essential role of matrix metalloproteinases in interleukin-1-induced myofibroblastic activation of hepatic stellate cell in collagen. J Biol Chem 279: 4820–4828.
67. Moreno M, Gonzalo T, Kok RJ, Sancho-Bru P, van Beuge M, et al. (2010) Reduction of advanced liver fibrosis by short-term targeted delivery of an angiotensin receptor blocker to hepatic stellate cells in rats. Hepatology 51: 942–952.

Hepatotoxicity or Hepatoprotection? Pattern Recognition for the Paradoxical Effect of the Chinese Herb *Rheum palmatum* L. in Treating Rat Liver Injury

Jia-bo Wang[1*❡], Hai-ping Zhao[1,2❡], Yan-ling Zhao[1], Cheng Jin[1], Dao-jian Liu[1], Wei-jun Kong[1,3], Fang Fang[1,3], Lin Zhang[1,3], Hong-juan Wang[1], Xiao-he Xiao[1]

1 Integrative Medicine Center, 302 Military Hospital, Beijing, People's Republic of China, **2** Key Laboratory of Modern Preparation of Traditional Chinese Medicine, Ministry of Education, Jiangxi University of Traditional Chinese Medicine, Nanchang, People's Republic of China, **3** Chengdu University of Traditional Chinese Medicine, Chengdu, People's Republic of China

Abstract

The hepatotoxicity of some Chinese herbs has been a cause for concern in recent years. However, some herbs, such as rhubarb, have been documented as having both therapeutic and toxic effects on the liver, leading to the complex problem of distinguishing the benefits from the risks of using this herb. To comparatively analyze the dose-response relationship between rhubarb and hepatic health, we administrated total rhubarb extract(RE) to normal and carbon tetrachloride(CCl_4)-treated rats for 12 weeks at 4 dosage levels(2.00, 5.40, 14.69 and 40.00 $g \cdot kg^{-1}$, measured as the quantity of crude material), followed by biochemical and histopathological tests of the rats' livers. A composite pattern was extracted by factor analysis, using all the biochemical indices as variables, into a visual representation of two mathematically obtained factors, which could be interpreted as the fibrosis factor and the cellular injury factor, according to the values of the variable loadings. The curative effect of administering the two lowest dosages of RE to CCl_4-treated rats was mainly expressed as a decrease in the extent of cellular injury. The hepatoprotective mechanism of RE might be related to its antioxidant effect, the antagonism of the free radical damage to hepatocytes caused by CCl_4. By contrast, the RE-induced liver damage was mainly expressed as a significant increase in the amount of fibrosis in both normal rats at all dosage levels and CCl_4-treated rats at the two highest dosage levels. Therefore, the hepatotoxic potential of RE could be attributable to the liver cell fibrosis induced by high doses of the herb. This study illustrates the bidirectional potential of rhubarb and demonstrates the feasibility of using factor analysis to study the dose-response relationships between herbal medicines and hepatotoxicity or the healing effects of these herbs by extracting the underlying interrelationships among a number of functional bio-indices in a holistic manner.

Editor: John E. Tavis, Saint Louis University, United States of America

Funding: This work was funded by the National Key Technologies R&D Program of China (No. 2009ZX09502-022) and by the National Natural Science Foundation of China (No. 30625042 and 30973947). The funders had no role in study design, data collection and analysis, decision to publish, or preparation of the manuscript.

Competing Interests: The authors have declared that no competing interests exist.

* E-mail: pharmacy302@126.com

❡ These authors contributed equally to this work.

Introduction

Traditional Chinese herbal medicines are used worldwide, but there are a number of concerns regarding their use. Some researchers believe that herbal medicines are effective and safe, while others doubt their effectiveness and safety. The latter group has increased in number, especially after consecutive reports of adverse hepatotoxic effects of a number of phytomedicines, including *Polygonum multiflorum* [1], Shou-Wu Pian [2], Xiao-Chai-Hu-Tang (Syo-saiko-to), [3] and some herbs containing anthraquinones, such as *Sennae fructus angustifoliae* [4] and *Rheum palmatum* L. (rhubarb) [5]. Chitturi et al. believe that herbal hepatotoxicity is an expanding but poorly defined problem [6].

These herbal medicines, especially rhubarb and its constituent components, are frequently used as treatments for chronic liver diseases and as laxatives in Asian countries, and a number of cases have demonstrated their affirmative effectiveness and safety [7,8]. In addition to the clinical evidence of the effectiveness of rhubarb in treating chronic hepatic diseases, [9,10] many experiments at the animal, cellular and molecular levels have revealed that rhubarb and its anthraquinone constituents exert a protective effect against hepatic injury by inhibiting the carbon tetrachloride (CCl_4)-induced elevation of serum alanine aminotransferase (ALT), aspartate aminotransferase (AST), hyaluronic acid (HA) and laminin (LN) levels. [11,12]

In vitro and in vivo studies focusing on the anthraquinone constituents of rhubarb, however, have revealed conflicting results. A two-year National Toxicology Program (NTP) study, conducted by the U.S. Department of Health and Human Services (DHHS) on emodin, one of the main anthraquinone derivatives contained within rhubarb, demonstrated the hepatotoxic potential of emodin on normal rats and mice. The toxic effects included elevations of ALT levels, total bile acids (TBIL) levels and organ-weight-to-body-weight ratios (relative weights) of the liver, as well as decreases in alkaline phosphatase (AP) and total protein levels (TP). [13] Other investigators have reported that administration of rhubarb extracts (REs) led to elevations of serum ALT and TBIL levels in patients and experimental animals, leading to hepatitis and nephritis. [14–17]

The conflicting results of these reports might be due to the heterogeneity and complexity of herbal medicines with respect to their geographic origin, harvest season, and discrepancy of constituent components. Herbal medicines, which usually contain hundreds of chemical components with broad pharmacological targets and effects, present difficulties in describing overall biological profiles in a simple manner with a few essential factors that can be readily comprehended. Many phytopharmacologists have dedicated themselves to solving this provlem for decades. In recent years, pattern recognition, [18] a type of multivariate analysis approach, has become a promising method for identifying and interpreting meaningful regularities in noisy or complex systems, by analyzing data from different perspectives and summarizing them as useful information or by mining potential interrelationships. The factor analysis used in this study is a common pattern recognition method that reduces a large number of disease parameters to a relatively small number of independent factors, by describing the covariance structure of the observed data variables in terms of a few underlying and independent but non-measurable features called "factors". [19]

The aim of this study was to determine the paradoxical effects of liver protection and hepatotoxicity of rhubarb in the treatment of rat experimental hepatitis induced by carbon tetrachloride by categorizing a number of functional bio-indices into separate complementary domains (protection or toxicity) with no *a priori* assumptions. We believe that our data will provide useful information for the safe evaluation and proper application of rhubarb and, furthermore, will help increase our understanding of the rational use of phytomedicines.

Materials and Methods

Ethics Statement

This study was conducted in strict accordance with the recommendations of the Guidelines for the Care and Use of Laboratory Animals of the Ministry of Science and Technology of China. The animal protocol was approved by the Committee on the Ethics of Animal Experiments of the 302 Military Hospital (Approval ID: 09-056).

Animals and reagents

Male and female Sprague- Dawley rats, aged 6-8 weeks and weighing 180 ± 30 g, were obtained from the Laboratory Animal Center of the Academy of Military Medical Sciences. The animals were raised separately by gender and had unlimited access to food and water in an environmentally controlled breeding room (temperature 22±2°C, humidity 60–80%). The breeding room was illuminated by an artificial light cycle with 12 hours of light and 12 hours of darkness every day and was disinfected regularly.

Carbon tetrachloride (CCl_4) was purchased from Beijing Beihua Fine Chemicals Co. Ltd (Cat. #20060525), and olive oil was purchased from Sinopharm Chemical Reagent Beijing Co. Ltd (Cat. #F20080219). Both reagents were of AR grade.

Herb extraction and UPLC-MS/MS analysis

Rhubarb is the peeled and dried root of *Rheum palmatum* L., *R. tanguticum Maxim. ex* Balf. or *R. officinale* Baill. (Polygonaceae family), as stipulated in the Chinese Pharmacopoeia[20]. Rhubarb is also officially listed in European and Japanese pharmacopoeias. [21,22] *R. palmatum* was used in this study because it is described in all three pharmacopoeias and is more commonly used than the other species. The dried root and rhizome of *R. palmatum* L. were collected in Lixian County of the Gansu Province of China and were identified by Professor Xiao-he Xiao, a taxonomist at the Military Institute of Chinese Materia Medica. In total, 100 kg rhubarb was added to 600 L of 90% ethanol and then heated and extracted 3 times for 1 hour each time. The residual compounds after extraction were added to 1000 L of water and then heated and extracted for 1 hour. The filtrate was merged and sprayed dry, producing a yield of 29.3%. The samples were preserved for further experiments.

Rhubarb extract (RE) was analyzed for quality control by ultra-performance liquid chromatography coupled with an ultraviolet-visible detector and electrospray ionization tandem mass spectrometry (UPLC-UV-ESI-MS/MS). [23] The experimental conditions and data are provided in Text S1.

Animal model and study groups

In this study, a CCl_4-induced liver injury model was used because it has been well documented and demonstrated to have good repeatability and reliability. One experiment cycle continued for 16 weeks, and the following procedure was used immediately prior to the experiment, 180 rats were randomized into 10 groups of 18 animals each, with equal distributions by gender. The groups shown in Tables 1 and 2 were differentiated based on the treatment group and extract dosage. The rats in the five model groups (groups M and M_1-M_4) were injected intraperitoneally (i.p.) with CCl_4 oil (containing 1 portion CCl_4 and 9 portions olive oil, 5 ml/kg) 2 times per week for 12 weeks to induce chronic liver injury, and the rats in the other groups received normal saline (N.S.). The rats in all medication groups (groups N_1-N_4 and M_1-M_4) were administered RE intragastrically once per day from the 4th week until the end of the 16th week. Rats in the control (group N) and model (group M) groups were administered normal saline intragastrically. The RE dosages were 2.00, 5.40, 14.69 and 40.00 g/kg (measured as the quantity of crude material) per kg of body weight once per day and were equivalent to between 4 and 80 times the human upper dosage limit stipulated in the Chinese Pharmacopoeia (0.5 g/kg). Food and water were available *ad libitum* for all rats throughout the experiment.

Histopathologic examination and biochemical analysis

Necropsies were performed on all the animals at the end of the experiment. Tissues for histopathologic examination were fixed and preserved in 10% neutral buffered formalin, processed and trimmed, embedded in paraffin, sectioned to a thickness of approximately 5μm, and stained with hematoxylin and eosin (HE).

Biochemical analyses were performed on all animals. The biochemical parameters of serum ALT, AST, AP, urea nitrogen (SUN), creatinine (CREA), TP, albumin (ALB), globulin (GLO), calcium, inorganic phosphate, total cholesterol (CHOL) and TBIL levels were measured by the Clinical Laboratory of 302 Military Hospital of China. The levels of HA, LN and transforming growth factor β_1 (TGF-β_1) in rat serum were quantitated by chemiluminescence using assay kits from Beijing Deyuan Biomedical Engineering Corporation, China.

Statistical analysis

The experimental values were expressed as means ± standard deviation (means ± SD). All data were analyzed using the Statistical Package for the Social Sciences for Windows, version 13.0 (SPSS Inc, Chicago, IL, USA). The groups were compared

Table 1. Liver toxicity induced by rhubarb extract in normal rats with regard to survival and biochemical indices.

Groups	N	ND_1	ND_2	ND_3	ND_4
Dosage (g/kg)	0	2	5.4	14.69	40
Survival[a]	18	18	17	15	14
ALT (U/L)	73.00±17.70	104.86±10.17	119.43±31.36△	125.43±19.86△	175.86±22.75△
AST (U/L)	149.57±27.78	187.00±37.46	207.86±71.81	268.00±57.83△	261.00±48.55△
AP (U/L)	53.71±21.26	73.00±28.14	89.29±18.31	97.29±21.48△	116.43±19.7△
TBIL (μmol/L)	1.09±0.32	1.01±0.59	1.24±0.30	1.50±0.53	1.66±0.75△
TP (g/L)	69.71±12.31	74.14±13.56	76.29±11.34	84.43±10.72	87.71±8.12△
GLO (g/L)	27.57±7.50	34.43±6.48	35.71±5.77	46.29±9.72	51.43±7.57△
HA (ng/L)	203.30±71.98	220.4±73.97	277.79±23.17△	281.46±44.08△	350.13±47.98△
LN (ng/L)	31.53±5.05	36.76±10.47	38.01±8.43	48.47±10.22△	54.19±9.78△
TGF-β_1 (pg/L)	18.23±1.42	20.87±1.95	19.09±3.38	29.82±6.27	39.19±7.76△

N, normal rat group without treatment; ND_1-ND_4, normal rat groups treated with rhubarb extract at dosages of 2.00, 5.40, 14.69 and 40.00 g kg^{-1}, respectively. ALT, serum alanine aminotransferase; AST, serum aspartate aminotransferase; AP, alkaline phosphatase; TBIL, total bile acids; TP, total protein; GLO, globulin; HA, hyaluronic acid; LN, laminin; TGF-β_1, transforming growth factor β_1.
[a] The initial number of animals in each group of the study was 18.
△ $P<0.05$ compared to the N group.

using ANOVA and multivariate statistical analysis, and the significance probability was set at $P=0.05$.

The factor analysis model was as follows:

$$y_c = l_{c1}F_1 + l_{c2}F_2 + l_{c3}F_3 + \ldots + l_{cn}F_n + \varepsilon_c$$

where y_c is the cth original variable, $c = 1, \ldots, p$, p is the number of original variables, $l_{c1}, l_{c2}, l_{c3}, \ldots, l_{cn}$ are the factor loadings, $F_1, F_2, F_3, \ldots, F_n$ are the (new) factors, n is the number of factors, and ε_c the error term related to y_c. [24] The correlation coefficients were analyzed by principal component analysis and subsequent rotation according to the standard varimax criterion. The correlation between parameters was attributed to their common dependence on independent entities called "factors." The coefficients that linked the parameters to factors were named "factor loadings".

Results

Study design

This study included two parts. First, a comparative experiment was designed to investigate the dose-responses of RE to normal and CCl_4-treated rats. Standard blood chemistry analyses were used to evaluate liver damage and histological changes were assessed. All doses were set at high levels to uncover potential toxicities to rigorously investigate the hepatic risks of RE.

Table 2. Protective effect of rhubarb extract against CCl_4-induced liver injury with regard to the survival and biochemical indices in the model groups.

Groups	M	MD_1	MD_2	MD_3	MD_4
Dosage (g/kg)	0	2	5.4	14.69	40
Survival[a]	16	18	15	13	11
ALT (U/L)	519.14±64.46△	261.14±46.52*	213.43±33.16*	183.14±33.26*	253.43±55.24*
AST (U/L)	775.14±119.95△	421.00±35.13*	234.71±43.18*	268.57±77.34*	367.57±104.59*
AP (U/L)	140.57±58.8△	58.86±15.55*	63.57±20.56*	83.00±18.35	103.57±27.67
TBIL (μmol/L)	2.34±0.24△	1.49±0.71*	1.24±0.72*	1.64±1.07	2.89±0.72*
TP (g/L)	92.43±14.12△	71.00±10.85*	71.00±6.68*	75.71±9.41	87.14±7.99
GLO (g/L)	58.43±9.36△	29.86±10.93*	33.00±3.51*	38.14±8.28	49.71±6.70
HA (ng/L)	362.17±36.88△	284.23±38.73*	310.29±70.63*	436.37±61.71*	508.10±62.38*
LN (ng/L)	53.31±23.25△	36.59±10.25	38.64±7.85	52.49±6.93	91.96±19.21*
TGF-β_1 (pg/L)	33.07±11.06△	30.69±6.75	32.48±5.73	34.08±6.71	53.77±10.45*

M, model rat group without treatment; MD_1-MD_4, model rat groups treated with rhubarb extract at dosages of 2.00, 5.40, 14.69 and 40.00 g kg^{-1}, respectively. ALT, serum alanine aminotransferase; AST, serum aspartate aminotransferase; AP, alkaline phosphatase; TBIL, total bile acids; TP, total protein; GLO, globulin; HA, hyaluronic acid; LN, laminin; TGF-β_1, transforming growth factor β_1.
[a] The initial number of animals in each group of the study was 18.
△ $P<0.05$ compared to the N group.
*$P<0.05$, compared to the M group.

Second, a factor analysis approach was utilized to mathematically illustrate the bidirectional effect of liver protection and hepatotoxicity of RE on subjects under different physiological conditions. The mathematical modeling process used a dimension reduction effect to convert the original dataset of numerous disease variables into a relatively small number of independent "factors" that are not measurable but are easy to comprehend, including the protection factor and the lesion factor.

Identification of the chemical constituents in rhubarb extract (RE)

In a previous study, it was demonstrated that the major components contained in RE are anthraquinone derivatives and tannin-related compounds. [25] Using liquid chromatography coupled with tandem mass spectrometry, seventeen compounds were identified in this study, and their structures were tentatively assigned as twelve anthraquinone derivatives and five tannin-related compounds. The identified chemical constituents (Table S1) and the contents of the index compounds in the RE (Table S2) are summarized in the supplementary materials to illustrate the chemical basis of the RE utilized in this study. The chemical structures of the identified constituents in RE are depicted in Figures S1 and S2. The chromatographic profile is depicted in Fig. 1.

Common changes

All the RE-treated rats had a dose-related fur color change patterns, ranging from yellow to red, that appeared early in the study with exposure to increasing concentrations of RE. Red-to-brown urine and reddish-brown staining of the anal area were also noted for all rats that were treated with RE. Marked and chronic diarrhea accompanied by emaciation and inactivity were observed in all model and normal rats that were treated with 40 g/kg, but not the lower doses, of RE. During RE administration, the rats in the CCl_4-treated groups had lower increases in weight than those in the normal groups at the same dosage. Rats in all the RE-administered groups had negative dose-related body weight changes, and the rats in the highest dosage group had the lowest increase in weight until cessation of RE administration.

Histopathology

Dosage-dependent vacuolar degeneration of the hepatic portal area and/or hyperplasia of interstitial fibrous tissue were observed in over 67% of animals in the ND_1-ND_4 groups.

In the control group (group N), all rats exhibited normal histology. By contrast, 16 out of 18 animals in the model group (group M) exhibited vacuolar degeneration, which was characterized by small or medium vacuole formation in hepatocytes accompanied by nuclear loss or dislocation to the margins of the vacuoles. Hepatocytes with large nuclei were occasionally observed. Small focal lymphocytic infiltration of the stroma and/or portal area was also observed in 12 out of 18 animals in group M. Moreover, an obviously thickened envelope and fibrosis of the portal area and/or stroma were observed in 11 out of 18 animals in group M. The animals in groups MD_1-MD_4 showed decreases in vacuolar degeneration and lymphocytic infiltration in hepatocytes with increasing RE dosages. Over 67% of the animals in both groups MD_1 and MD_2 exhibited notably alleviated fibrosis of the liver envelope, portal area, and/or stroma, whereas 67% of the animals in the MD_3 group and 88% of the animals in the MD_4 group exhibited obvious aggravation of fibrosis. Typical histopathologic changes are depicted in Fig. 2.

Biochemical indices

The biochemical indices that changed significantly in the study groups are shown in Tables 1 and 2.

In the control group (N) and RE-treated normal rat groups (ND_1-ND_4), the indices exhibited overall dose-dependent increasing trends (Table 1). Compared to the group N, serum ALT and HA values increased significantly in the ND_2, ND_3 and ND_4 groups ($P<0.05$) and AST, LN and TGF-β_1 values increased significantly in the ND_3 and ND_4 groups ($P<0.05$), whereas TBIL values increased significantly in the ND_4 group only ($P<0.05$).

The serum ALT and AST values of all RE-treated model groups (MD_1-MD_4) were significantly lower than those of group M without treatment ($P<0.05$). However, these two indices stopped declining and started to increase when the dosage increased from the second dosage (MD_2, 5.40 g/kg) to the third (MD_3, 14.69 g/kg). Regarding the TBIL, HA, LN and TGF-β_1 levels, the values

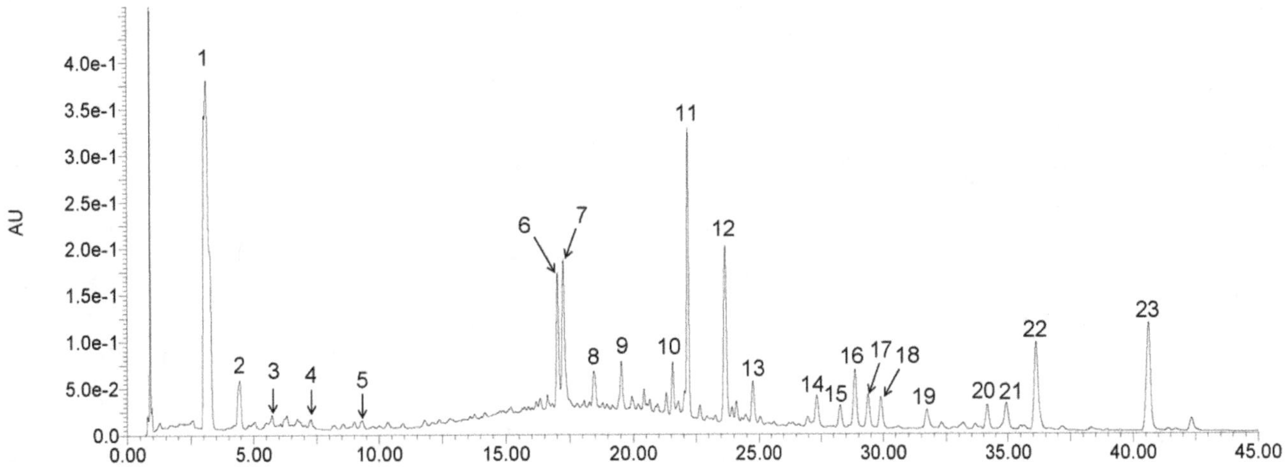

Figure 1. UPLC/UV chromatogram at 280 nm of the extract of *Rheum palmatum* L. Seventeen compounds were identified by electrospray ionization tandem mass spectrometry: galloyl glucose (1), glucopyranosyl-galloyl-glucose (3), catechin glucopyranoside (4), isomer of catechin glucopyranoside (5), aloe emodin *O*-glucoside (9), rhein *O*-glucoside (10), cinnamoyl-*O*-galloyl-glucose (11), laccaic acid D *O*-glucoside (13), dehydroxylaccaic acid D *O*-glucoside (14), chrysophanol *O*-glucoside (15), isomer of chrysophanol *O*-glucoside (16), emodin *O*-glucoside (17), laccaic acid D (19), physcion *O*-glucoside (20), emodin (21), acetyl- chrysophanol (22) and physcion (23). The other six chromatographic peaks (2, 6-8, 12 and 18) are unknown compounds.

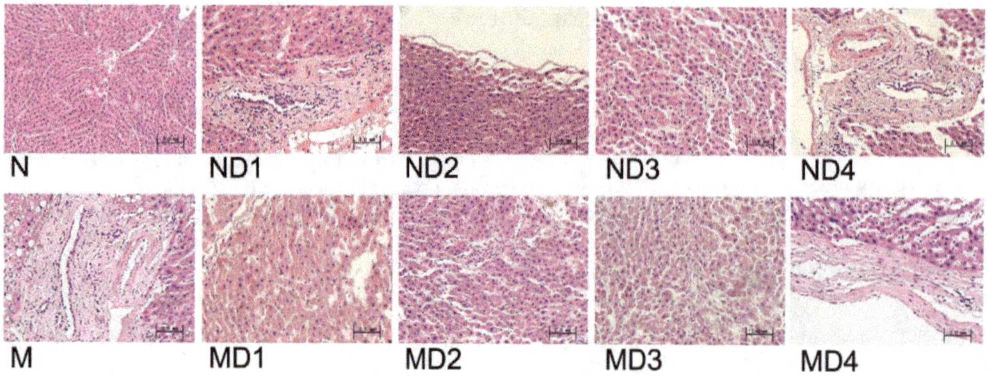

Figure 2. Typical histopathologic section photographs of rats in different groups (HE stained, 200× magnification). Dose-dependent vacuolar degeneration of the portal area and/or hyperplasia of the interstitial fibrous tissue were observed in the normal groups ND_1–ND_4. Obviously thickened envelopes and fibrosis of the portal area and/or stroma was observed in the animals of group M. This toxic degeneration caused by CCl_4 was improved after treatment with rhubarb extract in groups MD_1–MD_4. Notably, alleviation of fibrosis of the liver envelope, portal area, and/or stroma was observed in the animals in the MD_1 and MD_2 groups, whereas aggravation of fibrosis was found in over 67% of animals in the MD_3 and MD_4 groups. N, normal rat group without treatment; ND_1-ND_4, normal rat groups treated with rhubarb extract at dosages of 2.00, 5.40, 14.69 and 40.00 g kg^{-1}, respectively. M, model rat group without treatment; MD_1-MD_4, model rats groups treated with rhubarb extract at dosages of 2.00, 5.40, 14.69 and 40.00 g kg^{-1}, respectively.

of the maximum dosage group (MD_4 group) were even higher than those of group M without treatment ($P<0.05$) (Table 2).

Factor analysis using biochemical indices as variables

Bartlett's test of sphericity indicated a correlation between the currently used variables because the correlation matrix was significantly different from the identity matrix ($P<0.01$). The KMO measure of sampling adequacy was 0.789, which was higher than the acceptable criterion of 0.5. [26] The eigenvalues of the 9 factors are depicted in a scree plot in Fig. 3. Several methods were used to determine the number of meaningful factors that should be extracted. As a general rule, factors with an eigenvalue greater than 1.0 are retained. [27] The rationale for this rule is that the amount of variance accounted for by each factor should be at least equal to the variance of one variable. [24] This criterion indicated that two factors should be extracted in the present study. The first

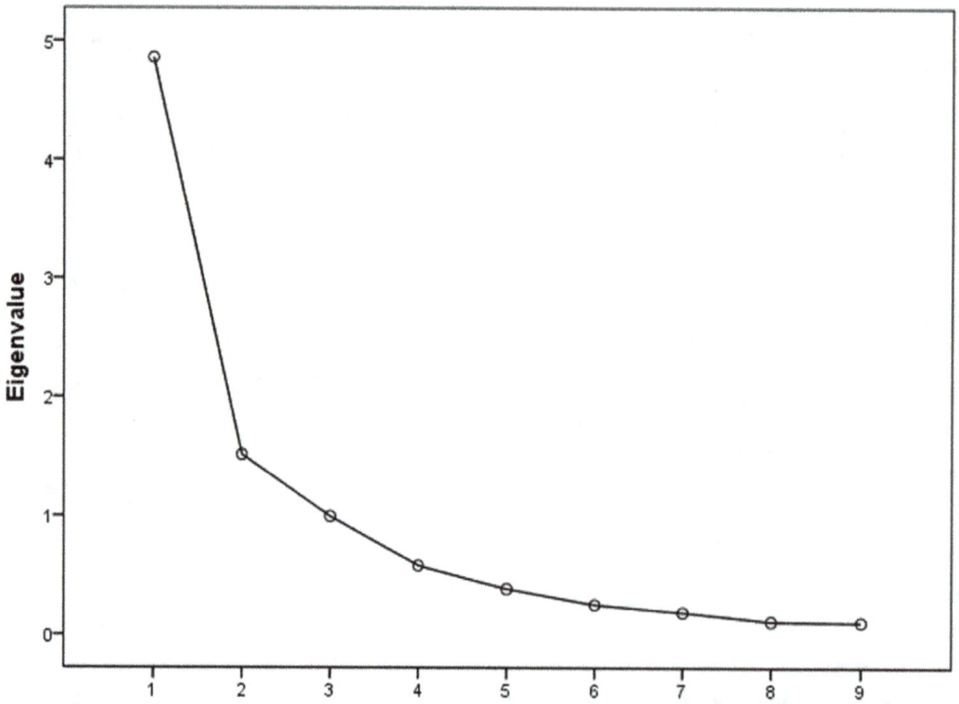

Figure 3. Scree plot depicting the eigenvalues of the factors extracted by factor analysis using biochemical indices as variables. The two factors with eigenvalue greater than 1.0 were retained in subsequent analyses.

and second factors accounted for 53.985% and 16.856% of the total variability, respectively. These two primary factors could explain 70.840% of the total variability in the dataset. The results of the factor analysis and a suggested interpretation are shown in Table 3. In interpreting the retained factors, we only selected variables with loadings above 0.5 or below -0.5 (i.e., variables with high influence).[28] According to this criterion, factor 1 could be labeled as "fibrosis" because the selected biochemical variables including HA, LN and TGF-β_1 (all loadings >0.85) are related to the fibrotic course[29-31] and factor 2 could be labeled as "cellular injury" because it was mainly affected by ALT and AST (both loadings >0.90), which were altered when the hepatocellular membrane was damaged.

The graphical representation of the dose-response relationship of RE, using these two statistically obtained factors as the axes to show the distribution pattern of different study groups in the plot, is depicted in Fig. 4. In the graphical representation, the toxicity- and pharmacologically induced variation patterns of the biochemical indices could be deduced from the ordered distribution of the studied groups. The untreated N group and the untreated M group are represented at the left lower side and upper right side of the diagram, respectively. The distance of group M away from group N illustrated certain hepatotoxic effects of both enzyme variations and fibrosis in rats with CCl_4-induced hepatitis compared to normal animals. The values of the fibrosis factor of the normal rat groups increased in all dosage groups (ND_1-ND_4, dosages from 2.00 to 40 g/kg), whereas their values of the cellular injury factor did not significantly increase. In the model rat groups, the values of the cellular injury factor of the first (MD_1, 2.00 g/kg) and second (MD_2, 5.40 g/kg) dosage groups decreased compared to the value of the untreated model group (M), whereas the values decreased by a smaller degree when the dosage was further increased. Although the values of the fibrosis factor of the MD_1 and MD_2 groups decreased slightly compared to the value of the M group, the values of the MD_3 (14.69 g/kg) and MD_4 (40.00 g/kg) groups shifted to an increasing trend with increasing dosage.

Table 3. Results of factor analysis after a varimax rotation[a].

Variable	Factor 1	Factor 2
AST	0.068	**0.910**
ALT	0.090	**0.901**
ALP	0.348	**0.620**
TP	0.448	**0.514**
GLO	**0.526**	**0.675**
TBIL	**0.685**	0.434
HA	**0.856**	0.264
TGF-β_1	**0.856**	0.121
LN	**0.896**	0.103
Eigenvalue	4.859	1.517
Cumulative proportion [b]	53.985	70.840
Suggested interpretation	Fibrosis	Cellular injury

ALT, serum alanine aminotransferase; AST, serum aspartate aminotransferase; AP, alkaline phosphatase; TBIL, total bile acids; TP, total protein; GLO, globulin; HA, hyaluronic acid; LN, laminin; TGF-β_1, transforming growth factor β_1.

[a] The loadings, eigenvalues, cumulative proportion of the total variance and a suggested interpretation are provided for the two factors. Only variables with loadings above 0.5 or below -0.5 were used in the interpretation (displayed in bold).

[b] The cumulative proportion is the cumulative proportion of the total variance in the data. Because the variables are standardized to a variance of 1, the total eigenvalue is equal to 9 (number of variables).

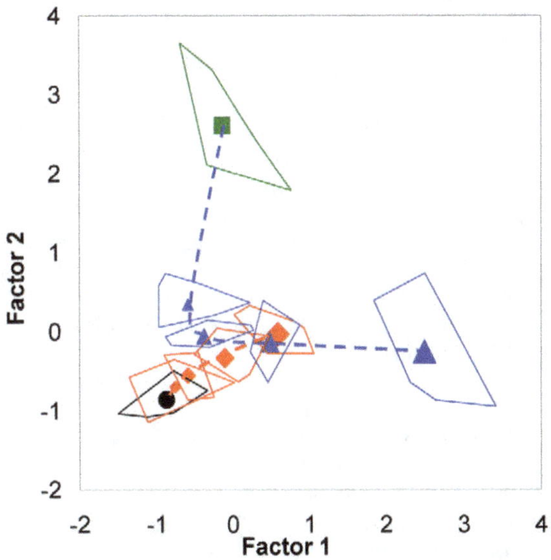

Figure 4. Dose-response relationships of rhubarb extract to both normal and model rats, as represented by a factor plot. The alteration pattern of the dose-response relationship between rhubarb extract and hepatic health in normal rats showed an almost linear variation: factor 1, considered in relation to fibrosis and called the "fibrosis factor", showed a notable increasing trend with increasing of dosage levels (ND_1-ND_4, dosages of 2.00, 5.40, 14.69 and 40.00 g kg^{-1}, respectively), whereas factor 2, considered in relation to cell membrane integrality and called the "cellular injury factor", revealed a nonsignificant increase. By contrast, the alteration pattern in the model rat groups assumed a parabolic shape with increasing dosages. The factor 1 values decreased in the MD_1 and MD_2 groups but decreased to a small degree when the dosage was further increased. The factor 2 values decreased slightly in the MD_1 and MD_2 groups and then shifted to a significant increasing trend with increasing dosages in the MD_3 and MD_4 groups. The center points of the different groups are labeled as follows: untreated normal rats group (N, ■ green square); normal rat groups treated with rhubarb extract at different dosages (ND_1-ND_4, ◆) (symbol size indicates dosage); untreated model rat group (M, ●); and model rat groups treated with rhubarb extract at different dosages (MD_1-MD_4, ▲ blue triangle) (symbol size indicates dosage). The border lines around the center points are presented for the range of original data points of the studied groups.

Discussion

It has been previously reported that the protective effect of rhubarb against CCl_4-induced liver lesions was largely attributed to the inhibition of the generation of free radicals and antioxidant activity. [32,33] The mechanism of CCl_4-induced liver injury is generally interpreted as follows: the compound is bioactivated by cytochrome P450 2E1 to the trichloromethyl free radical (•CCl_3) and then further converted to a peroxy radical (CCl_3O_2•), which leads to a chain reaction auto-oxidation of the fatty acids in the cytoplasmic membrane phospholipids causing functional and morphological changes to the cell membrane. [34] As a consequence, the cell membranes of hepatocytes become more permeable, and enzymes such as ALT and AST can leak out into the bloodstream, leading to increased levels of these enzymes in the blood. These increases reflect the degree of hepatocyte damage and necrosis [35] and vice versa. Therefore, it could be inferred that the pharmacological activity of rhubarb in treating liver injury is strongly related to its antioxidant effects via the protection of hepatic cells against free radical damage. This outcome manifested as a decrease in the cellular injury factor, (shown in Fig. 4), which was closely correlated with biomarkers such as ALT and AST (shown in Table 2).

The anti-oxidative effects [36] of rhubarb anthraquinone derivatives, along with their hepatoprotective effects, [11] have been reported. In addition, a series of tannin-related compounds with strong antioxidant effects have been identified in RE (see Supplementary Materials). In a previous report, the antioxidant activities of rhubarb tannins were verified. [37] Therefore, we believe that rhubarb tannins and anthraquinone derivatives may all contribute to the hepatoprotective effects of rhubarb against CCl_4-induced liver damage.

The hepatoprotective effect of rhubarb and its components has also been documented as antagonizing α-naphthylisothiocyanate (ANIT)-[38] and concanavalin A [39]- induced experimental liver injury. In a previous study, we found that free anthraquinones extracted from rhubarb, such as rhein and emodin, exhibited protective activity against ANIT-induced cholestatic liver injury by reducing the serum levels of glutamate-pyruvate transaminase, glutamic oxaloacetic transaminase and the serum total bilirubin, direct bilirubin, alkaline phosphatase, γ-glutamyltransferase and total bile acids. These effects were markedly different from the effects on CCl_4-induced liver injury. The morphological alterations induced by ANIT in rats, including the necrosis of hepatocytes and biliary epithelial cells, as well as neutrophil infiltration and sinusoid congestion, were also alleviated by concurrent intragastric administration of these free anthraquinones. [8] Some clinical evidence has also revealed a hepatoprotective effect of rhubarb against infantile cholestatic hepatitis[40] and acute icteric hepatitis [41]. The protective effect against CCl_4-induced liver damage reported in this study demonstrated only one aspect of the pharmacological potential of rhubarb to protect the liver. Although there is some evidence of the protective potential of this herb against liver injury due to multiple causes, the molecular mechanisms of this protection remain unclear. Rigorous clinical studies and in-depth experimental studies are needed to demonstrate rhubarb's hepatoprotective effects and mechanisms of action.

In our study, dose-dependent alterations of liver fibrosis associated with increases in the fibrosis factor were clearly observed in the rats in the normal groups (Figs 2 and 4). Although the occurrence of fibrosis of the liver tissues of normal rats that were treated with rhubarb has been reported infrequently, this phenomenon warrants further consideration. Elevation of TBIL, TP and GLO levels in serum have also been found in normal rat groups. These alterations usually occur along with hepatic impairment, indicating functional deterioration of the liver. Although the hepatoprotective effects of anthraquinone derivatives are well documented, it has also been reported that the total anthraquinone derivatives isolated from rhubarb show some hepatotoxic potential in rats in a six month-long experiment. [14] Therefore, the dose-response relationship between rhubarb anthraquinones and liver health warrants further investigation.

The alteration pattern of the fibrosis factor in the model rat groups assumed a parabolic shape with increasing dosages of RE (shown in Fig. 4). At lower dosages (MD_1, 2.00 g/kg and MD_2, 5.40 g/kg), rhubarb demonstrated some ameliorative effects on liver injury by decreasing the fibrosis caused by CCl_4; however, the fibrosis was aggravated rather than alleviated when the dosage was increased further (MD_3, 14.69 g/kg and MD_4, 40.00 g/kg). Therefore, we believe that the hepatotoxic potential of rhubarb is strongly related to liver fibrosis, although this effect is undetectable when the normal dosage recommended in the Chinese Pharmacopoeia (0.5 g/kg) is administered. [20]

The results of the factor analysis of biochemical indices indicated that the parallel histopathological changes arose coincidently. The vacuolar degeneration, and lymphocyte infiltration and fibrosis observed in the hepatocytes of CCl_4-treated rats were alleviated after treatment with RE, demonstrating the herb's effectiveness in protecting hepatocytes from the toxicant. However, the anti-fibrotic effect of RE that was observed in the lower dosage groups was reversed with further increases in the RE dosage. The dose-dependent hyperplasia of interstitial fibrous tissue was also observed in liver tissue sections from normal rats that were treated with RE, which was in accordance with the variations in the fibrosis factor.

A classical description of the understanding of such bidirectional effects of rhubarb and other herbal medicines, *You Gu Wu Yun*, was recorded in the Chinese Medical Treatise *Su Wen* (translated as *Plain Questions*, part of *The Yellow Emperor's Classic of Internal Medicine*), which was written 2,500 years ago.[42] The archaic and recondite wording of *You Gu Wu Yun* can be explained as follows. A drug will reveal its therapeutic effect when it is prescribed to patients with the correct indications; however, it may produce deleterious effects in both sick and healthy people as a result of incorrect indications. Another translation of the wording implies that the dosage of the drug is critical to its rational application in the clinic to balance the benefits and risks. Ancient Traditional Chinese Medicine (TCM) has effectively relied on the theory of *You Gu Wu Yun* as an important set of guidelines in the treatment of diseases and disorders. The dose-related bidirectional effect of TCM illustrated in this study supports the aforementioned theory. The pattern recognition approach proposed in this report opens an avenue to decode the ancient TCM theory and to elucidate its medical implications with the use of modern biochemical tools.

In conclusion, the findings of this study illustrate the bidirectional potential, both liver protection and hepatotoxicity, of rhubarb on CCl_4-treated and normal rats and demonstrate the feasibility of using a multivariate analysis approach factor analysis, to study the dose-response (therapeutic efficacy versus toxicity) relationships of traditional herbal medicines by revealing the underlying interrelationships within a number of functional bio-indices in a holistic manner. This study provides a paradigm for a better understanding and scientific assessment of the benefits and risks of herbal medicines to facilitate the rational clinical administration of these medicines.

Supporting Information

Figure S1 Chemical structures of the free anthraquinones in the rhubarb extract.

Figure S2 Chemical structures of the tannin-related compounds in the rhubarb extract.

Table S1 Identification of the chemical constituents in the rhubarb extract.

Table S2 The contents (%) of anthraquinones and tannins in the rhubarb extract.

Text S1 UPLC- ESI-MS/MS analysis.

Acknowledgments

We gratefully acknowledge Yuan-li Mao and her colleagues for performing biochemical analysis.

Author Contributions

Conceived and designed the experiments: XHX JBW. Performed the experiments: JBW HPZ WJK FF HJW. Analyzed the data: CJ JBW HPZ WJK YLZ LZ. Contributed reagents/materials/analysis tools: YLZ CJ. Wrote the paper: JBW YLZ HPZ DJL.

References

1. Medicines And Healthcare Products Regulatory Agency. *Polygonum multiflorum* and liver reactions. Available: http://www.mhra.gov.uk/Howweregulate/Medicines/Herbalmedicines/HerbalSafetyNews/Currentsafetyissues/CON2023590.
2. Mazzanti G, Battinelli L, Daniele C, Mastroianni CM, Lichtner M, et al. (2004) New case of acute hepatitis following the consumption of Shou Wu Pian, a Chinese Herbal product derived from *Polygonum multiflorum*. Ann Intern Med 140: W30.
3. Itoh S, Marutani K, Nishijima T, Matsuo S, Itabashi M (1995) Liver injuries induced by herbal medicine, Syo-saiko-to (xiao-chai-hu-tang). Digest Dis Sci 40: 1845–1848.
4. Vanderperren B, Rizzo M, Angenot L, Haufroid V, Jadoul M, et al. (2005) Acute liver failure with renal impairment related to the abuse of senna anthraquinone glycosides. Ann Pharmacother 39: 1353–1357.
5. Yuen MF, Tam S, Fung J, Wong DK, Wong BC, et al. (2006) Traditional Chinese medicine causing hepatotoxicity in patients with chronic hepatitis B infection: a 1-year prospective study. Aliment Pharmacol Ther 24: 1179–1186.
6. Chitturi S, Farrell GC (2000) Herbal hepatotoxicity: An expanding but poorly defined problem. J Gastroen Hepatol 15: 1093–1099.
7. World Health Organization (1999) WHO Monographs on Selected Medicinal Plants. Geneva: World Health Organization. pp 231–240.
8. Zhao YL, Wang JB, Zhou GD, Shan LM, Xiao XH (2009) Investigations of free anthraquinones from rhubarb against α- naphthylisothiocyanate- induced cholestatic liver injury in rats. Basic Clin Pharmacol Toxicol 104: 463–469.
9. Huang ZH, Dong YS, Ye WY (1997) Clinical observation on treatment of infantile cholestatic hepatitis syndrome by rhubarb. Chin J Integr Trad West Med 17: 459–461.
10. Wang GS (1985) Clinical and experimental study on the treatment of severe subacute hepatitis with traditional Chinese medicinal compounds. Chin J Integr Trad West Med 5: 329–331, 322.
11. Arosio B, Gagliano N, Fusaro LM, Parmeggiani L, Tagliabue J, et al. (2000) Aloe-Emodin quinone pretreatment reduces acute liver injury induced by carbon tetrachloride. Pharmacol Toxicol 87: 229–233.
12. Jin H, Sakaida I, Tsuchiya M, Okita K (2005) Herbal medicine Rhei rhizome prevents liver fibrosis in rat liver cirrhosis induced by a choline- deficient L-amino acid- defined diet. Life Sci 76: 2805–2816.
13. National Toxicology Program (2001) Technical report on the toxicology and carcinogenesis studies of emodin in F344/N rats and B6C3F1 mice. Series No. 493. NIH Publication No. 01-3952. U.S. Department of Health and Human Services, Public Health Service, National Institutes of Health, Research Triangle Park, NC.
14. Zhang LY, Jiang ZZ, Pu CH, Yan M (2004) Six- month oral toxicity study of total anthraquinone in radix et rhizoma rhei in SD rats. Chin J Biochem Pharm 25: 206–209.
15. Xu Y (2005) Clinical analysis of 30 cases of drug-induced liver injury by Chinese medicine. Modern J Integr Trad Chin West Med 14: 600–601.
16. Tian Y, Yang J, Lu JY (2008) Toxic effect of rhubarb overdose on mouse hepatocytes. Chin J Histochem Cytochem 17: 303–307.
17. Wang JB, Zhao YL, Xiao XH, Li HF, Zhao HP, et al. (2009) Assessment of the renal protection and hepatotoxicity of rhubarb extract in rats. J Ethnopharmacol 124: 18–25.
18. Wael ED (1997) Pattern recognition approaches in biomedical and clinical magnetic resonance spectroscopy: a review. NMR Biomed 10: 99–124.
19. Tafeit E, Möller R, Sudi K, Reibnegger G (2000) Artificial neural networks compared to factor analysis for low- dimensional classification of high-dimensional body fat topography data of healthy and diabetic subjects. Comput Biomed Res 33: 365–374.
20. (2005) Pharmacopoeia of the People's Republic of China, First Div. Beijing: China Chemical Industry Press. pp 17–18.
21. (2001) European Pharmacopoeia, 4th ed. Strasbourg: European Directorate for the Quality of Medicines, Council of Europe. 1858 p.
22. Japanese Pharmacopoeia, 15th ed (2006) Tokyo: Pharmaceutical and Food Safety Bureau, Ministry of Health, Labour and Welfare. 1344 p.
23. Ye M, Han J, Chen H, Zheng J, Guo D (2007) Analysis of phenolic compounds in rhubarbs using liquid chromatography coupled with electrospray ionization mass spectrometry. J Am Soc Mass Spectrom 18: 82–91.
24. Sharma S (1996) Applied Multivariate Techniques. New York: Wiley Press. pp 90–143.
25. Qin Y, Wang JB, Kong WJ, Zhao YL, Yang HY, et al. (2011) The diarrheogenic and antidiarrhoeal bidirectional effects of rhubarb and its potential mechanism. J Ethnopharmacol 133(3): 1096–1102.
26. Leung TF, Wong GW, Ko FW, Lam CW, Fok TF (2005) Clinical and atopic parameters and airway inflammatory markers in childhood asthma: a factor analysis. Thorax 60: 822–826.
27. Cattell RB (1966) The Scree test for the number of factors. Multivariate Behav Res 1: 245–276.
28. Thoefner MB, Ersbøll AK, Jensen AL, Hesselholt M (2001) Factor analysis of the interrelationships between clinical variables in horses with colic. Prev Vet Med 48: 201–214.
29. Tong Z, Chen R, Alt DS, Kemper S, Perbal B, et al. (2009) Susceptibility to liver fibrosis in mice expressing a connective tissue growth factor transgene in hepatocytes. Hepatology 50: 939–947.
30. Miele L, Forgione A, La Torre G, Vero V, Cefalo C, et al. (2009) Serum levels of hyaluronic acid and tissue metalloproteinase inhibitor-1 combined with age predict the presence of nonalcoholic steatohepatitis in a pilot cohort of subjects with nonalcoholic fatty liver disease. Transl Res 154: 194–201.
31. Attallah AM, Toson EA, Shiha GE, Omran MM, Abdel-Aziz MM, et al. (2007) Evaluation of serum procollagen aminoterminal propeptide III, laminin, and hydroxyproline as predictors of severe fibrosis in patients with chronic hepatitis C. J Immunoassay Immunochem 28: 199–211.
32. Liu L, Mei QB, Li BL, Zhou SY, Cao ZX (2001) Antioxidation of *Tanguticum* Maxim polysaccharide on acute liver injury mice. J Fourth Mil Med Univ 22: 530–533.
33. Wan SH, Ding YQ, Pu XH, Guo L, Kang TG (2006) Protective effect of hydroxy- anthroquinones from *Rheum Palmatum* L. on acute liver injure of rats induced by CCl_4. Chinese Pharmacological Bulletin 22: 1405–1406.
34. Jeong HG (1999) Inhibition of cytochrome P450 2E1 expression by oleanolic acid: hepatoprotective effects against carbon tetrachloride- induced hepatic injury. Toxicol Lett 105: 215–222.
35. Napoli J, Prentice D, Niinami C, Bishop GA, Desmond P, et al. (1997) Sequential increases in the intrahepatic expression of epidermal growth factor, basic fibroblast growth factor, and transforming growth factor beta in a bile duct ligated rat model of cirrhosis. Hepatology 26: 624–633.
36. Luo ZY, Huang X, Bao GR (2007) ESR study on the scavenging effects of the main ingredients in *Rheum palmatum* L. on superoxide anion radical. Chin Arch Tradit Chin Med 25: 612–614.
37. Iizuka A, Iijima OT, Kondo K, Itakura H, Yoshie F, et al. (2004) Evaluation of Rhubarb using antioxidative activity as an index of pharmacological usefulness. J Ethnopharmacol 91: 89–94.
38. Ding Y, Zhao L, Mei H, Zhang SL, Huang ZH, et al. (2008) Exploration of Emodin to treat alpha-naphthylisothiocyanate-induced cholestatic hepatitis via anti-inflammatory pathway. Eur J Pharmacol 590(1-3): 377–386.
39. Mase A, Makino B, Tsuchiya N, Yamamoto M, Kase Y, et al. (2010) Active ingredients of traditional Japanese (kampo) medicine, inchinkoto, in murine concanavalin A-induced hepatitis. J Ethnopharmacol 127(3): 742–749.
40. Huang ZH, Dong YS, Ye WY (1997) Clinical observation on treatment of infantile cholestatic hepatitis syndrome by rhubarb. Zhongguo Zhong Xi Yi Jie He Za Zhi 17(8): 459–461.
41. Wu CX (1984) A preliminary study on the effect of a single Rheum officinale in heavy doses in the treatment of acute icteric hepatitis. Zhong Xi Yi Jie He Za Zhi 4(2): 88–89.
42. Ni M (1995) The Yellow Emperor's Classic of Medicine: A New Translation of the Neijing Suwen with Commentary. Boston: Shambhala.

5

Total and High Molecular Weight Adiponectin and Hepatocellular Carcinoma with HCV Infection

Shuji Sumie[1]*, Takumi Kawaguchi[1,2], Ryoko Kuromatsu[1], Akio Takata[1], Masahito Nakano[1], Manabu Satani[1], Shingo Yamada[1], Takashi Niizeki[1], Takuji Torimura[3], Michio Sata[1,2]

1 Division of Gastroenterology, Department of Medicine, Kurume University School of Medicine, Kurume, Japan, 2 Department of Digestive Disease Information and Research, Kurume University School of Medicine, Kurume, Japan, 3 Liver Cancer Research Division, Research Center for Innovative Cancer Therapy, Kurume University, Kurume, Japan

Abstract

Background: Adiponectin is shown to be inversely associated with development and progression of various cancers. We evaluated whether adiponectin level was associated with the prevalence and histological grade of hepatocellular carcinoma (HCC), and liver fibrosis in patients with hepatitis C virus (HCV) infection.

Methods: A case-control study was conducted on 97 HCC patients (cases) and 97 patients (controls) matched for sex, Child-Pugh grade and platelet count in patients with HCV infection. The serum total and high molecular weight (HMW) adiponectin levels were measured by enzyme-linked immunosorbent assays and examined in their association with the prevalence of HCC. In addition, the relationship between these adiponectin levels and body mass index (BMI), progression of liver fibrosis, and histological grade of HCC was also evaluated. Liver fibrosis was assessed using the aspartate aminotransferase to platelet ratio index (APRI).

Results: There were no significant differences in the serum total and HMW adiponectin levels between cases and controls. Moreover, there were no inverse associations between serum total and HMW adiponectin levels and BMI in both cases and controls. On the other hand, serum total and HMW adiponectin levels are positively correlated with APRI in both cases ($r = 0.491$, $P < 0.001$ and $r = 0.485$, $P < 0.001$, respectively) and controls ($r = 0.482$, $P < 0.001$ and $r = 0.476$, $P < 0.001$, respectively). Interestingly, lower serum total (OR 11.76, 95% CI: 2.97–46.66 [$P < 0.001$]) and HMW (OR 10.24, CI: 2.80–37.40 [$P < 0.001$] adiponectin levels were independent risk factors of worse histological grade of HCC.

Conclusions: Our results suggested that serum total and HMW adiponectin levels were predictors of liver fibrosis, but not prevalence of HCC in patients with HCV infection. Moreover, low these adiponectin levels were significantly associated with worse histological grades.

Editor: Maria Tsokos, National Cancer Institute, United States of America

Funding: This research was supported by a Grant-in-Aid for Young Scientists (B) from the Ministry of Education, Culture, Sports, Science and Technology of Japan (No. 22790874). The funder had no role in study design, data collection and analysis, decision to publish, or preparation of the manuscript. No additional external funding received for this study.

Competing Interests: The authors have declared that no competing interests exist.

* E-mail: sumie_shyuuji@kurume-u.ac.jp

Introduction

Hepatocellular carcinoma (HCC) is one of the most common malignancies in the world. The incidence of HCC has increased in Eastern Asia and Africa during the past several decades, and has also increased in the United States [1]. In many countries, this trend is attributed to hepatitis C virus (HCV) infections, and in Japan, over 70% of all HCC are related to chronic liver disease with HCV infection [2]. In order to prevent and treat this malignancy, it is important to understand the pathogenesis of HCC in patients with HCV infection.

Obesity is widely recognized as a significant risk factor for the development of various cancers [3]. It also is suggested that obesity is associated with the progression of chronic liver disease [4,5] and with HCC [6]. Especially, nonalcoholic fatty liver disease is recognized to be a hepatic manifestation of the metabolic syndrome and obesity and insulin resistance play a major role in the pathogenesis [7]. Nonalcoholic fatty liver disease represents a spectrum of conditions that are histologically characterized from simple steatosis to nonalcoholic steatohepatits, which is associated with increased risk of advanced liver fibrosis, cirrhosis and development of HCC [8]. Similarly, in patients with HCV infection, several studies have shown that obesity was associated with disease progression [4,5] and with HCC development [9,10]. However, it is unclear how obesity is linked to development of HCC in patients with HCV infection.

Adiponectin is a peptide hormone secreted by adipocyte and hepatocyte [11]. Adiponectin exists primarily in three forms: low molecular weight trimers, medium molecular weight hexamers, and high molecular weight (HMW) multimers [12]. Among three forms, HMW adiponectin is thought to have more biological activity than other forms of adiponectin [12,13]. Adiponectin has antiatherogenic, antiinflamatory and insulin-sensitizing actions and is inversely associated with body mass index (BMI); therefore it is also linked to the various metabolic abnormalities associated with obesity [14]. Recently, hypoadiponectinemia has been shown to be an important risk factor for the development of various cancers associated with obesity such as breast cancer [15], endometrial cancer [16], colorectal cancer [17], and gastric cancer [18]. However, it is still unknown whether adiponectin contribute to the development of HCC in patients with HCV infection. Moreover, adiponectin has been shown to be associated with progression of liver fibrosis in patients with chronic liver disease [19,20,21]. However, in patients with HCV infection, the association between adiponectin and liver fibrosis is uncertain.

Histological grade is known to be one of the most important risk factor for patients with HCC. Several studies have shown that histological grade affected recurrence and survival after curative resection and liver transplantation for HCC [22,23]. Although it is known that worse histological grade is associated with high cell proliferation and angiogenesis of HCC, these molecular mechanisms is not unclear. Several clinical studies have demonstrated that serum adiponectin levels were negatively associated with increasing of histological grades of several cancers [15,24,25].

Therefore, in case-control study, we investigated the association of serum total and HMW adiponectin levels with prevalence of HCC in chronic liver disease with HCV infections. In addition, the associations between these adiponectin levels and BMI, progression of liver fibrosis, and histological grades of HCC were also examined.

Materials and Methods

Ethics Statement

The study protocol was approved by The Ethical Committee of Kurume University, and written informed consent for participation in the study was obtained from each subject and conformed to the guidelines of the 1995 Declaration of Helsinki.

Patients

Between January 1997 and December 2007, 97 Japanese cases with chronic HCV infection at the Kurume University School of Medicine were diagnosed with HCC and enrolled in this study. All cases had no medical history of previous or present neoplastic disease at any other site. The case patients were histologically confirmed with HCC by needle biopsy, and with a single tumor ≤5 cm or three or fewer tumors each ≤3 cm seen on ultrasonography and computed tomography. Histological classification was based on Liver Cancer Study Group of Japan [26]. According to Edmondson-Steiner classification [27], well differentiated corresponds to grade I and a part of grade II, and moderately differentiated corresponds to grade II and grade III with a clear trabecular pattern, and poorly differentiated corresponds to grade III with an indistinct trabecular pattern and part of grade IV. Tumor sizes were determined based on the largest dimension of the tumor. Between January 2005 and December 2007, 97 patients with chronic HCV infection, who matched for sex, Child-Pugh grade and platelet count ($\pm 20\times10^9$/L), were randomly selected as controls at the same hospital. The control patients had no medical history of previous or present neoplastic disease, including HCC. In all cases and controls, hepatic functional reserve was determined using the Child-Pugh scoring system. Diabetes was defined as a fasting blood glucose ≥126 mg/dl, and/or a random blood glucose ≥200 mg/dl. BMI was calculated as body weight in kg divided by the square of the height in meters (kg/m^2).

Assessment of liver fibrosis

Liver fibrosis was assessed using the aspartate aminotransferase (AST) to platelet ratio index (APRI) in this study. APRI has been recognized as a noninvasive test to characterize the degree of liver fibrosis in chronic liver disease with HCV infection [28]. APRI was calculated for all study subjects as follows: AST/upper limit of normal (45 IU/L)×100/platelet count (10^9/L).

Markers of hepatic virus

HCV infection was evaluated using anti-HCV antibody (HCV-Ab). The diagnosis of HBV infection was also based on detection of hepatitis B surface antigen (HBsAg). The presence of HCV-Ab and HBsAg was determined using standard clinical methods (Department of Clinical Laboratory, Kurume University Hospital). All cases and controls were positive for HCV-Ab and negative for HBsAg in this study.

Measurement of serum adiponectin

Fasting morning blood samples were obtained from all subjects and stored at −20°C for later analysis. Blood samples were collected by all cases before HCC therapy was initiated. Serum total and HMW adiponectin levels were measured by enzyme-linked immunosorbent assays using the Human Adiponectin Latex Kit (Eiken Chemical Co., Ltd., Tokyo, Japan) and High Molecular Weight Adiponectin Assay Kit (Fujirebio Inc., Tokyo, Japan), respectively.

Statistical Analysis

Continuous variables were expressed as mean ± standard deviation. Comparisons between the 2 groups were performed using the Mann-Whitney U test for continuous variables, and the chi-square test for discrete variables. Pearson correlation test was used to evaluate the association between plasma total and HMW adiponectin levels and BMI and APRI in each cases and controls. Comparison analysis between histological grades was performed by the one-way ANOVA with Bonferroni corrections for post hoc comparisons. The relationships between total and HMW adiponectin and HCC histological grades of were determined using multiple logistic regression models. Data were reported as odds ratios (ORs) and 95% confidence intervals (95% CIs). All P values were 2-tailed, and $P<0.05$ was considered to be statistically significant. Statistical analysis was performed using SPSS software (SPSS Inc., Chicago, IL).

Results

Serum adiponectin levels and prevalence of HCC

The baseline clinical characteristics of the 97 cases and 97 controls were shown in Table 1. No significant differences were found between cases and controls according to AST level, alanine transaminase (ALT) level, APRI, diabetes mellitus, or BMI. The mean age of the cases was significantly higher than the mean age of the controls. The associations between serum total and HMW adiponectin levels and prevalence of HCC were shown in Figure 1. There were no significant differences between the mean total adiponectin levels of the cases and controls (15.5±10.4 µg/ml and 16.6±12.8 µg/ml, respectively, $P=0.670$) (Figure 1A), or the mean HMW adiponectin levels (10.1±7.4 µg/ml and 10.8±9.0 µg/ml, respectively, $P=0.752$) (Figure 1B).

Association between serum adiponectin levels and BMI

We examined the associations between serum total and HMW adiponectin levels and BMI in cases and controls. In controls,

Table 1. Baseline clinical characteristics in case and control.

	Case	Control	P value
Number	97	97	
Age (years)	67.4±8.3	61.2±11.4	<0.001
Gender (Female/Male)	30/67	30/67	Matched variable
AST (U/L)	61.8±28.3	60.0±28.5	0.632
ALT (U/L)	58.4±33.4	60.0±31.8	0.513
Platelet (×10^9/L)	115.0±51.4	115.5±52.5	Matched variable
APRI	1.5±1.0	1.5±1.1	0.863
Child-Pugh grade (A/B+C)	82/15	82/15	Matched variable
Diabetes mellitus (Absent/Present)	64/33	71/26	0.275
BMI (kg/m^2)	22.5±3.2	23.1±3.3	0.228
Total adiponectin (μg/ml)	15.5±10.4	16.6±12.8	0.670
HMW adiponectin (μg/ml)	10.1±7.4	10.8±9.0	0.752

Continuous variables presented as mean ± standard deviation.
Abbreviation: AST = aspartate aminotransferase; ALT = alanine aminotransferase; APRI = aspartate aminotransferase-to-platelet ratio index; BMI = body mass index; HMW = high molecular weigh.

there were no inverse associations between serum total and HMW adiponectin levels and BMI (r = −0.142, P = 0.166 for total adiponectin [Figure 2A] and r = −0.144, P = 0.160 for HMW adiponectin [Figure 2B]). Similarly, in cases, there were also no inverse associations between serum total or HMW adiponectin levels and BMI (r = −0.129, P = 0.208 for total adiponectin [Figure 2C] and r = −0.131, P = 0.201 for HMW adiponectin [Figure 2D]).

Association between serum adiponectin levels and APRI

We also evaluated the associations between serum total and HMW adiponectin levels and APRI in cases and controls. In controls, serum levels of total and HMW adiponectin were positively associated with APRI (r = 0.482, P<0.001 for total adiponectin [Figure 3A] and r = 0.476, P<0.001 for HMW adiponectin [Figure 3B]). Similarly, in cases, serum levels of total and HMW adiponectin were positively associated with APRI (r = 0.491, P<0.001 for total adiponectin [Figure 3C] and r = 0.485, P<0.001 for HMW adiponectin [Figure 3D]).

Comparison of serum adiponectin levels according to HCC histological grades

The baseline clinical characteristics of 97 HCC cases were also separately evaluated according to the histological grades (Table 2). No significant differences were found between HCC histological grades and age, gender, AST level, ALT level, platelet count, APRI, Child-Pugh grade, diabetes mellitus, BMI, alpha-fetoprotein (AFP) level, des-gamma-carboxy prothrombin (DCP) level, and number of tumor. Patients with moderately and poorly differentiated HCC had significantly larger tumor sizes than patients with well-differentiated HCC. The associations between serum total and HMW adiponectin levels and HCC histological grades were shown in Figure 4. The mean total adiponectin levels in patients with moderately (13.4±6.9 μg/ml, P = 0.001) and

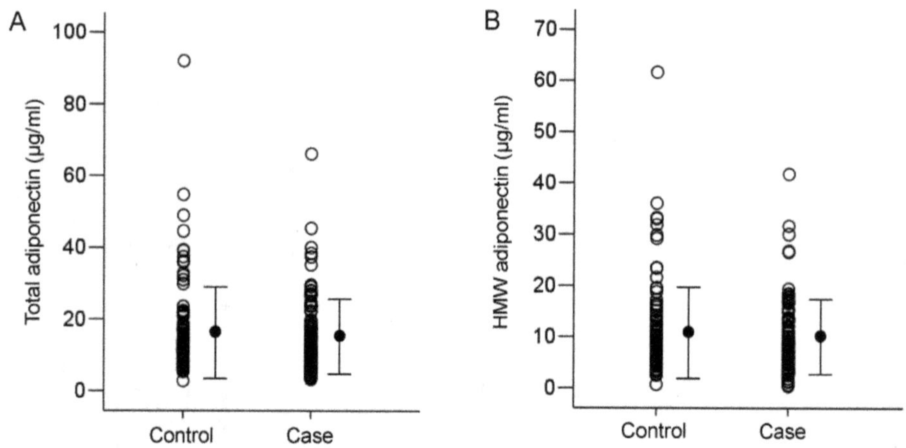

Figure 1. Comparison of adiponectin levels between 97 controls and 97 cases. A. Comparison of total adiponectin levels between patients with cases and controls (P = 0.670). B. Comparison of HMW adiponectin levels between patients with cases and controls (P = 0.752).

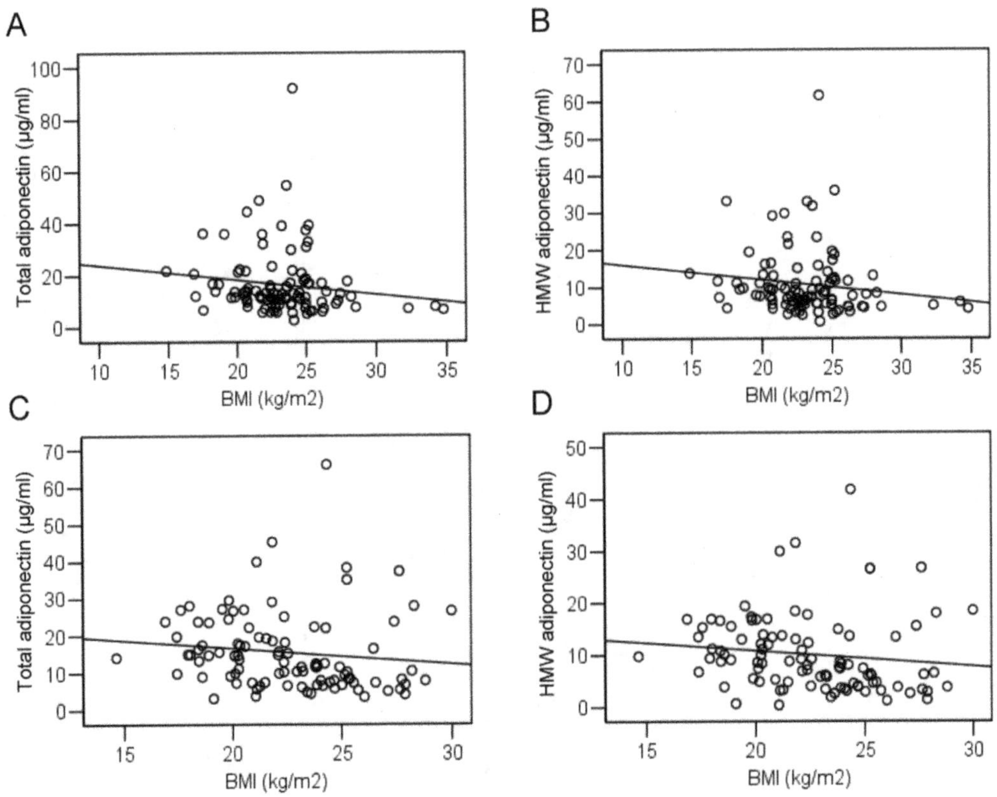

Figure 2. Serum adiponectin levels and body mass index (BMI). A. Correlation between serum total adiponectin levels and BMI in controls (r = −0.142, P = 0.166). B. Correlation between serum high molecular adiponectin (HMW) adiponectin levels and BMI in controls (r = −0.144, P = 0.160). C. Correlation between serum total adiponectin levels and BMI in cases (r = −0.129, P = 0.208). D. Correlation between serum HMW adiponectin levels and BMI in cases (r = −0.131, P = 0.201).

poorly (11.5±7.3 μg/ml, P<0.001) differentiated HCC were significantly lower compared to those in patients with well-differentiated HCC (22.0±13.6 μg/ml). The mean HMW adiponectin levels in patients with moderately (8.6±4.7 μg/ml, P<0.001) and poorly (6.9±5.0 μg/ml, P<0.001) differentiated HCC were significantly lower compared to those in patients with well-differentiated HCC (14.9±9.5 μg/ml). In addition, multiple logistic regression analyses were performed to determine whether the serum total and HMW adiponectin levels were independently associated with HCC histological grades (Table 3). In the analysis adjusted for other variables, lower serum total adiponectin levels (12–24 μg/ml; OR: 9.33, 95% CI: 2.27–38.43 [P = 0.002], <12 μg/ml; OR 11.76, 95% CI: 2.97–46.66 [P<0.001]) and serum HMW adiponectin levels (7–14 μg/ml; OR: 5.67, 95% CI: 1.66–19.33 [P = 0.006], <7 μg/ml; OR 10.24, CI: 2.80–37.40 [P<0.001]) were independent risk factors for worse HCC histological grades.

Discussion

Obesity is known to be associated with various cancers and hypoadiponectinemia has been also shown to be a risk factor for these obesity-associated cancers [15,16,17,18]. Epidemiological evidence of the association between obesity and HCC is also rapidly increasing including patients with HCV infection. In a community-based cohort study, Chen et al. reported that obesity was an independent risk factor for HCC development in anti-HCV-seropositive subjects [9]. Therefore, we hypothesized that serum adiponectin level may be associated with the prevalence of HCC in patients with HCV infection. However, in this case-control study, serum total and HMW adiponectin levels were not significantly and inversely associated with the prevalence of HCC. Similarly, Nkontchou et al. also demonstrated that serum level of adiponectin is not predictive of HCC development in patients with compensated HCV cirrhosis [29]. In patients with HCV infection, it is well known that metabolic abnormalities such as obesity and diabetes are closely associated with hepatic steatosis [4] and severe fibrosis [5]; as a result, obesity affect as a partial factor of HCC development. On the other hand, several recent reports have shown that hypoadiponectinemia was associated with hepatic steatosis only in limited genotype [30] and association between hypoadiponectinemia and fibrosis progression was not found in patients with HCV infection [31]. In addition, we assessed the association between BMI and serum adiponectin levels in cases and controls. Our results showed that these adiponectin levels were not inversely associated with BMI, suggesting that adiponectin is not a cofactor in the development of HCC associated with obesity in patients with HCV infection.

Recently, several studies have been reported that serum adiponectin level was associated with progression of liver fibrosis in patients with chronic liver disease [19,20,21]. We also evaluated the association between serum total and HMW adiponectin levels and progression of liver fibrosis. APRI is a useful noninvasive marker for the prediction of liver fibrosis in chronic liver disease with HCV infection [28] and we assessed the degree of liver fibrosis by APRI in this study. As a result, serum total and HMW adiponectin levels were positively and significantly associated with APRI in both cases and controls. Tietge et al. reported that circulating adiponectin level increased in patients with liver

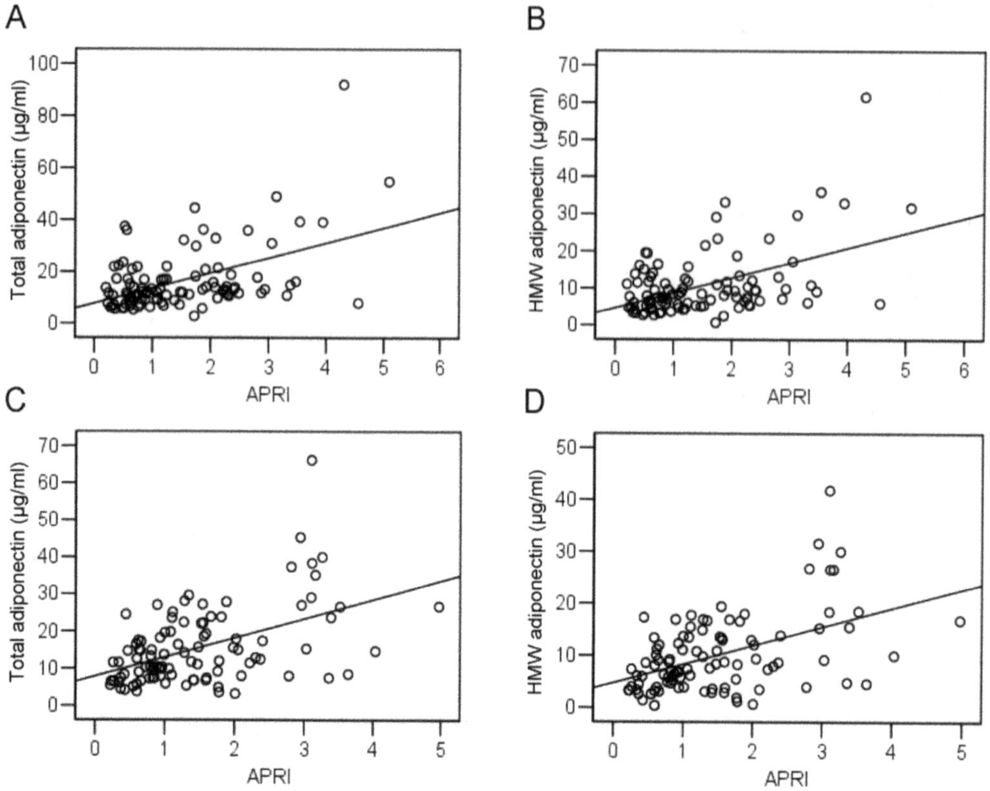

Figure 3. Serum adiponectin levels and aspartate aminotransferase-to-platelet ratio index (APRI). A. Correlation between serum total adiponectin levels and APRI in controls (r = 0.482, $P<0.001$). B. Correlation between serum high molecular adiponectin (HMW) adiponectin levels and APRI in controls (r = 0.476, $P<0.001$). C. Correlation between serum total adiponectin levels and APRI in cases (r = 0.491, $P<0.001$). D. Correlation between serum HMW adiponectin levels and APRI in cases (r = 0.485, $P<0.001$).

Table 2. Association between clinical characteristics and histological grade in patients with hepatocellular carcinoma.

	Well	Moderate	Poor	*P* value
Number	30	39	28	
Age (years)	67.5±6.9	67.3±8.2	67.1±9.9	0.942
Gender (Female/Male)	11/19	12/27	7/21	0.630
AST (U/L)	67.2±23.8	59.5±28.8	59.3±25.9	0.409
ALT (U/L)	61.0±35.5	60.0±33.1	53.5±32.1	0.647
Platelet count (×10^9/L)	103.1±46.5	116.9±47.6	125.1±54.0	0.228
APRI	1.8±1.1	1.3±0.9	1.3±0.9	0.213
Child-Pugh grade (A/B+C)	22/8	36/3	24/4	0.095
Diabetes mellitus (Absent/Present)	24/6	21/18	19/9	0.073
BMI (kg/m^2)	22.5±3.2	22.4±3.0	22.6±3.5	0.949
AFP (ng/ml)	51.3±74.4	165.0±448.4	560.1±1508.8	0.065
DCP (mAU/ml)	65.5±139.5	464.2±978.8	276.1±586.4	0.070
Tumor size (mm)	21.0±4.9	26.8±10.0†	26.6±11.8†	0.027
Tumor number (single/2–3)	19/11	29/10	19/9	0.609
Total adiponectin (μg/ml)	22.0±13.6	13.4±6.9†	11.5±7.3†	<0.001
HMW adiponectin (μg/ml)	14.9±9.5	8.6±4.7†	6.9±5.0†	<0.001

Continuous variables presented as mean ± standard deviation.
Abbreviation: AST = aspartate aminotransferase; ALT = alanine aminotransferase;
APRI = aspartate aminotransferase-to-platelet ratio index; BMI = body mass index;
AFP = alpha-fetoprotein; DCP = des-gamma-carboxy prothrombin; HMW = high molecular weigh.
†P<0.05 for Bonferroni corrected post hoc comparison with well-differentiated hepatocellular carcinoma.

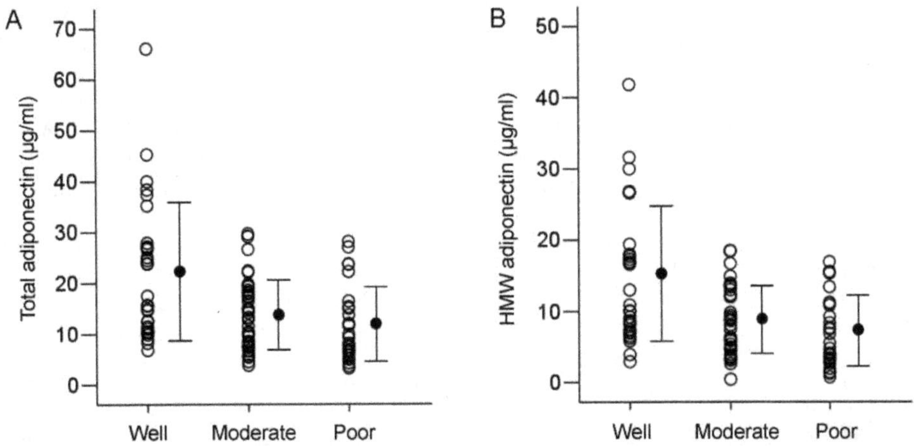

Figure 4. Comparison of adiponectin levels according to histological grades in 97 cases. A. The serum total adiponectin levels in patients with moderately ($P=0.001$) and poorly ($P<0.001$) differentiated hepatocellular carcinoma (HCC) were significantly lower compared to those in patients with well-differentiated HCC. B. The serum high molecular weight (HMW) adiponectin levels in patients with moderately ($P<0.001$) and poorly ($P<0.001$) differentiated HCC were significantly lower compared to those in patients with well-differentiated HCC.

cirrhosis, because of reduced liver function as a major source of adiponectin extraction and altered hepatic hemodynamics [20]. Taken together serum total and HMW adiponectin levels may be a predictors of liver fibrosis in patients with HCV infection.

Next, we examined the relationship between serum adiponectin levels and HCC histological grades. Interestingly, low total and HMW adiponectin levels were independent risk factors for worse HCC histological grades. It is generally known that majority of HCC arises as very well-differentiated cancers and proliferate in a stepwise process of dedifferentiation. When small HCC of the early-stage reach around 1.5–2.0 cm, moderately or poorly differentiated cancer tissues develops within the well-differentiated cancer tissue, and well-differentiated cancer tissue are replaced by less differentiated cancer tissue in so-called advanced HCC [32]. In this study, the mean tumor size of well-differentiated HCC was 14.2±3.2 mm, which was significantly smaller than the mean size of moderately and poorly differentiated HCC. This result indicated that a dedifferentiation of HCC is associated with tumor proliferation.

This is a cross-sectional study and causal relationship between serum adiponectin level and dedifferentiation of HCC is unclear. One would think that dedifferentiation of HCC may trigger a mechanism which leads to decreased serum adiponectin level. However, it seems that hypoadiponectinemia may trigger dedifferentiation of HCC because of followings: Saxena et al. showed that adiponectin increased the phosphorylation of AMP-activated protein kinase (AMPK) and the TSC2 tumor suppressor, and inhibited phosphorylation of the mammalian target of rapamycin (mTOR) in vitro assay using Huh7 and HepG2 HCC cells [11]. Moreover, microarray analysis of tissue adiponectin expression levels in human HCC patients revealed that adiponectin expression was inversely correlated with tumor size [11]. Miyazaki et al. showed that adiponectin stimulated c-Jun NH2-terminal kinase (JNK) activation and suppressed signal transducer and activator of transcription 3 (STAT3) activation in HepG2 HCC cells [33]. Thus, these studies support that adiponectin level may inhibit proliferation and differentiation of HCC.

Table 3. Association between total and HMW adiponectin and histological grade in patients with hepatocellular carcinoma by multiple logistic regression analysis.

	Model 1		**Model 2**	
	OR (95%CI)	***P* value**	**OR (95%CI)**	***P* value**
Total adiponectin (μg/ml)				
24<	Reference		Reference	
12–24	6.67 (1.83–24.3)	0.004	9.33 (2.27–38.43)	0.002
<12	9.87 (2.76–35.2)	<0.001	11.76 (2.97–46.66)	<0.001
HMW adiponectin (μg/ml)				
14<	Reference		Reference	
7–14	4.38 (1.40–13.64)	0.011	5.67 (1.66–19.33)	0.006
<7	9.92 (2.91–33.85)	<0.001	10.24 (2.80–37.40)	<0.001

Abbreviation: OR = odds ratio; 95% CI = confidence interval; HMW = high molecular weigh.
Model 1: adiponectin only.
Model 2: adiponectin and covariates in Table 2.

Angiogenesis is also an important process for proliferation, dedifferentiation, and metastasis of HCC. In small sized and well-differentiated HCCs, artery-like vessels are not well developed [34]. On the other hand, in moderately or poorly differentiated HCCs with 2 cm or larger, artery-like vessels are well developed [35], and these tumors display high proliferation and metastasis so-called advanced stage. Vascular endothelial growth factor (VEGF) is an endothelial cell-specific mitogen, and is the most important factor in tumor angiogenesis [36]. Yamaguchi et al. showed that VEGF expression in well-differentiated HCC was higher than expression in moderately and poorly differentiated HCC [37]. Well-differentiated HCCs that are 1.0–1.5 cm would be in the transitioning from the portal blood supply to an arterial blood supply, which would result in increased VEGF expression because of relative hypoxia from low blood flow. Therefore, high VEGF expression in small-sized and Well-differentiated HCCs suggests that VEGF plays an important role during relatively early angiogenesis stages in HCC. Previous studies have reported on the the molecular mechanisms involved in the negative association of adiponectin with tumor angiogenesis [38,39]. Man et al. showed in an orthotopic liver tumor nude mouse model that adiponectin suppresses tumor growth through inhibition of tumor angiogenesis [39]. The molecular mechanism involves adiponectin downregulation of VEGF expression through inhibition of tumor-associated macrophages in tumor tissue. Moreover, the nude mice administrated adiponectin had significantly lower circulating VEGF levels than the control. This result suggests that adiponectin may inhibit dedifferentiation in well-differentiated HCC by inhibition of tumor angiogenesis-related VEGF.

Adiponectin exists mainly in three forms [12]. HMW adiponectin is thought to have higher biological activity than the other forms of adiponectin, especially in the liver [12,13]. Several studies have reported that HMW adiponectin levels or the ratio of HMW to total adiponectin is inversely and more strongly associated with metabolic risk factors than total adiponectin levels [40,41]. However, it remains unknown whether HMW adiponectin has more strongly potential actions on cancer pathophysiology than total adiponectin. In this study, we demonstrated that total and HMW adiponectin were independent risk factors for HCC histological grade. However, odds ratio of these factors were similar and serum total adiponectin levels were significantly associated with serum HMW adiponectin levels in this study (data not shown). Thus, one would think that impact of HMW adiponectin may be equal to total adiponectin for predicting HCC histological grade and testing for either total or HMW adiponectin levels may be as effective as testing both levels.

In conclusion, our data suggested that serum total and HMW adiponectin levels were predictors of liver fibrosis, but not prevalence of HCC in patients with chronic HCV infection. Moreover, we showed that low total and HMW adiponectin levels were independent risk factors for worse histological grades of HCC. Further study will be focused on the causal relationship between hypoadiponectinemia and dedifferentiation of HCC.

Author Contributions

Conceived and designed the experiments: SS TK M. Sata. Performed the experiments: SS MN. Analyzed the data: SS AT M. Satani. Contributed reagents/materials/analysis tools: MN M. Satani SY TN. Wrote the paper: SS TK RK M. Sata TT.

References

1. Bosch FX, Ribes J, Diaz M, Cleries R (2004) Primary liver cancer: worldwide incidence and trends. Gastroenterology 127: S5–S16.
2. Kiyosawa K, Umemura T, Ichijo T, Matsumoto A, Yoshizawa K, et al. (2004) Hepatocellular carcinoma: recent trends in Japan. Gastroenterology 127: S17–26.
3. Bergstrom A, Pisani P, Tenet V, Wolk A, Adami HO (2001) Overweight as an avoidable cause of cancer in Europe. Int J Cancer 91: 421–430.
4. Monto A, Alonzo J, Watson JJ, Grunfeld C, Wright TL (2002) Steatosis in chronic hepatitis C: relative contributions of obesity, diabetes mellitus, and alcohol. Hepatology 36: 729–736.
5. Jonsson JR, Barrie HD, O'Rourke P, Clouston AD, Powell EE (2008) Obesity and steatosis influence serum and hepatic inflammatory markers in chronic hepatitis C. Hepatology 48: 80–87.
6. Marrero JA, Fontana RJ, Fu S, Conjeevaram HS, Su GL, et al. (2005) Alcohol, tobacco and obesity are synergistic risk factors for hepatocellular carcinoma. J Hepatol 42: 218–224.
7. Marchesini G, Bugianesi E, Forlani G, Cerrelli F, Lenzi M, et al. (2003) Nonalcoholic fatty liver, steatohepatitis, and the metabolic syndrome. Hepatology 37: 917–923.
8. Ascha MS, Hanouneh IA, Lopez R, Tamimi TA, Feldstein AF, et al. (2010) The incidence and risk factors of hepatocellular carcinoma in patients with nonalcoholic steatohepatitis. Hepatology 51: 1972–1978.
9. Chen CL, Yang HI, Yang WS, Liu CJ, Chen PJ, et al. (2008) Metabolic factors and risk of hepatocellular carcinoma by chronic hepatitis B/C infection: a follow-up study in Taiwan. Gastroenterology 135: 111–121.
10. Ohki T, Tateishi R, Sato T, Masuzaki R, Imamura J, et al. (2008) Obesity is an independent risk factor for hepatocellular carcinoma development in chronic hepatitis C patients. Clin Gastroenterol Hepatol 6: 459–464.
11. Saxena NK, Fu PP, Nagalingam A, Wang J, Handy J, et al. (2010) Adiponectin Modulates C-Jun N-Terminal Kinase and Mammalian Target of Rapamycin and inhibits hepatocellular carcinoma. Gastroenterology.
12. Waki H, Yamauchi T, Kamon J, Ito Y, Uchida S, et al. (2003) Impaired multimerization of human adiponectin mutants associated with diabetes. Molecular structure and multimer formation of adiponectin. J Biol Chem 278: 40352–40363.
13. Ouchi N, Kobayashi H, Kihara S, Kumada M, Sato K, et al. (2004) Adiponectin stimulates angiogenesis by promoting cross-talk between AMP-activated protein kinase and Akt signaling in endothelial cells. J Biol Chem 279: 1304–1309.
14. Adachi M, Brenner DA (2008) High molecular weight adiponectin inhibits proliferation of hepatic stellate cells via activation of adenosine monophosphate-activated protein kinase. Hepatology 47: 677–685.
15. Miyoshi Y, Funahashi T, Kihara S, Taguchi T, Tamaki Y, et al. (2003) Association of serum adiponectin levels with breast cancer risk. Clin Cancer Res 9: 5699–5704.
16. Dal Maso L, Augustin LS, Karalis A, Talamini R, Franceschi S, et al. (2004) Circulating adiponectin and endometrial cancer risk. J Clin Endocrinol Metab 89: 1160–1163.
17. Wei EK, Giovannucci E, Fuchs CS, Willett WC, Mantzoros CS (2005) Low plasma adiponectin levels and risk of colorectal cancer in men: a prospective study. J Natl Cancer Inst 97: 1688–1694.
18. Ishikawa M, Kitayama J, Kazama S, Hiramatsu T, Hatano K, et al. (2005) Plasma adiponectin and gastric cancer. Clin Cancer Res 11: 466–472.
19. Hui CK, Zhang HY, Lee NP, Chan W, Yueng YH, et al. (2007) Serum adiponectin is increased in advancing liver fibrosis and declines with reduction in fibrosis in chronic hepatitis B. J Hepatol 47: 191–202.
20. Tietge UJ, Boker KH, Manns MP, Bahr MJ (2004) Elevated circulating adiponectin levels in liver cirrhosis are associated with reduced liver function and altered hepatic hemodynamics. Am J Physiol Endocrinol Metab 287: E82–89.
21. Kaser S, Moschen A, Kaser A, Ludwiczek O, Ebenbichler CF, et al. (2005) Circulating adiponectin reflects severity of liver disease but not insulin sensitivity in liver cirrhosis. J Intern Med 258: 274–280.
22. Wayne JD, Lauwers GY, Ikai I, Doherty DA, Belghiti J, et al. (2002) Preoperative predictors of survival after resection of small hepatocellular carcinomas. Ann Surg 235: 722–730.
23. Jonas S, Bechstein WO, Steinmuller T, Herrmann M, Radke C, et al. (2001) Vascular invasion and histopathologic grading determine outcome after liver transplantation for hepatocellular carcinoma in cirrhosis. Hepatology 33: 1080–1086.
24. Seker M, Bilici A, Sonmez B, Ustaalioglu BB, Gumus M, et al. (2010) The association of serum adiponectin levels with histopathological variables in gastric cancer patients. Med Oncol 27: 1319–1323.
25. Barresi V, Tuccari G, Barresi G (2009) Adiponectin immunohistochemical expression in colorectal cancer and its correlation with histological grade and tumour microvessel density. Pathology 41: 533–538.
26. Liver Cancer Study Group of Japan (2010) General rules for the clinical and pathological study of primary liver cancer. 3nd English ed. Tokyo: Kanehara & Co., Ltd. 96 p.

27. Edmondson HA, Steiner PE (1954) Primary carcinoma of the liver: a study of 100 cases among 48,900 necropsies. Cancer 7: 462–503.
28. Wai CT, Greenson JK, Fontana RJ, Kalbfleisch JD, Marrero JA, et al. (2003) A simple noninvasive index can predict both significant fibrosis and cirrhosis in patients with chronic hepatitis C. Hepatology 38: 518–526.
29. Nkontchou G, Bastard JP, Ziol M, Aout M, Cosson E, et al. (2010) Insulin resistance, serum leptin, and adiponectin levels and outcomes of viral hepatitis C cirrhosis. J Hepatol 53: 827–833.
30. Zografos TA, Liaskos C, Rigopoulou EI, Togousidis E, Makaritsis K, et al. (2008) Adiponectin: a new independent predictor of liver steatosis and response to IFN-alpha treatment in chronic hepatitis C. Am J Gastroenterol 103: 605–614.
31. Liu CJ, Chen PJ, Jeng YM, Huang WL, Yang WS, et al. (2005) Serum adiponectin correlates with viral characteristics but not histologic features in patients with chronic hepatitis C. J Hepatol 43: 235–242.
32. Kojiro M (2005) Histopathology of liver cancers. Best Pract Res Clin Gastroenterol 19: 39–62.
33. Miyazaki T, Bub JD, Uzuki M, Iwamoto Y (2005) Adiponectin activates c-Jun NH2-terminal kinase and inhibits signal transducer and activator of transcription 3. Biochem Biophys Res Commun 333: 79–87.
34. Nakashima O, Sugihara S, Kage M, Kojiro M (1995) Pathomorphologic characteristics of small hepatocellular carcinoma: a special reference to small hepatocellular carcinoma with indistinct margins. Hepatology 22: 101–105.
35. Himeno H, Enzan H, Saibara T, Onishi S, Yamamoto Y (1994) Hitherto unrecognized arterioles within hepatocellular carcinoma. J Pathol 174: 217–222.
36. Leung DW, Cachianes G, Kuang WJ, Goeddel DV, Ferrara N (1989) Vascular endothelial growth factor is a secreted angiogenic mitogen. Science 246: 1306–1309.
37. Yamaguchi R, Yano H, Iemura A, Ogasawara S, Haramaki M, et al. (1998) Expression of vascular endothelial growth factor in human hepatocellular carcinoma. Hepatology 28: 68–77.
38. Brakenhielm E, Veitonmaki N, Cao R, Kihara S, Matsuzawa Y, et al. (2004) Adiponectin-induced antiangiogenesis and antitumor activity involve caspase-mediated endothelial cell apoptosis. Proc Natl Acad Sci U S A 101: 2476–2481.
39. Man K, Ng KT, Xu A, Cheng Q, Lo CM, et al. (2010) Suppression of liver tumor growth and metastasis by adiponectin in nude mice through inhibition of tumor angiogenesis and downregulation of Rho kinase/IFN-inducible protein 10/matrix metalloproteinase 9 signaling. Clin Cancer Res 16: 967–977.
40. Pajvani UB, Du X, Combs TP, Berg AH, Rajala MW, et al. (2003) Structure-function studies of the adipocyte-secreted hormone Acrp30/adiponectin. Implications fpr metabolic regulation and bioactivity. J Biol Chem 278: 9073–9085.
41. Aso Y, Yamamoto R, Wakabayashi S, Uchida T, Takayanagi K, et al. (2006) Comparison of serum high-molecular weight (HMW) adiponectin with total adiponectin concentrations in type 2 diabetic patients with coronary artery disease using a novel enzyme-linked immunosorbent assay to detect HMW adiponectin. Diabetes 55: 1954–1960.

6

Role of Alcohol Metabolism in Non-Alcoholic Steatohepatitis

Susan S. Baker[1], Robert D. Baker[1], Wensheng Liu[1], Norma J. Nowak[2,3], Lixin Zhu[1]*

1 Digestive Diseases and Nutrition Center, Department of Pediatrics, The State University of New York, Buffalo, New York, United States of America, **2** Department of Biochemistry and the New York State Center of Excellence in Bioinformatics and Life Sciences, The State University of New York at Buffalo, Buffalo, New York, United States of America, **3** Microarray and Genomics Facility, Roswell Park Cancer Institute, Buffalo, New York, United States of America

Abstract

Background: Non-alcoholic steatohepatitis (NASH) is a serious form of non-alcoholic fatty liver disease (NAFLD), associated with obesity and insulin resistance. Previous studies suggested that intestinal bacteria produced more alcohol in obese mice than lean animals.

Methodology/Principal Findings: To investigate whether alcohol is involved in the pathogenesis of NASH, the expression of inflammation, fibrosis and alcohol metabolism related genes in the liver tissues of NASH patients and normal controls (NCs) were examined by microarray (NASH, n = 7; NC, n = 4) and quantitative real-time PCR (NASH, n = 6; NC, n = 6). Genes related to liver inflammation and fibrosis were found to be elevated in NASH livers compared to normal livers. The most striking finding is the increased gene transcription of alcohol dehydrogenase (ADH) genes, genes for catalase and cytochrome P450 2E1, and aldehyde dehydrogenase genes. Immunoblot analysis confirmed the increased expression of ADH1 and ADH4 in NASH livers (NASH, n = 9; NC, n = 4).

Conclusions/Significance: The augmented activity of all the available genes of the pathways for alcohol catabolism suggest that 1) alcohol concentration was elevated in the circulation of NASH patients; 2) there was a high priority for the NASH livers to scavenge alcohol from the circulation. Our data is the first human evidence that suggests alcohol may contribute to the development of NAFLD.

Editor: Christian Gluud, Copenhagen University Hospital, Denmark

Funding: This work was supported by an unrestricted grant from the Peter and Tommy Fund, Inc., Buffalo, New York. The funder had no role in study design, data collection and analysis, decision to publish, or preparation of the manuscript.

Competing Interests: The authors have declared that no competing interests exist.

* E-mail: lixinzhu@buffalo.edu

Introduction

Non-alcoholic steatohepatitis (NASH) is a serious form of non-alcoholic fatty liver disease (NAFLD), characterized by hepatic steatosis associated with evidence of inflammation and variable degrees of fibrosis [1]. The prevalence of NASH is increasing with the ever-growing problem of obesity in the general population. Up to 20% of the population may have fatty liver, and up to 3% may have NASH as estimated in 2004 [2].

According to the current "two-hit" hypothesis, NASH patients first develop fatty liver before a second hit initiates inflammation in the liver [3]. Studies with NASH patients and various animal models in the last decade have revealed insights into liver fat infiltration, damage, inflammation and fibrosis. Insulin resistance (IR) seems to be a major reason for fat deposition in liver by way of uncontrolled lipolysis in adipose tissue leading to increased levels of circulating free fatty acids [4]. Measurement with stable isotopes in NAFLD patients indicated that free fatty acids are the major source for fat accumulation in liver. De novo lipogenesis and dietary fatty acids are also significant sources of fat [5]. Other studies suggested that insufficient fatty acid utilization could also cause fat desposition in hepatocytes. Peroxisome proliferator-activated receptors are transcriptional factors regulating lipid metabolism in liver and therefore believed to play a central role in hepatic fat accumulation [6]. Lipotoxicity may cause mitochondrial dysfunction and subsequent liver damage and trigger inflammation [7]. Oxidative stress is possibly a potent thrust in this process and in subsequent activation of hepatic stellate cells [8].

Despite these efforts, the exact mechanism of the development of NASH is unclear. And it remains a puzzle that NASH and alcoholic steatohepatitis share many histological features [9]. Both NASH and alcoholic steatohepatitis patients exhibit macrovesicular and microvesicular fat in hepatocytes. The number and size of Mallory bodies, and the pattern of pericellular fibrosis are also indistinguishable between two disease groups. Previous studies suggested that intestinal bacteria produced more alcohol in obese mice than lean animals [10]. Therefore, we hypothesize that alcohol is involved in the pathogenesis of NASH.

In this report, gene expression in NASH livers was examined by a whole-genome DNA microarray and quantitative real-time PCR (qRT-PCR). We found that all the available genes of the pathways for alcohol catabolism exhibited elevated expression levels in NASH livers, among which the elevated protein levels of ADH1

Table 1. Characteristics of study groups.

	Microarray		Real-time PCR		Western blot	
	NASH	**Normal control**†	**NASH**	**Normal control**†	**NASH**	**Non-NASH control**‡
Sex (F : M)	F2 : M5	F1 : M3	F2 : M3	F2 : M4	F4 : M5	F3 : M1
Age (years)	9–16	1–19	9–14	1–9	11–18	4–12
Body Mass Index	35.0±2.9§	19.1±1.6¶	38.4±5.9§	16.5±0.8¶	32.7±1.6§	20.6±2.9¶
Fasting Insulin (mU/ml)	27.0±2.2	NA	31.2±2.3	NA	20.7±5.1	<2
Fasting glucose (mmol/L)	5.0±0.2	NA	5.1±0.3	NA	5.7±0.4	4.7±0.2
IR (HOMA)††	6.0±0.5	NA	7.0±0.5	NA	5.7±1.7	<1

†Normal healthy liver intended for transplantation, no liver disease reported.
‡Liver biopsies from patients with hepatitis C, autoimmune hepatitis, gall stones or cystic fibrosis, respectively. They were free from steatosis.
§Patients are all above 95 percentile of the population.
¶Normal controls are all below 80 pencentile of the population.
††IR (HOMA) for healthy subjects is around 1.
NA: Not available.

and ADH4 in NASH livers were confirmed by Western blot analysis. Our results suggest a key role for intestinal alcohol in the pathogenesis of NASH.

Methods

Patients

The human studies have been approved by the Institutional Review Board (IRB) of the State University of New York at Buffalo. Only children and adolescents were included in this study to ensure that our patients were not sustained alcohol users. All NASH patients included in this study (Table 1) exhibited significant insulin resistance (IR). IR was calculated based on the "homeostasis model assessment (HOMA)" method [11]. Liver biopsies were obtained, with prior written consent, from parents of patients suspected of having NASH as part of regular medical care. Patients from 7 to 18 years of age signed an assent to the research. Diagnosis of NASH was based on hepatic fat infiltration, inflammation and fibrosis as revealed by liver biopsy, following Kleiner's criteria [12].

For non-steatosis controls, total RNA was purchased from Admet Technologies (Durham, NC). These samples were derived from liver grafts of normal controls with normal body mass index (Table 1). The ages of these normal controls were similar to our NASH patients. No liver diseases were diagnosed with these normal controls. The healthy status of these livers was ascertained by the lower transcription levels of marker genes for inflammation and fibrosis, as detailed in the Results section. The non-NASH controls used in Western blot analysis were liver biopsies from patients with hepatitis C, autoimmune hepatitis, gall stones or cystic fibrosis, respectively. They were free from steatosis.

Table 2. Primer pairs for real-time quantitative PCR analysis.

Symbol	Description	Sequence	
GAPD	glyceraldehyde-3-phosphate dehydrogenase	AGCCTCAAGATCATCAGCAATG	(Forward)
		ATGGACTGTGGTCATGAGTCCTT	(Reverse)
CXCL10	chemokine (C-X-C motif) ligand 10	TTCCTGCAAGCCAATTTTGT	(Forward)
		ATGGCCTTCGATTCTGGATT	(Reverse)
ADH1C	alcohol dehydrogenase 1C (class I)	GGCTTGACACCATGATGGCT	(Forward)
		GGAGGTACCCCTACAATGACA	(Reverse)
ADH4	alcohol dehydrogenase 4 (class II)	CTGAAACCATGAAAGCAGCC	(Forward)
		GCCGATTATTAGCTCCTCTGG	(Reverse)
ADH6	alcohol dehydrogenase 6 (class V)	CAATACTGCCAAGGTGACTCC	(Forward)
		GCTCCTGCTGCTTTACAACC	(Reverse)
ALDH2	aldehyde dehydrogenase 2	TGGTTACTTCATCCAGCCCAC	(Forward)
		GCTCTCCCAACAACCTCCTCTAT	(Reverse)
ALDH8A1	aldehyde dehydrogenase 8 family, member A1	TGGGAGTCGCTGGTCTGAT	(Forward)
		CTGGGCTTGGCTATCACAGT	(Reverse)
TLR4	toll-like receptor 4	AATCCCCTGAGGCATTTAGG	(Forward)
		CCCCATCTTCAATTGTCTGG	(Reverse)

RNA Extraction and Microarray Hybridization

Liver biopsies were stored in RNAlater before total RNA was extracted with RNeasy and treated with RNase-free DNase I set (Qiagen, Valencia, CA). RNA samples obtained from Admet were also treated with RNase free DNase before downstream experiments. Quality of the RNA samples was assured with Bioanalyzer (Agilent Technologies) before downstream biotin-labeling and hybridization to the CodeLink Human Whole Genome Bioarray (GE Health care-Amersham Biosciences, Piscataway, NJ) following the manufacturer's manual. The original microarray data have been uploaded to Gene Expression Omnibus (GEO) website: http://www.ncbi.nlm.nih.gov/geo/index.cgi. All data is MIAME compliant. The accession numbers for NASH liver datasets are GSM435821 to GSM435827, and for normal control datasets: GSM435828, GSM435833 to GSM435835.

Quantitative RT-PCR

Specific primers (Table 2) were designed with the assistance of Primer 3 [13]. Complementary DNA was synthesized from 0.8 μg of RNA in a volume of 20 μl, using the iScript cDNA synthesis kit (Bio-Rad Laboratories, Hercules, CA). Real-time PCR was performed on an iCycler iQ real-time detection system (Bio-Rad Laboratories, Hercules, CA), using Sybergreen (iQ™ SYBR® Green Supermix; Bio-Rad Laboratories, Hercules, CA) for real-time monitoring of the PCR. GAPD RNA level were tested in parallel with the genes of interest. The presence of a single specific PCR product was verified by melting curve analysis and confirmed on agarose gels.

Threshold cycles (Ct) for each sample were determined by Bio-rad iQ5 optical system software (Bio-Rad Laboratories). The concentration of mRNA ([mRNA]) is represented by the following equation: $[mRNA] = M/E^{Ct}$, where constant M is an arbitrary threshold, E is the efficiency of PCR, Ct is the threshold cycle. All PCR reactions had efficiencies higher than 1.9, as determined experimentally with 4-times serial diluted samples. The relative mRNA concentration of each target gene was calculated as the mRNA concentration of target gene normalized against that of GAPD, as represented by the following equation:

$$[mRNA]_{target}/[mRNA]_{GAPD} = E_{GAPD}{}^{Ct.GAPD}/E_{target}{}^{Ct.target}$$

Western Blot Analysis

Liver biopsies stored in RNAlater were homogenized in PBS, and then boiled for 5 min in SDS-PAGE loading buffer. Samples

Table 3. Comparison of the gene expressions between liver tissues and breast cancer tissues.†

	GenBank Accession #	Gene Description	NASH Liver (n = 7)	Normal Liver (n = 4)	Breast Cancer (n = 4)	NASH Liver/Breast Cancer‡
House-keeping genes	NM_000402.2	glucose-6-phosphate dehydrogenase (G6PD)	1.58±0.10§	1.53±0.27	1.37±0.64	1.16
	NM_001101.2	actin, beta (ACTB)	18.19±2.91	16.07±4.88	20.38±19.35	0.89
	NM_000034.2	aldolase A, fructose-bisphosphate (ALDOA)	9.02±1.63	19.02±4.34	6.91±6.18	1.30
	NM_003379.3	villin 2 (ezrin) (VIL2)	1.78±0.42	4.02±1.28	1.38±0.84	1.29
	AL133626.1	H2A histone family, member J	1.66±0.12	1.81±0.22	1.88±0.20	0.88
	NM_002954.3	ribosomal protein S27a (RPS27A)	171.21±46.00	184.38±33.35	91.67±61.77	1.87
	NM_006951.2	TAF5 RNA polymerase II, TATA box binding protein-associated factor	1.64±0.24	1.04±0.25	1.46±0.20	1.13
	NM_001190.1	branched chain aminotransferase precursor (BCATm)	1.32±0.42	1.40±0.64	1.44±0.39	0.92
Liver specific genes¶	NM_000777.2	cytochrome P450, family 3, subfamily A, polypeptide 5 (CYP3A5)	4.91±1.83	8.08±3.40	0.00±0.21	10177.97
	NM_000040.1	apolipoprotein C-III (APOC3)	625.93±126.08	312.83±67.97	0.40±0.00	1579.62
	NM_001443.1	fatty acid binding protein 1, liver (FABP1)	605.55±80.67	250.15±51.55	0.42±0.25	1458.34
	NM_000039.1	apolipoprotein A-I (APOA1)	557.21±58.12	306.33±52.72	0.52±0.16	1071.00
	NM_006744.2	retinol binding protein 4, plasma (RBP4)	606.95±83.36	295.00±43.11	0.68±0.30	888.88
	NM_145740.1	glutathione S-transferase A1 (GSTA1)	312.50±33.64	25.17±14.02	0.42±0.22	742.18
	NM_000667.2	alcohol dehydrogenase 1A (class I), alpha polypeptide (ADH1A)	470.96±40.68	82.50±34.30	0.64±0.11	735.11
	NM_000483.3	apolipoprotein C-II (APOC2)	501.93±30.57	288.10±49.95	1.20±0.75	419.61
	NM_000236.1	hepatic triglyceride lipase (HTGL)	289.35±47.50	142.52±10.06	0.76±0.23	383.05
	NM_000670.2	alcohol dehydrogenase 4 (class II), pi polypeptide (ADH4)	257.14±38.38	6.53±2.17	0.80±0.44	323.14
	NM_000041.1	apolipoprotein E (APOE)	353.83±49.92	258.38±53.30	1.81±0.63	195.99

†Microarray data for breast cancer were downloaded from PubMed, accession #: GSE6304.
‡Fold difference of gene expression levels (sample mean) between NASH liver tissues and breast cancer tissues.
§Median normalized gene expression signal as detected by the Codelink microarray. Sample mean ± standard error.
¶For all the liver specific genes listed, significant differences in gene expression were detected between liver tissues and breast cancer tissues ($P<0.05$).

(4μg total protein each) were separated on 10% SDS PAGE gels. After blotting onto nitrocellulose membranes, ADH1 (cat#sc-137091, Santa Cruz Biotechnology Inc., CA), ADH4 (cat#sc-134249, Santa Cruz Biotechnology Inc.) and β-actin (Clone C4, MP Biomedicals, LLP, Ohio) were probed on separate blots, as all these proteins are of similar sizes. The results were visualized using

Table 4. Comparison of gene expressions between NASH livers and normal controls: house-keeping genes, inflammation and fibrosis related genes.†

	GenBank Accession#	Gene Description	NASH Liver (n = 7)	Normal Liver (n = 4)	NASH/ Normal‡	P value§
House-keeping genes	NM_000402.2	glucose-6-phosphate dehydrogenase (G6PD)	1.58±0.10	1.53±0.27	1.03	0.875
	NM_001101.2	actin, beta (ACTB)	18.19±2.91	16.07±4.88	1.13	0.723
	NM_000034.2	aldolase A, fructose-bisphosphate (ALDOA), transcript variant 1	9.02±1.63	19.02±4.34	0.47	0.100
	NM_003379.3	villin 2 (ezrin) (VIL2)	1.78±0.42	4.02±1.28	0.44	0.179
	AL133626.1	H2A histone family, member J	1.66±0.12	1.81±0.22	0.91	0.560
	NM_002954.3	ribosomal protein S27a (RPS27A)	171.21±46.00	184.38±33.35	0.93	0.822
	NM_006951.2	TAF5 RNA polymerase II, TATA box binding protein (TBP)-associated factor	1.64±0.24	1.04±0.25	1.59	0.122
	NM_001190.1	branched chain aminotransferase precursor (BCATm)	1.32±0.42	1.40±0.64	0.94	0.922
Inflammation related genes	NM_002121.4	major histocompatibility complex, class II, DP beta 1 (HLA-DPB1)	70.94±8.30	3.49±1.96	20.31	0.000
	NM_006120.2	major histocompatibility complex, class II, DM alpha (HLA-DMA)	24.91±3.39	4.77±1.41	5.22	0.001
	NM_002121.4	major histocompatibility complex, class II, DP beta 1 (HLA-DPB1)	15.86±2.85	1.01±0.28	15.64	0.002
	NM_002127.3	HLA-G histocompatibility antigen, class I, G (HLA-G)	27.88±2.00	7.97±0.71	3.50	0.000
	NM_019111.2	major histocompatibility complex, class II, DR alpha (HLA-DRA)	153.26±18.42	15.67±4.81	9.78	0.000
	NM_033554.2	major histocompatibility complex, class II, DP alpha 1 (HLA-DPA1)	122.95±15.12	10.77±3.51	11.41	0.000
	X02902.1	mRNA for HLA class II DR-beta 1 (Dw14)	26.29±5.05	2.08±0.74	12.64	0.003
	NM_001565.1	chemokine (C-X-C motif) ligand 10 (CXCL10)	26.04±6.78	1.21±0.47	21.55	0.010
	NM_004887.3	chemokine (C-X-C motif) ligand 14 (CXCL14)	62.97±8.44	3.78±1.79	16.64	0.000
	NM_000609.3	chemokine (C-X-C motif) ligand 12 (stromal cell-derived factor 1) (CXCL12)	13.99±2.63	2.56±1.46	5.47	0.005
	NM_005409.3	chemokine (C-X-C motif) ligand 11 (CXCL11)	0.82±0.10	0.27±0.10	3.08	0.004
	NM_001250.3	tumor necrosis factor receptor superfamily, member 5 (TNFRSF5), transcript variant 1	8.00±1.16	1.57±0.69	5.08	0.001
	NM_000043.3	tumor necrosis factor receptor superfamily, member 6 (TNFRSF6), transcript variant 1	7.22±0.80	2.59±0.76	2.79	0.003
Fibrosis related genes	NM_000072.1	CD36 antigen (collagen type I receptor, thrombospondin receptor) (CD36)	16.55±3.10	2.87±1.63	5.76	0.004
	NM_005505.3	CD36 antigen (collagen type I receptor, thrombospondin receptor)-like 1 (CD36L1)	1.84±0.41	0.76±0.15	2.42	0.041
	NM_030582.2	collagen, type XVIII, alpha 1 (COL18A1), transcript variant 1	29.30±3.83	9.69±2.14	3.02	0.002
	NM_001853.2	collagen, type IX, alpha 3 (COL9A3)	6.00±1.94	1.15±0.66	5.20	0.049
	NM_004369.1	RNA for type VI collagen alpha3 chain	4.73±0.79	1.41±0.73	3.36	0.014
	X52022.1	RNA for type VI collagen alpha3 chain	1.10±0.10	0.28±0.17	3.95	0.011
	NM_001850.3	collagen, type VIII, alpha 1 (COL8A1), transcript variant 1	1.50±0.15	0.43±0.04	3.49	0.000
	NM_015719.2	collagen, type V, alpha 3 (COL5A3)	0.98±0.26	0.17±0.05	5.73	0.019

†The gene expression levels (sample mean ± standard error) shown were median normalized.
‡Fold difference of gene expression levels (sample mean) between NASH liver tissues and normal liver controls.
§Two tailed student t test.

the SuperSignal West Dura Extended Duration Substrate (Invitrogen) and recorded with an image reader LAS-1000 (Fujifilm).

Statistical Analysis

All analysis for statistically significant differences was performed with Student's t test with a two-tailed distribution. P values smaller than 0.05 were considered significant.

Results

The Integrity of the Microarray Datasets

To compare the global gene expression profiles between NASH livers and normal livers, total RNA samples from both populations (NASH, n = 7; NC, n = 4) were analyzed on CodeLink Human Whole Genome Bioarray. To ascertain the quality of RNA used in microarray analysis, similar datasets of breast cancer tissue generated with the same CodeLink platform were downloaded (GEO accession numbers: GSM144855 to GSM144858) and compared with the liver microarray datasets. As represented by the housekeeping genes listed in Table 3 (upper part), the majority of the genes showed similar expression levels among NASH livers, normal livers and breast cancer tissues. In contrast, drastically elevated expression was detected in liver tissues for the liver-specific genes including apolipoproteins, fatty acid binding protein, hepatic triglyceride lipase, glutathione S-transferase, and alcohol dehydrogenase (Table 3, lower part).

Elevated Expression of Inflammation and Fibrosis Related Genes in NASH Livers

The expression levels of genes involved in the process of inflammation and fibrosis were of immediate attention, as the activities of these genes would provide an ultimate evaluation of the quality of the datasets. Listed in Table 4, most of the chosen housekeeping genes showed similar transcription levels between NASH livers and normal controls (Table 4, upper panel). In contrast, significant differences were observed for many genes known to be involved in inflammation (Table 4, middle panel). These include several members of the HLAs, C-X-C motif containing chemokines and members of the TNF receptor superfamily.

The NASH patients included in this study all had certain degrees of fibrosis. It was therefore of great interest to see if the NASH microarray dataset could characterize the disease status. The abnormal deposition of collagen is a structural basis of liver fibrosis. From the datasets, it was noted that several types of collagen and collagen receptor exhibited elevated transcription activity in NASH livers (Table 4, lower panel). The activation of stellate cells from their resting state to myofibroblasts was also suggested by the elevated transcription for genes specific for smooth muscle functions (data not shown).

To confirm the observations made with the microarray technique, cDNA was synthesized from liver RNA and subjected to qRT-PCR analysis (NASH, n = 6; NC, n = 6) with gene specific primer pairs for GAPD and CXCL10 (Table 2). CXCL10 was chosen because it was the most highly activated inflammatory gene based on the microarray datasets. The real-time PCR result (Figure 1) indicated that the transcription level of CXCL10 in NASH liver was 21.86 times of that in normal healthy liver (P = 0.003), which is consistent with the microarray data (in which, NASH/normal = 21.55).

Overall, the elevated transcription of inflammation and fibrosis related genes validated both the NASH and normal control samples for further investigation on the gene expression patterns of NASH livers.

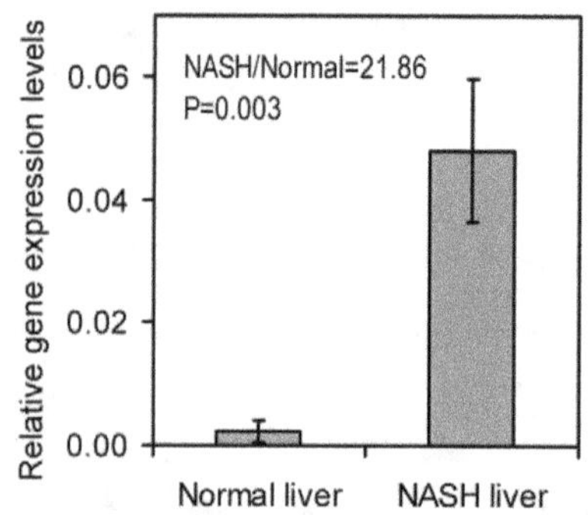

Figure 1. Quantitative RT-PCR analysis of CXCL10 in NASH livers and normal controls (NCs). Quantitative RT-PCR analysis were performed as described in Methods. CXCL10 and GAPD (housekeeping gene) specific primer pairs are specified in Table 2. The complementary DNAs prepared from NASH livers (n = 6) and NCs (n = 6) were analyzed in duplicate. CXCL10 expression level of each sample was normalized with that of GAPD. Sample means of the CXCL10 gene expression levels were plotted with error bars indicating the standard errors.

Elevated Expression of Genes Responsible for Alcohol Catabolism

When comparing the microarray datasets between NASH livers and normal livers, alcohol dehydrogenase 4 (ADH4) stands out as even more elevated than the inflammation related genes with an almost 40 fold increase in NASH livers (Table 5, upper panel). This observation prompted us to examine other genes in the ADH family. Of the 7 well established members of ADH family, ADH1A, ADH1B, ADH1C, ADH4, ADH5 and ADH6 showed significantly elevated transcription activity in NASH livers compared with normal livers (Table 5, upper panel). ADH7 also seemed to be highly elevated in NASH livers. However, the absolute signal for ADH7 gene transcription is low in both liver samples and the difference is statistically insignificant (P>0.05). This is consistent with the fact that ADH7 is usually expressed in stomach; less in liver [14].

Besides ADH, the liver has two additional enzymatic systems to remove alcohol: microsomal ethanol oxidizing system (MEOS) in endoplasmic reticulum and catalase in the peroxisomes. Significant elevation in gene transcription was observed for catalase and cytochrome P450 2E1 (CYP2E1), the major functional component of MEOS. Together with the augmented transcriptional activities of ADH genes, these results indicated a high demand for removing alcohols from the circulations of NASH patients.

The immediate products from the aforementioned alcohol oxidizing systems are aldehydes, which are more toxic than alcohol and therefore need to be removed immediately, usually by aldehyde dehydrogenases (ALDHs). The fact that there are many isoforms of ALDH encoded in human genome reflects the importance of these genes. Except ALDH3, 4, 6 and 9, all other isoforms of ALDH were found to be transcribed significantly higher in NASH livers compared to normal livers (Table 5, middle panel).

Since none of the patients had any history of alcohol consumption, these results were considered extraordinary and therefore real-time PCR was performed to confirm the microarray data. As ADH is the major mechanism for alcohol metabolism, several ADH genes were targeted. Again, with GAPD as internal reference, these ADH genes showed greater transcriptional activity

Table 5. Comparison of gene expressions between NASH livers and normal controls: alcohol metabolism and TLR4 related genes.†

Group	GenBank Accession#	Gene Description	NASH Liver (n = 7)	Normal Liver (n = 4)	NASH/ Normal‡	P value§
Alcohol oxidation related	NM_000667.2	alcohol dehydrogenase 1A (class I), alpha polypeptide (ADH1A)	470.96±40.68	82.50±34.30	5.71	0.000
	NM_000668.3	alcohol dehydrogenase IB (class I), beta polypeptide (ADH1B)	95.00±21.68	34.23±9.89	2.78	0.034
	NM_000669.2	alcohol dehydrogenase 1C (class I), gamma polypeptide (ADH1C)	76.58±16.72	18.75±5.60	4.08	0.013
	NM_000670.2	alcohol dehydrogenase 4 (class II), pi polypeptide (ADH4)	257.14±38.38	6.53±2.17	39.40	0.001
	NM_000671.2	alcohol dehydrogenase 5 (class III), chi polypeptide (ADH5)	10.95±1.97	2.71±1.16	4.04	0.006
	NM_000672.2	alcohol dehydrogenase 6 (class V) (ADH6)	36.68±5.09	3.56±1.14	10.30	0.000
	NM_000673.2	alcohol dehydrogenase 7 (class IV), mu or sigma polypeptide (ADH7)	0.34±0.08	0.01±0.11	26.96	0.053
	NM_000773.2	cytochrome P450, family 2, subfamily E, polypeptide 1 (CYP2E1)	423.85±42.84	194.97±50.22	2.17	0.010
	NM_001752.1	catalase (CAT)	12.27±2.16	0.97±0.39	12.70	0.002
Aldehyde oxidation related	NM_000689.3	aldehyde dehydrogenase 1 family, member A1 (ALDH1A1)	45.47±9.70	5.61±2.18	8.11	0.006
	NM_003888.2	aldehyde dehydrogenase 1 family, member A2 (ALDH1A2)	0.70±0.13	0.27±0.09	2.57	0.023
	NM_000692.3	aldehyde dehydrogenase 1 family, member B1 (ALDH1B1)	63.79±5.52	15.01±2.81	4.25	0.000
	NM_000690.2	aldehyde dehydrogenase 2 family (mitochondrial) (ALDH2)	4.47±1.07	0.71±0.24	6.30	0.012
	NM_000695.2	aldehyde dehydrogenase 3 family, member B2 (ALDH3B2)	0.37±0.10	0.24±0.09	1.55	0.354
	NM_003748.2	aldehyde dehydrogenase 4 family, member A1 (ALDH4A1)	25.86±3.87	16.25±2.08	1.59	0.058
	NM_001080.3	aldehyde dehydrogenase 5 family, member A1 (ALDH5A1)	3.79±0.41	1.31±0.45	2.89	0.004
	NM_000693.1	aldehyde dehydrogenase 6 mRNA, complete cds	0.49±0.12	0.33±0.08	1.48	0.280
	NM_000694.1	aldehyde dehydrogenase ALDH7	8.17±0.52	3.26±0.21	2.51	0.000
	NM_022568.2	aldehyde dehydrogenase 8 family, member A1 (ALDH8A1)	24.43±1.84	5.46±0.57	4.47	0.000
	NM_000696.2	aldehyde dehydrogenase 9 family, member A1 (ALDH9A1)	89.27±11.55	75.57±16.01	1.18	0.513
TLR4 related	NM_003266.2	toll-like receptor 4 (TLR4), transcript variant 3	1.34±0.12	0.99±0.08	1.35	0.034
	NM_000591.1	CD14 antigen (CD14)	17.47±5.34	14.85±6.85	1.18	0.772
	NM_004139.2	lipopolysaccharide binding protein (LBP)	66.88±11.71	167.76±15.77	0.40	0.002
	NM_015364.2	MD-2, lymphocyte antigen 96 (LY96)	5.21±0.97	4.24±2.77	1.23	0.758

†The gene expression levels (sample mean ± standard error) shown were median normalized.
‡Fold difference of gene expression levels (sample mean) between NASH liver tissues and normal liver controls.
§Two tailed student t test.

in NASH livers than in normal livers (Figure 2, A, B and C). In NASH livers, the ADH1C transcription was 12.5 times that of normal livers. For ADH4 and ADH6, it was 30.89 and 9.81 times, respectively. Note that these numbers showed a similar pattern given by microarray data, in which NASH/normal = 4.08 (ADH1C), 39.40 (ADH4), and 10.30 (ADH6). Significantly higher transcriptional activities of ALDH2 and ALDH8A1 were also observed by qRT-PCR in NASH livers compared to normal livers (Figure 2, D and E), confirming the previously described microarray data.

NASH Liver Did Not Exhibit Elevated Gene Transcription for TLR4 and Related Genes

Studies with rodent models suggested that TLR4 mediated pathway is elevated in NASH liver[15,16]. From our microarray data, the gene transcription of TLR4 was slightly elevated in NASH patients (NASH/normal = 1.35, $P<0.05$). Yet the transcription of TLR4 related genes CD14, LBP and MD-2 were not elevated (Table 5, lower panel). In fact, a significant decrease in LBP transcription was detected with these patients (NASH/normal = 0.4,

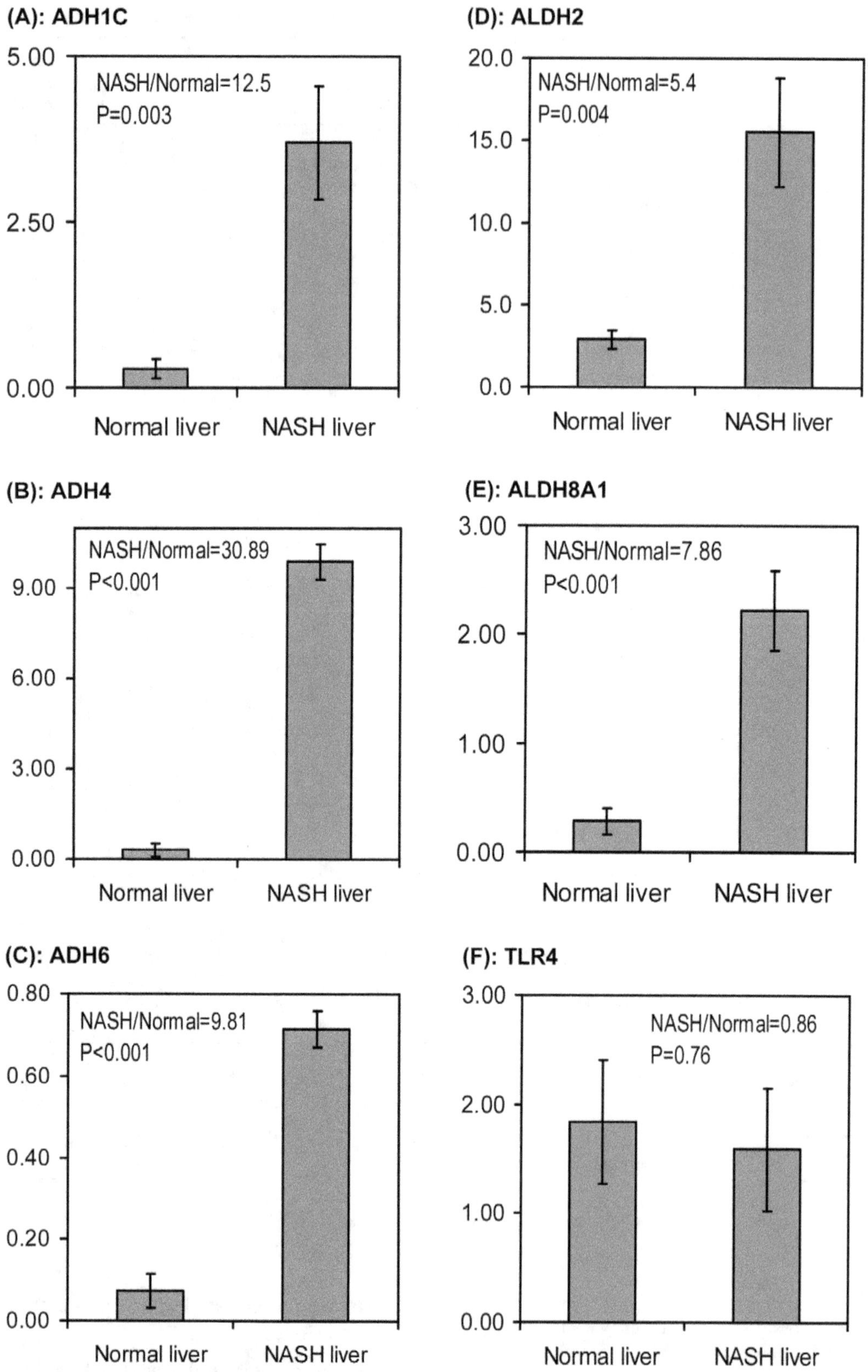

Figure 2. Quantitative RT-PCR analysis with NASH livers and NCs. Gene expression levels of (A) ADH1C, (B) ADH4, (C) ADH6, (D) ALDH2, (E) ALDH8A1 and (F) TLR4 were examined by qRT-PCR as described in Methods. The complementary DNAs prepared from NASH livers (n = 6) and NCs (n = 6) were analyzed in duplicate. PCR primer pairs are specified in Table 2. Gene expression levels of each sample were normalized with those of GAPD. Sample means were plotted with error bars indicating the standard errors.

P = 0.002). Real-time PCR analysis with an overlapping but different subgroup of NASH samples indicated that TLR4 gene transcription was not elevated in NASH livers (Figure 2F). Therefore, the small elevation in TLR4 gene transcription observed with microarray analysis may not be a universal phenomenon in NASH liver.

Elevated Protein Expression of ADH1 and ADH4 in NASH Livers

To examine the expression of ADH at protein level, Western blot analyses were performed with the lysates made from NASH liver biopsies (NASH, n = 9; Control, n = 4). As normal healthy liver tissue from adolescent is not available, non-NASH liver biopsies free from steatosis were used as controls. Blots were probed with antibodies specific for ADH1 and ADH4, respectively. Separate blot was also probed for β-actin as loading controls. While all samples had similar signals for actin, NASH patients exhibited higher expression of ADH1 and ADH4 (Figure 3A). Quantitation of the results with NIHimage software indicated that there were significant increases in ADH1 and ADH4 proteins in NASH livers: for ADH1, NASH/normal control = 2.8, $P<0.001$; for ADH4, NASH/normal control = 4.1, $P<0.001$ (Figure 3B).

Discussion

Liver Specific Genes, Inflammation and Fibrosis Related Genes

Gene transcription of NASH livers was examined by a whole genome DNA microarray and qRT-PCR techniques. Although the sample size in the microarray analysis (NASH, n = 7; NC, n = 4) is relatively small, convincing results were observed with a larger sample size (NASH, n = 6; NC, n = 6) in qRT-PCR analysis. The similar gene expression patterns detected by both techniques testify to the reliability of the techniques and the results. We acknowledge that the clinical information of the normal liver RNA purchased from Admet is limited. However, we are confident that these samples are appropriate to serve as controls, not only because Admet guaranteed that these samples were derived from normal healthy livers intended for transplantation, but also for the following reasons: 1) each of the normal controls had a moderate BMI, therefore they were not likely to have NASH (Table 1); 2) comparison with similar gene transcription datasets of human breast cancer showed that both the normal control RNA and NASH RNA exhibited similar good quality, that is, liver specific genes were highly expressed in both groups of liver tissue (Table 3);

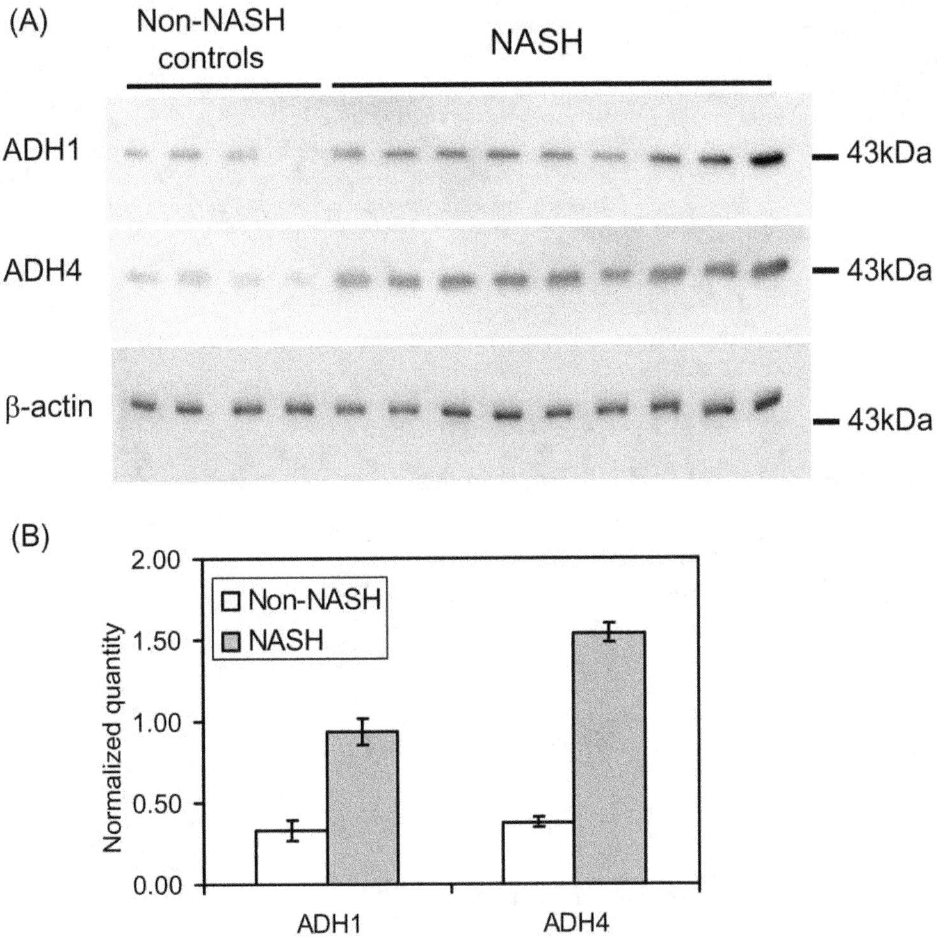

Figure 3. Elevated expression of ADH1 and ADH4 proteins in NASH livers. (A) Western blot analyses were performed with lysates prepared from NASH livers and NCs. The NCs were of normal BMI and free from steatosis. Separate blots were probed for ADH1, ADH4 and β-actin as these proteins all migrate at about 43 kDa. While similar signals for actin were detected for all samples, the NASH livers exhibited stronger signals for both ADH1 and ADH4. (B) The Western blot results were quantitated with NIHimage software. The normalized quantities of the ADH1 and ADH4 signals were the densities of the ADH bands divided by that of the β-actin bands, respectively. The mean values for NASH and NC were plotted with error bars representing the standard errors of the means.

and 3) these normal liver samples showed lower transcription of inflammation and fibrosis related genes as compared to NASH liver samples, in the context of similar gene transcription for housekeeping genes between these two groups (Table 4 and Figure 1).

Genes Responsible for Alcohol Catabolism

Alcohol is promptly removed from circulation via three cellular mechanisms mainly found in liver: alcohol dehydrogenases in the cytosol; MEOS (with cytochrome P450 2E1 as the major component) in endoplasmic reticulum and catalase in peroxisomes. All known ADH genes except ADH7, together with cytochrome P450 2E1 and catalase genes, showed elevated transcription in NASH livers. The different behavior of ADH7 from other alcohol oxidizing enzymes is predicted by the fact that ADH7 is not a liver enzyme [17]. The elevated expression for ADH1 and ADH4 at protein level were also observed in NASH livers (NASH, n = 9; NC, n = 4), consistent with the elevated mRNA levels for these genes. The significant elevation of the activity of these enzymes indicated that 1), alcohol concentration was elevated in the circulation and 2), it is a high priority for NASH patients to remove alcohol from the circulation.

All our adolescent patients claimed that they were not regular drinkers of alcoholic beverages. We also were assured by their parents that these adolescent patients had no access to alcoholic beverages. Even, in the event that some of our patients did ingest alcohol, it was certainly not consistent long-term alcohol use. In considering other possible sources of alcohol (aspartame, fruit), we also did a three day food record before any biopsy was performed. We found no significant sources for alcohol.

Where did the alcohol come from? For people who do not have access to alcoholic beverages, circulating alcohol mainly comes from diet and intestinal bacteria. For instance, the concentration of methanol in the human body could increase by an order of magnitude after consumption of fruit [18]. Alcohol production by intestinal bacteria was observed long ago in rodents and humans [19,20]. Studies with obese ob/ob mice indicated that intestinal bacteria are the largest source of circulating alcohol in obese animals [10]. When intestinal bacterial growth was inhibited with neomycin, a 50% decrease of circulating alcohol was observed in obese mice. Based on this observation, Diehl and her colleagues hypothesized that intestinal production of alcohol may contribute to the genesis of non-alcoholic liver diseases [10]. Coincidently, our microarray data provided molecular biological evidence in support of this hypothesis. To pursue this avenue, the immediate future directions are 1) to examine the enzymatic activities of the enzymes related to alcohol catabolism, and 2) to measure the concentrations of circulating alcohol in NASH patients and healthy subjects. If these studies come to the same conclusion as the mRNA data suggest, oral antibiotics, lactobacillus or other means of altering colonic bacteria might be a treatment for NASH.

Our results are also consistent with two interesting discoveries. First, it was observed that cytochrome P450 2E1 is ethanol inducible, with a 4–10 fold increase in liver biopsies of recently drinking subjects [21]. Second, increased P450 2E1 was detected in NASH patients [22].

Alcohol and Steatosis

The pathomechanisms of alcohol in liver disease have been intensively studied in alcoholic liver disease. It has long been observed that ethanol stimulates hepatic fatty acid synthesis [23].

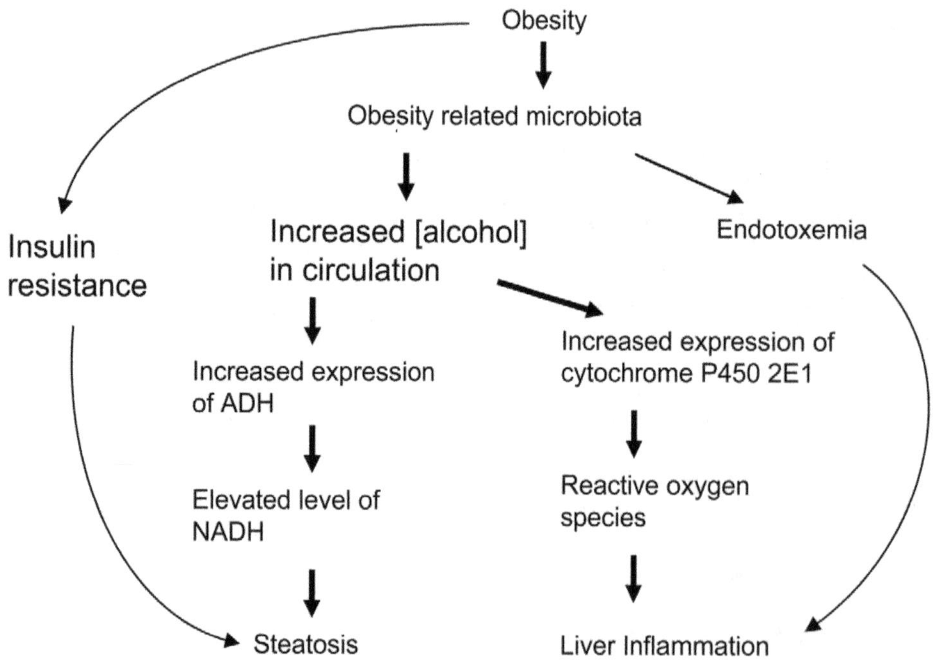

Figure 4. The alcohol hypothesis of non-alcoholic liver diseases. Non-alcoholic fatty liver diseases are commonly associated with obesity. In addition to the well-known mechanisms that obesity leads to steatosis via insulin resistance, and obesity related bacteria facilitate liver inflammation, the gene transcription data reported here support a central role for alcohol in the pathogenesis of NAFLD. Overgrowth of alcohol-producing bacteria in the intestine of obese patients likely causes increased alcohol in the circulation, which in turn induced the expression of genes for alcohol catabolism, including ADH and cytochrome P450 2E1. The increased activity of ADH results in the elevated level of NADH, which favors fatty acid synthesis and opposes its break down, leading to steatosis; the elevated P450 2E1 could generate excessive ROS, a known cause for liver inflammation.

The oxidation of alcohol to aldehyde by ADH concomitantly reduces NAD to NADH. The increased NADH promotes fatty acid synthesis and opposes lipid catabolism, leading to fat accumulation in hepatocytes [23,24]. Elevated ADH level as suggested by our microarray data strengthens the connection between alcohol metabolism and steatosis.

Alcohol and Liver Inflammation

One possible mechanism for alcohol induced liver inflammation begins with mucosal injury in the upper gastrointestinal tract induced by alcohol. This leads to increased permeability for macromolecules like LPS endotoxin. The resulting endotoxemia would then activate TLR4 mediated signaling and culminate in the release of pro-inflammatory cytokines (reviewed in [25]). If the intestinal bacteria could cause elevated production of alcohol, it is conceivable that the NASH patients may suffer from endotoxemia. However, for all the TLR4 related genes examined (TLR4, LBP, CD14, and MD-2), the microarray and real-time PCR analysis did not show significant activation at the mRNA level in NASH patients. Although more convincing conclusion awaits studies of TLR4 signaling at the protein level in NASH patients, our data suggest an emphasis on direct toxicity of alcohol per se.

Szabo and her colleagues reported that alcohol directly suppressed the NF-κB activity in monocytes [26]. Their results are in concert with a previous report that ethanol suppressed TNF activity [27]. However, McClain's group reported the opposite. They found that peripheral blood monocytes from patients who had alcoholic hepatitis have spontaneous TNF production and enhanced LPS-stimulated TNF production [28]. Their finding was confirmed with an in vivo experiment using rats chronically fed alcohol [29]. Work in Nagy's lab further revealed that ERK1/2 and Egr-1 are important mediators in elevated TNF-α production after chronic ethanol exposure [30,31]. The reality of the ethanol effect on TNF-α production was made clear by Kolls' group. In a time-series alcohol experiment, they demonstrated that acute ethanol exposure suppressed TNF production, while long-term treatment significantly up-regulated TNF production [32]. More importantly, the increase in TNF production was associated with increased generation of reactive oxygen species (ROS).

Therefore, ROS could be the important mediator between alcohol and TNF. Alcohol is known to induce cytochrome P450, mainly CYP2E1 [33]. Metabolism by CYP2E1 generates superoxide and other free radicals collectively known as ROS. There are two possible mechanisms for ROS to induce TNF production. Firstly, ROS could serve as signaling molecules to activate NF-κB, leading to elevated transcription of TNF-α [34]; Secondly, ROS could activate TNF-α converting enzyme, the enzyme responsible for the processing of the transmembrane TNF-α precursor [35].

In summary, the gene expression studies of NASH livers revealed elevated transcription of enzymes in ALL the alcohol metabolism pathways: ADH pathway, catalase pathway and the MEOS pathway. Elevated expression of ADH1 and ADH4 at protein level were also observed in NASH livers. These results support a central role for alcohol in the development of NASH in obese patients, as summarized in Figure 4 and for the first time, provide molecular evidence in support of Diehl et al.'s hypothesis that alcohol is an important mediator for the development of non-alcoholic fatty liver diseases [10]. Our findings suggest a mechanism that offers a single explanation for the similar histological findings in alcoholic liver disease and NASH [3]. Our findings might provide a basis for studies on the prevention and treatment of NASH.

Acknowledgments

The authors thank Chaoyan Liu, Cuiling Shu and Gian Visentin for their excellent technical assistance in RNA preparation and primer design for real-time quantitative PCR.

Author Contributions

Conceived and designed the experiments: SSB RDB LZ. Performed the experiments: SSB RDB WL NN LZ. Analyzed the data: SSB RDB WL NN LZ. Wrote the paper: SSB RDB WL NN LZ.

References

1. Ludwig J, Viggiano TR, McGill DB, Oh BJ (1980) Nonalcoholic steatohepatitis: Mayo Clinic experiences with a hitherto unnamed disease. Mayo Clin Proc 55: 434–438.
2. Browning JD, Szczepaniak LS, Dobbins R, Nuremberg P, Horton JD, et al. (2004) Prevalence of hepatic steatosis in an urban population in the United States: impact of ethnicity. Hepatology 40: 1387–1395.
3. Day CP, James OF (1998) Steatohepatitis: a tale of two "hits"? Gastroenterology 114: 842–845.
4. Sanyal AJ, Campbell-Sargent C, Mirshahi F, Rizzo WB, Contos MJ, et al. (2001) Nonalcoholic steatohepatitis: association of insulin resistance and mitochondrial abnormalities. Gastroenterology 120: 1183–1192.
5. Donnelly KL, Smith CI, Schwarzenberg SJ, Jessurun J, Boldt MD, et al. (2005) Sources of fatty acids stored in liver and secreted via lipoproteins in patients with nonalcoholic fatty liver disease. J Clin Invest 115: 1343–1351.
6. Gervois P, Fruchart JC, Staels B (2007) Drug Insight: mechanisms of action and therapeutic applications for agonists of peroxisome proliferator-activated receptors. Nat Clin Pract Endocrinol Metab 3: 145–156.
7. Begriche K, Igoudjil A, Pessayre D, Fromenty B (2006) Mitochondrial dysfunction in NASH: causes, consequences and possible means to prevent it. Mitochondrion 6: 1–28.
8. Parola M, Robino G (2001) Oxidative stress-related molecules and liver fibrosis. J Hepatol 35: 297–306.
9. Diehl AM, Goodman Z, Ishak KG (1988) Alcohollike liver disease in nonalcoholics. A clinical and histologic comparison with alcohol-induced liver injury. Gastroenterology 95: 1056–1062.
10. Cope K, Risby T, Diehl AM (2000) Increased gastrointestinal ethanol production in obese mice: implications for fatty liver disease pathogenesis. Gastroenterology 119: 1340–1347.
11. Matthews DR, Hosker JP, Rudenski AS, Naylor BA, Treacher DF, et al. (1985) Homeostasis model assessment: insulin resistance and beta-cell function from fasting plasma glucose and insulin concentrations in man. Diabetologia 28: 412–419.
12. Kleiner DE, Brunt EM, Van Natta M, Behling C, Contos MJ, et al. (2005) Design and validation of a histological scoring system for nonalcoholic fatty liver disease. Hepatology 41: 1313–1321.
13. Rozen S, Skaletsky H (2000) Primer3 on the WWW for general users and for biologist programmers. Methods Mol Biol 132: 365–386.
14. Yokoyama S, Matsuo Y, Ramsbotham R, Yokoyama R (1994) Molecular characterization of a class IV human alcohol dehydrogenase gene (ADH7). FEBS Lett 351: 411–415.
15. Szabo G, Velayudham A, Romics L, Jr., Mandrekar P (2005) Modulation of non-alcoholic steatohepatitis by pattern recognition receptors in mice: the role of toll-like receptors 2 and 4. Alcohol Clin Exp Res 29: 140S–145S.
16. Kawaratani H, Tsujimoto T, Kitazawa T, Kitade M, Yoshiji H, et al. (2008) Innate immune reactivity of the liver in rats fed a choline-deficient L-amino-acid-defined diet. World J Gastroenterol 14: 6655–6661.
17. Yokoyama H, Baraona E, Lieber CS (1994) Molecular cloning of human class IV alcohol dehydrogenase cDNA. Biochem Biophys Res Commun 203: 219–224.
18. Lindinger W, Taucher J, Jordan A, Hansel A, Vogel W (1997) Endogenous production of methanol after the consumption of fruit. Alcohol Clin Exp Res 21: 939–943.
19. Baraona E, Julkunen R, Tannenbaum L, Lieber CS (1986) Role of intestinal bacterial overgrowth in ethanol production and metabolism in rats. Gastroenterology 90: 103–110.
20. Nosova T, Jokelainen K, Kaihovaara P, Jousimies-Somer H, Siitonen A, et al. (1996) Aldehyde dehydrogenase activity and acetate production by aerobic bacteria representing the normal flora of human large intestine. Alcohol Alcohol 31: 555–564.
21. Tsutsumi M, Lasker JM, Shimizu M, Rosman AS, Lieber CS (1989) The intralobular distribution of ethanol-inducible P450IIE1 in rat and human liver. Hepatology 10: 437–446.

22. Weltman MD, Farrell GC, Hall P, Ingelman-Sundberg M, Liddle C (1998) Hepatic cytochrome P450 2E1 is increased in patients with nonalcoholic steatohepatitis. Hepatology 27: 128–133.
23. Lieber CS, Schmid R (1961) The effect of ethanol on fatty acid metabolism; stimulation of hepatic fatty acid synthesis in vitro. J Clin Invest 40: 394–399.
24. Galli A, Price D, Crabb D (1999) High-level expression of rat class I alcohol dehydrogenase is sufficient for ethanol-induced fat accumulation in transduced HeLa cells. Hepatology 29: 1164–1170.
25. Bode C, Bode JC (2005) Activation of the innate immune system and alcoholic liver disease: effects of ethanol per se or enhanced intestinal translocation of bacterial toxins induced by ethanol? Alcohol Clin Exp Res 29: 166S–171S.
26. Mandrekar P, Catalano D, Szabo G (1999) Inhibition of lipopolysaccharide-mediated NFkappaB activation by ethanol in human monocytes. Int Immunol 11: 1781–1790.
27. Nelson S, Bagby G, Summer WR (1989) Alcohol suppresses lipopolysaccharide-induced tumor necrosis factor activity in serum and lung. Life Sci 44: 673–676.
28. McClain CJ, Cohen DA (1989) Increased tumor necrosis factor production by monocytes in alcoholic hepatitis. Hepatology 9: 349–351.
29. Honchel R, Ray MB, Marsano L, Cohen D, Lee E, et al. (1992) Tumor necrosis factor in alcohol enhanced endotoxin liver injury. Alcohol Clin Exp Res 16: 665–669.
30. Kishore R, Hill JR, McMullen MR, Frenkel J, Nagy LE (2002) ERK1/2 and Egr-1 contribute to increased TNF-alpha production in rat Kupffer cells after chronic ethanol feeding. Am J Physiol Gastrointest Liver Physiol 282: G6–15.
31. Shi L, Kishore R, McMullen MR, Nagy LE (2002) Chronic ethanol increases lipopolysaccharide-stimulated Egr-1 expression in RAW 264.7 macrophages: contribution to enhanced tumor necrosis factor alpha production. J Biol Chem 277: 14777–14785.
32. Zhang Z, Bagby GJ, Stoltz D, Oliver P, Schwarzenberger PO, et al. (2001) Prolonged ethanol treatment enhances lipopolysaccharide/phorbol myristate acetate-induced tumor necrosis factor-alpha production in human monocytic cells. Alcohol Clin Exp Res 25: 444–449.
33. Lieber CS (1999) Microsomal ethanol-oxidizing system (MEOS): the first 30 years (1968–1998)–a review. Alcohol Clin Exp Res 23: 991–1007.
34. Schreck R, Rieber P, Baeuerle PA (1991) Reactive oxygen intermediates as apparently widely used messengers in the activation of the NF-kappa B transcription factor and HIV-1. EMBO J 10: 2247–2258.
35. Zhang Z, Kolls JK, Oliver P, Good D, Schwarzenberger PO, et al. (2000) Activation of tumor necrosis factor-alpha-converting enzyme-mediated ectodomain shedding by nitric oxide. J Biol Chem 275: 15839–15844.

7

Interference with Oligomerization and Glycosaminoglycan Binding of the Chemokine CCL5 Improves Experimental Liver Injury

Andreas Nellen[1], Daniel Heinrichs[1], Marie-Luise Berres[1], Hacer Sahin[1], Petra Schmitz[1], Amanda E. Proudfoot[2], Christian Trautwein[1], Hermann E. Wasmuth[1]*

1 Medical Department III, University Hospital Aachen, Aachen, Germany, **2** Merck Serono, Geneva Research Centre, Geneva, Switzerland

Abstract

Background: The chemokine CCL5 is involved in the recruitment of immune cells and a subsequent activation of hepatic stellate cells (HSC) after liver injury. We here investigate whether inhibition of CCL5 oligomerization and glycosaminoglycan binding by a mutated CCL5 protein (^{44}AANA^{47}-CCL5) has the potential to ameliorate liver cell injury and fibrosis in vivo.

Methodology: Liver injury was induced in C57BL/6 mice by intraperitoneal injection of carbon tetrachloride (CCl_4) in an acute and a chronic liver injury model. Simultaneously, mice received either ^{44}AANA^{47}-CCL5 or vehicle. Liver cell necrosis and fibrosis was analyzed by histology, and measurement of serum transaminases and hydroxyproline. Intrahepatic mRNA expression of fibrosis and inflammation related genes were determined by quantitative RT-PCR and infiltration of immune cells was assessed by FACS analysis and immunocytochemistry. In vitro, HSC were stimulated with conditioned media of T-cell enriched splenocytes.

Principal Findings: ^{44}AANA^{47}-CCL5 treated mice displayed a significantly reduced degree of acute liver injury (liver cell necrosis, transaminases) and fibrosis (Sirus red positive area and hydroxyproline content) compared to vehicle treated mice. Ameliorated fibrosis by ^{44}AANA^{47}-CCL5 was associated with a decreased expression of fibrosis related genes, decreased α-smoth muscle antigen (αSMA) and a reduction of infiltrating immune cells. In the acute model, ^{44}AANA^{47}-CCL5 treated mice displayed a reduced immune cell infiltration and mRNA levels of TNF, IL-1 and CCL3 compared to vehicle treated mice. In vitro, conditioned medium of T-cell enriched splenocytes of ^{44}AANA^{47}-CCL5 treated mice inhibited the chemotaxis and proliferation of HSC.

Conclusions: The results provide evidence that inhibition of oligomerization and glycosaminoglycan binding of the chemokine CCL5 is a new therapeutic strategy for the treatment of acute and chronic liver injuries and represents an alternative to chemokine receptor antagonism.

Editor: Wing-Kin Syn, Institute of Hepatology London, United Kingdom

Funding: The study was supported by grants from the Deutsche Forschungsgemeinschaft (SFB-TRR57, WA2557/2-1) and the Else Kröner-Freseniusstiftung to HEW. The funders had no role in study design, data collection and analysis, decision to publish, or preparation of the manuscript.

Competing Interests: AEP is an employee of Merck Serono.

* E-mail: hwasmuth@ukaachen.de

Introduction

Acute and chronic liver diseases are a major cause of morbidity and mortality worldwide. In most diseases an inflammatory response within the liver is a mainstay of tissue damage [1]. After acute injury, an overwhelming immune response can lead to massive hepatocyte damage and subsequent liver failure [2]. On the other hand a continuous, low-level inflammation is a central pathophysiological aspect of liver fibrogenesis which ultimately leads to the development of liver cirrhosis in a significant number of cases [3]. Therefore, elucidation of pivotal inflammatory pathways in liver disease models might of great clinical interest as interference with these pathways bears the potential for new therapeutic options in diverse acute and chronic liver diseases.

The inflammatory infiltrate within the damaged liver consists of different immune cells subsets, including macrophages, dendritic cells, T cells, NK cells, NKT-cells and B-cells. Most of these cells are recruited into the liver along a chemotactic gradient. Classical chemoattractant molecules are chemokines, which are long known to govern the directed migration of leukocytes to sites of inflammation. In recent years, an important role of chemokines has also been deciphered in liver diseases [4]. Chemokines bind with high affinity to classical G-protein coupled receptors on the cell membrane of target cells and with lower affinity to glycosaminoglycans (GAG) of the extracellular matrix and endothelial cell surfaces [5]. Interaction of chemokines with GAG appears to be essential for the *in vivo* activity of certain chemokines and is considered as a prerequisite for establishing a chemotactic gradient across endothelial barriers [6]. Another

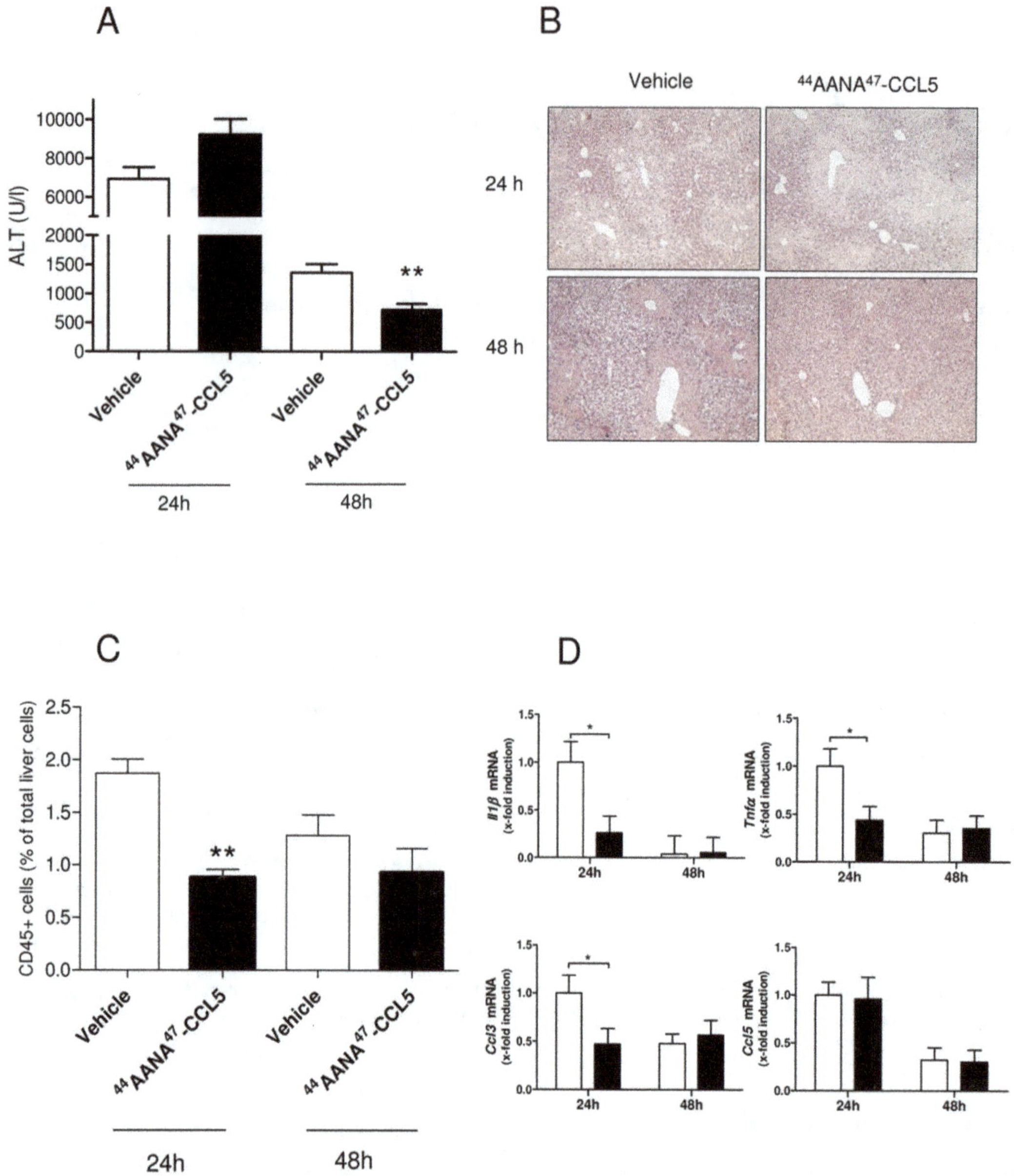

Figure 1. In vivo effects of treatment with [[44]AANA[47]]-CCL5 on acute liver cell injury. (**A**) Mice treated with [[44]AANA[47]]-CCL5 have reduced serum transaminases 48 hours after CCl_4 application compared to vehicle treated mice. (**B**) Reduced liver cell damage is also evidenced by reduced necrotic areas 48 h hours after injury (HE staining, ×100). (**C**) The ameliorated damage after 48 h in [[44]AANA[47]]-CCL5 treated mice is preceded by a significantly reduced infiltration of CD45+ immune cells. (**D**) Reduced inflammatory liver damage in [[44]AANA[47]]-CCL5 is also associated with significantly repressed pro-inflammatory mRNA expression (black bars: [[44]AANA[47]]-CCL5, open bars: vehicle). * $P<0.05$, ** $P<0.01$.

biochemical characteristic of chemokines is their ability to form higher order oligomers what appears to be essential for their GAG binding and chemotactic activity *in vivo* [7].

CCL5 (traditional name: regulated upon activation, normally T cell expressed and secreted, RANTES) belongs to the CC family of inflammatory chemokines and is expressed by many liver resident and infiltrating cells [8]. In humans, CCL5 expression is up-regulated in acute and chronic liver damage [9,10,11] and functional *Ccl5* gene variants have been associated with inflammatory liver damage [12,13] and treatment response [14]. Notably, in murine models of experimental fibrosis, CCL5 and its receptors CCR1 and CCR5 have been shown to be essential for fibrosis progression [9,15]. Furthermore, antagonism of the CCL5 receptors with Met-CCL5 ameliorated liver fibrosis and accelerated the regression of scar formation in vivo [9]. Thus, this particular chemokine might be an attractive candidate for anti-inflammatory or anti-fibrotic therapies of liver diseases. However, chemokine receptor antagonism bears the potential for numerous unwanted side effects [16]. Therefore, other therapeutic strategies of chemokine antagonism should be systematically investigated.

Based on this background, we here investigate a novel therapeutic approach to interfere with the chemokine CCL5 in experimental liver damage models. We show that administration of the CCL5 mutant [44][AANA][47]-CCL5, which loses the ability to oligomerise, but forms inactive heterodimers with wild-type CCL5

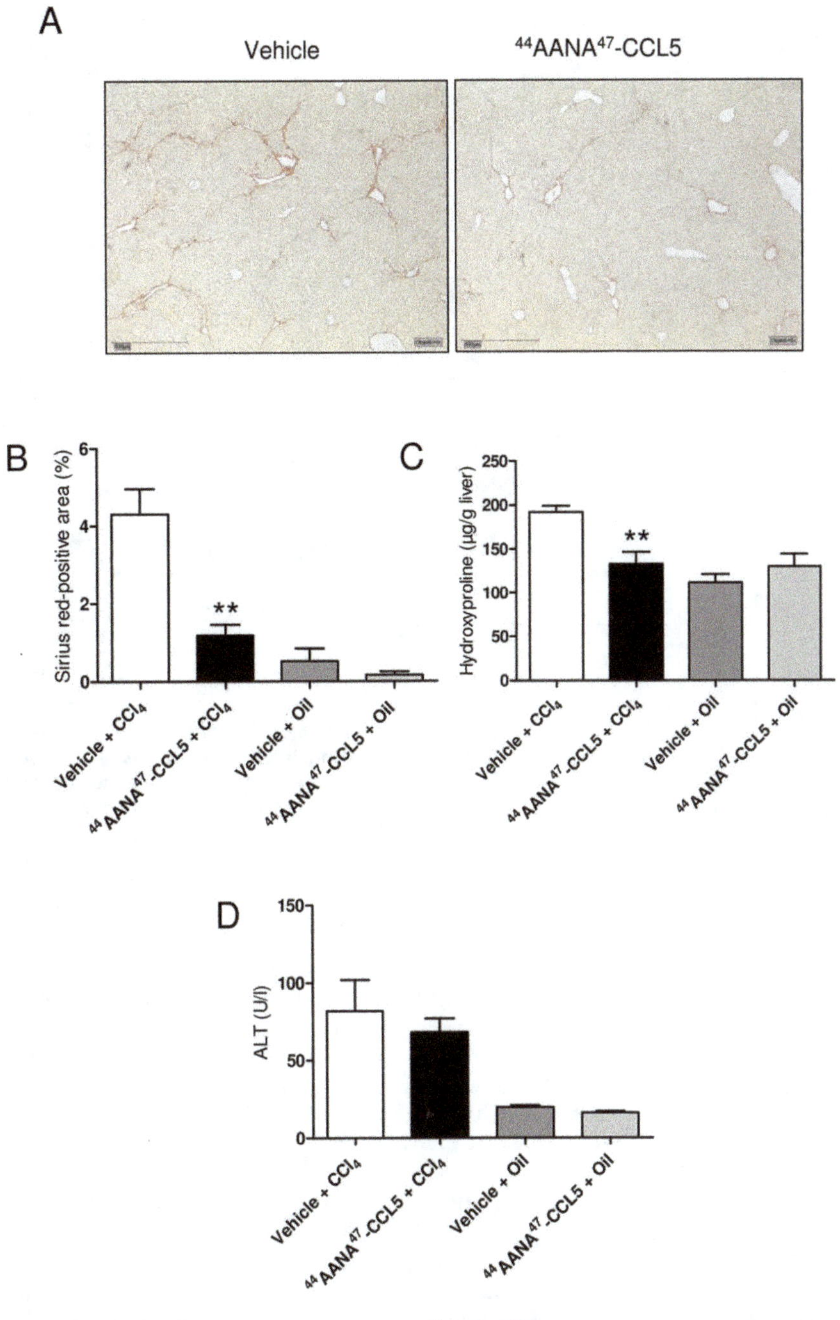

Figure 2. In vivo effects of treatment with [44AANA47]-CCL5 on chronic liver injury. (**A**) Treatment of mice with [44AANA47]-CCL5 in parallel to chronic CCl_4 intoxication reduced scar formation in the liver compared to vehicle (representative Sirius red stainings, ×100). Ameliorated liver fibrosis in [44AANA47]-CCL5 treated mice is quantified by a reduced Sirius red positive area (**B**) and a decreased hepatic concentration of the collagen specific amino acid hydroxyproline (**C**). ALT levels were not significantly changed in [44AANA47]-CCL5 treated mice compared to vehicle treated mice when taken 72 h after the last CCl_4 injection (**D**). ** $P<0.01$.

and loses 80% of its capacity to bind to GAG [17], strongly reduces acute liver injury and tissue fibrosis *in vivo*.

Materials and Methods

Murine *in vivo* experiments

Male wild-type (WT) mice on the C57BL/6 background (purchased from Charles River Laboratories) were subjected at the age of 8 weeks to two different liver damage models. In the first model, WT mice received a single intraperitoneal (i.p.) injection of carbon tetrachloride (CCl_4, 0.8 mg/kg bodyweight) to induce acute liver injury. Animals were treated with the CCL5 antagonist [44AANA47]-CCL5 [17] or vehicle (PBS) i.p. before as well as 12 and 24 hours after liver damage. Mice were sacrificed 24 or 48 hours (n = 6/group) after the CCl_4 administration for further analysis. In the second model, mice received repeated i.p. injections CCl_4 for 6 weeks (0.6 mg/kg bodyweight in 1:1 mineral oil, twice weekly) to induce liver fibrosis. Mice were sacrificed three days after the last CCl_4 injection when the peek of fibrosis is expected [9]. [44AANA47]-CCL5 (10 µg daily) or vehicle (PBS,

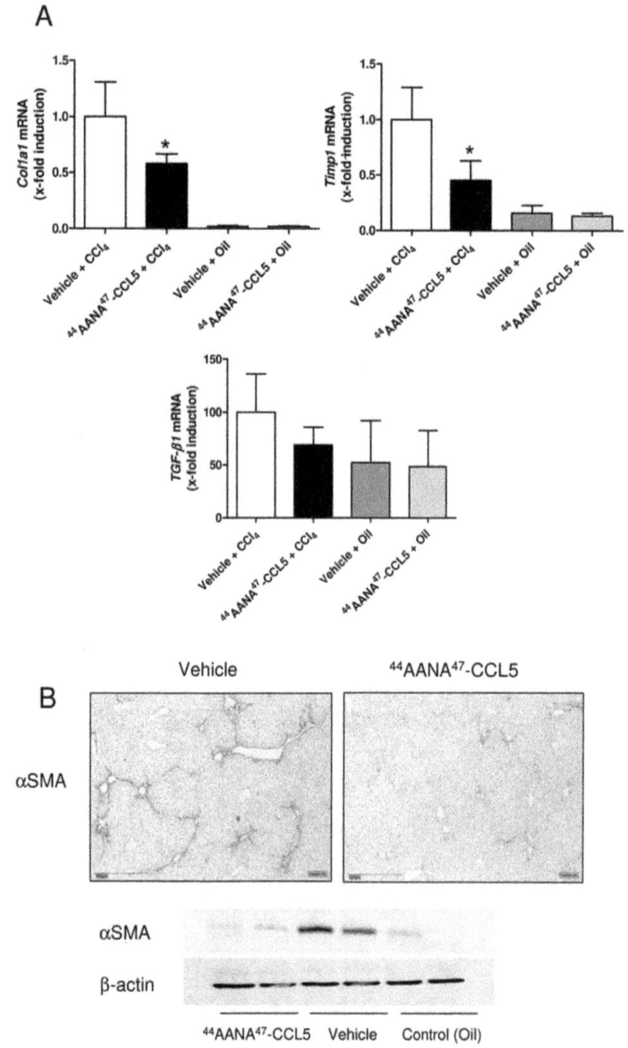

Figure 3. Treatment with [44AANA47]-CCL5 is associated with reduced stellate cell activation. (**A**) Mice treated with [44AANA47]-CCL5 concomitantly to CCl4 display repressed mRNA expressions of the pivotal stellate cell genes *Col1a1* and *Timp1* compared to vehicle treated animals, while the mRNA of Tgf-β showed only a trend to lower expression. (**B**) Reduced activation of stellate cells in [44AANA47]-CCL5 treated mice is further evidenced by decreased protein expression of the stellate cell activation marker αSMA by immunohistochemistry (upper panels) and western bot of total liver extracts (lower panel). * $P<0.05$.

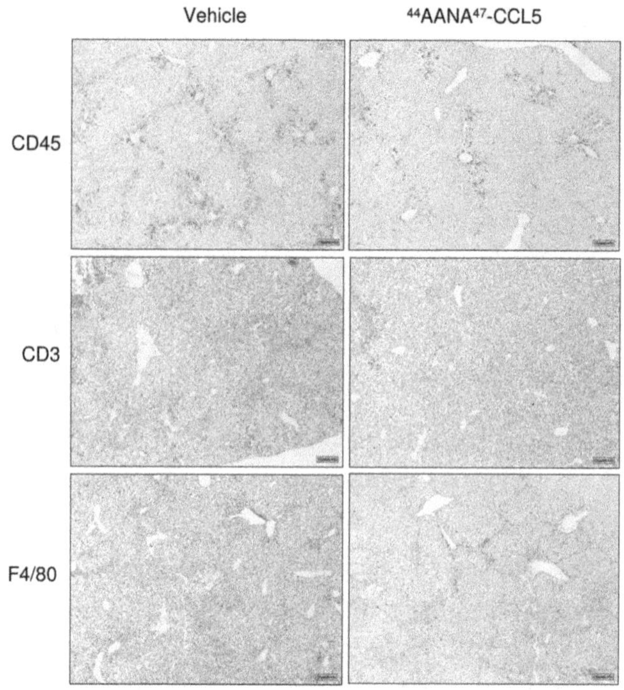

Figure 4. Treatment with [44AANA47]-CCL5 leads to altered immune cell infiltration during liver fibrogenesis. The photomicrographs show representative liver sections of mice treated with [44AANA47]-CCL5 or vehicle after staining for CD45 (total leukocytes), CD3 (T-cells) and macrophages (F4/80). Magnification ×100.

n = 12/group) were administered i.p. concomitantly to CCl_4. In all mice, serum samples were obtained via cardiac puncture and livers were harvested for histological and biochemical analysis.

All animals were housed under specific-pathogen-free conditions in the animal facility of the RWTH University hospital Aachen. The experiments were carried out after approval by the animal welfare board at the Bezirksregierung Cologne, Germany (permit number 50.203.2-AC 5a, 51/06).

Histological and biochemical evaluation of liver damage

Liver fibrosis was assessed histologically by quantification of the Sirius-red positive area on 10 low power (40×) fields/slide by use of the NIH software Image J, which is available from http://rsbweb.nih.gov/. Hepatic collagen content was analyzed biochemically by photometric measurement of the collagen specific amino acid hydroxyproline as recently described [9]. The intrahepatic expression of α-smooth muscle antigen (α-SMA) was assessed histologically with a mouse anti-SMA (Clone1A4, Dako) antibody. Immunohistochemical stainings for immune cell infiltration were performed in cooperation with the Institute of Pathology of University Hospital Bonn, Germany. The following antibodies were used: CD45, rat Clone30-F11 (BD Sciences); CD3, rabbit Clone SP7 (LabVision); F4/80, rat Clone BM8 (Dianova).

Hepatic immune cell isolation and flow cytometry analysis

Single-cell suspensions were isolated from freshly harvested livers using mechanical and enzymatic digestion. Viable white blood cells were purified from the suspension by centrifugation for 20 min at 800× g with a density gradient separation medium (Lymphocyte, PAA Laboratories). PBMCs were collected from the gradient/supernatant interface and then washed in Hank's balanced salt solution (PAA Laboratories) supplemented with 1% bovine serum albumin and 2 mM ethylene diamine tetraacetic acid (EDTA). For flow cytometry analysis, cells were stained with fluorochrome-conjugated antibodies for CD3, CD4, CD8, CD45 and NK1.1 (all antibodies from Bioscience) and the relative numbers were quantified using the FACSCanto II (Becton Dickinson). Data were analyzed using FlowJo software (Tree Star).

α-SMA Western blot

Snap-frozen liver samples were homogenised in 1 ml RIPA buffer (20 mM Tris-HCl, 150 mM NaCl, 2% Nonidet P40, 0.1% SDS, 0.5% Na-deoxycholate) with proteinase inhibitor (Mini Complete Protease Inhibitor Cocktail Tablets, Roche Applied

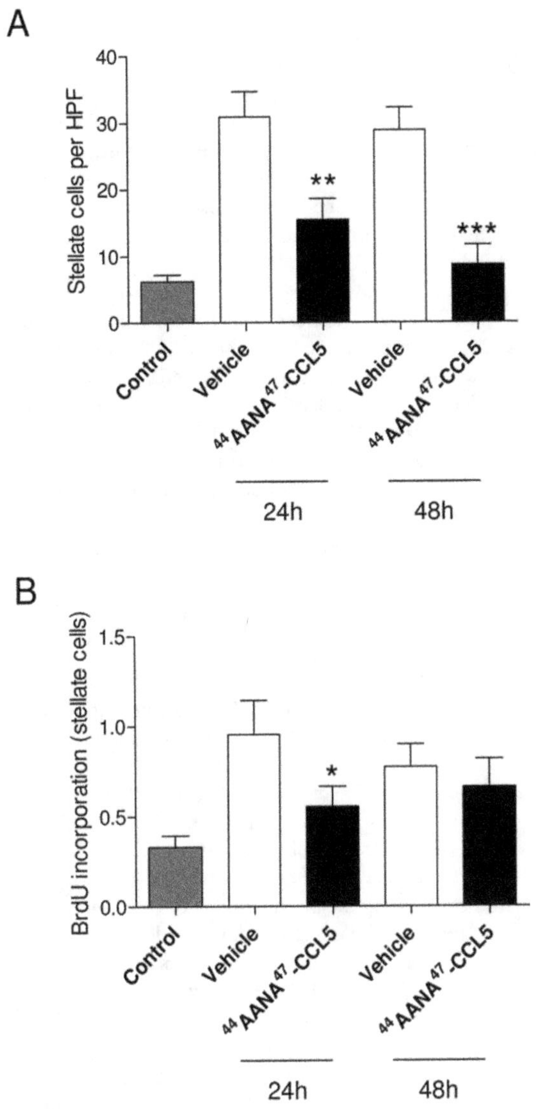

Figure 5. Treatment with [^{44}AANA^{47}]-CCL5 leads to qualitative changes in splenocytes. (**A**) Splenocytes were isolated from [^{44}AANA^{47}]-CCL5 and vehicle treated mice and conditioned mediate of splenocyte cultures were assessed for stellate cells migration in a Boyden chamber. Conditioned medium of splenocytes isolated from [^{44}AANA^{47}]-CCL5 treated mice (24 and 48 h after CCl_4 application) was significantly less effective in inducing stellate cell migration compared to splenocytes isolated from vehicle treated mice. (**B**) Conditioned medium from mice treated [^{44}AANA^{47}]-CCL5 was also less effective in inducing stellate cell proliferation as assessed by BrdU incorporation. * $P<0.05$, ** $P<0.01$.

Science) for isolation of total protein. Western blotting of α-SMA was performed from total liver protein, using a monoclonal mouse anti-mouse α-SMA antibody (Millipore). The primary antibody was visualized using horseradish peroxidase–conjugated anti-mouse IgG (DAKO) and the PIERCE ECL Western Blotting Substrate (Thermo Scientific). β-actin was used as loading control.

mRNA expression analysis of murine fibrogenic and inflammatory genes

Total RNA was isolated from livers with peqGold TriFast (Peqlab) and reversely transcribed using RevertAid Premium FS cDNA Synthesis Kit (Fermentas) following the manufacturer's instructions. Quantitative RT-PCR was carried out for *Col1a1, Timp1, Tgf-β, IL-1β, TNF-α, Ccl3 and Ccl5* with Assays on Demand obtained from http://www.appliedbiosystems.com.

Splenocyte isolation and preparation of conditioned media

Splenocytes from CCl_4 alone or CCl_4 plus [^{44}AANA^{47}]-CCL5 treated WT mice (see above) were isolated using standard protocols. Cells were cultured for 24 hours in RPMI-1640 medium (PAA Laboratories) and transferred to another tissue culture flask. The cell concentration was adjusted to 8×10^5 cells per ml. For conditioned media, splenocyte suspensions were incubated for 48 hours with 10 μg/ml Concanavalin A (Sigma-Aldrich). The supernatant was centrifuged for 10 min at 900× g to remove cells and debris.

Cell migration assay

A cell migration assay was performed using a modified Boyden Chamber. The stellate cell line GRX [18][9] (2.5×10^5 cells/ml) was placed in the upper chamber in RPMI-1640 medium with 10% fetal calf serum (FCS) and exposed to conditioned media of splenocytes isolated from CCl_4 or CCl_4 plus [^{44}AANA^{47}]-CCL5 treated WT mice in the lower chamber. After 4 hours of incubation at 37°C, cells that migrated to the lower chamber were counted in 6 randomly chosen (magnification, ×100) fields. All experiments were replicated at least twice in quadruplicates.

Cell proliferation assay

GRX cells were starved for 16 hours in RPMI-1640 medium without FCS and stimulated for 24 hours with conditioned media from splenocytes of treated and untreated WT mice (see above). As controls RPMI-1640 medium with 10% FCS respectively without FCS was used. Proliferation of cells was measured by colorimetric immunoassay (Cell Proliferation Elisa, Roche Applied Science) following the manufacturer's instructions.

Statistical analysis

Data are given as means ± SEM. Continuous variables were compared by two-sided *t*-tests with Welch's correction in case of unequal variances. *P*-values less than 0.05 were considered significant in all analyses. Statistical tests were performed by GraphPad Prism 5.

Results

[^{44}AANA^{47}]-CCL5 ameliorates acute liver injury through reduced immune cell infiltration

We first subjected mice to a single toxic insult with CCl_4 to induce acute liver injury. Mice were treated with either [^{44}AANA^{47}]-CCL5 or vehicle to assess the effects of interfering with CCL5 oligomerization and glycosaminoglycan binding on the severity of acute liver damage in this model. As depicted in figure 1A, administration [^{44}AANA^{47}]-CCL5 concomitantly to CCl_4 resulted in reduced ALT levels 48 h after injury compared to vehicle treated mice ($P<0.01$). Interestingly, [^{44}AANA^{47}]-CCL5 did not modulate the ALT levels at 24 h what might mirror a direct cytotoxic effect of CCl_4 which is not modifiable by immune interventions. Furthermore, it should be noted that the ALT levels 48 h after CCl_4 administration are still much higher that the ALT levels in naïve animals. The same results were obtained for AST levels (data not shown). Decreased hepatocellular damage at 48 h was also reflected by a lower extend of hepatic necrosis as assessed by histology (Fig. 1B). Since

[^{44}AANA^{47}]-CCL5 is thought to mainly inhibit the recruitment of leukocytes by reduced CCL5 binding to endothelial cells [19], we next analyzed the overall inflammatory infiltrate in the damaged livers. Indeed, treatment of the mice with [^{44}AANA^{47}]-CCL5 significantly reduced the overall inflammatory cell infiltration 24 h after CCl_4 administration, as assessed by FACS counting of CD45+ cells, compared to vehicle treated animals (Fig. 1C, $P<0.01$). Reduced inflammatory liver damage was further evidenced by RT-PCRs for pivotal inflammation-related genes in mice with or without [^{44}AANA^{47}]-CCL5 treatment (Fig. 1D). Specifically, a significantly reduced hepatic mRNA expression of *IL-1β*, *Tnf-α* and the chemokine *Ccl3* preceded the ameliorated ALT levels in [^{44}AANA^{47}]-CCL5 compared to vehicle treated mice. Interestingly, the mRNA expression of CCL5 was not different between the two groups, supporting that compensatory CCL5 synthesis is not induced by [^{44}AANA^{47}]-CCL5.

Liver fibrosis is strongly reduced in [^{44}AANA^{47}]-CCL5 treated animals

After having shown that treatment with [^{44}AANA^{47}]-CCL5 has a strong impact on the extent of acute inflammatory liver damage, we next evaluated whether this antagonistic strategy does also inhibit progression of liver fibrosis induced by repetitive CCl_4 intoxications. As depicted in figure 2A, mice treated with [^{44}AANA^{47}]-CCL5 indeed showed a reduced extend of scar formation compared to vehicle treated animals. The improved severity of fibrosis in the [^{44}AANA^{47}]-CCL5 treated animals was quantified by a significant decrease in the Sirius red-positive area ($P<0.01$, Fig. 2B) and a reduced hepatic concentration of the collagen-specific amino acid hydroxyproline (reduction of 30.1%, $P<0.01$, Fig. 2C), respectively. Although there was also a trend towards lower ALT levels, Furthermore, the mRNA expression of the fibrosis-associated genes *Col1a1* and *Timp1* was significantly reduced in the livers of [^{44}AANA^{47}]-CCL5 compared to vehicle treated mice (both $P<0.05$, Fig. 3A). In addition, the mRNA expression of the important fibrogenic cytokine *Tgf-β* was reduced by 32% in [^{44}AANA^{47}]-CCL5 treated mice compared to vehicle treated mice, although this difference did not reach statistical significane due to the high variation of expression within the groups. Since *Timp1* is mainly expressed by hepatic stellate cells, we also assessed the activation status of these pivotal pro-fibrogenic cells [20] by determination of αSMA expression. As shown in figure 3B, treatment of mice with [^{44}AANA^{47}]-CCL5 resulted in a reduced expression of αSMA as assessed by immunohistochemistry and western blot analysis of total αSMA protein in the liver. Thus, the reduced fibrosis phenotype in [^{44}AANA^{47}]-CCL5 treated mice appeared to be associated with a strongly reduced activation of hepatic stellate cells.

[^{44}AANA^{47}]-CCL5 leads to quantitative and qualitative changes in the immune response following CCl_4 administration

We and others have recently shown that hepatic stellate cells are a main target of CC chemokines during liver fibrogenesis which are mainly secreted by liver infiltrating immune cells [9,15]. Thus, we next analysed whether treatment with [^{44}AANA^{47}]-CCL5 also leads to reduced immune cell infiltration during chronic liver injury with CCl_4. Indeed, the infiltration of CD45+ leukocytes was strongly reduced in [^{44}AANA^{47}]-CCL5 compared to vehicle treated mice (Fig. 4, upper panel). Since chemokines, including CCL5, are mainly secreted by T-cells and monocytes/macrophages during liver fibrogenesis [21], we specifically determined the recruitment of these cells into the liver at peak of fibrosis. As depicted in figure 4, the infiltration of both cell populations was indeed reduced in [^{44}AANA^{47}]-CCL5 treated mice as assessed by immunohistochemistry for CD3 and F4/80, respectively. As CCL5 is a main chemoattractant for both of these cell populations [22], these results are well in line with the proposed action of [^{44}AANA^{47}]-CCL5 which has abrogated glycosaminoglycan binding and forms inactive heterodimers with WT-CCL5 thereby inhibits transendothelial migration of immune cells induced by CCL5.

Apart from these quantitative changes in immune cell subsets, we also assessed whether [^{44}AANA^{47}]-CCL5 has an impact on qualitative aspects of the immune response. To this end, splenocytes of [^{44}AANA^{47}]-CCL5 or vehicle treated mice were isolated and the direct effects of conditioned media of these cells after ConA stimulation on hepatic stellate cells were analyzed. The results are presented in figure 5. Compared to vehicle treated mice, conditioned medium from [^{44}AANA^{47}]-CCL5 treated mice significantly reduced the migration (Fig. 5A) and the proliferation (Fig. 5B) of hepatic stellate cells *in vitro*. As both aspects are important parameters of these cells during fibrogenesis [20], [^{44}AANA^{47}]-CCL5 appears to also impact the biology of these cells by modulating qualitative changes of the immune response outside the liver.

Discussion

The findings presented in the current study further establish an important role of the CC chemokine CCL5 in acute and chronic liver diseases. There is now ample evidence that this particular chemokine and its receptors play a functional role in murine models of acute [23] and chronic liver diseases [9,15]. Furthermore, expression data and genetic analysis also suggest that CCL5 is involved in the pathogenesis of liver diseases in humans [12,13,14,24]. Thus, CCL5 might be an attractive candidate for antagonistic studies to inhibit the progression and/or accelerate the regression of chronic liver diseases. Indeed, we could recently show that administration of an amino-terminally modified CCL5 molecule (Met-CCL5 [25]), which is an antagonist of the CCL5 receptors CCR1 and CCR5, is able to ameliorate experimental liver damage in mice [9]. However, this particular antagonist blocks not only the action of CCL5 but also of other ligands of these chemokine receptors, including CCL3 and CCL4, which might have differential effects within and outside the liver [16]. We therefore investigated another principle of interference with the chemokine system in the current study which is not based on receptor antagonism, and might exhibit another pattern of side effects. The mutated chemokine [^{44}AANA^{47}]-CCL5 is known to interfere with heparin binding and oligomerization of CCL5, which are both important biological aspects of it's activity *in vivo* [26,27]. This antagonist has been shown to limit inflammatory cell recruitment into the peritoneal cavity, bronchoalveolar air space and the CNS in mice, thereby ameliorating the phenotype of inflammation in these organs [17]. Furthermore, [^{44}AANA^{47}]-CCL5 is able to ameliorate myocardial reperfusion injury in atherosclerotic mice [19]. We here extend these earlier findings by showing that systemic administration of [^{44}AANA^{47}]-CCL5 is also able to strongly inhibit the infiltration of immune cells into the damaged liver. This therapeutical effect was true for an acute model of liver injury as well as a chronic model leading to liver fibrosis. As it is now well established that infiltrating immune cells play a pivotal role in both phenotypes of liver disease [28], these effects of [^{44}AANA^{47}]-CCL5 might be considered as the driving force behind the observed reduction of liver damage. Since T-cells and macrophages are known to carry receptors for CCL5 [29], we systematically addressed the infiltration of these cells into the liver by immunocytochemistry. As depicted in figure 4, the infiltration of both of these cell populations was indeed reduced in [^{44}AANA^{47}]-CCL5 compared to vehicle treated mice. As T-cells [30] and monocytes/macrophages [31] are considered as pivotal pro-fibrogenic cell populations, these results might largely explain the phenotype observed in our models. In support of this hypothesis immune cell populations which do not carry CCL5 receptors (e.g. B-cells) were not changed by treatment with [^{44}AANA^{47}]-CCL5 (data not shown). In the acute model of liver injury the reduced infiltration of immune cells was associated with a strong reduction of pivotal inflammatory genes, while in the chronic model reduced cell recruitment was linked to diminished HSC activation. This finding further emphasizes the important interplay between immune cells and HSCs during different types of liver injury [32].

Nevertheless, we also observed qualitative differences of immune mediated HSC activation in mice treated with [^{44}AANA^{47}]-CCL5. To this end, we isolated splenocytes from mice treated with [^{44}AANA^{47}]-CCL5 or vehicle and used the supernatant of these cultures for assessing the migration and proliferation of HSCs *in vitro*. Indeed, splenocyte supernatants obtained from mice treated with [^{44}AANA^{47}]-CCL5 were significantly less potent in inducing migration and proliferation of HSCs. Thus, the effects of [^{44}AANA^{47}]-CCL5 in our liver disease models appears to be mediated not only by quantitative effects of immune cell infiltration into the liver, but also by qualitative changes outside the liver. Whether this is due to the function of [^{44}AANA^{47}]-CCL5 to sequester endogenous CCL5 by forming non-functional heterodimers [17] needs to be analyzed in further studies. Furthermore, other cytokines might be involved in the modulation of stellate cell behaviour. In a first attempt to identify these cytokines, we determined a subset of these molecules in the conditioned media of activated splenocytes, but could not detect major differences between cells isolated [^{44}AANA^{47}]-CCL5 and vehicle treated mice (data not shown). Thus, the identification of the molecules involved in the modulation of HSC behaviour in our models is still warranted but beyond the scope of the current study.

In summary, the current results suggest that interference with oligomerization and glycosaminoglycan binding of the chemokine CCL5 is able to ameliorate experimental liver injury and fibrosis *in vivo*. Although we cannot decide from our data that this approach is associated with fewer side effects than direct chemokine receptor antagonism, this strategy of immune intervention might be further evaluated as a novel option for the treatment of liver diseases.

Author Contributions

Conceived and designed the experiments: AN CT HEW. Performed the experiments: AN DH MLB HS PS. Analyzed the data: AN AEP HEW. Contributed reagents/materials/analysis tools: AEP. Wrote the paper: AN HEW.

References

1. Holt AP, Salmon M, Buckley CD, Adams DH (2008) Immune interactions in hepatic fibrosis. Clin Liver Dis 12: 861–882, x.
2. Wu Z, Han M, Chen T, Yan W, Ning Q (2010) Acute liver failure: mechanisms of immune-mediated liver injury. Liver Int 30: 782–794.
3. Friedman SL (2008) Mechanisms of hepatic fibrogenesis. Gastroenterology 134: 1655–1669.
4. Wasmuth HE, Tacke F, Trautwein C (2010) Chemokines in liver inflammation and fibrosis. Semin Liver Dis 30: 215–225.
5. Colditz IG, Schneider MA, Pruenster M, Rot A (2007) Chemokines at large: in-vivo mechanisms of their transport, presentation and clearance. Thromb Haemost 97: 688–693.
6. Proudfoot AE, Handel TM, Johnson Z, Lau EK, LiWang P, et al. (2003) Glycosaminoglycan binding and oligomerization are essential for the in vivo activity of certain chemokines. Proc Natl Acad Sci U S A 100: 1885–1890.
7. Fernandez EJ, Lolis E (2002) Structure, function, and inhibition of chemokines. Annu Rev Pharmacol Toxicol 42: 469–499.
8. Sahin H, Trautwein C, Wasmuth HE (2010) Functional role of chemokines in liver disease models. Nat Rev Gastroenterol Hepatol 7: 682–690.
9. Berres ML, Koenen RR, Rueland A, Zaldivar MM, Heinrichs D, et al. (2010) Antagonism of the chemokine Ccl5 ameliorates experimental liver fibrosis in mice. J Clin Invest 120: 4129–4140.
10. Haybaeck J, Zeller N, Wolf MJ, Weber A, Wagner U, et al. (2009) A lymphotoxin-driven pathway to hepatocellular carcinoma. Cancer Cell 16: 295–308.
11. Nischalke HD, Nattermann J, Fischer HP, Sauerbruch T, Spengler U, et al. (2004) Semiquantitative analysis of intrahepatic CC-chemokine mRNAs in chronic hepatitis C. Mediators Inflamm 13: 357–359.
12. Hellier S, Frodsham AJ, Hennig BJ, Klenerman P, Knapp S, et al. (2003) Association of genetic variants of the chemokine receptor CCR5 and its ligands, RANTES and MCP-2, with outcome of HCV infection. Hepatology 38: 1468–1476.
13. Promrat K, McDermott DH, Gonzalez CM, Kleiner DE, Koziol DE, et al. (2003) Associations of chemokine system polymorphisms with clinical outcomes and treatment responses of chronic hepatitis C. Gastroenterology 124: 352–360.
14. Wasmuth HE, Werth A, Mueller T, Berg T, Dietrich CG, et al. (2004) Haplotype-tagging RANTES gene variants influence response to antiviral therapy in chronic hepatitis C. Hepatology 40: 327–334.
15. Seki E, De Minicis S, Gwak G-Y, Kluwe J, Inokucki A, et al. (2009) CCR1 and CCR5 promote hepatic fibrosis in mice. J Clin Invest 119: 1858–1870.
16. Schall TJ, Proudfoot AE (2011) Overcoming hurdles in developing successful drugs targeting chemokine receptors. Nat Rev Immunol 11: 355–363.
17. Johnson Z, Kosco-Vilbois MH, Herren S, Cirillo R, Muzio V, et al. (2004) Interference with heparin binding and oligomerization creates a novel anti-inflammatory strategy targeting the chemokine system. J Immunol 173: 5776–5785.
18. Borojevic R, Monteiro AN, Vinhas SA, Domont GB, Mourao PA, et al. (1985) Establishment of a continuous cell line from fibrotic schistosomal granulomas in mice livers. In Vitro Cell Dev Biol 21: 382–390.
19. Braunersreuther V, Pellieux C, Pelli G, Burger F, Steffens S, et al. (2010) Chemokine CCL5/RANTES inhibition reduces myocardial reperfusion injury in atherosclerotic mice. J Mol Cell Cardiol 48: 789–798.
20. Friedman SL (2008) Hepatic stellate cells: protean, multifunctional, and enigmatic cells of the liver. Physiol Rev 88: 125–172.
21. Karlmark KR, Wasmuth HE, Trautwein C, Tacke F (2008) Chemokine-directed immune cell infiltration in acute and chronic liver disease. Expert Rev Gastroenterol Hepatol 2: 233–242.
22. Appay V, Rowland-Jones SL (2001) RANTES: a versatile and controversial chemokine. Trends Immunol 22: 83–87.
23. Ajuebor MN, Wondimu Z, Hogaboam CM, Le T, Proudfoot AE, et al. (2007) CCR5 deficiency drives enhanced natural killer cell trafficking to and activation within the liver in murine T cell-mediated hepatitis. Am J Pathol 170: 1975–1988.
24. Schwabe RF, Bataller R, Brenner DA (2003) Human hepatic stellate cells express CCR5 and RANTES to induce proliferation and migration. Am J Physiol Gastrointest Liver Physiol 285: G949–958.
25. Proudfoot AE, Power CA, Hoogewerf AJ, Montjovent MO, Borlat F, et al. (1996) Extension of recombinant human RANTES by the retention of the initiating methionine produces a potent antagonist. J Biol Chem 271: 2599–2603.
26. Proudfoot AE, Fritchley S, Borlat F, Shaw JP, Vilbois F, et al. (2001) The BBXB motif of RANTES is the principal site for heparin binding and controls receptor selectivity. J Biol Chem 276: 10620–10626.
27. Rot A (2010) Chemokine patterning by glycosaminoglycans and interceptors. Front Bioscience 15: 645–660.
28. Adams DH, Ju C, Ramaiah SK, Uetrecht J, Jaeschke H (2010) Mechanisms of immune-mediated liver injury. Toxicol Sci 115: 307–321.
29. Charo IF, Ransohoff RM (2006) The many roles of chemokines and chemokine receptors in inflammation. N Engl J Med 354: 610–621.
30. Safadi R, Ohta M, Alvarez CE, Fiel MI, Bansal M, et al. (2004) Immune stimulation of hepatic fibrogenesis by CD8 cells and attenuation by transgenic interleukin-10 from hepatocytes. Gastroenterology 127: 870–882.
31. Karlmark KR, Weiskirchen R, Zimmermann HW, Gassler N, Ginhoux F, et al. (2009) Hepatic recruitment of the inflammatory Gr1+ monocyte subset upon liver injury promotes hepatic fibrosis. Hepatology 50: 261–274.
32. Bataller R, Brenner DA (2005) Liver fibrosis. J Clin Invest 115: 209–218.

8

Hepatocyte IKK2 Protects Mdr2$^{-/-}$ Mice from Chronic Liver Failure

Hanno Ehlken[1], Vangelis Kondylis[1], Jan Heinrichsdorff[1¤a], Laura Ochoa-Callejero[1¤b], Tania Roskams[2], Manolis Pasparakis[1]*

1 Institute for Genetics, Centre for Molecular Medicine (CMMC), Cologne Excellence Cluster on Cellular Stress Responses in Aging-Associated Diseases (CECAD), University of Cologne, Cologne, Germany, **2** Department of Pathology, Catholic University of Leuven, Leuven, Belgium

Abstract

Mice lacking the Abc4 protein encoded by the multidrug resistance-2 gene (*Mdr2*$^{-/-}$) develop chronic periductular inflammation and cholestatic liver disease resulting in the development of hepatocellular carcinoma (HCC). Inhibition of NF-κB by expression of an IκBα super-repressor (IκBαSR) transgene in hepatocytes was shown to prevent HCC development in *Mdr2*$^{-/-}$ mice, suggesting that NF-κB acts as a tumour promoter in this model of inflammation-associated carcinogenesis. On the other hand, inhibition of NF-κB by hepatocyte specific ablation of IKK2 resulted in increased liver tumour development induced by the chemical carcinogen DEN. To address the role of IKK2-mediated NF-κB activation in hepatocytes in the pathogenesis of liver disease and HCC in *Mdr2*$^{-/-}$ mice, we generated Mdr2-deficient animals lacking IKK2 specifically in hepatocytes using the Cre-loxP system. Mdr2$^{-/-}$ mice lacking IKK2 in hepatocytes developed spontaneously a severe liver disease characterized by cholestasis, major hyperbilirubinemia and severe to end-stage fibrosis, which caused muscle wasting, loss of body weight, lethargy and early spontaneous death. Cell culture experiments showed that primary hepatocytes lacking IKK2 were more sensitive to bile acid induced death, suggesting that hepatocyte-specific IKK2 deficiency sensitized hepatocytes to the toxicity of bile acids under conditions of cholestasis resulting in greatly exacerbated liver damage. Mdr2$^{-/-}$ IKK2$^{Hep\text{-}KO}$ mice remarkably recapitulate chronic liver failure in humans and might be of special importance for the study of the mechanisms contributing to the pathogenesis of end-stage chronic liver disease or its implications on other organs.

Conclusion: IKK2-mediated signaling in hepatocytes protects the liver from damage under conditions of chronic inflammatory cholestasis and prevents the development of severe fibrosis and liver failure.

Editor: Thierry Tordjmann, Université Paris Sud, France

Funding: This work was funded by European Commission FP7 program grant "INFLA-CARE" (EC contract number 223151) to MP. The funders had no role in study design, data collection and analysis, decision to publish, or preparation of the manuscript.

Competing Interests: The authors have declared that no competing interests exist.

* E-mail: pasparakis@uni-koeln.de

¤a Current address: Division of Endocrinology and Metabolism, Department of Medicine, University of California San Diego, La Jolla, California, United States of America

¤b Current address: Oncology Area, Center for Biomedical Research of La Rioja (CIBIR), Logroño, Spain

Introduction

In humans, liver fibrosis is caused by a variety of different diseases such as chronic viral hepatitis, autoimmune liver disease and other disorders characterized by chronic liver inflammation [1]. Although the quality of the fibrosis may be different depending on the underlying pathology, in all cases fibrosis is caused by the activation of specialized stellate cells, which differentiate into active myofibroblasts that remodel the extracellular matrix of the liver [2], [3]. Under normal conditions myofibroblasts reside in a quiescent state and need to become stimulated in order to proliferate and differentiate into motile collagen-producing cells. In humans, almost all patients with chronic liver injury will develop fibrosis, which in many individuals will ultimately result in liver cirrhosis and end-stage liver disease, a condition that has a high morbidity and mortality and is discussed to favor initiation and progression of hepatocellular carcinoma [4]. Therefore, there is an urgent need to study the molecular and cellular mechanisms by which inflammatory signals regulate myofibroblast activation in order to better understand the mechanisms that control the pathogenesis of liver fibrosis and its detrimental consequences.

The multidrug resistance-2 knockout (Mdr2$^{-/-}$) mouse provides a model for the study of liver fibrosis and hepatocarcinogenesis in the context of chronic inflammation. In contrast to other multidrug resistance proteins of the Mdr family, Mdr2 does not facilitate resistance towards specific chemicals (as for human Mdr1) by directly shuttling metabolites out of the cell [5]. Instead, studies in Mdr2$^{-/-}$ mice suggest that Mdr2 mediates the flipping of phospholipids (phosphatidylcholine) from the cytosol of the hepatocyte into the bile canaliculi [5]. Phospholipids are thought to potently emulsify hydrophobic molecules such as certain bile acids and thereby attenuate their toxicity. Although the mechanisms controlling the pathogenesis of liver disease in Mdr2$^{-/-}$ mice are still under discussion, several studies have demonstrated that mice lacking Mdr2 develop a chronic inflammatory liver condition, which is characterized by periductular inflammatory cell infiltration and periportal fibrosis typically bridging adjacent portal fields [6], [7], [8]. Additionally, in the FVB/N genetic background, 100% of Mdr2 deficient mice develop hepatocellular carcinoma at the age of 16 months [8].

The transcription factor Nuclear Factor kappa B (NF-κB) regulates immune and inflammatory responses by controlling the expression of genes with important immunoregulatory functions. In resting cells NF-κB dimers are sequestered in the cytoplasm by association with inhibitory proteins belonging to the IκB family. When the cell is activated by a variety of stress-inducing stimuli, the IκB kinase complex (IKK), consisting of two catalytic subunits, IKK1 (or IKKα) and IKK2 (or IKKβ) and a regulatory subunit named NEMO (or IKKγ), phosphorylates IκBs on specific serine residues triggering their polyubiquitination and degradation through the proteasome. Consequently, NF-κB homo- and heterodimers are set free and translocate into the nucleus where they transactivate target genes, among them survival factors and inflammatory mediators [9], [10]. NF-κB is activated by a large number of stress-inducing stimuli, including cytokines, microbial products and conditions that impose threat on the cell such as radiation, hypoxia, mechanical stress [9]. With particular relevance to bile duct disease, cytotoxic bile acids are also potent activators of the NF-κB pathway [11], [12].

Studies in genetic mouse models revealed important functions of the IKK/NF-κB pathway in the regulation of liver physiology and the pathogenesis of liver diseases [9]. Mice lacking NEMO in liver parenchymal cells spontaneously develop chronic liver disease due to increased death of NEMO-deficient hepatocytes, which triggers liver inflammation and compensatory hepatocyte proliferation resulting in hepatocellular carcinoma (HCC) [13]. In addition, IKK2 has been shown to protect mice from chemically induced liver cancer mainly by inhibiting carcinogen-induced hepatocyte death and preventing compensatory proliferation of hepatocytes [14]. Moreover, recent studies showed that mice lacking both IKK1 and IKK2 in liver parenchymal cells develop severe jaundice and fatal cholangitis, demonstrating that IKK1 and IKK2 cooperate to maintain the integrity of the small bile ducts in the liver. Importantly, ablation of solely NEMO, IKK1 or IKK2 could not provoke this phenotype [15], indicating that the individual IKK subunits show a degree of functional redundancy in the liver.

NF-κB inhibition in hepatocytes by expression of an IκB super-repressor (IκBαSR) transgene did not affect liver inflammation in Mdr2$^{-/-}$ mice but strongly reduced the development of hepatocellular carcinoma, suggesting that NF-κB activation promotes the survival of premalignant cells facilitating liver cancer development in this model [7]. To unveil the role of IKK2 in liver cancer development in Mdr2$^{-/-}$ mice, we generated and analyzed Mdr2$^{-/-}$ animals that lack IKK2 expression specifically in hepatocytes (Mdr2$^{-/-}$IKK2$^{Hep\text{-}KO}$). Surprisingly, we found that hepatocyte-specific deletion of IKK2 severely aggravated liver pathology of Mdr2$^{-/-}$ mice. Mdr2$^{-/-}$IKK2$^{Hep\text{-}KO}$ mice developed severe jaundice at young age and failed to thrive remaining considerably smaller compared to their wild-type or *Mdr2*$^{-/-}$ littermates. In addition, Mdr2$^{-/-}$IKK2$^{Hep\text{-}KO}$ mice developed severe liver fibrosis accompanied by massive bile duct proliferation as compared to Mdr2$^{-/-}$ mice. Finally, we show that IKK2 deficient hepatocytes were more sensitive to bile acid induced cytotoxicity, suggesting that IKK2 signaling has an important function to protect hepatocytes from bile acid toxicity and prevent severe liver damage in conditions of primary biliary disease.

Results

Mdr2$^{-/-}$IKK2$^{Hep\text{-}KO}$ mice develop severe wasting due to liver disease

To study the hepatocyte-specific role of IKK2 mediated NF-κB activation in liver disease and cancer induced by Mdr2 deficiency, we crossed Mdr2$^{-/-}$ mice with mice carrying loxP-flanked IKK2 alleles [16] and the Albumin-Cre transgene [17]. These double Mdr2$^{-/-}$IKK2$^{Hep\text{-}KO}$ mice lack Mdr2 expression in all cells and additionally have a hepatocyte-specific ablation of IKK2 (Fig. 1A). Mdr2$^{-/-}$IKK2$^{Hep\text{-}KO}$ mice were born at the expected Mendelian ratio but were already distinguishable from their littermates in the first two weeks of life as they were considerably smaller. Although Mdr2$^{-/-}$IKK2$^{Hep\text{-}KO}$ mice showed an initial phase of growth till they reached 4 weeks of age, they subsequently lost about 30% of their body weight and at the age of 8 weeks weighed 50% less compared to their heterozygous Mdr2$^{+/-}$IKK2$^{Hep\text{-}KO}$ but also single Mdr2$^{-/-}$ littermates (Fig. 1B, 1C). These results suggested that Mdr2$^{-/-}$IKK2$^{Hep\text{-}KO}$ mice suffer from liver disease resulting in poor growth and prompted us to investigate in detail the liver function in these animals.

Mdr2$^{-/-}$IKK2$^{Hep\text{-}KO}$ mice appeared severely jaundiced and their limbs and trunk showed varying degrees of muscle wasting and loss of fat mass (Fig. 1C). Necropsy of Mdr2$^{-/-}$, Mdr2$^{+/-}$IKK2$^{Hep\text{-}KO}$ and Mdr2$^{-/-}$IKK2$^{Hep\text{-}KO}$ mice confirmed major jaundice of organs and serosae and substantial loss of body fat (Fig. 1D) only in the double knockout animals. The livers of Mdr2$^{-/-}$IKK2$^{Hep\text{-}KO}$ mice appeared yellow - green tainted and were harder to cut compared to the livers of Mdr2$^{-/-}$ or Mdr2$^{+/-}$IKK2$^{Hep\text{-}KO}$ mice (Fig. 1D). Mdr2$^{-/-}$IKK2$^{Hep\text{-}KO}$ mice also showed massively enlarged gallbladders that were filled with bile (Fig. 1D). In contrast, single Mdr2$^{-/-}$ and heterozygous Mdr2$^{+/-}$IKK2$^{Hep\text{-}KO}$ mice were indistinguishable from wild type mice (Fig. 1C, 1D) arguing that the lack of IKK2 in hepatocytes only culminates in the observed phenotype when Mdr2 is completely absent.

Mdr2$^{-/-}$IKK2$^{Hep\text{-}KO}$ mice show increased liver damage

To further characterize the liver disease developing in Mdr2$^{-/-}$IKK2$^{Hep\text{-}KO}$ mice we measured the levels of serum alanine amino transferase (ALT) in young adult mice (aged 2–6 months). We could not analyze a statistically meaningful number of mice in older age as most Mdr2$^{-/-}$IKK2$^{Hep\text{-}KO}$ mice died or showed very severe disease and had to be sacrificed before the age of 30 weeks. We found that Mdr2$^{-/-}$IKK2$^{Hep\text{-}KO}$ mice had about six-fold elevated serum ALT levels compared to their control littermates, indicating that these animals showed increased spontaneous liver damage (Fig. 2A). At this age, Mdr2$^{-/-}$ mice did not show elevated serum ALT levels compared to heterozygous Mdr2$^{+/-}$IKK2$^{Hep\text{-}KO}$ mice. In line with the increased ALT levels, we found that liver sections from Mdr2$^{-/-}$IKK2$^{Hep\text{-}KO}$ mice contained increased numbers of dying hepatocytes as compared to Mdr2$^{-/-}$ mice or Mdr2$^{+/-}$IKK2$^{Hep\text{-}KO}$ mice (Fig. 2D). In addition, liver sections from Mdr2$^{-/-}$IKK2$^{Hep\text{-}KO}$ also showed more PCNA positive cells in comparison to Mdr2$^{-/-}$ mice or Mdr2$^{+/-}$IKK2$^{Hep\text{-}KO}$ mice indicating a higher level of compensatory proliferation (Fig. 2E). The observation that Mdr2$^{-/-}$IKK2$^{Hep\text{-}KO}$ mice were severely jaundiced prompted us to further investigate potential bile duct related complications. We therefore measured the levels of serum Alkaline Phosphatase (AP), a widely used marker for bile flow obstruction [18], in Mdr2$^{-/-}$IKK2$^{Hep\text{-}KO}$ and their control littermates. Indeed, serum AP levels were massively elevated in Mdr2$^{-/-}$IKK2$^{Hep\text{-}KO}$ mice compared to either Mdr2$^{-/-}$ or Mdr2$^{+/-}$IKK2$^{Hep\text{-}KO}$ littermates (Fig. 2B). Additionally, Mdr2$^{-/-}$IKK2$^{Hep\text{-}KO}$ mice showed strongly elevated levels of total bilirubin in the serum compared to their littermate controls (Fig. 2C). These results suggest that Mdr2$^{-/-}$IKK2$^{Hep\text{-}KO}$ mice suffer from obstructive biliary disease. Mdr2$^{-/-}$ mice showed slightly elevated AP levels compared to heterozygous Mdr2$^{+/-}$IKK2$^{Hep\text{-}KO}$ mice but the levels of bilirubin were within the normal range in both control groups. Collectively, these results showed that Mdr2$^{-/-}$IKK2$^{Hep\text{-}KO}$ mice

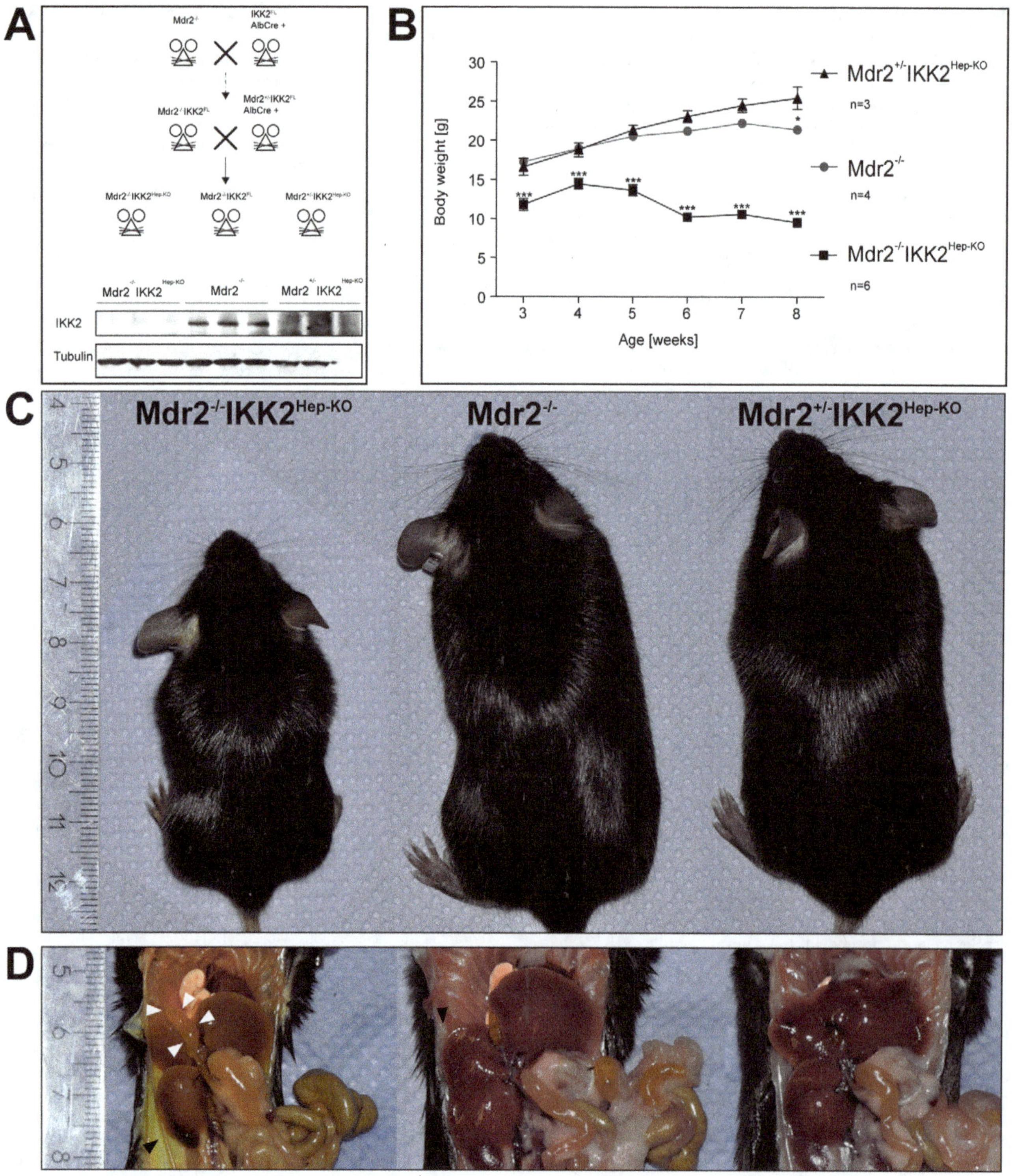

Figure 1. Mdr2$^{-/-}$IKK2$^{\text{Hep-KO}}$ mice show impaired growth and signs of jaundice. (A) Immunoblot of whole liver lysates from 3 representative mice for each depicted genotype. Tubulin serves as loading control. (B) Weight curve of male mice for the denoted genotypes. * $p<0{,}05$ for Mdr2$^{+/-}$ IKK2$^{\text{Hep-KO}}$ vs. Mdr2$^{-/-}$, ** $p<0{,}001$ for Mdr2$^{-/-}$ IKK2$^{\text{Hep-KO}}$ vs. Mdr2$^{-/-}$. (C) Macroscopic appearance of littermate male mice at 12 weeks of age. Genotypes as specified in the picture. (D) Necropsy of littermate mice from (C). White arrowheads: enlarged gall bladder in double knockout mouse. Black arrowhead: jaundiced peritoneal serosa in double knockout mouse vs. normal appearance of serosa in Mdr2$^{-/-}$ and Mdr2$^{+/-}$ IKK2$^{\text{Hep-KO}}$ mice. The ruler indicates centimeters in C and D.

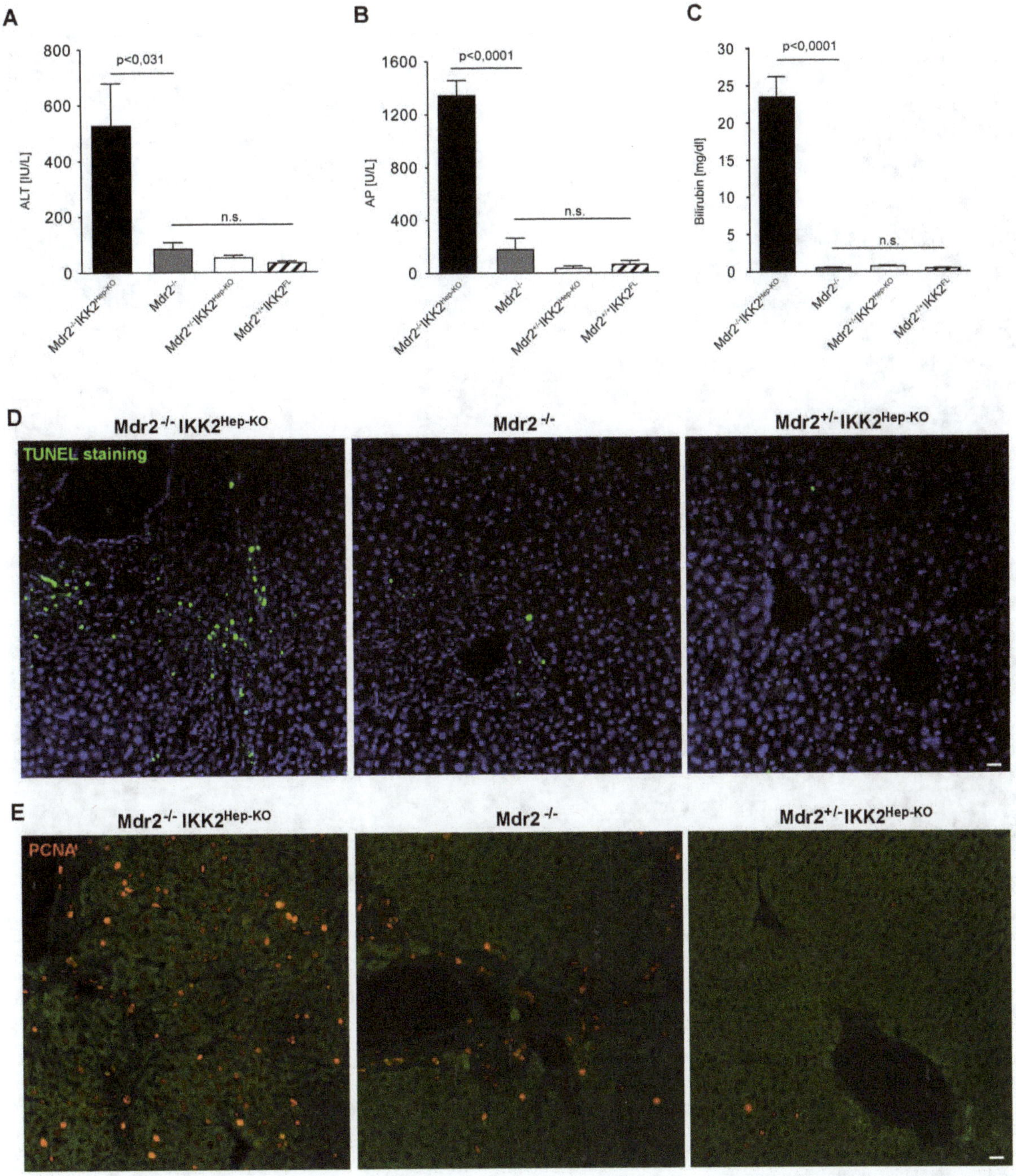

Figure 2. Mdr2$^{-/-}$IKK2^{Hep-KO} mice exhibit increased liver damage, hepatocyte death and cholestasis. (A) Alanine aminotransferase (ALT), (B) alkaline phosphatase (AP), and (C) bilirubin levels in serum of adult male mice (8–26 weeks) with the indicated genotypes. Error bars indicate SEM. Number of mice: Mdr2$^{-/-}$IKK2^{Hep-}KO: n = 10, Mdr2$^{-/-}$: n = 7, Mdr2$^{+/-}$IKK2^{Hep-KO}: n = 7 and Mdr2$^{+/+}$IKK2^{FL}: n = 2. (D–E) Representative pictures of TUNEL (D) and PCNA staining (E) on sections of paraffin-embedded livers from mice with the indicated genotypes. The green signal in E corresponds to background auto-fluorescence and was used to visualize the general morphology of the liver tissues. Scale bars: 20 μm.

spontaneously developed an obstructive bile duct-related disease resulting in liver damage and severe jaundice.

Increased cholangiocyte proliferation and severe liver fibrosis in Mdr2$^{-/-}$IKK2^{Hep-KO} mice

To further characterize the liver pathology developing in Mdr2$^{-/-}$IKK2^{Hep-KO} mice we performed immunohistochemical analysis of liver sections from these animals and from littermate controls. Consistent with previous reports [6], [8], [7], the livers of Mdr2$^{-/-}$ mice showed immune cell infiltration around the bile ducts already at young age, which was more pronounced in older animals (Fig. 3A). Analysis of liver sections from Mdr2$^{-/-}$IKK2^{Hep-KO} mice showed a more severe pathology with strong immune cell infiltration in the portal areas and massive expansion of the bile ducts in older animals (Fig. 3A). Immunostaining for cytokeratin 19, a marker of bile duct epithelial cells in the liver, revealed that Mdr2$^{-/-}$IKK2^{Hep-KO} mice showed more pronounced expansion and hyperproliferation of biliary epithelial cells

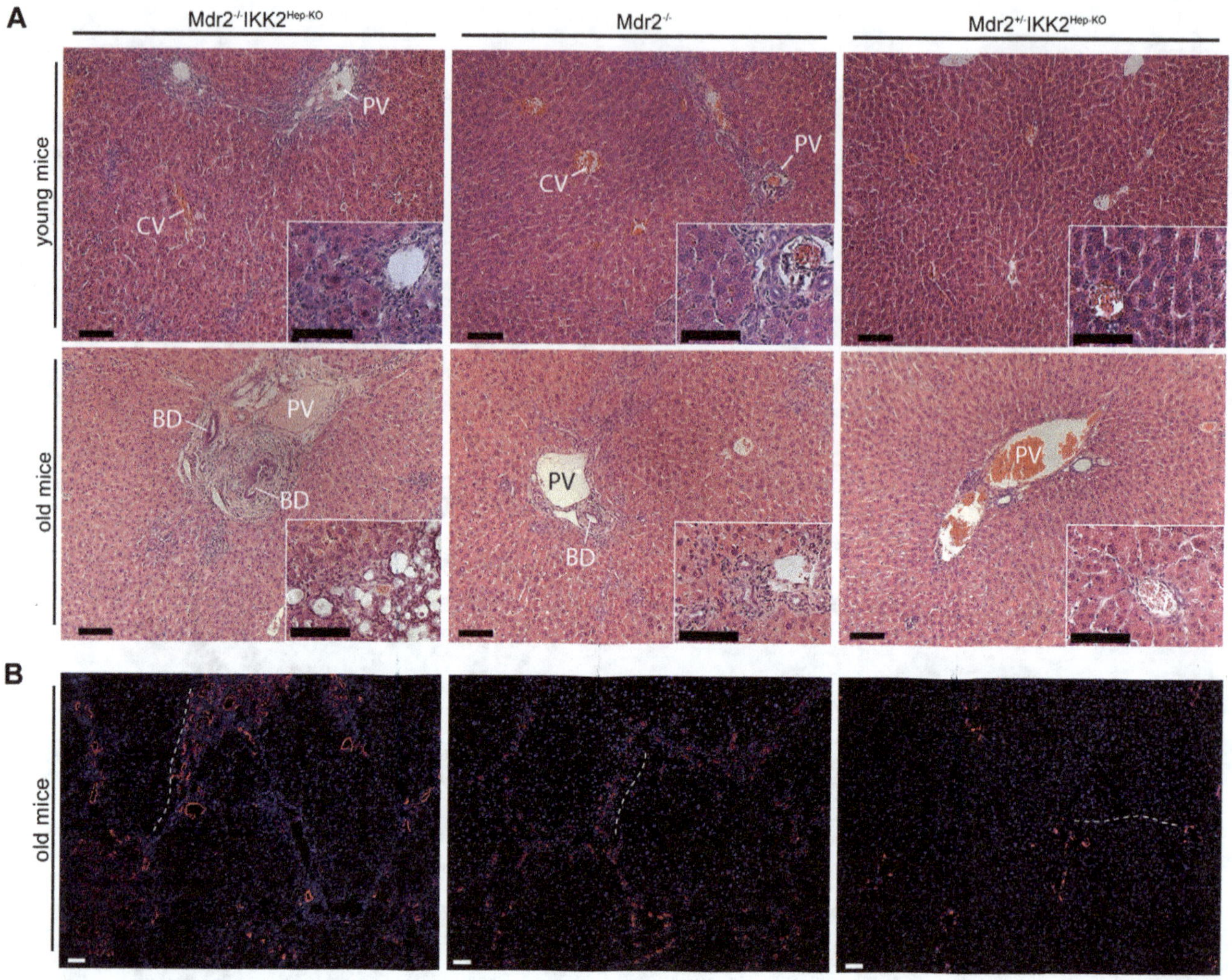

Figure 3. Histological analysis of the liver pathology in Mdr2$^{-/-}$IKK2$^{Hep\text{-}KO}$ mice. (A) Representative images of Hematoxylin & Eosin (HE) stained livers from young (12-week-old) littermate male mice and old (27–30 weeks) mice with the specified genotypes. Insert: High magnification of corresponding liver sections. (B) Immunofluorescence staining of cytokeratin 19 (CK19) in old male mice. DNA was stained with DAPI. The dashed line marks the distance from one portal field to the next, showing extreme abundance of CK19 positive cells in the Mdr2$^{-/-}$ IKK2$^{Hep\text{-}KO}$ as compared to Mdr2$^{-/-}$ or Mdr2$^{+/-}$IKK2$^{Hep\text{-}KO}$ mice. PV portal vein. CV central vein. BD bile duct. Scale bars, 100 μm.

compared to Mdr2 deficient mice (Fig. 3B). Whereas the livers from Mdr2$^{-/-}$ mice presented with hyperproliferating bile ducts close to or connecting the portal fields (Fig. 3A, 3B), Mdr2$^{-/-}$ IKK2$^{Hep\text{-}KO}$ mice had strongly enlarged bile duct lumina and showed hyperproliferating bile ducts spanning from one portal field to the next also affecting more central areas (Fig. 3B and 4A). We did not detect histological signs of pathology in the livers of heterozygous *Mdr2*$^{+/-}$IKK2$^{Hep\text{-}KO}$ control mice (Fig. 3A and 3B).

The livers from Mdr2$^{-/-}$IKK2$^{Hep\text{-}KO}$ mice were hard to cut, indicating the presence of fibrosis. We therefore stained liver sections with Masson's trichrome and with Sirius red to visualize fibrotic areas. As reported previously, livers from Mdr2$^{-/-}$ mice showed bridging fibrosis with connective tissue fibers concentrating in the periportal and periductular area as shown by Masson Trichrome and Sirius Red staining (Fig. 4A and 4B respectively). Interestingly, fibers were more abundant in the liver of Mdr2$^{-/-}$IKK2$^{Hep\text{-}KO}$ mice already at younger age compared to Mdr2 knockouts, while Mdr2$^{+/-}$IKK2$^{Hep\text{-}KO}$ animals did not show any fibrosis (Fig. 4A and 4B). Furthermore, already at young age fibrosis in Mdr2$^{-/-}$ IKK2$^{Hep\text{-}KO}$ mice followed also a pericellular distribution (Fig. 4B). This latter pattern of fiber deposition is sometimes referred to as chicken-wire fibrosis and in humans can help to distinguish between causes of liver injury [19]. Only in Mdr2$^{-/-}$IKK2$^{Hep\text{-}KO}$ animals fibrosis reached a stage where macroscopically and microscopically the liver surface became uneven (data not shown). Quantification of the fibrotic area in Sirius red stained liver sections revealed that Mdr2$^{-/-}$IK-K2$^{Hep\text{-}KO}$ mice have significantly more fibrosis as compared to Mdr2$^{-/-}$ and Mdr2$^{-/-}$IKK2$^{Hep\text{-}KO}$ mice (Fig. 4C).

Mdr2$^{-/-}$ mice in the FVB/N genetic background were shown to spontaneously develop hepatocellular carcinoma with 100% penetrance by the age of 16 months [8]. Due to the severe phenotype and early lethality of Mdr2$^{-/-}$IKK2$^{Hep\text{-}KO}$ mice we could not analyze animals older than 9–10 months to evaluate HCC development. However, we did not observe any malignant or premalignant lesions in livers from Mdr2$^{-/-}$IKK2$^{Hep\text{-}KO}$ at 2 to 10 months of age. In addition, we could not detect any malignant or premalignant areas in the livers of Mdr2$^{-/-}$ mice up to 14 months of age (data not shown). These findings are consistent with a recent report demonstrating that when Mdr2$^{-/-}$ mice were crossed into the C57Bl/6 background tumor development was suppressed [20].

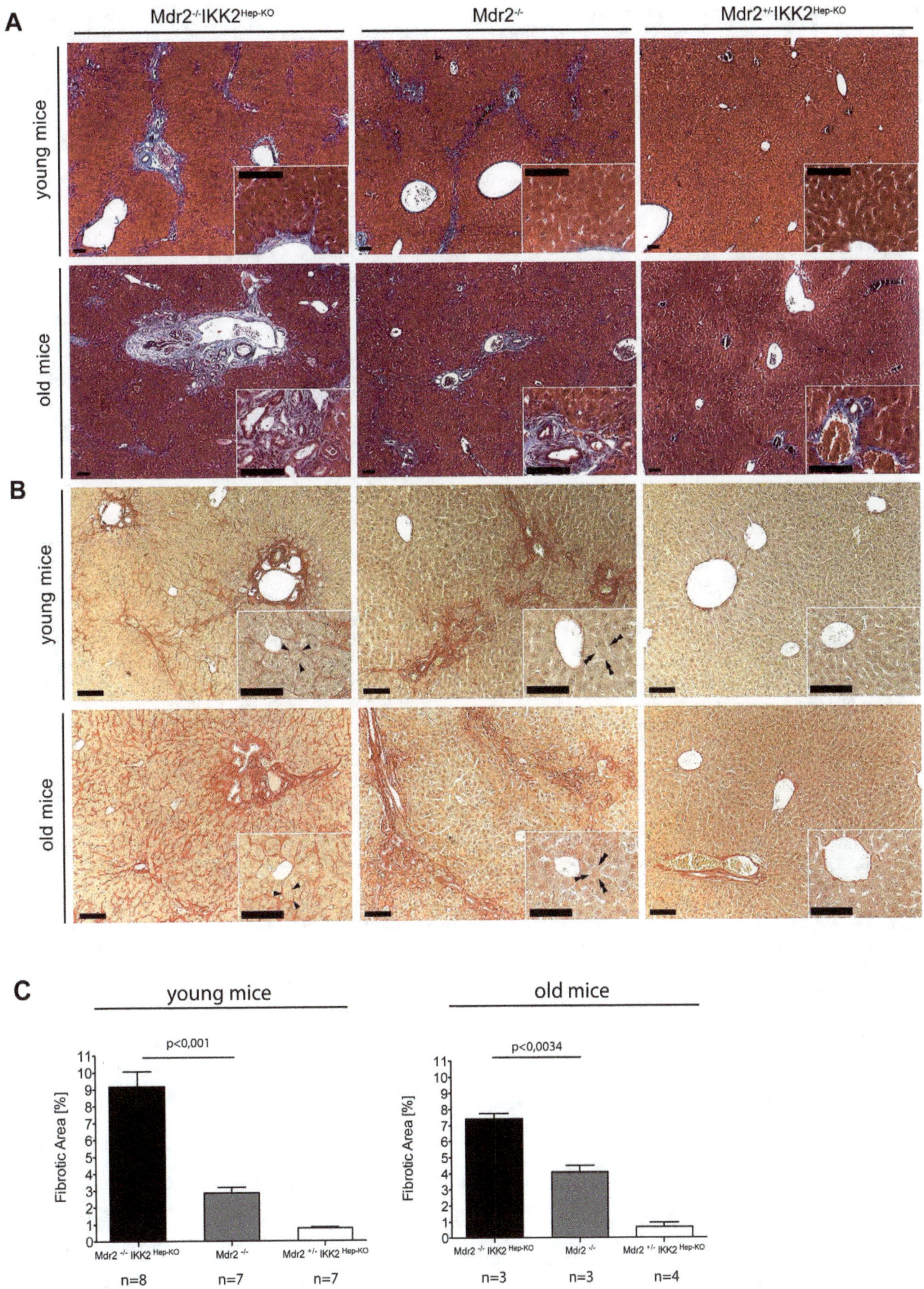
A
Mdr2-/-IKK2Hep-KO
Mdr2-/-
Mdr2+/-IKK2Hep-KO
young mice
old mice
B
young mice
old mice
C
young mice
old mice
p<0,001
p<0,0034
Fibrotic Area [%]
Mdr2 -/- IKK2 Hep-KO
Mdr2 -/-
Mdr2 +/- IKK2 Hep-KO
n=8
n=7
n=7
n=3
n=3
n=4

Figure 4. Mdr2$^{-/-}$IKK2^{Hep-KO} mice develop severe fibrosis. (A) Representative images of Masson trichrome stained livers from 12-week-old littermate male mice and from 27–30 week-old male mice. (B) Representative images of Sirius Red stained livers from 12-week-old littermate male mice and from old adult male mice (27–30 weeks). Insert: High magnification of corresponding liver sections. Arrowhead: Pericellular fibers. Double arrowhead: Pericellular space free of stained fibers. Genotypes as in (A). (C) Quantification of fibrosis in mice with the depicted genotypes measured as percentage of Sirius Red positive area as a fraction of the total area of at least 10 high power fields per mouse. Left: young adult mice (males, 8–19 weeks), right: old adult mice (males, 20–42 weeks). Error bars indicate SEM. Scale bars, 100 μm.

IKK2 protects primary hepatocytes from bile acid induced apoptosis

Our results presented above showed that hepatocyte-specific ablation of IKK2 severely affected liver function in Mdr2-deficient animals resulting in chronic obstructive bile duct disease, severe jaundice, liver fibrosis and early death.

Mdr2-deficiency impairs the enrichment of bile with phospholipids, which are important to emulsify and thus reduce the toxicity of bile acids. Therefore the bile of Mdr2$^{-/-}$ mice is more toxic. We hypothesized that IKK2 ablation in hepatocytes strongly aggravated the liver pathology of Mdr2-deficient mice by sensitizing hepatocytes to bile acid toxicity. Indeed, bile acids have been shown to activate the NF-κB pathway in obstructive cholestasis suggesting that NF-κB might have a protective function in cholestatic liver disease, although the exact mechanism remains poorly understood [12]. It has been shown that hydrophobic bile acids can induce apoptosis in primary cultured hepatocytes of mouse or rat origin [21]. We therefore chose to compare the toxicity of glycochenodeoxycholate (GCDC) and taurolithocholylsulfate (TLCS), both of which have been reported to induce apoptosis in primary hepatocytes from rat and mouse [11,12,22,23,24], in wild-type and IKK2-deficient primary hepatocytes. TLCS treatment of wild-type and IKK2-deficient primary hepatocytes resulted in markedly increased numbers of apoptotic/dead cells as revealed after DAPI staining by the detection of small highly fluorescent nuclei with condensed chromatin [25] (Fig. 5A). We observed about two-fold increase of apoptotic/dead cells in the IKK2-deficient as compared to the wild-type hepatocytes at 12, 24 and 48 hours of stimulation with TLCS (Fig. 5B). To assess differences in the early apoptotic response we stimulated wild type and IKK2-deficient primary mouse hepatocytes with TLCS or GCDC and examined caspase-3 activation by immunoblotting with antibodies recognizing the cleaved/active version of caspase-3. These experiments revealed a stronger and earlier activation of caspase-3 in TLCS and GCDC stimulated IKK2-deficient primary hepatocytes, suggesting that NF-κB inhibition by ablation of IKK2 sensitized hepatocytes to bile acid-induced apoptosis (Fig. 5C). Taken together, these results show that IKK2-mediated signaling protects primary hepatocytes from the toxicity of hydrophobic bile acids, suggesting that NF-κB activation in hepatocytes is critical for the prevention of liver damage in obstructive biliary disease.

Discussion

In humans, chronic cholestatic liver diseases constitute a major risk for the development of liver cirrhosis and end-stage liver disease culminating in liver failure. Obstruction of the bile flow in bile ducts and bile canaliculi can damage both bile duct epithelial cells and hepatocytes. Our knowledge about the mechanisms regulating the cross-talk between hepatocytes and bile duct epithelial cells in the normal liver and also under conditions of cholestasis remains limited. The Mdr2 knockout mouse is an excellent model for the study of chronic inflammatory biliary liver disease, liver fibrosis and hepatocarcinogenesis. Abc4, the product of the Mdr2 gene, is expressed in hepatocytes and functions to flip phospholipids into the bile canaliculi. Phospholipids emulsify hydrophobic bile acids reducing their toxic effects, therefore enrichment of the bile with phospholipids is important to reduce bile toxicity. The increased toxicity of the bile in Mdr2-deficient mice is thought to induce bile duct inflammation and the liver disease in these animals [6], [5]. Here we show that hepatocyte-specific ablation of IKK2 in the context of disturbed bile homeostasis induced by Mdr2 deficiency results in severe cholestatic liver disease in young age, suggesting that activation of the IKK2/NF-κB pathway in hepatocytes constitutes an essential regulator of liver function under conditions of bile duct inflammation.

In older Mdr2$^{-/-}$ mice, bile duct inflammation progresses to fibrosis especially around the periportal area of the liver lobule. Ultimately, as a result of the chronic inflammation, Mdr2$^{-/-}$ mice in the FVB genetic background develop hepatocellular carcinoma by the age of 16 months [26]. Mdr2$^{-/-}$IKK2^{Hep-KO} mice showed more severe bile duct inflammation and biliary epithelial cell hyperproliferation, and also they presented with more severe fibrosis in all areas of the liver, i.e. periportal and pericentral areas compared to Mdr2$^{-/-}$ animals. At early stages, Mdr2$^{-/-}$IKK2^{Hep-KO} mice also showed more prominent fibrosis in the periportal area as compared to the central area of the liver lobule. It seems plausible that while in Mdr2$^{-/-}$ mice hepatocyte damage is restrained in the vicinity of the bile ducts, the absence of IKK2 in Mdr2$^{-/-}$IKK2^{Hep-KO} hepatocytes facilitates the extension of parenchymal damage spreading into more centrally located areas of the liver lobule. Our experiments showing that IKK2-deficient primary hepatocytes were more sensitive to apoptosis induced by hydrophobic bile acids, suggest that low concentrations of toxic bile acids, which might not reach the threshold required to damage wild-type hepatocytes, could trigger the death of IKK2-deficient cells. This increased sensitivity of IKK2-deficient hepatocytes to bile acid toxicity could explain the spreading of the damage and the severe liver disease in the Mdr2$^{-/-}$IKK2^{Hep-KO} mice.

The original aim of our experiments was to address the role of IKK2-mediated NF-κB activation in hepatocytes in HCC development in Mdr2$^{-/-}$ mice, prompted by the study of Pikarsky et al. [7] who showed that NF-κB inhibition in hepatocytes by expression of an IκBα super-repressor could prevent or delay HCC development in Mdr2-deficient mice. In particular since IKK2^{Hep-KO} mice were shown to develop more liver tumors than wild type mice in response to administration of the chemical carcinogen diethylnitrosamine (DEN), we were curious to test whether IKK2 deficiency would ameliorate or aggravate HCC development in Mdr2$^{-/-}$ mice. However, we found that hepatocyte-specific IKK2 ablation caused a severe cholestatic liver disease already in very young Mdr2$^{-/-}$ mice resulting in poor growth and early lethality, which prevented the study of HCC development as the double knockout mice did not live long enough to analyze tumor development. The oldest Mdr2$^{-/-}$IKK2^{Hep-KO} mouse we obtained was 42 week old and had no signs of HCC development. Moreover, histological evaluation failed to reveal even the earliest premalignant lesions that have been described to occur in the liver of Mdr2$^{-/-}$ mice at

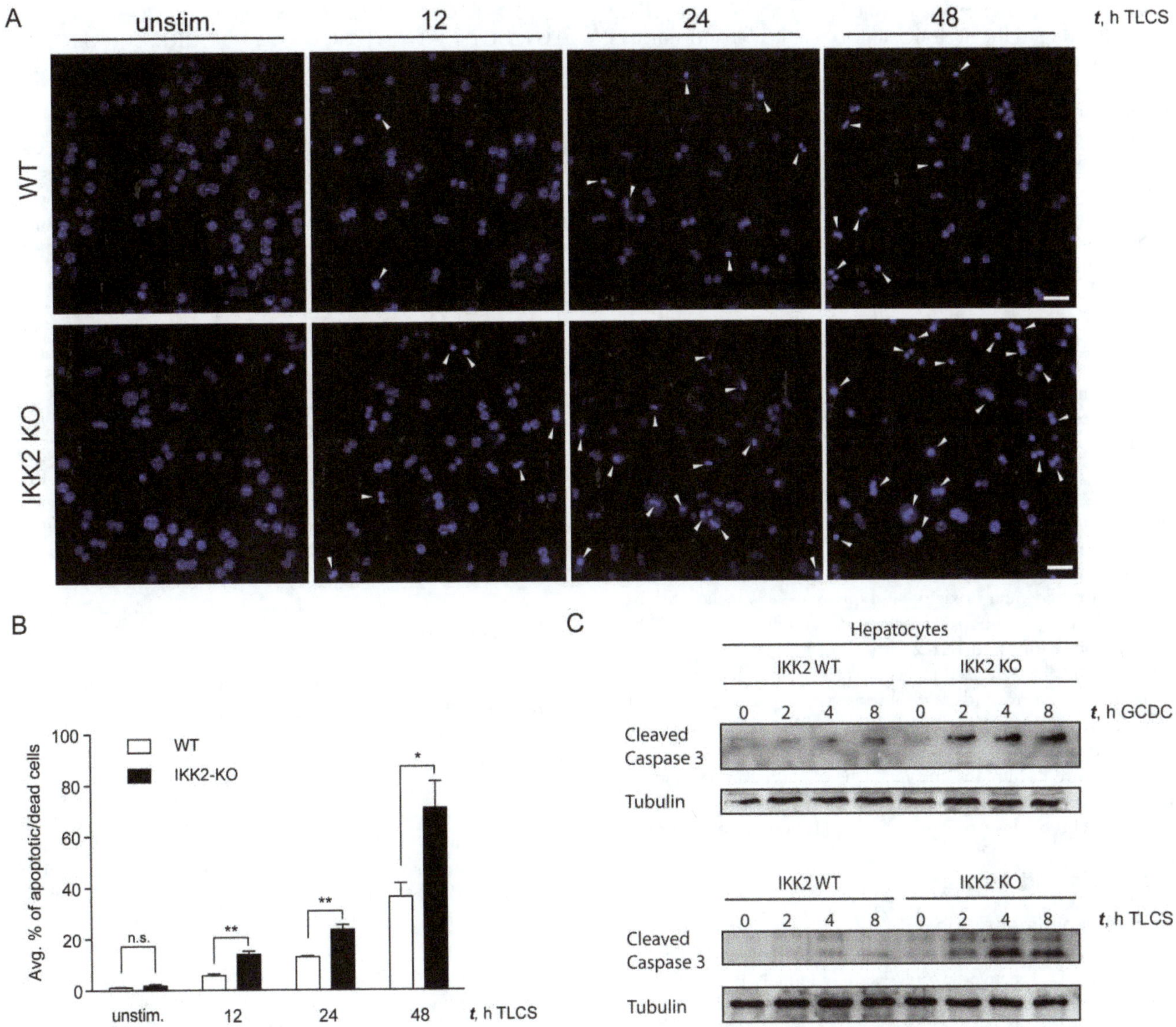

Figure 5. IKK2-deficient hepatocytes are more sensitive to bile acid induced apoptosis compared to wild type cells. (A) Representative images of DAPI stained primary WT and IKK2-KO hepatocyte cultures. Cells were left untreated or were stimulated with taurolithocholic acid 3-sulfate disodium salt (TLCS, 100 μM) for the indicated time periods. Arrowheads show apoptotic hepatocytes as indicated by smaller highly fluorescent nuclei with condensed chromatin. Scale bars, 100 μm. (B) Graphs showing the average proportion of apoptotic hepatocytes from 3 independent experiments. Mean values ± SEM shown. * $p<0,05$; ** $p<0,01$; n.s.: not statistically significant. (C) Immunoblot detection of cleaved Caspase-3. Primary hepatocytes were stimulated with glycochenodeoxy-cholate (GCDC, 50 μM, top) or TLCS (100 μM, bottom) for the indicated time periods. Tubulin serves as loading control.

younger age [6] in our Mdr2$^{-/-}$IKK2$^{Hep\text{-}KO}$ mice (data not shown). However, histological examination of Mdr2$^{-/-}$ mice up to 14 months of age failed to reveal any evidence of malignant or premalignant lesions (data not shown). As the *Mdr2*$^{-/-}$ mice in our colony were backcrossed for at least 4 generations in the C57BL/6 genetic background, it is likely that the C57Bl/6 genetic background prevents HCC development in these mice in contrast to the FVB/N strain in which the malignant phenotype was described [6]. The absence of tumors in our *Mdr2*$^{-/-}$ mice (having more than 90% C57Bl/6 genetic background) is consistent with the results of Klopstock et al, who observed strong reduction in HCC development in *Mdr2*$^{-/-}$ mice having 75% FVB/N and 25% C57Bl/6 genetic background [20]. The C57Bl/6 genetic background does not prevent HCC development only in the *Mdr2*$^{-/-}$ but also in the HCV/ATX mouse model as first described by Keasler et al. [27].

Curiously, Pikarsky et al. showed that NF-κB inhibition in hepatocytes did not affect the early liver disease in Mdr2$^{-/-}$ mice [7]. In contrast, our results presented here show that IKK2-ablation strongly aggravated the liver pathology of Mdr2$^{-/-}$ mice already at a very young age. This apparent discrepancy could be due to the different genetic background of the animals, as our studies were performed in mice backcrossed into the C57Bl/6 genetic background while Pikarsky et al. studied animals in the FVB/N background. Alternatively, qualitative or quantitative differences in the NF-κB inhibition achieved by the two different models could also affect the phenotype. IKK2-ablation may have a stronger inhibitory effect as compared to the expression of the

IκBα super-repressor transgene. Another possibility is that IKK2 knockout prevents the nuclear translocation of a broader range of NF-κB dimers compared to the IκBα-SR transgene, which potently inhibits p50/p65 heterodimers but may be less efficient to prevent nuclear translocation of other dimers. Finally, we cannot exclude the possibility that additional non-NF-κB related functions of IKK2 might also contribute to the observed phenotype in $Mdr2^{-/-}IKK2^{Hep\text{-}KO}$ mice. Further experiments will be required to resolve the differential effect of IKK2 ablation versus IκBα super-repressor expression in *Mdr2*$^{-/-}$ mice.

Interestingly, Mair et al. recently demonstrated that $Mdr2^{-/-}$ mice with liver parenchymal cell specific deficiency of STAT3 developed an aggravated liver disease compared to $Mdr2^{-/-}$ mice. $Mdr2^{-/-}$ mice lacking STAT3 or STAT5 in hepatocytes strikingly resemble the phenotype of $Mdr2^{-/-}IKK2^{Hep\text{-}KO}$ mice [28,29]. In one study the absence of STAT3 rendered primary hepatocytes more vulnerable to apoptosis induced by bile acids as we have observed in our experiments with IKK2 deficient hepatocytes [28]. Thus, NF-κB, STAT3 and STAT5 are important to protect hepatocytes from bile acid toxicity and prevent early liver damage in the $Mdr2^{-/-}$ genetic background.

In conclusion, our results revealed a previously unrecognized essential function of IKK2-mediated signaling to protect hepatocytes from bile acid toxicity and prevent or ameliorate liver damage under conditions of inflammatory biliary disease. Mice lacking both Mdr2 and IKK2 in hepatocytes developed a severe liver disease characterized by cholestasis, major hyperbilirubinemia and severe to end-stage fibrosis, which resulted in muscle wasting, loss of body weight, lethargy and spontaneous death. Thus, $Mdr2^{-/-}IKK2^{Hep\text{-}KO}$ mice remarkably recapitulate chronic liver failure in humans and might be of special importance for the study of the mechanisms contributing to the pathogenesis of end-stage chronic liver disease or its implications on other organs.

Materials and Methods

Animal experimentation

All animal procedures were conducted in accordance with European (EU directive 86/609/EEC), national (TierSchG), and institutional guidelines, and protocols and were approved by local governmental authorities (Landesamt für Natur, Umwelt und Verbraucherschutz Nordrhein-Westfalen) under the license 8.87–50.10.37.09.242.

The general health status of the mice was monitored regularly and assessed by the following criteria: body weight, posture, signs of pain, distress or discomfort and insufficient grooming. In order to minimize suffering, mice were sacrificed when showing deterioration in their general health. C57Bl/6 mice carrying loxP-site flanked ikk2 alleles ($IKK2^{FL}$) [16] were crossed to Albumin-Cre transgenic mice [17] to obtain mice with a hepatocyte specific deletion of IKK2 ($IKK2^{Hep\text{-}KO}$). $IKK2^{Hep\text{-}KO}$ mice were crossed to $Mdr2^{-/-}$ mice to generate double knockout mice ($Mdr2^{-/-}IKK2^{Hep\text{-}KO}$), mice heterozygous for Mdr2 carrying liver-specific deletion of IKK2 ($Mdr2^{+/-}IKK2^{Hep\text{-}KO}$) and also *Mdr2*$^{-/-}$ mice carrying the IKK2 loxP-flanked alleles but not expressing Cre recombinase ($Mdr2^{-/-}IKK2^{FL/FL}$, referred to as $Mdr2^{-/-}$ in the text and figures).

Genotyping

Genotyping-PCR was performed on DNA prepared from tail biopsies of mice. The following primers were used for typing of $IKK2^{floxed}$ and $Mdr2^{-/-}$ and $Mdr2^{+/-}$ mice: Mdr2: 5′-CGGCGAGGATCTCGTCGTGACCCA-3′, 5′-TGATGAAT-ATTGGCGTTGTG-3′, 5′-AATAGGGCAAACAGTCTACA-G-3′. IKK2: 5′ - GTT CAG AGG TTC AGT CCA TTA TC - 3′, 5′ - TAG CCT GCA AGA GAC AAT ACG - 3′, 5′ - TCC TCT CCT CGT CAT CCT TCG - 3′. CRE: 5′ – GTC CAA TTT ACT GAC CGT ACA C - 3′, 5′- CTG TCA CTT GGT CGT GGC AGC - 3′.

Histochemistry and Immunofluorescent Liver stainings

Hematoxylin/Eosin (HE), Masson's trichrome and Sirius red staining of liver sections were performed as recommended by the manufacturer of the respective chemicals or staining kits (Sigma Aldrich). Immunofluorescent detection of Cytokeratin 19 (CK19) was performed on 10–12 μm thick freshly cut cryosections from liver pieces previously kept on −80°C in tissue freezing medium (Jung, Leica Microsystems Nussloch GmbH, Germany). After fixation for 10 min in 4°C acetone and washing in PBS, sections were incubated in blocking buffer (PBS, 3% BSA, 5% FCS) for 60 min. The sections were then incubated overnight at 4°C with Cytokeratin 19 antibody (goat, Santa Cruz, 1:180 in blocking solution). After washing, the secondary antibody (Alexa Fluor 594 donkey anti goat, molecular probes) was applied (1:1000 in PBS, 0.5% BSA) at room temperature for 60 minutes. After washing, sections were incubated with DAPI and mounted with fluoromount. All images were analyzed and acquired on a Leica DM 5500 B microscope system.

TUNEL staining

Dying hepatocytes were detected by the terminal deoxynucleotidyl transferase-mediated nick-end labeling (TUNEL) staining kit according to the manufacturer's instructions (Promega).

PCNA staining

Paraffin-embedded 5 μm sections were used for PCNA staining after antigen retrieval by heating in citrate buffer [13]. The mouse anti-PCNA antibody (Invitrogen) was used at a 1:200 dilution followed by a goat anti-mouse secondary antibody coupled to Alexa 594 (Molecular probes) at a 1:300 dilution. The samples were visualized under a Zeiss LSM510 confocal microscope.

Biochemical analysis

Alanine aminotransferase, bilirubin and alkaline phosphatase were measured on a Cobas chemical analyzer unit according to the manufacturer (Roche Diagnostics, Mannheim, Germany). Whole blood was collected by direct puncture of the heart and the serum was obtained by 20-minute centrifugation at 13000 rpm.. The samples were diluted 1:6 (NaCl 0,9%) for measurements. The results in graphs are depicted multiplied by 6.

Quantification of fibrotic area

The fibrotic area was measured by quantification of Sirius red stained liver tissue relative to the section area. Therefore, at least 10 liver sections per mouse (at 100× magnification) from 2–3 liver lobes were cut at 5 μm and stained with Sirius red. The imageJ software was utilized to measure Sirius red positive tissue area.

Isolation of primary hepatocytes and cell culture experiments

Anesthetized mice were perfused via the vena cava with solution I (EBSS without Ca^{2+} and Mg^{2+}, 0,5 mM EGTA). Subsequently, perfusion with 50 ml of collagenase solution (EBSS with Ca^{2+} and Mg^{2+}, 10 mM Hepes, 3810 U collagenase and 2 mg Trypsin inhibitor) was performed and single cell suspensions of perfused liver were generated using a 70 μm nylon mesh. Hepatocytes were washed twice in high glucose DMEM supplemented with 1% FCS. $2{,}5\times10^6$ cells were seeded on collagen coated 10 cm dishes and after 4 hours the medium was renewed. Cells were stimulated the day after plating for 2, 4 and 8 hours with hydrophobic bile acids. Sodium glycochenodeoxy-cholate (Sigma G0759) was prepared as 1000× Stock in DMSO and added to the hepatocytes in DMEM/1% FCS to a final concentration of 50 μM. Taurolithocholic acid 3-sulfate disodium salt (Sigma T0512) was prepared as 1000× Stock in Methanol and added to the hepatocytes in DMEM/1% FCS to a final concentration of 100 μM. For dead cell counts after stimulation with bile acids primary hepatocytes were plated on fibronectin (BD Bioscience) covered Menzel glasses in 6 well plates and stimulated with taurolithocholic acid 3-sulfate disodium salt (TLCS, Sigma) for the indicated time periods. Apoptotic nuclei were identified by DAPI staining (as indicated by smaller highly fluorescent nuclei with condensed chromatin) [25]. Three independent experiments were performed and apoptotic/dead and total number of cells were counted in 3 random non-overlapping high power fields per timepoint. Unstimulated primary hepatocytes were changed to fresh DMEM/1% FCS medium and kept until the 48 h time point and then further processed as the stimulated cells.

Immunoblot analysis

Cells were lysed with NP40 buffer supplemented with protease- and phosphatase inhibitors (both Roche, Mannheim Germany). 5× SDS sample buffer was added, extracts were boiled for 10 minutes and run on standard 10% or 15% SDS polyacrylamid gels. The following antibodies were used in this study: α-IKK2: cell signaling #2684, 1:1000, α-cleaved caspase-3 (Asp175): cell signaling, #9664, 1:1000, α-Tubulin: Sigma, #T6074, 1:1000, Alkaline phosphatase conjugated anti-rabbit (NA934V) and anti-mouse (NA9310V) antibodies were both from GE Healthcare and were used 1:10.000 and 1:5000 respectively.

Acknowledgments

We are grateful to Elza Mahlberg and Jennifer Buchholz for excellent technical assistance.

Author Contributions

Conceived and designed the experiments: HE MP. Performed the experiments: HE VK JH LO-C. Analyzed the data: HE VK TR MP. Wrote the paper: HE MP.

References

1. Poynard T, Mathurin P, Lai C-L, Guyader D, Poupon R, et al. (2003) A comparison of fibrosis progression in chronic liver diseases. Journal of hepatology 38: 257–265.
2. Iredale JP (2007) Models of liver fibrosis: exploring the dynamic nature of inflammation and repair in a solid organ. The Journal of clinical investigation 117: 539–548.
3. Bataller R, Brenner DA (2005) Liver fibrosis. The Journal of clinical investigation 115: 209–218.
4. Elsharkawy AM, Mann DA (2007) Nuclear factor-kappaB and the hepatic inflammation-fibrosis-cancer axis. Hepatology (Baltimore, Md) 46: 590–597.
5. Trauner M, Fickert P, Wagner M (2007) MDR3 (ABCB4) defects: a paradigm for the genetics of adult cholestatic syndromes. Semin Liver Dis 27: 77–98.
6. Mauad TH, van Nieuwkerk CM, Dingemans KP, Smit JJ, Schinkel AH, et al. (1994) Mice with homozygous disruption of the mdr2 P-glycoprotein gene. A novel animal model for studies of nonsuppurative inflammatory cholangitis and hepatocarcinogenesis. Am J Pathol 145: 1237–1245.
7. Pikarsky E, Porat RM, Stein I, Abramovitch R, Amit S, et al. (2004) NF-kappaB functions as a tumour promoter in inflammation-associated cancer. Nature 431: 461–466.
8. Katzenellenbogen M, Mizrahi L, Pappo O, Klopstock N, Olam D, et al. (2007) Molecular mechanisms of liver carcinogenesis in the mdr2-knockout mice. Mol Cancer Res 5: 1159–1170.
9. Pasparakis M (2009) Regulation of tissue homeostasis by NF-kappaB signalling: implications for inflammatory diseases. Nat Rev Immunol 9: 778–788.
10. Vallabhapurapu S, Karin M (2009) Regulation and function of NF-kappaB transcription factors in the immune system. Annu Rev Immunol 27: 693–733.
11. Schoemaker MH, Gommans WM, Conde de la Rosa L, Homan M, Klok P, et al. (2003) Resistance of rat hepatocytes against bile acid-induced apoptosis in cholestatic liver injury is due to nuclear factor-kappa B activation. Journal of hepatology 39: 153–161.
12. Miyoshi H, Rust C, Guicciardi ME, Gores GJ (2001) NF-kappaB is activated in cholestasis and functions to reduce liver injury. Am J Pathol 158: 967–975.
13. Luedde T, Beraza N, Kotsikoris V, van Loo G, Nenci A, et al. (2007) Deletion of NEMO/IKKgamma in liver parenchymal cells causes steatohepatitis and hepatocellular carcinoma. Cancer Cell 11: 119–132.
14. Maeda S, Kamata H, Luo JL, Leffert H, Karin M (2005) IKKbeta couples hepatocyte death to cytokine-driven compensatory proliferation that promotes chemical hepatocarcinogenesis. Cell 121: 977–990.
15. Luedde T, Heinrichsdorff J, de Lorenzi R, De Vos R, Roskams T, et al. (2008) IKK1 and IKK2 cooperate to maintain bile duct integrity in the liver. Proc Natl Acad Sci U S A 105: 9733–9738.
16. Pasparakis M, Courtois G, Hafner M, Schmidt-Supprian M, Nenci A, et al. (2002) TNF-mediated inflammatory skin disease in mice with epidermis-specific deletion of IKK2. Nature 417: 861–866.
17. Postic C, Magnuson MA (2000) DNA excision in liver by an albumin-Cre transgene occurs progressively with age. Genesis 26: 149–150.
18. Kamath PS (1996) Clinical approach to the patient with abnormal liver test results. Mayo Clin Proc 71: 1089–1094; quiz 1094–1085.
19. Angulo P (2002) Nonalcoholic fatty liver disease. N Engl J Med 346: 1221–1231.
20. Klopstock N, Katzenellenbogen M, Pappo O, Sklair-Levy M, Olam D, et al. (2009) HCV tumor promoting effect is dependent on host genetic background. PLoS One 4: e5025.
21. Reinehr R, Becker S, Keitel V, Eberle A, Grether-Beck S, et al. (2005) Bile salt-induced apoptosis involves NADPH oxidase isoform activation. Gastroenterology 129: 2009–2031.
22. Faubion WA, Guicciardi ME, Miyoshi H, Bronk SF, Roberts PJ, et al. (1999) Toxic bile salts induce rodent hepatocyte apoptosis via direct activation of Fas. The Journal of clinical investigation 103: 137–145.
23. Becker S, Reinehr R, Graf D, vom Dahl S, Haussinger D (2007) Hydrophobic bile salts induce hepatocyte shrinkage via NADPH oxidase activation. Cell Physiol Biochem 19: 89–98.
24. Reinehr R, Graf D, Haussinger D (2003) Bile salt-induced hepatocyte apoptosis involves epidermal growth factor receptor-dependent CD95 tyrosine phosphorylation. Gastroenterology 125: 839–853.
25. Najimi M, Smets F, Sokal E (2009) Hepatocyte apoptosis. Methods Mol Biol 481: 59–74.
26. Katzenellenbogen M, Pappo O, Barash H, Klopstock N, Mizrahi L, et al. (2006) Multiple adaptive mechanisms to chronic liver disease revealed at early stages of liver carcinogenesis in the Mdr2-knockout mice. Cancer Res 66: 4001–4010.
27. Keasler VV, Lerat H, Madden CR, Finegold MJ, McGarvey MJ, et al. (2006) Increased liver pathology in hepatitis C virus transgenic mice expressing the hepatitis B virus X protein. Virology 347: 466–475.
28. Mair M, Zollner G, Schneller D, Musteanu M, Fickert P, et al. Signal transducer and activator of transcription 3 protects from liver injury and fibrosis in a mouse model of sclerosing cholangitis. Gastroenterology 138: 2499–2508.
29. Blaas L, Kornfeld JW, Schramek D, Musteanu M, Zollner G, et al. Disruption of the growth hormone–signal transducer and activator of transcription 5–insulinlike growth factor 1 axis severely aggravates liver fibrosis in a mouse model of cholestasis. Hepatology (Baltimore, Md) 51: 1319–1326.

9

β-Catenin Loss in Hepatocytes Promotes Hepatocellular Cancer after Diethylnitrosamine and Phenobarbital Administration to Mice

Prince Kwaku Awuah[1], Byung Han Rhieu[1], Sucha Singh[1], Amalea Misse[1], Satdarshan P. S. Monga[1,2*]

1 Department of Pathology, University of Pittsburgh, Pittsburgh, Pennsylvania, United States of America, **2** Department of Medicine, University of Pittsburgh, Pittsburgh, Pennsylvania, United States of America

Abstract

Hepatocellular Carcinoma (HCC) is the fifth most common cancer worldwide. β-Catenin, the central orchestrator of the canonical Wnt pathway and a known oncogene is paramount in HCC pathogenesis. Administration of phenobarbital (PB) containing water (0.05% w/v) as tumor promoter following initial injected intraperitoneal (IP) diethylnitrosamine (DEN) injection (5 μg/gm body weight) as a tumor inducer is commonly used model to study HCC in mice. Herein, nine fifteen-day male β-catenin knockout mice (KO) and fifteen wild-type littermate controls (WT) underwent DEN/PB treatment and were examined for hepatic tumorigenesis at eight months. Paradoxically, a significantly higher tumor burden was observed in KO ($p<0.05$). Tumors in KO were β-catenin and glutamine synthetase negative and HGF/Met, EGFR & IGFR signaling was unremarkable. A significant increase in PDGFRα and its ligand PDGF-CC leading to increased phosphotyrosine-720-PDGFRα was observed in tumor-bearing KO mice ($p<0.05$). Simultaneously, these livers displayed increased cell death, stellate cell activation, hepatic fibrosis and cell proliferation. Further, PDGF-CC significantly induced hepatoma cell proliferation especially following β-catenin suppression. Our studies also demonstrate that the utilized DEN/PB protocol in the WT C57BL/6 mice did not select for β-catenin gene mutations during hepatocarcinogenesis. Thus, DEN/PB enhanced HCC in mice lacking β-catenin in the liver may be due to their ineptness at regulating cell survival, leading to enhanced fibrosis and regeneration through PDGFRα activation. β-Catenin downregulation also made hepatoma cells more sensitive to receptor tyrosine kinases and thus may be exploited for therapeutics.

Editor: William B. Coleman, University of North Carolina School of Medicine, United States of America

Funding: This work was supported by National Institutes of Health grants 1R01DK62277 (National Institute of Digestive Diseases and Kidney) and 1R01CA124414 (National Cancer Institute) to S.P.S.M. and by Rango's Fund for the Enhancement of Pathology Research. P.K.A. was funded in part by T32 EB001026 (National Institute of Biomedical Imaging and Bioengineering). The funders had no role in study design, data collection and analysis, decision to publish, or preparation of the manuscript.

Competing Interests: The authors have declared that no competing interests exist.

* E-mail: smonga@pitt.edu

Introduction

Hepatocellular Carcinoma (HCC) is the fifth most common cancer and the third cause of cancer death worldwide [1]. There is a strong need to delineate the molecular alterations responsible for the initiation and exacerbation of this disease. In order to study the cellular and molecule perturbations in HCC, many preclinical strategies employ the use of genetic and chemical models of carcinogenesis. Administration of diethylnitrosamine (DEN) alone or in conjunction with phenobarbital (PB) in mice is frequently used to induce HCC in mice.

One pathway of critical importance in HCC is the Wnt/β-catenin signaling. β-Catenin is the central effector of the canonical Wnt signaling, which is a highly conserved pathway regulating critical cellular processes such as proliferation, differentiation, survival and self-renewal [2,3,4,5]. In the absence of Wnt, β-catenin is phosphorylated at amino-terminal serine and threonine residues and targeted for ubiquitination [6]. Upon binding of Wnt protein to its cell surface receptor Frizzled and co-receptor low-density lipoprotein– related protein 5/6 (LRP5/6), a signal is transduced through disheveled that allows for inactivation of degradation complex comprised of glycogen synthase kinase 3β (GSK3β), adenomatous polyposis coli gene product (APC) and casein kinase Iα, which allows β-catenin to dissociate and translocate to the nucleus to bind to lymphoid enhancer-binding factor/T cell factor (LEF/TCF) family of proteins to transactivate target genes. The Wnt/β-catenin pathway has been implicated in a subset of HCC where activating mutations in the β-catenin gene (*CTNNB1*) have been reported in 20%–40% of patients [7,8]. Knockdown of β-catenin in hepatoma cells leads to decreased growth and survival. For the aforementioned reasons, β-catenin is a well-recognized oncogene and considered a valuable therapeutic target.

With this background, we hypothesized that lack of β-catenin in hepatocytes might protect against chemical-induced carcinogenesis especially in a model where HCC is conceived through tumor induction by DEN and tumor promotion through the continuous use of PB [9,10]. We used male conditional hepatocyte-specific β-catenin knockout (KO) mice and sex-matched wild-type littermate controls (WT) to study tumorigenesis in response to DEN/PB. We report a paradoxical increase in hepatic tumorigenesis in the absence of β-catenin that was attributable to enhanced injury, fibrosis and ensuing regeneration, which appear to be driven by a rather non-classical epithelial receptor tyrosine kinase receptor PDGFRα. We also demonstrate that utilizing the commonly employed DEN/PB protocol in C57BL/6 mice, the tumorigenesis does not occur through β-catenin mutations as is observed in C3H mice. Lastly, β-catenin inhibition lead to PDGFRα activation and thus may make the hepatoma cells more amenable to receptor tyrosine kinases inhibition for therapies.

Results

β-Catenin loss in hepatocytes engenders enhanced hepatocarcinogenesis in mice in response to DEN/PB

WT and KO male mice (C57BL/6) were given a single dose (5 μg/gram) of DEN injection at postnatal day 14 days and two weeks later allowed *ad libitum* access to PB containing drinking water for 8 months at which time mice were examined for liver tumors (Fig. 1A). Intriguingly, the mice lacking β-catenin in hepatocytes displayed significantly enhanced tumorigenesis than WT mice that was grossly appreciable as larger and greater numbers of tumors (Fig. 1B). H&E staining was employed to also determine the microscopic tumor foci in both groups of animals (Fig. 1C). The total numbers of foci were counted in representative sections from four lobes from the KO and WT, which show significantly more tumors in KO as compared to the WT ($p<0.05$) (Fig. 1D).

β-Catenin KO livers after DEN/PB treatment shows increased cell death, stellate cell activation and fibrosis and tumor proliferation

Next, we addressed the cellular mechanisms that may be the basis of enhanced tumorigenesis in KO. We identify higher numbers of TUNEL-positive hepatocytes in KO at 8 months after DEN/PB as compared to similarly treated WT, suggesting greater cell death (Fig. 2A). There was an accompanying increase in hepatic parenchymal cell proliferation in KO that exceeded that of WT (Fig. 2A). In addition, KO mice exhibited a dramatic increase in the numbers of α-smooth muscle actin, which identifies activated stellate cells that are responsible for collagen deposition and fibrosis (Fig. 2A). Concomitant to stellate cell activation, we observed enhanced fibrosis by Masson Trichrome staining in the KO as compared to the WT (Fig. 2B). In fact only one of the 15 WT animals after DEN/PB challenge showed fibrosis, which was comparable to fibrosis in the KO. All together, our results suggest that greater tumorigenesis in KO livers was associated with significantly greater cell death and proliferation (Fig. 2C), and hepatic fibrosis as well.

Tumors in KO livers after DEN/PB are not composed of β-catenin-positive hepatocytes

Since there have been reports from our lab and others that in response to specific injuries, there is pressure on hepatocytes that may have escaped cre-mediated deletion, our first goal was to ascertain if livers exposed to DEN/PB from KO group showed any reappearance of β-catenin especially when compared to the WT. A representative WB showed that all KO livers from DEN/PB exposed mice expressed dramatically lower levels of β-catenin as compared to WT by western blots (Fig. 3A). This was also verified by a detailed immunohistochemical analysis included in a forthcoming section (Table 1 and Fig. 4). The low level of β-catenin in KO livers represents its presence in the non-parenchymal cells of the liver that show no albumin cre-mediated recombination. Similarly analysis presented from representative KO and WT livers also showed absence of glutamine synthetase, a surrogate target gene of β-catenin signaling in the KO (Fig. 3A). Cyclin-D1, another prominent target of β-catenin in liver and elsewhere was increased in most WT, whereas 8/9 KO showed very low or absent cyclin-D1 in response to DEN/PB (Fig. 3A and not shown). C-Myc, another target of β-catenin, was ironically higher in KO as compared to WT mice after DEN/PB exposure as shown in a representative western blot (Fig. 3A). Thus KO livers after DEN/PB continue to be negative for β-catenin after 8 months.

Tumors in KO livers after DEN/PB are not associated with activation of traditional HCC associated receptor tyrosine kinases. Due to a paradoxical increase in DEN/PB-induced tumorigenesis in KO, we next explored possible molecular mechanisms. Both epidermal growth factor (EGF) signaling and hepatocyte growth factor (HGF) signaling are critical players in the development and exacerbation of HCC [11]. We explored both total and phosphorylated status of receptors of these receptor tyrosine kinases (RTKs) in livers from DEN/PB-treated KO and WT mice. Interestingly we noted a decrease in total and phosphorylated levels of c-Met, the HGF receptor in KO animals as compared to WT (Fig. 3B). Both total and phosphorylated levels of EGFR between WT and KO animals remain unaltered (Fig. 3B). We also examined insulin like growth factor receptor, another signaling pathway implicated in HCC [11]. We noted higher levels of its phosphorylation in the WT as compared to KO (Fig. 3B). Thus, classical RTKs do not appear to be responsible for enhanced HCC in KO but p-Met and P-IGFR are prominently induced in tumor bearing WT mice indicating their important role in HCC.

Immunohistochemical characterization of KO and WT liver tumors for β-catenin and PDGFRα

We next characterized the tumors observed in the WT and KO by immunohistochemistry for β-catenin localization. Around 31% of total tumor foci in WT mice showed nuclear β-catenin (Table 1, Fig. 4). Out of 63 observed foci in 9 KO mice, only two were composed of β-catenin-positive tumor cells that exhibited its nuclear/cytoplasmic localization (data not shown) while others were negative (Fig. 4). This substantiated the observations in Fig. 3A and also demonstrates that almost all tumors in this group were comprised by β-catenin-negative hepatocytes and cannot be due to expansion of cells, which may have retained β-catenin due to incomplete albumin-cre recombination.

We next investigated PDGFRα signaling, which has been implicated in HCC and is involved in tumor growth, angiogenesis, and maintenance of tumor microenvironment [12,13,14]. 54.5% of all tumor foci in the WT mice showed cytoplasmic PDGFRα expression (Table 1). We found around 94% of tumor foci in KO to be strongly positive for PDGFRα in the cytoplasm of tumor cells (Table 1, Fig. 4). Only four foci were negative for PDGFRα. The two tumor foci that were β-catenin-positive in the KO livers were simultaneously positive for PDGFRα.

In an additional analysis, 9 of the 55 tumors observed in the WT were concomitantly positive for both PDGFRα and nuclear β-catenin, while others were positive for either one of the two (Table 1, Fig. 4). A small fraction of tumors were negative for both these proteins. The two tumors that were composed of β-catenin-positive hepatocytes in the KO were also positive for PDGFRα signaling (Table 1). Overall, PDGFRα expression was higher and also in greater numbers of tumor foci in the KO as compared to the WT 8 months after DEN/PB exposure.

DEN/PB induced increased tumorigenesis is associated with activation of PDGFRα signaling. To further verify PDGFRα increase in the KO over WT after DEN/PB, we utilized western blots analysis.

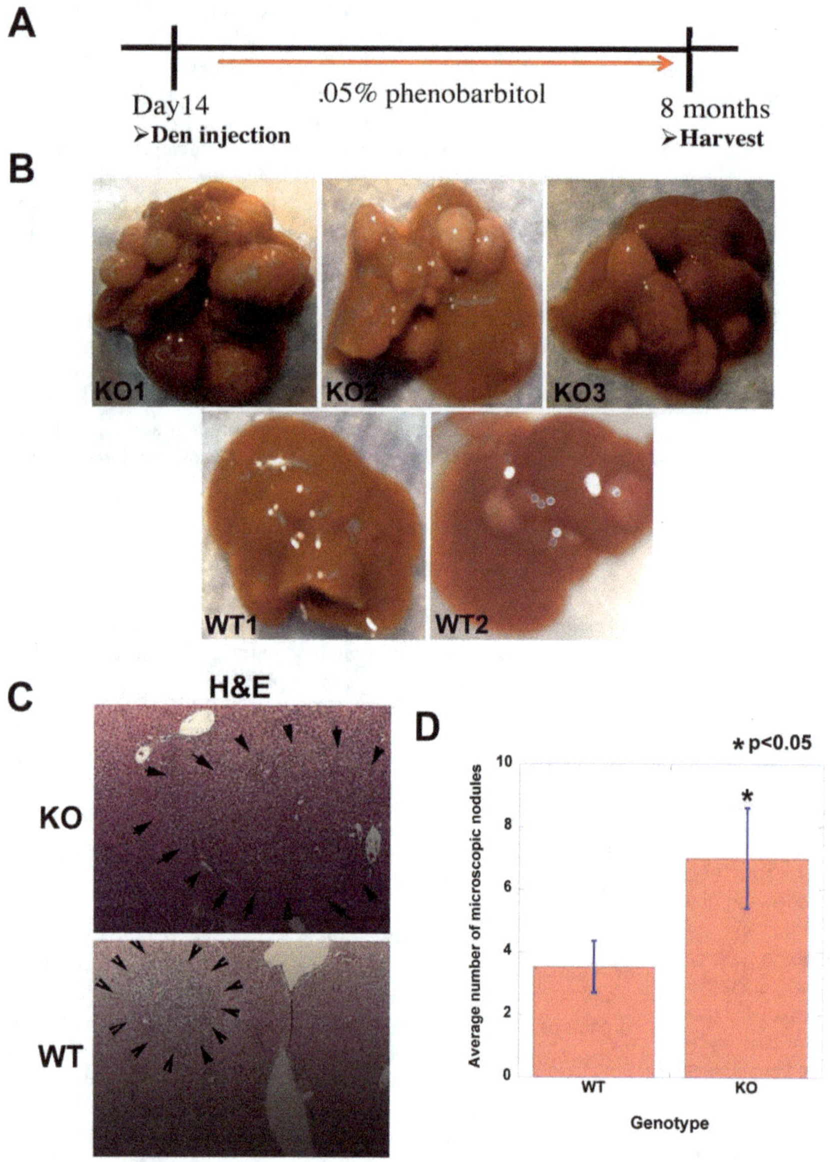

Figure 1. Enhanced tumorigenesis in β-catenin KO mice exposed to DEN/PB regimen. Experimental strategy summarizing DEN/PB treatment in KO and WT mice. A. Representative photographs of tumor-bearing livers in DEN/PB treated KO and WT mice at the time of harvest at 8 months of age. B. DEN/PB induced microscopic tumor foci (outlined by arrowheads) visualized by H&E in WT and KO livers at 8 months of age. C. A significant increase in microscopic tumor foci in KO as compared to WT ($p<0.05$). Tumors were counted from H&E stained sections representing 4 liver lobes from each KO and WT animals on DEN/PB protocol.

PDGFRα protein levels were higher in the KO than the WT livers (Fig. 5A), and this difference was statistically significant (Fig. 5B). There was a modest increase in PDGFRβ levels in the KO livers (Fig. 5A). We also identified a noteworthy increase in total protein levels of selective PDGFRα ligand PDGF-CC while PDGF-AA or PDGF-BB remained unaltered between the two groups (Fig. 5C).

To determine consequences of enhanced PDGF-CC/PDGFRα levels in KO we assessed levels of PDGFRα phosphorylation at several specific tyrosine residues using antibodies listed in methods. As shown in densitometric analyses, a significant increase in Tyr720-PDGFRα ($p<0.05$) (Fig. 5D) but not in Tyr849-PDGFRα (Fig. 5E) or Tyr572/574- and Tyr754-PDGFRα (not shown) was observed in the KO. These observations demonstrate PDGFRα activation in KO, which may be playing an important role in hepatocarcinogenesis.

PDGFRα ligand stimulates hepatoma cell proliferation only upon β-catenin suppression

To further ascertain the relevance of PDGFRα signaling in absence of β-catenin, we utilized human hepatoma cells. PDGF-CC was unable to induce any significant increase in Hep3B cell DNA synthesis when compared to HCl, which was utilized to reconstitute PDGF in almost confluent cell cultures (Fig. 6). β-Catenin knockdown when compared to control siRNA transfection, significantly lowered thymidine incorporation in Hep3B cells ($p<0.0005$) (Fig. 6). Only upon β-catenin silencing, was PDGF-CC treatment able to induce significant DNA synthesis in Hep3B cells as compared to HCl ($p<0.005$). Thus β-catenin suppression enabled PDGF-CC to be mitogenic to Hep3B cells.

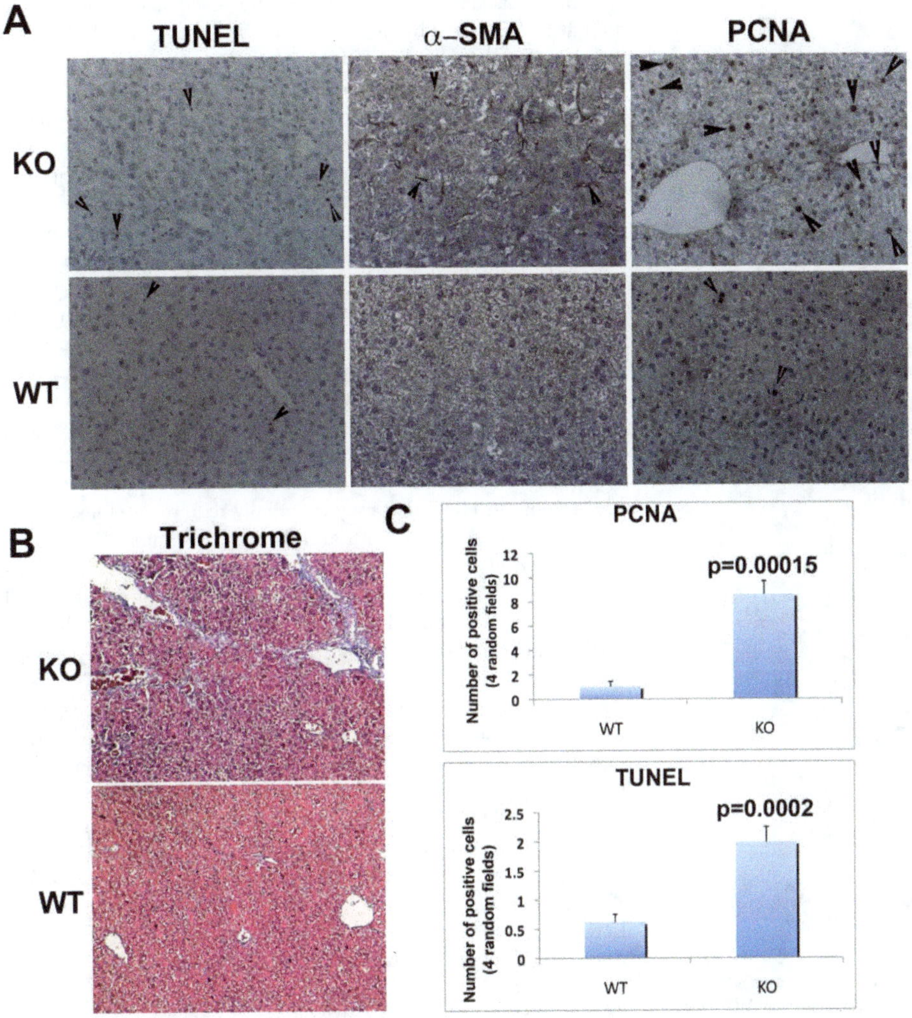

Figure 2. Tumorigenesis in KO mice following DEN/PB treatment is associated with greater injury, fibrosis and regeneration. A. Representative tumor-bearing KO livers show increased parenchymal cell death (TUNEL), greater stellate cell activation (α-SMA) and increased parenchymal cell proliferation (PCNA) as compared to WT. B. Increased hepatic fibrosis (blue) in tumor-bearing KO livers is evident by Masson Trichrome staining as compared to control. C. PCNA- and TUNEL-positive cells were counted in 4 random sections of 5 representative KO and WT livers. A significant increase in both PCNA and TUNEL positive parenchymal cells was evident in KO livers as compared to WT after DEN/PB treatment.

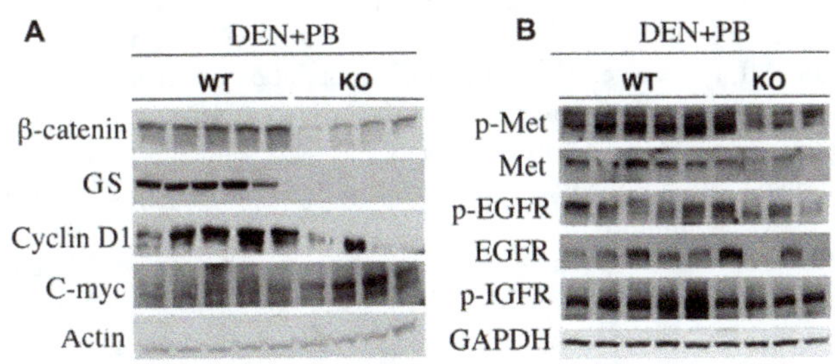

Figure 3. Molecular signaling in tumor-bearing KO and WT mice. A. Representative western blot analysis from 5 WT and 4 KO tumor-bearing livers shows low β-catenin, absent GS and dramatically lower cyclin-D1 in KO whereas c-Myc levels were increased. Actin verifies equal loading. B. Examination of RTK in the same sets of animals shows notably lower phospho-Met and phospho-IGFR and only marginally lower phospho-EGFR, in KO than WT livers by western blots. GAPDH verifies comparable loading.

Discussion

To understand the molecular and cellular basis of HCC in patients, several preclinical models are in use including DEN or DEN/PB regimens in rodents. DEN is a commonly used carcinogen to induce HCC in rodent models, however it has high strain specificity. In C57BL/129Sv×C3H/He mice, a strain more susceptible to hepatocarcinogenesis, DEN injection at around 6 weeks of age at a dose of 90 μg/gm body weight, induces HCC through Ha-Ras mutations, while inclusion of PB in drinking water after 3 weeks of DEN, promotes tumorigenesis due to *CTNNB1* mutations. [15]. However, another study in male B6C3F1 mice, obtained by interbreeding female C57BL/6J and male C3H/HeJ mice, injected DEN at 10 μg/gm body weight at 3 weeks of age without PB, showed HCC via *CTNNB1* mutations [16]. Another model utilizes DEN at a dose of 5 μg/gm body in C57BL/6 mice, a strain relatively resistant to HCC. Here, DEN induces DNA adducts in hepatocytes undergoing cell division, and eventually leads to development of HCC [17,18]. Inclusion of PB enhances tumorigenesis via its tumor promoting ability [9,10]. In

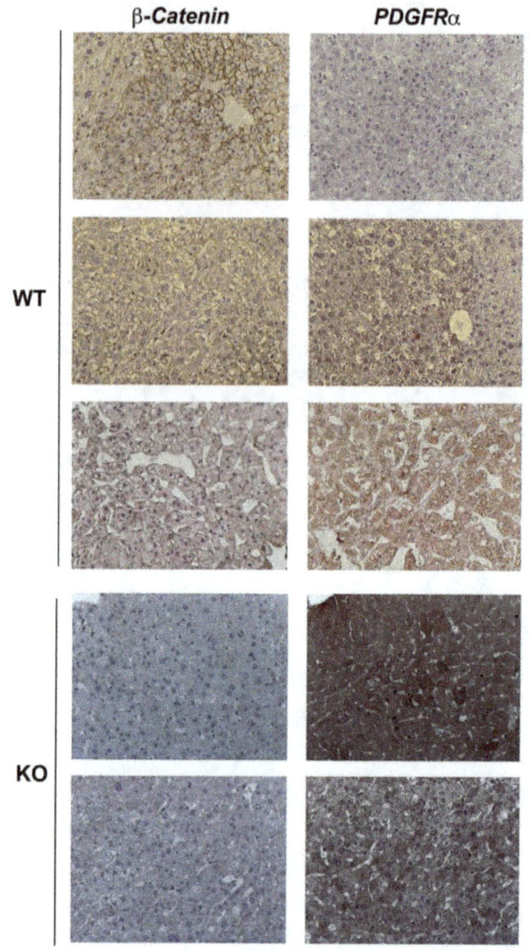

Figure 4. β-Catenin and PDGFRα immunohistochemistry in tumors in WT and KO exposed to DEN/PB. Tumors in WT were heterogeneous and were either positive for both β-catenin and PDGFRα, or for either one of them. In KO, almost all tumors lacked any β-catenin and showed intense PDGFRα-positivity.

our study, we show that unlike C57BL/129Sv×C3H/He mice, DEN/PB induced liver tumors in the C57BL/6 mice did not exhibit nuclear/cytoplasmic localization of β-catenin and hence does not selectively cause HCC via *CTNNB1* mutations. Thus mouse strain consideration for studying tumorigenesis in response to specific protocols is highly relevant.

Many pathways broadly categorized into Ras/MAPK, PIK3CA/AKT, and Wnt/β-catenin signaling, have been shown to be of significance in HCC [11,19]. β-Catenin, the central orchestrator of Wnt signaling, is a known oncogene due to its implications in a variety of cancers, including 20%–40% of all HCCs [20]. Intriguingly though, overexpression of either wild-type or mutant form of β-catenin in murine livers is unable to induce spontaneous HCC [21,22,23,24]. However, in the presence of another 'hit' in the form of a transgene or a chemical carcinogen, these various mice show enhanced tumorigenesis [23,25,26]. Paradoxically, conditional loss of β-catenin in hepatocytes in C57BL/6 mice led to an unexpectedly higher susceptibility to DEN-induced HCC [27]. Another group also recently showed demonstrated increased tumorigenesis in KO mice in response to DEN/PB, *albeit* in C3H/N mice [28]. In the current study, we provide evidence that β-catenin KO mice in C57BL/6 background subjected to DEN-mediated tumor induction at P14 followed by tumor promotion 2 weeks later by PB also led to a dramatically higher tumor burden.

DEN or DEN/PB induced HCC in any strain of mice is not typically associated with any hepatic fibrosis. However, in the β-catenin conditional null mice DEN/PB exposure led to development of HCC, which was associated with hepatic fibrosis and is in line with recent studies by others and us [27,28]. We also saw an increase in cell death and resulting increase in cell proliferation. In fact we identified increased stellate cell activation, a modest increase in PDGFRβ and ensuing hepatic fibrosis. These data indicate that β-catenin loss makes livers more prone to genotoxic injury and eventually tumorigenesis mimicking the predominant scenario of human HCC where tumors often occurs in cirrhotic background [29]. Role of β-catenin in regulating redox state has been implied in many recent studies where its interactions with HIF1α, FOXO3 and others may be critical [30,31]. It will thus be important to understand the basis of such 'tumor suppressive' roles of β-catenin in HCC that may eventually require careful selection of patients to be treated with anti-β-catenin therapies [32].

To ascertain the molecular basis of HCC in the absence of β-catenin, we were interested in signaling pathways that are well known in the development and exacerbation of HCC. C-Met and IGFR phosphorylation was increased in WT but not in KO mice while EGFR activation was only mildly elevated in WT. Thus while these RTK's may be playing an important role in tumorigenesis in the WT exposed to DEN/PB, their participation in KO is unlikely. Based on our previous findings in DEN-induced tumorigenesis in KO [27] and independent studies showing an important role of PDGFR signaling in HCC [12,13,14], we investigated its expression and activation in DEN/PB studies. PDGFRα levels were significantly upregulated in KO after DEN/PB-exposure. In addition, PDGF-CC a selective ligand of PDGFRα, whose overexpression in liver-specific transgenic mice has been shown to induce cirrhosis and HCC [33], was also increased in KO. In fact PDGF-CC was localized to hepatocytes in KO exposed to DEN/PB (data not shown) suggesting an autocrine loop of signaling. The results obtained from thymidine incorporation assay in the Hep3B cells, corroborates *in vivo* findings. While decreased cell proliferation was observed in hepatoma cells after β-catenin knockdown [34], PDGF-CC promoted their mitogenesis more robustly only after β-catenin suppression that leads to PDGFRα upregulation [27]. This also verifies PDGFRα signaling as a means of escape from β-catenin therapeutic inhibition.

PDGFRα overexpression in the presence of increased PDGF-CC led to increased Tyr720-PDGFRα in tumor bearing KO but not WT livers after DEN/PB. Phosphorylation at tyrosine 720 is known to activate phosphatase SHP2, which in turn dephosphorylates Src, leading to its activation [35]. Src activation has been shown to induce c-Myc, an important proto-oncogene [36], which was concomitantly elevated in KO. Other tyrosine sites in PDGFRα showed inconspicuous changes in phosphorylation between the KO and WT and thus may be of lesser relevance in the current tumorigenesis model.

Only around 3% of all tumors in the 9 KO's at 8 months after the DEN/PB regimen were β-catenin-positive tumors that may be due to 'leaky' cre-recombinase. β-Catenin-negative tumors were also negative for GS and mostly negative for cyclin-D1. We have not followed any animals in this study beyond 8 months. Others have recently reported extensive spontaneous repopulation in KO livers *albeit* at 18–20 months of age [37]. One group has reported a more robust spontaneous repopulation and hepatic adenomatosis in KO, which has not been reported by any other group working

Table 1. Summary of immunohistochemical findings of microscopic tumor foci for β-catenin and PDGFRα.

SAMPLE	NUMBER OF TUMOR FOCI	β-CATENIN-POSITIVE FOCI		PDGFRα-POSITIVE FOCI	NUMBER OF FOCI POSITIVE FOR BOTH N/C	FIGURE 4
		N/C	M	C	β-CATENIN & PDGFRα	
WT1	2	0	1	0	0	
WT2	2	0	0	2	0	
WT3	0	0	0	0	0	
WT4	4	4	3	2	2	
WT5	0	0	0	0	0	
WT6	9	2	1	6	1	
WT7	2	0	1	0	0	
WT8	6	5	5	3	3	
WT9	4	1	4	1	0	X
WT10	2	2	2	2	2	X
WT11	6	0	6	4	0	
WT12	2	0	2	1	0	
WT13	2	1	2	2	1	
WT14	11	2	8	7	1	X
WT15	1	0	1	0	0	
	55	*17*	*36*	*30*	*9*	
KO1	17	1	0	17	1	X
KO2	11	0	0	10	0	
KO3	3	0	0	3	0	X
KO4	4	0	0	4	0	
KO5	2	0	0	2	0	
KO6	6	0	0	6	0	
KO7	6	1	0	4	1	
KO8	10	0	0	10	0	
KO9	4	0	0	3	0	
	63	*2*	*0*	*59*	*2*	

Abbreviations: WT-wildtype; KO-knockout; N/C- nuclear/cytoplasmic; M-membranous; C-cytoplasmic.

with the β-catenin conditional knockout mice [38]. The only instance of extensive repopulation in the KO mice in our experience was observed after continuous administration of diet containing 0.1% 3,5-diethoxycarbonyl-1,4-dihydrocollidine (DDC) for 5 months [39]. In fact KO mice have been studied after partial hepatectomy, methionine-choline deficient diet, alcohol diet or DEN and have exhibited lack of hepatic repopulation with β-catenin-positive hepatocytes [27,31,40,41].

Materials and Methods

Animal studies

All animal experiments were performed under the guidelines of the National Institutes of Health and the Institutional Animal Use and Care Committee at the University of Pittsburgh. The studies performed in the current report were approved by the Institutional Animal Use and Care Committee at the University of Pittsburgh. Mice with conditional deletion of β-catenin in hepatocytes with genotype- $Ctnnb1^{loxp/loxp}$;$Alb\text{-}Cre^{+/-}$ are refered to as knockout mice (KO) and have been described previously [41]. Littermates with any of the following genotypes- $Ctnnb1^{loxp/loxp}$;$Alb\text{-}Cre^{-/-}$, $Ctnnb1^{loxp/WT}$;$Alb\text{-}Cre^{+/-}$, $Ctnnb1^{loxp/WT}$;$Alb\text{-}Cre^{-/-}$ are referred to as wild-type or WT. These mice are in C57BL/6 background.

Male KO (n = 9) and WT (n = 15) mice were injected intraperitoneally with DEN (Sigma-Aldrich, Inc.) at a dose of 5 μg/gram body weight at postnatal day 14 and from day 28 onwards the drinking water available *ad libitum* contained phenobarbital (PB) (0.05% w/v). Water containing fresh PB was prepared weekly for the duration of the studies. Mice were sacrificed at 8 months and liver collected for histology and protein analysis.

Western blot Analysis: Total tissue lysates prepared in radio immuno-precipitation assay (RIPA) buffer containing 1% IgePAL CA-630, 0.5% Sodium Deoxycholate, 0.1% SDS in 1 × PBS along with protease & phosphate inhibitor (1:100) (Thermo Scientific). Proteins were resolved on sodium dodecyl sulfate polyacrylamide gel electrophoresis in 4–15% gels and then transferred to Immobilon-P membranes (Millipore, Bedford, MA) in transfer buffer containing 10% methanol. Membranes were probed with primary antibodies (see below) in Tris-buffered saline with Tween-20 containing 5% nonfat milk or BSA. Horseradish peroxidase–conjugated secondary antibodies were used at 1:50,000 dilution and signal assessed with Super Signal West Pico chemiluminescence substrate (Pierce, Rockford, IL) and autoradiography. The

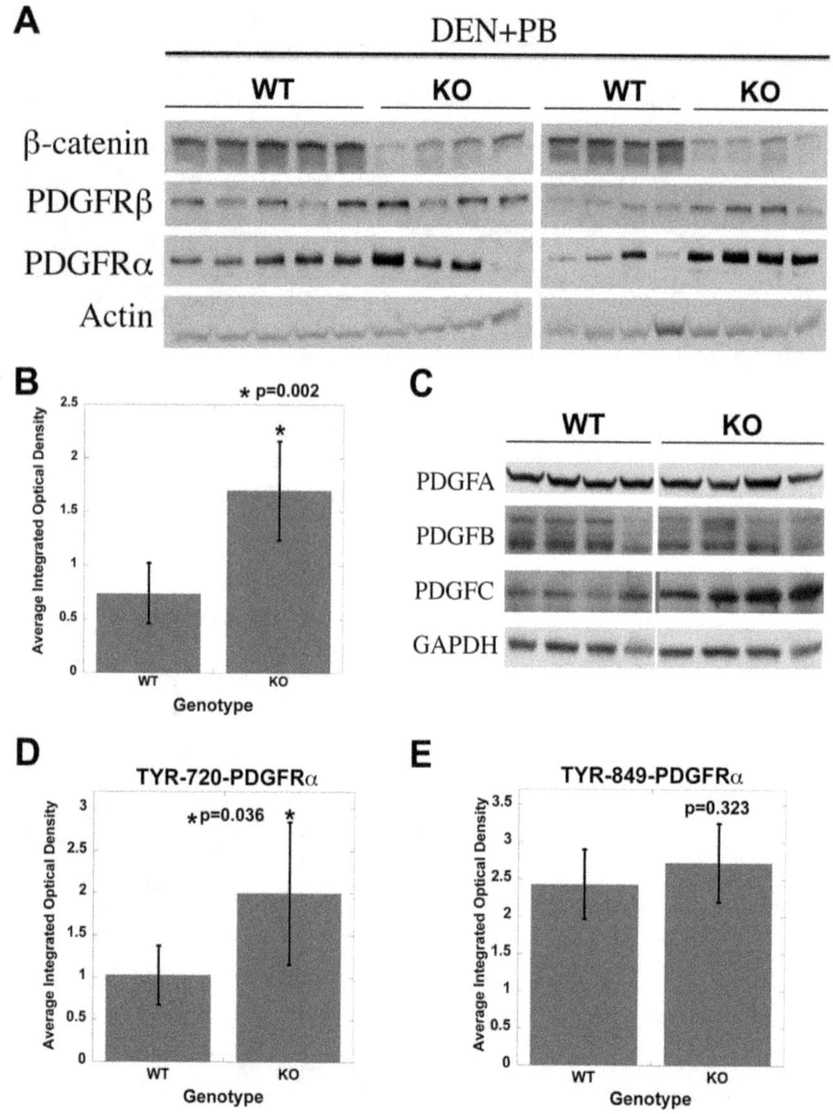

Figure 5. Tumor-bearing KO mice display active PDGFRα signaling when compared to WT. A. Representative western blots from 8 KO and 9 WT show a dramatic increase in total levels of PDGFRα and modest increase in PDGFRβ in the KO. Actin loading verifies equal loading. B. Average integrated optical density (IOD) obtained from scanned autoradiographs shown in Fig. 5A revealed significantly higher PDGFRα levels in KO ($p = 0.002$). C. Western blot from representative samples shows a dramatic increase in PDGF-CC, a ligand for PDGFRα in KO whereas PDGF-AA and BB remained unremarkable between the two groups. D. Bar graph depicts a significant increase in Tyr720-PDGFRα in KO as compared to WT ($p<0.05$). E. Insignificant differences were evident in Tyr-849-PDGFRα between the WT and KO.

films (Molecular Technology Sales, St. Louise, MI) were scanned to obtain integrated optic densitomery (IOD) using NIH Imager software. The average IOD for a protein was compared between the KO and WT groups and assessed for statistical significance by student *t* test and $p<0.05$ was considered significant.

Antibodies. Primary antibodies used for Western blotting included: c-Met (1:500), phospho-Met Tyr1234/1235 (1:1000), EGFR (1:1000), phospho-PDGFRα Tyr849 (1:1000), phospho-IGFR (1:1000) all from Cell Signaling Technology; β-catenin (1:1000) from BD Biosciences; PDGFRα (1:180), PDGFRβ (1:500), phospho-EGFR (1:500), phospho-PDGFRα Tyr720 (1:200), c-myc (1:200), PDGFA (1:200), PDGFB (1:200), PDGFC (1:200), phospho-PDGFRα Tyr754 (1:200), Glutamine Synthethase (1:200), and GAPDH (1:1000) all from Santa Cruz Biotechnology; phospho-PDGFRα Tyr572/574 (1:800, Invitrogen); Cyclin D1(1:200, Neomarkers); alpha smooth muscle actin (1:300, Abcam); and β-actin (1:2000, Millipore).

Histology and immunohistochemistry

Four-micron sections of paraffin-embedded liver tissues were used for histology and immunohistochemical staining. Hematoxylin and Eosin (H&E) staining was employed to identify tumor foci. Typically four representative lobes from each mouse were included on each slide. Tumor foci were identified based on characteristic attributes such as basophilic cytoplasm and mitotic figures. For comparison, total number of microscopic nodules were counted and average numbers compared for statistical significant by student *t* test with $p<0.05$ considered significant.

For immunohistochemistry, antigen retrieval was achieved both by steam cooking or boiling the slides in microwave in citrate buffer for 20 minutes or 10 minutes, respectively. The sections

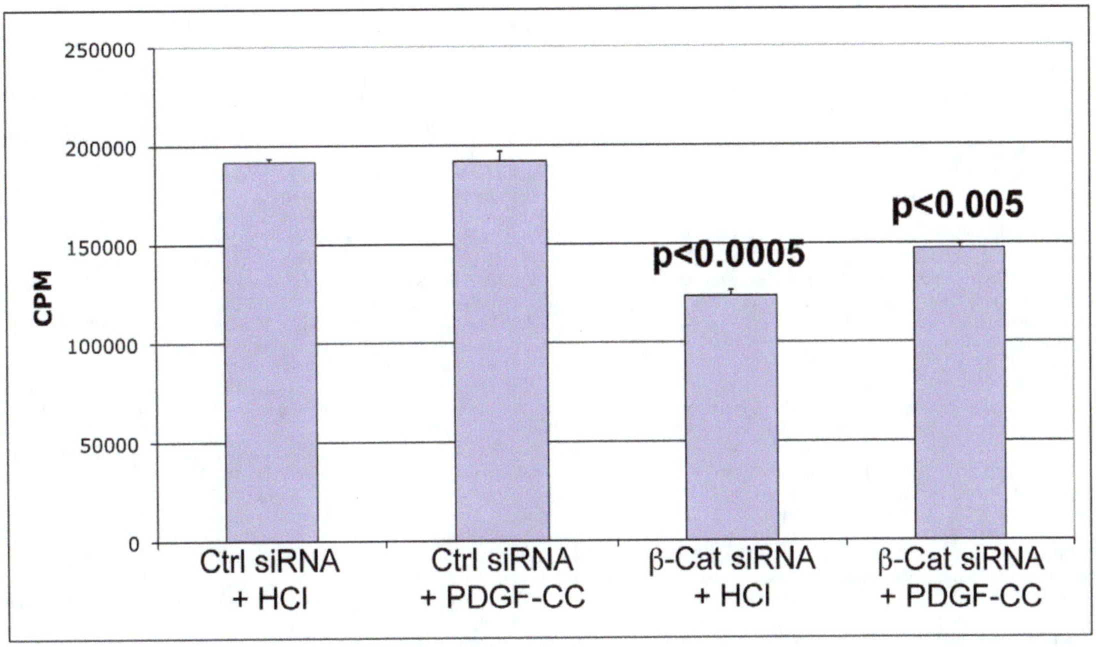

Figure 6. β-Catenin suppression engenders mitogenicity to PDGF-CC in hepatoma cell culture. PDGF-CC (10 ng/ml) treatment does not increase DNA synthesis as compared to HCl treatment of Hep3B cells. β-Catenin knockdown led to significant decrease in thymidine incorporation as compared to control siRNA ($p<0.0005$). However PDGF-CC treatment led to a significant increase in thymidine incorporation in β-catenin-suppressed as compared to control siRNA-transfected cells ($p<0.005$).

were inactivated for endogenous peroxide, blocked and incubated with primary antibody overnight at room temperature or for one hour at room temperature, washed and incubated with appropriate biotin-conjugated secondary antibody for 30 minutes. Sections were washed, incubated with ABC reagent, washed and incubated with DAB. Sections were next counterstained with Shandon hematoxylin solution (Sigma) and cover slipped using Cytoseal XYL (Richard Allen Scientific, Kalamazoo, MI). For negative control, the primary antibody was omitted in the protocol. Slides were viewed under an Axioskop 40 (Zeiss) upright research microscope and digital images obtained. Collages were prepared using Adobe Photoshop CS4 software. For PCNA and TUNEL, numbers of positive cells were counted in four random 400× fields in five representative livers from each group and averages compared for significance between groups by student *t* test. P value of less than 0.05 was considered significant. For quantitative analysis of β-catenin- and PDGFRα-positivity in tumors, all microscopic foci in KO and WT livers were assessed. Any tumor foci showing cytoplasmic and/or nuclear β-catenin staining were labeled as being β-catenin-positive and any foci exhibiting cytoplasmic staining for PDGFRα as compared to surrounding non-tumor areas were labeled as being PDGFRα-positive. This enabled us to calculate percentage of β-catenin and/or PDGFRα-positive tumors in each group after DEN/PB treatment.

Cell culture and treatment

Hep3B cells (ATCC) were grown to 100% confluence in 10% FBS and EMEM media. Cells were trypsinized and plated in 6 well plates containing 2 ml of 10% FBS EMEM media and serum-starved overnight. Transfection was performed using pre-validated β-catenin and control siRNA (Ambion) using lipofectamine as described previously [34]. 24 hours after transfection, cells were treated with 10 ng/ml of recombinant PDGF-CC (R&D systems) or HCl (used to reconstitute PDGF-CC) in 4% media containing tritiated thymidine. After 24 hours, the media was discarded and 1 ml of 5% trichloroacetic acid (TCA) was added to each well and plates placed in 4°C for 15 minutes. Cells were washed, dried and suspended in 1 ml of 0.33 M NaOH for 20 minutes, and 300 µl of total mixture from each well was added to 3 ml of scintillation fluid and then placed in scintillation counter. Experiment was repeated at least twice and each condition was done in triplicates. Average counts per minute (CPM) were compared between different conditions for statistical significance by student t test with value of less than 0.05 considered significant.

Author Contributions

Conceived and designed the experiments: SPSM. Performed the experiments: PKA BHR SS AM. Analyzed the data: PKA BHR SPSM. Contributed reagents/materials/analysis tools: PKA SPSM. Wrote the paper: PKA SPSM.

References

1. Parkin DM (2001) Global cancer statistics in the year 2000. Lancet Oncol 2: 533–543.
2. Lustig B, Behrens J (2003) The Wnt signaling pathway and its role in tumor development. J Cancer Res Clin Oncol 129: 199–221.
3. Clevers H (2006) Wnt/beta-catenin signaling in development and disease. Cell 127: 469–480.
4. Peifer M, Polakis P (2000) Wnt signaling in oncogenesis and embryogenesis–a look outside the nucleus. Science 287: 1606–1609.
5. Willert K, Brown JD, Danenberg E, Duncan AW, Weissman IL, et al. (2003) Wnt proteins are lipid-modified and can act as stem cell growth factors. Nature 423: 448–452.
6. Nelson WJ, Nusse R (2004) Convergence of Wnt, beta-catenin, and cadherin pathways. Science 303: 1483–1487.
7. de La Coste A, Romagnolo B, Billuart P, Renard CA, Buendia MA, et al. (1998) Somatic mutations of the beta-catenin gene are frequent in mouse and human hepatocellular carcinomas. Proc Natl Acad Sci U S A 95: 8847–8851.

8. Wong CM, Fan ST, Ng IO (2001) beta-Catenin mutation and overexpression in hepatocellular carcinoma: clinicopathologic and prognostic significance. Cancer 92: 136–145.
9. Kalinichenko VV, Major ML, Wang X, Petrovic V, Kuechle J, et al. (2004) Foxm1b transcription factor is essential for development of hepatocellular carcinomas and is negatively regulated by the p19ARF tumor suppressor. Genes Dev 18: 830–850.
10. Matsumoto K, Huang J, Viswakarma N, Bai L, Jia Y, et al. (2010) Transcription coactivator PBP/MED1-deficient hepatocytes are not susceptible to diethylnitrosamine-induced hepatocarcinogenesis in the mouse. Carcinogenesis 31: 318–325.
11. Kudo M (2011) Signaling pathway and molecular-targeted therapy for hepatocellular carcinoma. Dig Dis 29: 289–302.
12. Oseini AM, Roberts LR (2009) PDGFRalpha: a new therapeutic target in the treatment of hepatocellular carcinoma? Expert Opin Ther Targets 13: 443–454.
13. Stock P, Monga D, Tan X, Micsenyi A, Loizos N, et al. (2007) Platelet-derived growth factor receptor-alpha: a novel therapeutic target in human hepatocellular cancer. Mol Cancer Ther 6: 1932–1941.
14. Zhang T, Sun HC, Xu Y, Zhang KZ, Wang L, et al. (2005) Overexpression of platelet-derived growth factor receptor alpha in endothelial cells of hepatocellular carcinoma associated with high metastatic potential. Clin Cancer Res 11: 8557–8563.
15. Aydinlik H, Nguyen TD, Moennikes O, Buchmann A, Schwarz M (2001) Selective pressure during tumor promotion by phenobarbital leads to clonal outgrowth of beta-catenin-mutated mouse liver tumors. Oncogene 20: 7812–7816.
16. Ogawa K, Yamada Y, Kishibe K, Ishizaki K, Tokusashi Y (1999) Beta-catenin mutations are frequent in hepatocellular carcinomas but absent in adenomas induced by diethylnitrosamine in B6C3F1 mice. Cancer Res 59: 1830–1833.
17. Diwan BA, Meier H (1976) Carcinogenic effects of a single dose of diethylnitrosamine in three unrelated strains of mice: genetic dependence of the induced tumor types and incidence. Cancer Lett 1: 249–253.
18. Goldfarb S, Pugh TD, Koen H, He YZ (1983) Preneoplastic and neoplastic progression during hepatocarcinogenesis in mice injected with diethylnitrosamine in infancy. Environ Health Perspect 50: 149–161.
19. Villanueva A, Newell P, Chiang DY, Friedman SL, Llovet JM (2007) Genomics and signaling pathways in hepatocellular carcinoma. Semin Liver Dis 27: 55–76.
20. Monga SP (2011) Role of Wnt/beta-catenin signaling in liver metabolism and cancer. Int J Biochem Cell Biol 43: 1021–1029.
21. Cadoret A, Ovejero C, Saadi-Kheddouci S, Souil E, Fabre M, et al. (2001) Hepatomegaly in transgenic mice expressing an oncogenic form of beta-catenin. Cancer Res 61: 3245–3249.
22. Harada N, Miyoshi H, Murai N, Oshima H, Tamai Y, et al. (2002) Lack of tumorigenesis in the mouse liver after adenovirus-mediated expression of a dominant stable mutant of beta-catenin. Cancer Res 62: 1971–1977.
23. Nejak-Bowen KN, Thompson MD, Singh S, Bowen WC Jr., Dar MJ, et al. (2010) Accelerated liver regeneration and hepatocarcinogenesis in mice overexpressing serine-45 mutant beta-catenin. Hepatology 51: 1603–1613.
24. Tan X, Apte U, Micsenyi A, Kotsagrelos E, Luo JH, et al. (2005) Epidermal growth factor receptor: a novel target of the Wnt/beta-catenin pathway in liver. Gastroenterology 129: 285–302.
25. Harada N, Oshima H, Katoh M, Tamai Y, Oshima M, et al. (2004) Hepatocarcinogenesis in mice with beta-catenin and Ha-ras gene mutations. Cancer Res 64: 48–54.
26. Miyoshi H, Deguchi A, Nakau M, Kojima Y, Mori A, et al. (2009) Hepatocellular carcinoma development induced by conditional beta-catenin activation in Lkb1+/− mice. Cancer Sci 100: 2046–2053.
27. Zhang XF, Tan X, Zeng G, Misse A, Singh S, et al. (2011) Conditional beta-catenin loss in mice promotes chemical hepatocarcinogenesis: role of oxidative stress and platelet-derived growth factor receptor alpha/phosphoinositide 3-kinase signaling. Hepatology 52: 954–965.
28. Rignall B, Braeuning A, Buchmann A, Schwarz M (2011) Tumor formation in liver of conditional beta-catenin-deficient mice exposed to a diethylnitrosamine/phenobarbital tumor promotion regimen. Carcinogenesis 32: 52–57.
29. Farazi PA, DePinho RA (2006) Hepatocellular carcinoma pathogenesis: from genes to environment. Nat Rev Cancer 6: 674–687.
30. Lehwald N, Tao GZ, Jang KY, Sorkin M, Knoefel WT, et al. (2011) Wnt-beta-catenin signaling protects against hepatic ischemia and reperfusion injury in mice. Gastroenterology 141: 707–718, 718 e701–705.
31. Liu S, Yeh TH, Singh VP, Shiva S, Krauland L, et al. (2011) beta-catenin is essential for ethanol metabolism and protection against alcohol-mediated liver steatosis in mice. Hepatology.
32. Nejak-Bowen KN, Monga SP (2011) Beta-catenin signaling, liver regeneration and hepatocellular cancer: sorting the good from the bad. Semin Cancer Biol 21: 44–58.
33. Campbell JS, Hughes SD, Gilbertson DG, Palmer TE, Holdren MS, et al. (2005) Platelet-derived growth factor C induces liver fibrosis, steatosis, and hepatocellular carcinoma. Proc Natl Acad Sci U S A 102: 3389–3394.
34. Zeng G, Apte U, Cieply B, Singh S, Monga SP (2007) siRNA-mediated beta-catenin knockdown in human hepatoma cells results in decreased growth and survival. Neoplasia 9: 951–959.
35. Heldin CH, Ostman A, Ronnstrand L (1998) Signal transduction via platelet-derived growth factor receptors. Biochim Biophys Acta 1378: F79–113.
36. Barone MV, Courtneidge SA (1995) Myc but not Fos rescue of PDGF signalling block caused by kinase-inactive Src. Nature 378: 509–512.
37. Wang EY, Yeh SH, Tsai TF, Huang HP, Jeng YM, et al. (2011) Depletion of beta-catenin from mature hepatocytes of mice promotes expansion of hepatic progenitor cells and tumor development. Proc Natl Acad Sci U S A 108: 18384–18389.
38. Sekine S, Ogawa R, Kanai Y (2011) Hepatomas with activating Ctnnb1 mutations in 'Ctnnb1-deficient' livers: a tricky aspect of a conditional knockout mouse model. Carcinogenesis 32: 622–628.
39. Thompson MD, Wickline ED, Bowen WB, Lu A, Singh S, et al. (2011) Spontaneous repopulation of beta-catenin null livers with beta-catenin-positive hepatocytes after chronic murine liver injury. Hepatology 54: 1333–1343.
40. Behari J, Yeh TH, Krauland L, Otruba W, Cieply B, et al. (2010) Liver-specific beta-catenin knockout mice exhibit defective bile acid and cholesterol homeostasis and increased susceptibility to diet-induced steatohepatitis. Am J Pathol 176: 744–753.
41. Tan X, Behari J, Cieply B, Michalopoulos GK, Monga SP (2006) Conditional deletion of beta-catenin reveals its role in liver growth and regeneration. Gastroenterology 131: 1561–1572.

10

Interleukin-8 is Activated in Patients with Chronic Liver Diseases and Associated with Hepatic Macrophage Accumulation in Human Liver Fibrosis

Henning W. Zimmermann[1], Sebastian Seidler[1], Nikolaus Gassler[2], Jacob Nattermann[3], Tom Luedde[1], Christian Trautwein[1], Frank Tacke[1]*

1 Department of Medicine III, University Hospital, Aachen, Germany, 2 Institute of Pathology, University Hospital, Aachen, Germany, 3 Department of Medicine I, University of Bonn, Bonn, Germany

Abstract

Background: Interleukin-8 (IL-8, CXCL8) is a potent chemoattractant for neutrophils and contributes to acute liver inflammation. Much less is known about IL-8 in chronic liver diseases (CLD), but elevated levels were reported from alcoholic and hepatitis C-related CLD. We investigated the regulation of IL-8, its receptors CXCR1 and CXCR2 and possible IL-8 responding cells in CLD patients.

Methodology: Serum IL-8 levels were measured in CLD patients (n = 200) and healthy controls (n = 141). Intrahepatic IL-8, CXCR1 and CXCR2 gene expression was quantified from liver samples (n = 41), alongside immunohistochemical neutrophil (MPO) and macrophage (CD68) stainings. CXCR1 and CXCR2 expression was analyzed on purified monocytes from patients (n = 111) and controls (n = 31). *In vitro* analyses explored IL-8 secretion by different leukocyte subsets.

Principal Findings: IL-8 serum levels were significantly increased in CLD patients, especially in end-stage cirrhosis. Interestingly, patients with cholestatic diseases exhibited highest IL-8 serum concentrations. IL-8 correlated with liver function, inflammatory cytokines and non-invasive fibrosis markers. Intrahepatically, IL-8 and CXCR1 expression were strongly up-regulated. However, intrahepatic IL-8 could only be associated to neutrophil infiltration in patients with primary biliary cirrhosis (PBC). In non-cholestatic cirrhosis, increased IL-8 and CXCR1 levels were associated with hepatic macrophage accumulation. In line, CXCR1, but not CXCR2 or CXCR3, expression was increased on circulating monocytes from cirrhotic patients. Moreover, monocyte-derived macrophages from CLD patients, especially the non-classical $CD16^+$ subtype, displayed enhanced IL-8 secretion *in vitro*.

Conclusions: IL-8 is strongly activated in CLD, thus likely contributing to hepatic inflammation. Our study suggests a novel role of IL-8 for recruitment and activation of hepatic macrophages via CXCR1 in human liver cirrhosis.

Editor: Antonio Bertoletti, Singapore Institute for Clinical Sciences, Singapore

Funding: This work was supported by the German Research Foundation (DFG Ta434/2-1, DFG SFB/TRR 57), and by the Start-Program for Young Investigators and Interdisciplinary Centre for Clinical Research (IZKF) at RWTH-Aachen University. The funders had no role in study design, data collection and analysis, decision to publish, or preparation of the manuscript.

Competing Interests: The authors have declared that no competing interests exist.

* E-mail: frank.tacke@gmx.net

Introduction

Patients with chronic liver disease independent of its origin are prone to develop liver fibrosis and cirrhosis resulting in potentially lethal complications like esophageal varices or hepatic decompensation [1]. Inflammation is a key factor in the initiation and maintenance of fibrotic processes within the liver [2,3]. During recent years, compelling evidence emerged that cellular components of the innate immune system such as monocytes and NK cells play major roles in perpetuating and modulating chronic liver inflammation [4,5,6]. Neutrophils, another important cell population of the innate immune response, have been intensively studied in acute liver damage such as alcoholic hepatitis [7,8] or ischemia-reperfusion injury [9]. Increased endotoxemia, observed in patients with high ethanol intake, or ischemia-reperfusion lead to neutrophil accumulation in hepatic sinusoids and post-sinusoidal venules, resulting in extravasation and tissue infiltration. Furthermore, the degree of neutrophil infiltration in alcoholic hepatitis appears to be indicative of disease severity [10]. Yet, the contribution of neutrophils to chronic liver damage is less clear. For instance, it is controversial whether neutrophils are functionally intact or dysfunctional in patients with established cirrhosis [11,12,13,14].

Apart from 'classical' inflammatory mediators like IL-1, TNFα and LPS, CXC-motif chemokines are critically involved in directing neutrophil trafficking towards sites of tissue injury [15]. IL-8 (CXCL8) is one important member of the CXC chemokine family with an additional characteristic glutamate-leucine-arginine (ELR) motif near the N-terminus of the molecule [16]. A key function of these ELR^+ chemokines, such as CXCL8/IL-8, is the attraction of polymorphonuclear cells to sites of tissue injury and inflammation. Cytokines like IL-1 and TNFα are strong inducers of ELR^+ chemokines [17]. IL-8 is synthesized by a vast number of different cells. Virtually all cell subsets possessing toll-like-receptors (TLR) are able to produce IL-8, among them monocytes and macrophages [18,19]. CXCR1 and CXCR2 represent the cellular targets of IL-8 [20]. While CXCR1 binds almost exclusively IL-8, CXCR2 also shows high affinity to other CXC-chemokines (Gro-α/β/γ, NAP-2, ENA-78) [21]. Both, CXCR1 and CXCR2 can be found on neutrophils, monocytes/macrophages and other leukocyte subsets like T-cells [22,23].

Several observations suggested that IL-8 pathways might be also involved in the pathogenesis of chronic liver disease. For instance, IL-8 levels are increased intrahepatically and in the serum of patients with alcoholic liver disease, probably contributing to hepatic neutrophil accumulation and also exerting systemic actions [24,25]. In patients with chronic hepatitis C, IL-8 serum levels are associated with disease progression and relate to interferon unresponsiveness [26]. Interestingly, experimental work raised the possibility that IL-8 may not only act as a mere chemoattractant protein in the liver, but also exerts direct profibrogenic functions. As such, HCV core transduced Huh-7 cells were able to stimulate hepatic stellate cells (HSC) in an IL-8 dependent manner [27]. Likewise, IL-8 signalling has been linked to organ fibrosis in the prostate gland, pancreas and lung [28,29,30].

In this study, we investigated whether the IL-8 pathway is activated in patients with chronic liver disease (CLD). We demonstrate that IL-8 is upregulated in the circulation as well as in the liver of CLD patients, depending on disease severity and etiology. Activation of IL-8 is linked to progression of liver fibrosis in patients. Interestingly, monocytes/macrophages, and not neutrophils, appear to be main responders to IL-8 in liver fibrosis/cirrhosis via CXCR1. Moreover, the non-classical $CD16^+$ monocyte subset is also a potent producer of this chemokine in humans.

Materials and Methods

Ethics Statement

Written informed consent was obtained from all participants. The study protocol conformed to the ethical guidelines of the 1975 Declaration of Helsinki as reflected in *a priori* approval by the local ethics committee of the University Hospital Aachen. The ethics committee of the University Hospital Aachen, RWTH-University, Aachen, Germany, specifically approved this study.

Patients and controls

We investigated CLD patients with or without liver cirrhosis [4]. The presence of liver cirrhosis was assessed according to various imaging techniques (liver ultrasound, CT- or MRI-scan), biopsy or laparoscopy findings and if typical complications of liver cirrhosis (e.g. esophageal varices, ascites, hepatic encephalopathy) were present in conjunction with the history of chronic liver disease (Table 1). As controls, healthy volunteers with normal aminotransferases and negative serology for HBV, HCV and HIV were recruited from the local blood transfusion department.

In a subgroup of patients, liver tissue samples were available from routine liver biopsies. Cirrhotic tissue was obtained from explanted livers due to transplantation. Grading and staging of all liver specimens was performed according to Desmet-Scheuer score by a pathologist who was blinded for experimental data [4]. Normal liver samples were obtained from unaffected areas of liver resections for secondary liver malignancy (mostly metastasis of colorectal cancer).

IL-8 protein measurements

IL-8 protein in serum and cell culture supernatant was assessed using the FlowCytomix System (eBioscience) according to manufacturer's instructions.

Purification of circulating $CD14^+$ monocytes

EDTA whole blood from patients and healthy controls was directly subjected to peripheral blood mononuclear cell (PBMC) purification by FICOLL density gradient (LSM-1077, PAA) as previously described [31]. Monocytes were isolated by positive selection with CD14 microbeads by MACS (Miltenyi Biotec). A ≥95% purity of isolated monocytes was confirmed by flow-cytometry using antibody staining for CD14, CD16, CD3, CD4, CD8, CD19 and CD56 (BD). CXCR1 and CXCR2 staining was performed by specific antibodies (R&D); staining protocols were adapted from procedures previously established for different chemokine receptors in our laboratory [32].

RNA isolation and gene expression analysis

RNA isolation from purified blood $CD14^+$ monocytes or snap frozen whole liver tissue was conducted by pegGOLD (pegLAB). Complementary cDNA was generated with 1 μg (blood monocytes) and 2 μg RNA (liver specimen) by cDNA synthesis kit (Roche). Real-time PCR was performed with SYBR green (Invitrogen) in duplicates with β-actin as housekeeping gene [33,34]. Primer sequences are available upon request.

Immunohistochemistry

Frozen liver sections were stained with polyclonal rabbit anti-human MPO or monoclonal anti-human CD68 (Dako) by indirect immunoperoxidase reaction in an autostainer system (Dako). Ten visual-fields per slide were analysed at 200× magnification by a blinded investigator.

In vitro secretion of IL-8

Monocyte-derived macrophages were obtained as described before, cultured in autologous serum and stimulated with 1 mg/ml LPS for 24 h [31].

Analyses of macrophages derived from distinct monocyte subpopulations were performed by pooling PBMC from three buffy coats of healthy blood donors. For subsequent monocyte subpopulation isolation either "monocyte-isolation-kit-II" or "$CD16^+$ monocytes-isolation-kit" (Miltenyi) were used for separation of $CD14^+CD16^-$ and $CD14^+CD16^+$ monocytes respectively [4]. Isolation accuracy was confirmed by FACS analysis revealing purities >90%. Lymphocytes were obtained after removal of $CD14^+$ cells as a control population. 1×10^6 cells/petri dish were allowed to culture in RPMI medium containing 10% BSA and 1% penicillin-streptomycin (PAA) for 5 days. IL-8 concentrations in the supernatant were measured as described above.

Statistical analysis

Statistical comparisons between two groups were performed by Mann-Whitney-U-test, multiple comparisons by ANOVA-test followed by U-test for post hoc analysis using GraphPad Prism. A p-value<0.05 was considered statistically significant. The levels of significance are indicated in the figures as followed: *$p<0.05$; **$p<0.01$; ***$p<0.001$. Data are depicted as bar graphs representing mean and standard error of the mean (SEM). Correlation analysis was performed by Spearman rank correlation test (SPSS).

Table 1. Characteristics of the study population.

	all patients	Stage of cirrhosis			
		no cirrh.	Child A	Child B	Child C
n	200	75	45	37	43
sex male/female n	124/76	46/29	24/21	20/17	34/9
age median (range) yrs	53 (17–82)	43 (17–73)	62 (30–82)	59.5 (28–77)	53 (21–81)
disease etiology n					
virus hepatitis	75	43	18	10	4
biliary/autoimmune	27	14	7	4	2
alcohol	60	5	13	14	28
other origin	38	13	7	9	9
MELD score median (range)	n.a.	n.a.	8 (6–17)	12 (7–21)	17 (9–28)
ALT median (range) U/L	46 (7–2103)	68 (10–2103)	41 (8–1247)	40.5 (7–437)	46 (11–261)
bilirubin median (range) mg/dl	1.3 (0.2–43.2)	0.7 (0.3–23.9)	0.9 (0.2–8.9)	2.05 (0.4–12.2)	4.7 (0.6–43.2)
albumin median (range) mg/dl	38 (12–61)	44.9 (29–61)	39 (28–49)	30.7 (12–43)	26 (12–60)
hyaluronic acid median (range) µg/l	190 (11–800)	31 (10–530)	240 (28–800)	500 (140–800)	740 (55–800)
procollagen-III-peptide median (range) µg/l	1160 (414–10400)	910 (414–1750)	1010 (456–3140)	1960 (639–10400)	2120 (696–6560)
IL-8 median (range) pg/ml	14 (14–1986)	15 (14–588)	28 (14–2530)	53 (14–1533)	88 (14–1533)

n.a., not applicable.

Results

Serum IL-8 levels are significantly elevated in chronic liver disease, increase with stage of cirrhosis and vary between different disease etiologies

To comprehensively address the general significance of IL-8 in the progression of chronic liver diseases (CLD), IL-8 serum levels were measured in a large cohort of patients ($n = 200$) in comparison to healthy volunteers ($n = 147$). IL-8 serum concentrations were significantly increased in CLD patients compared to controls ($p<0.0001$, Fig. 1A, Table 1). Of note, patients with established liver cirrhosis displayed significantly higher IL-8 levels than CLD patients without cirrhosis ($p<0.0001$, Fig. 1B). At all stages of liver disease (no cirrhosis, Child A, B, C), patients revealed significantly higher IL-8 concentrations than controls (Fig. 1C). Highest IL-8 concentrations were found in patients with decompensated, Child C-staged liver cirrhosis (Fig. 1C).

Interestingly, besides the clear association of IL-8 with disease progression, there were striking variations in IL-8 serum levels between the different etiologies of CLD. Patients with alcoholic, but surprisingly also with cholestatic liver diseases were found to have highest IL-8 serum concentrations (Fig. 1D), while patients with viral hepatitis (hepatitis B or C) had much lower circulating IL-8. These differences between the disease etiologies remained significant, even if IL-8 levels were adjusted to the stage of cirrhosis, which was achieved by the ratio of serum IL-8 and Child-Pugh score points (Fig. 1E). In a small subgroup of patients with PBC ($n = 8$) we detected by far the highest serum levels of IL-8. These findings were corroborated by correlations (Table 2) between IL-8 serum levels and parameters indicating cholestasis like total conjugated bilirubin ($r = 0.394$, $p<0.001$), gamma-glutamyl-transpeptidase ($r = 0.308$, $p<0.001$) and alkaline phosphatase ($r = 0.402$; $p<0.001$).

IL-8 had been functionally linked to hepatic neutrophil infiltration, liver inflammation and to activation of profibrogenic, collagen-producing hepatic stellate cells [10,27]. In fact, our correlation analysis revealed that IL-8 levels were closely linked to non-invasive markers of liver fibrosis (pro-collagen-III-peptide $r = 0.349$, $p<0.001$; hyaluronic acid $r = 0.314$, $p<0.001$) and inversely to markers of the hepatic biosynthetic capacity (prothrombin time $r = -0.236$, $p = 0.001$; pseudocholinesterase $r = -0.337$, $p<0.001$). IL-8 did not correlate with alanine aminotransferase activity (ALT), but with inflammatory cytokines and chemokines (TNFα $r = 0.258$, $p<0.001$; IL-6 $r = 0.340$, $p<0.001$; IP-10 [CXCL10] $r = 0.357$, $p<0.001$; MIG [CXCL9] $r = 0.340$, $p<0.001$; IL-4 $r = 0.243$, $p = 0.001$). Noteworthy, the counts of circulating neutrophils, that are targeted by IL-8, were also correlated with this chemokine, although the correlation was rather weak (absolute neutrophil count: $r = 0.163$; $p = 0.004$). In line with this data, we detected a significant increase of neutrophils in peripheral blood between non-cirrhotic and cirrhotic patients ($p = 0.005$), while neutrophil counts did not differ among the various stages of liver cirrhosis (data not shown). These findings showed that IL-8 is significantly elevated in CLD patients dependent on disease etiology and severity, indicating that increased circulating IL-8 may contribute to proinflammatory and profibrogenic cascades during the progression of chronic liver diseases.

IL-8 and its receptor CXCR1 are up-regulated intrahepatically in chronic liver disease according to fibrosis severity and underlying pathology

Based on previous findings that several parenchymal (injured hepatocytes, biliary epithelial cells) and non-parenchymal (endothelium) liver cells as well as infiltrating immune cells are the primary sources of IL-8 in liver damage [27,35,36], we hypothesized that the elevated circulating IL-8 in CLD patients reflected increased hepatic IL-8 expression in liver disease. *IL-8* gene expression was significantly up-regulated in diseased liver in comparison to healthy control liver tissue by a mean of 12.4-fold (Fig. 2A). Interestingly, hepatic *IL-8* expression from CLD patients exceeded by far conditions of acute liver failure (ALF), in which

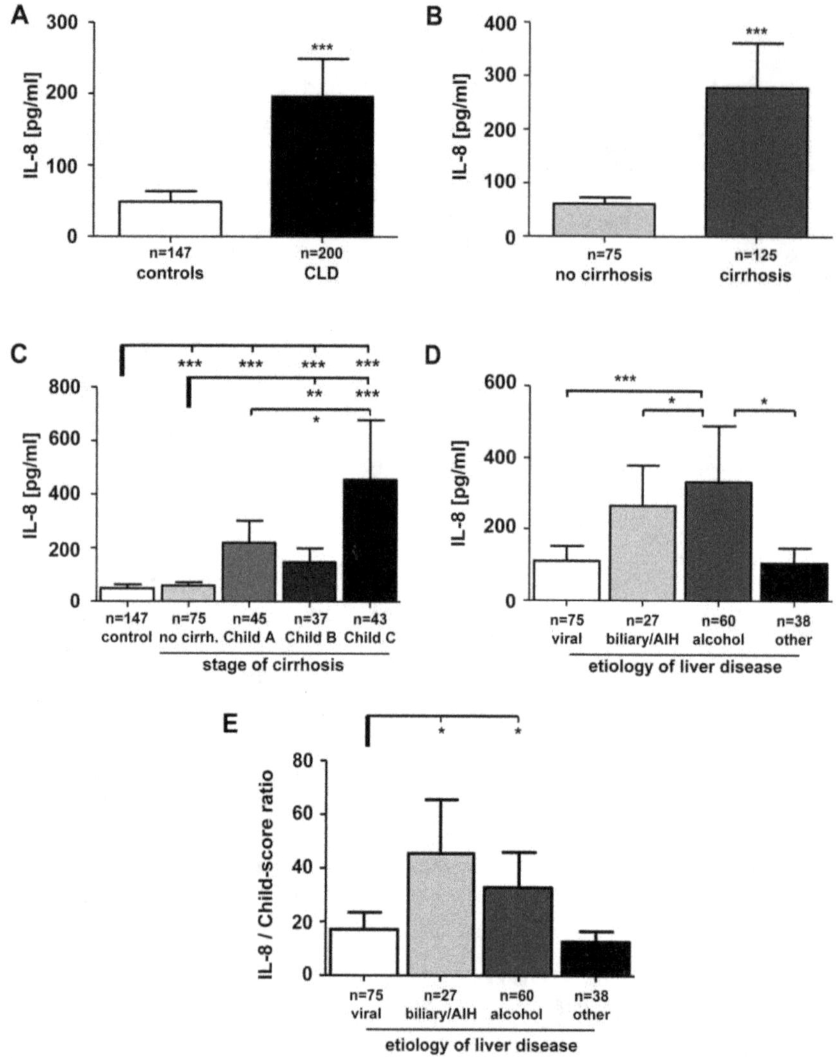

Figure 1. Serum IL-8 levels in healthy controls and patients with chronic liver disease. (A) Serum IL-8 levels are significantly increased in patients compared to healthy controls. (B) Cirrhotic patients show higher IL-8 serum levels than non-cirrhotics. (C) Dissecting the various stages of CLD revealed that IL-8 levels are highest in end-stage liver disease. (D) Patients with underlying alcoholic and biliary/autoimmune liver diseases showed higher IL-8 serum concentrations than viral hepatitis or other causes of CLD. (E) To normalize for the stage of cirrhosis, IL-8 serum levels were divided by the Child-Pugh score points. Elevated IL-8 in cholestatic and alcoholic liver diseases remained significant. CLD, chronic liver disease; AIH, autoimmune hepatitis.

IL-8-mediated neutrophil attraction has been described as an important mechanism of injury [15]. Highest *IL-8* mRNA levels were found in samples from cirrhotic livers (F4 fibrosis score), while *IL-8* induction at earlier fibrosis stages was more variable. Among the different etiologies tested, patients with primary biliary cirrhosis (PBC) exhibited highest *IL-8* mRNA expression (Fig. 2A).

We next investigated the intrahepatic expression of IL-8 receptors *CXCR1* and *CXCR2* to analyze if hepatic *IL-8* expression drives activation or infiltration of responsive cells in CLD. In full agreement with *IL-8* expression, *CXCR1* mRNA levels were significantly increased in samples from CLD patients, especially in advanced fibrosis/cirrhosis and in PBC patients (Fig. 2B). In contrast, *CXCR2* mRNA was not generally induced in CLD versus control livers, confirming prior observations [34]. However, *CXCR2* expression was increased in PBC patients (Fig. 2C). These data showed that intrahepatic expression of *IL-8* and its main receptor *CXCR1* was significantly induced in chronic liver injury, indicating that this pathway might be an important factor in driving hepatic inflammation and disease progression.

Intrahepatic accumulation of neutrophils and macrophages in chronic liver diseases

Neutrophils have been described as a major target of IL-8 in inflammatory diseases [37]. To better understand the biological relevance of IL-8 and its receptors CXCR1 and CXCR2 in CLD we stained the liver sections for myeloperoxidase (MPO), a common marker for activated neutrophils. Although MPO$^+$ neutrophils could be regularly found in livers from CLD patients by immunohistochemistry, the clear increase of *IL-8* and *CXCR1* mRNA in cirrhotic samples was not associated with increased neutrophil counts in livers with cirrhosis compared to non-cirrhotic livers (Fig. 3A). Nevertheless, there was a distinct rise of intrahepatic neutrophils in PBC, indicating that neutrophils might be specifically involved in this disease entity.

Table 2. Correlation analysis of serum IL-8 concentrations with other laboratory parameters.

	all patients (n = 200)		cirrhotic patients (n = 123)	
	r	*p*	r	*p*
Inflammation				
white blood cell count	0.163	*0.04*	-	*n.s.*
neutrophil count	0.155	*0.034*	-	*n.s.*
C-reactive protein	0.315	*<0.001*	0.268	*0.003*
IL-6	0.340	*<0.001*	0.350	*<0.001*
IL-10	0.220	*0.002*	0.245	*0.018*
IL-1β	0.267	*<0.001*	0.238	*0.008*
IL-4	0.243	*0.001*	-	*n.s.*
IL-2R	0.245	*0.026*	-	*n.s.*
TNFα	0.258	*<0.001*	0.342	*<0.001*
IFNy	0.241	*0.003*	0.345	*0.001*
Chemokines				
MCP-1 (CCL2)	0.345	*<0.001*	0.308	*<0.001*
MIP-1α (CCL3)	0.344	*<0.001*	0.334	*0.003*
MIP-1β (CCL4)	0.720	*<0.001*	0.734	*<0.001*
MIG (CXCL9)	0.340	*<0.001*	0.238	*0.008*
IP-10 (CXCL10)	0.357	*<0.001*	-	*n.s.*
Liver function				
MELD score	n.a.	*n.a.*	0.242	*0.008*
Child-Pugh-score	n.a.	*n.a.*	0.321	*<0.001*
albumin	−0.338	*<0.001*	−0.213	*0.020*
pseudocholinesterase	−0.337	*<0.001*	−0.235	*0.011*
prothrombin time	−0.236	*0.001*	−0.240	*0.008*
Cholestasis				
bilirubin (conjugated)	0.394	*<0.001*	0.368	*<0.001*
gamma-glutamyl-transferase	0.308	*<0.001*	0.220	*0.016*
alkaline phosphatase	0.402	*<0.001*	0.285	*0.002*
Fibrosis markers				
procollagen-III-peptide	0.349	*<0.001*	0.397	*<0.001*
hyaluronic acid	0.314	*<0.001*	-	*n.s.*

Correlations of serum interleukin-8 with other laboratory parameters were assessed by Spearman rank correlation test, and data are presented for all patients as well as for the subgroup of patients with liver cirrhosis. Only significant ($p<0.05$) results are shown.

Recent studies revealed that also monocytes/macrophages may respond to IL-8, because monocytic expression of the IL-8 receptors CXCR1 and CXCR2 can be induced by several mediators like the Th2 cytokines IL-4 and IL-13 [38]. In fact, the numbers of macrophages significantly increased with progression of liver fibrosis, as evidenced by immunohistochemistry for CD68 (Fig. 3B). This finding suggested that monocytes/macrophages might be the primary responders to IL-8 in liver diseases.

Circulating monocytes from patients with liver cirrhosis up-regulate CXCR1 expression

Following the hypothesis that monocytes/macrophages are an important target of elevated IL-8 in CLD, we analyzed the expression of CXCR1 and CXCR2 by monocytes in peripheral blood. We purified circulating monocytes from healthy controls (n = 31) and CLD patients (n = 111) by CD14-labelled microbeads at a >95% purity (Fig. 4A). *CXCR1* and *CXCR2* gene expression was assessed by quantitative real-time PCR. Monocytes isolated from patients with established cirrhosis (n = 69) expressed significantly higher *CXCR1* mRNA than from non-cirrhotic patients (n = 42) (Fig. 4B). In contrast, monocytic *CXCR2* expression was moderately down-regulated in patients compared to healthy controls, independent of the presence of cirrhosis (Fig. 4C). We confirmed these findings for a subgroup of study participants on a protein level as well. In patients with liver cirrhosis, monocytic CXCR1 expression was significantly upregulated compared to healthy controls (Fig. 4D–F). CXCR2 was only barely detectable on circulating monocytes from healthy volunteers or patients (Fig. 4D). These data demonstrated that CXCR1 is upregulated on peripheral monocytes from patients with liver cirrhosis, corroborating that monocytes might be an important target of IL-8 in chronic liver diseases. Furthermore, these findings paralleled the intrahepatic expression patterns of up-regulated *CXCR1*, but not *CXCR2* (Fig. 2), in patients with liver cirrhosis. Gene expression of *CXCR3*, the receptor for CXCL9 (MIG), CXCL10 (IP-10) and CXCL11 (I-TAC), was only detected at very

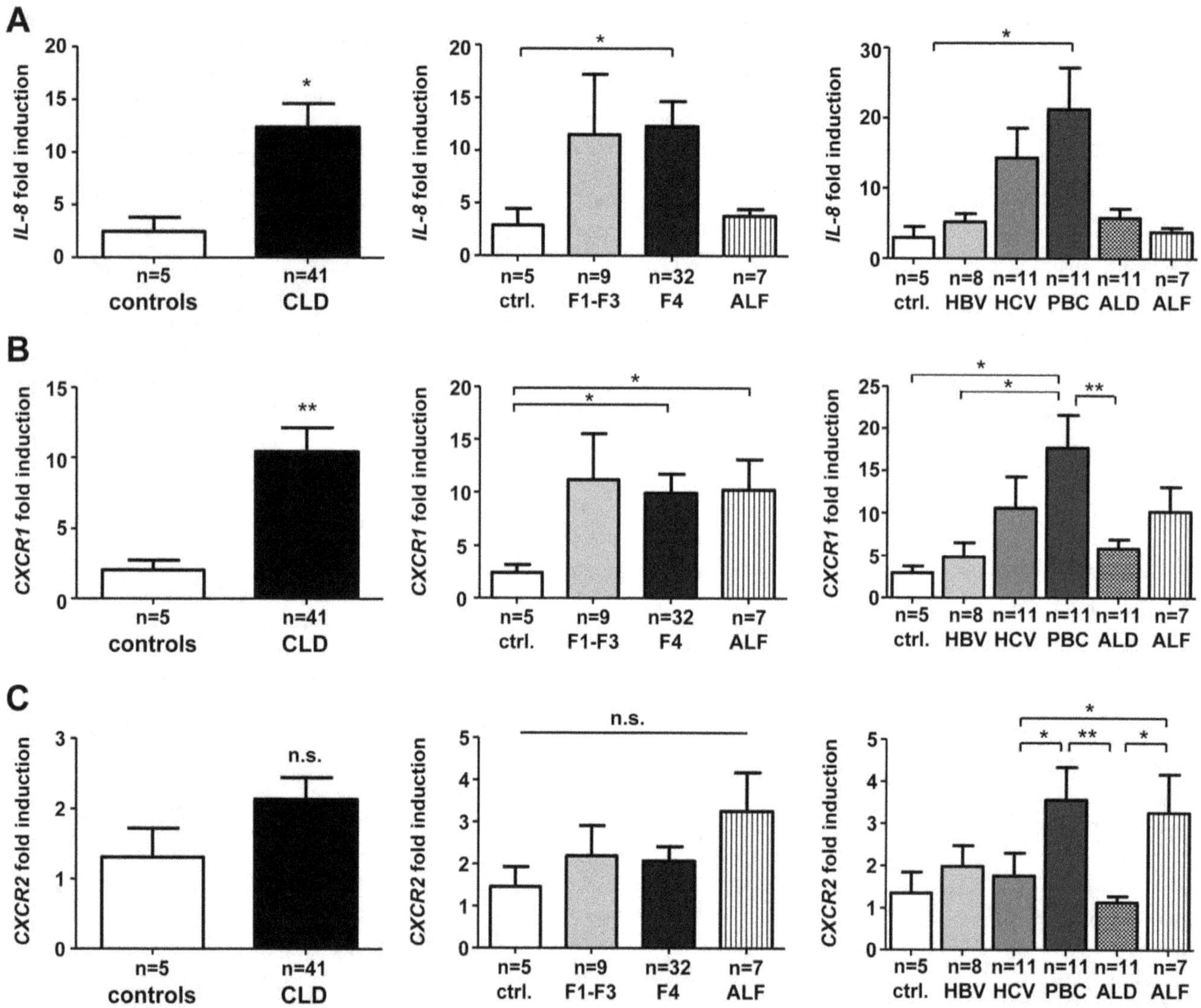

Figure 2. Intrahepatic IL-8 and IL-8 receptor gene expression. Gene expression levels of *IL-8* (A) and the IL-8 receptors *CXCR1* (B) and *CXCR2* (C) were assessed from liver tissue by real-time qPCR and are displayed as fold induction. Samples from CLD patients were divided according to fibrosis stage (middle graphs) and to disease etiology (right graphs). Tissue from acute liver failure (ALF) was analyzed in parallel for comparison. CLD, chronic liver disease; ctrl, control; PBC, primary biliary cirrhosis; ALD, alcoholic liver disease; ALF, acute liver failure.

low levels on monocytes from healthy volunteers and even further downregulated in CLD patients (data not shown). Thus, we could exclude that macrophage infiltration was primarily driven by CXCR3 ligands, which are also upregulated during liver disease progression [39].

Proinflammatory CD16$^+$ monocyte-derived macrophages are potent producers of IL-8

To this point, our data demonstrated that IL-8 expression is induced systemically and intrahepatically in patients with CLD and that monocytes might be important responders to IL-8 during liver disease progression. However, macrophages have also been described as important IL-8 producing cells [40]. We therefore investigated whether macrophages from CLD patients may contribute to elevated IL-8 by an increased capacity to secrete IL-8. Macrophages from healthy volunteers (n = 20) and patients with liver cirrhosis (n = 15) were obtained by isolating peripheral monocytes and subsequent culture of adherent cells with autologous serum for 48 h. Macrophages from cirrhotic patients showed a significantly higher IL-8 synthesis *in vitro* (Fig. 5A). Of note, the production of other cytokines or chemokines like MCP-1, IL-10, IL-6, TNFα, MIP-1α, MIP-1β and IL-1β did not differ between patients and controls [4]. Also in contrast to other inflammatory cytokines, IL-8 production by monocyte-derived macrophages could not be further stimulated by LPS (Fig. 5A).

We had previously reported that 'non-classical' CD14$^+$CD16$^+$ monocytes, in contrast to 'classical' CD14^{++}CD16$^-$ monocytes, are critically involved in liver fibrosis progression in humans, by perpetuating a pro-inflammatory hepatic cytokine microenvironment and directly activating collagen-producing hepatic stellate cells [4]. Thus, we also compared these two major monocyte subsets for their IL-8 secretion capacity. In line with their described pro-inflammatory phenotype [31], CD14$^+$CD16$^+$ monocytes secreted significantly higher amounts of IL-8 *in vitro* compared to CD14^{++}CD16$^-$ monocytes upon LPS stimulation (Fig. 5B). Interestingly, this difference did not reach statistical significance without LPS stimulation, suggesting that endotox-

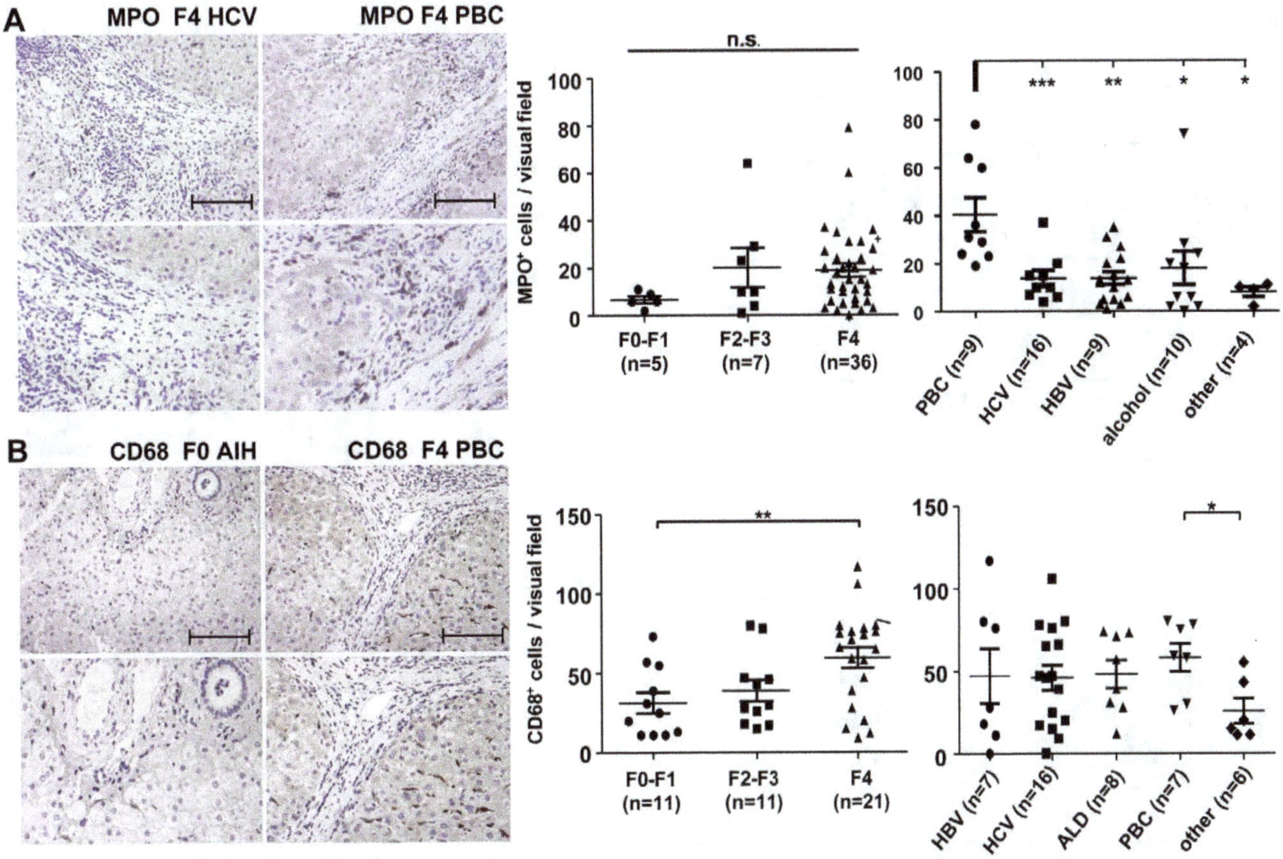

Figure 3. Immunohistochemical analysis of neutrophil and macrophage accumulation in chronic liver disease. (A) Myeloperoxidase (MPO) staining was performed to detect neutrophils within the liver. Upper panels depict representative images of neutrophil accumulation in PBC (left column) and HCV (right column) with F4 fibrosis at 200× magnification, lower panels magnify the periportal region of upper panels. MPO-positive neutrophils accumulate in PBC in comparison to ALD, HCV and HBV, whereas degree of fibrosis was not indicative for neutrophil count within the liver. Neutrophil cell infiltrate predominate within the cirrhotic fibres in periportal regions whereas remaining parenchyma was absent for neutrophil invasion. (B) $CD68^+$ cells indicating macrophages accumulate according to severity of liver disease irrespective of underlying etiology. Images represent exemplarily distribution of $CD68^+$ in F0 fibrosis (AIH) and F4 fibrosis (PBC). Scale bars represent 100 μm. AIH, autoimmune hepatitis; PBC, primary biliary cirrhosis; ALD, alcoholic liver disease.

emia, as often observed in advanced liver diseases [41], supports monocytic IL-8 secretion. Both monocyte subtypes were much more potent to synthesize IL-8 than lymphocytes (T-, B- and NK-cells) that were cultured as control cells (Fig. 5B). Taken together, these experiments revealed that monocytes not only respond to IL-8 in liver disease, but are also potent producers of IL-8. This indicates that IL-8, especially from 'non-classical' $CD14^+CD16^+$ monocytes, might contribute to amplify inflammatory signals in liver fibrosis.

Discussion

The CXC chemokine IL-8 (CXCL8) has long been identified as a major factor of acute inflammation, acting as a potent chemoattractant and activator of neutrophils by two receptors, CXCR1 and CXCR2 [37]. High IL-8 levels in the liver and the circulation have been found in patients with acute liver injury, such as alcoholic hepatitis or ischemia-reperfusion injury [9,10,42]. While these conditions are clearly associated with neutrophil-mediated tissue damage [15], less data exist about the involvement of IL-8 and/or neutrophils in chronic liver injury. By comprehensively analyzing a large cohort of patients with various liver diseases, we here show that serum IL-8 levels were significantly elevated in CLD patients. IL-8 serum levels were closely associated with the progression of fibrosis/cirrhosis, as reflected by clinical scores (e.g. Child-Pugh, MELD) and laboratory tests indicating deteriorated liver function or progressed fibrosis. Thus, our data expand prior studies that were restricted to patients with HCV infection or alcoholic disease [24,25,26]. Moreover, our data implicate that the source of elevated circulating IL-8 in patients with chronic liver diseases is likely the injured liver, because intrahepatic *IL-8* gene expression was strongly (about 12-fold) induced in patient in comparison to control tissue.

Besides the clear association of IL-8 with disease progression, we noticed distinct differences in IL-8 serum and intrahepatic expression dependent on the underlying disease etiology. Patients with alcoholic, but surprisingly also with cholestatic liver diseases had highest IL-8 levels. Interestingly, hepatic *IL-8* expression was exceptionally high in patients with PBC. In line, IL-8 expression had been previously detected specifically in injured biliary epithelial cells in patients with cholestatic liver diseases and linked to neutrophilic infiltration around reactive bile ducts [35]. Such a specific chemoattractive role of IL-8 for neutrophil infiltration to

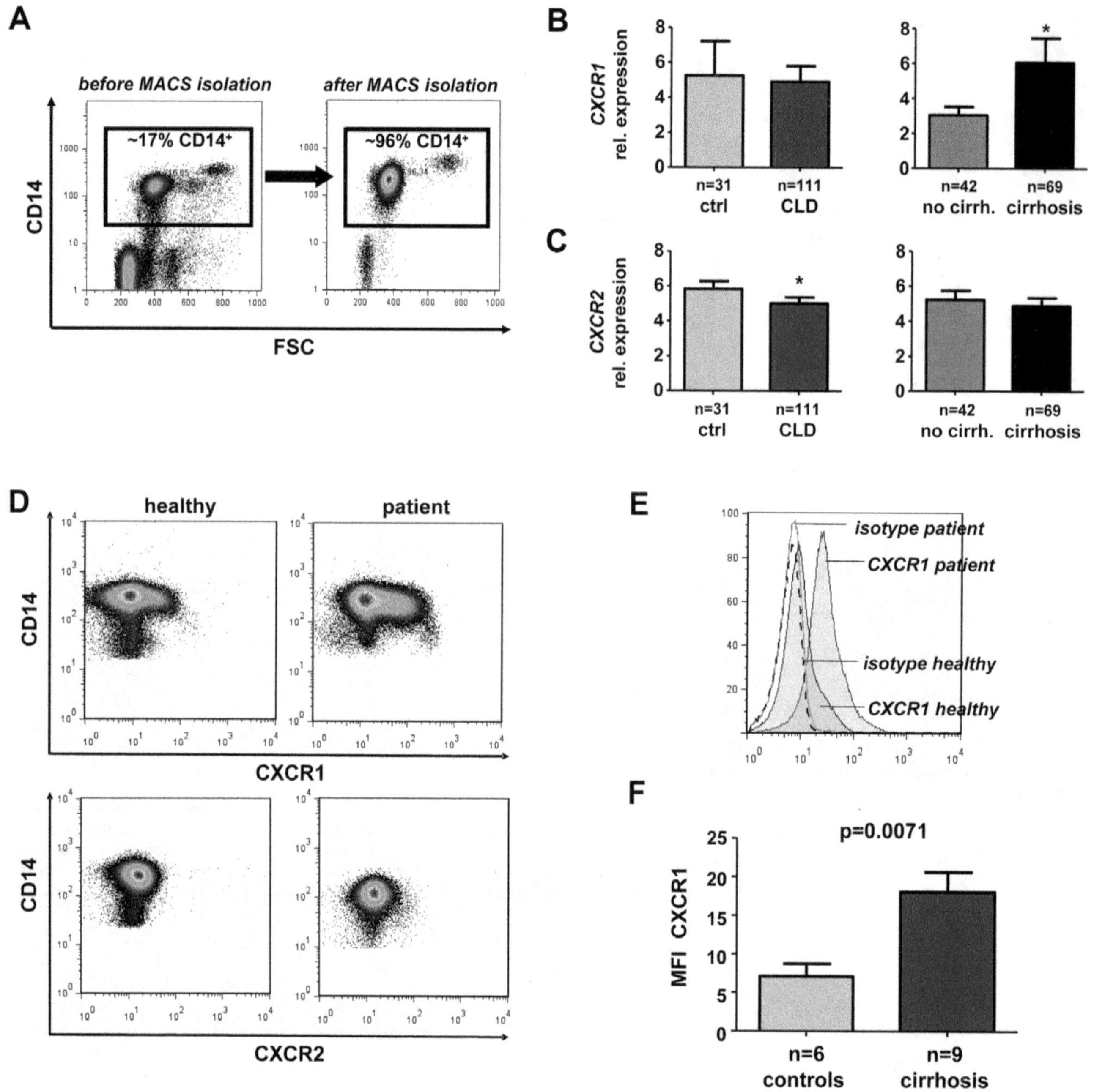

Figure 4. CXCR1 and CXCR2 mRNA and protein expression on circulating monocytes. (A) Monocytes were purified from whole blood by MACS with anti-CD14 antibodies, revealing purities above 95%. Representative FACS analysis before and after purification is shown. (B–C) Gene expression levels of the IL-8 receptors *CXCR1* (B) and *CXCR2* (C) were assessed from purified circulating monocytes of patients and controls and are displayed as relative expression levels. CLD, chronic liver disease. (D) CXCR1 and CXCR2 expression was also measured on a protein level by FACS. Representative plots from a healthy control (left) and patients with alcoholic Child C cirrhosis (right) are shown; pre-gating on $CD14^+$ monocytes to exclude CXCR1 expression by neutrophils. (E) Representative histograms showing how mean fluorescence intensity (MFI) was assessed: isotype control staining was subtracted from CXCR1 expression on circulating $CD14^+$ monocytes from healthy controls or patients. (F) Comparison of monocytic CXCR1 protein expression between healthy controls and patients with liver cirrhosis. Peripheral blood neutrophils served as a positive control for CXCR1 and CXCR2 staining (not shown).

injured bile ducts would very well explain our findings, and it would also fit to the prominent accumulation of MPO^+ neutrophils that we noticed in livers of PBC patients.

On the other hand, the high IL-8 expression in non-biliary cirrhosis could not be attributed to a clear hepatic neutrophil accumulation in progressing fibrosis *per se*. In fact, we observed that fibrosis progression was paralleled by increasing intrahepatic *CXCR1* levels and increasing $CD68^+$ hepatic macrophages. This indicated that monocytes/macrophages might be the main IL-8 responding cells in chronic liver disease patients. It has been reported previously that the Th2-cytokines IL-4 and IL-13 promote the up-regulation of CXCR1 and CXCR2 on human monocytes, thereby 'converting' IL-8 and related ELR^+ chemokines, prototypic neutrophil attractants, into monocyte chemotac-

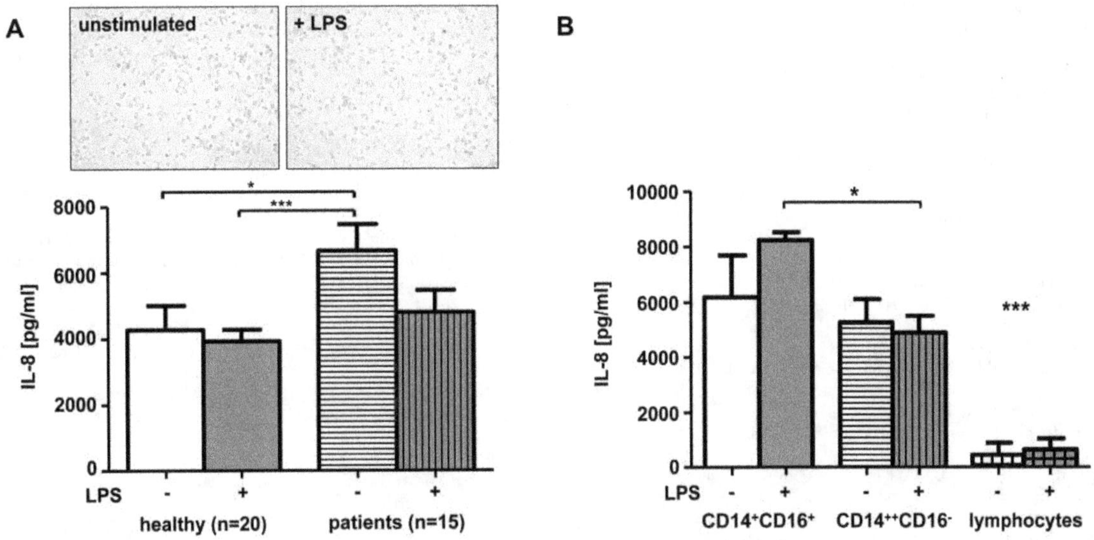

Figure 5. IL-8 secretion by monocyte-derived macrophages. (A) Macrophages were derived from blood monocytes of healthy donors (n = 20) and patients with Child B or C liver cirrhosis (n = 15). IL-8 secretion was measured in supernatant after 2 days of culture with autologous serum (white bars) as well as after stimulation with LPS (grey). Representative bright field microscopy pictures of cultured macrophages are displayed. (B) $CD14^{+}CD16^{+}$ monocytes, $CD14^{++}CD16^{-}$ monocytes and lymphocytes were isolated from healthy donors. IL-8 secretion was measured in supernatant after 5 days of culture with autologous serum (white bars) as well as after stimulation with LPS (grey).

tic agonists [38]. Interestingly, circulating monocytes from cirrhotic patients indeed had increased *CXCR1* expression, both on a gene and protein level. The enhanced monocytic CXCR1 expression could likely result from induction by Th2-cytokines, because IL-4 was found increase with progression of liver disease (not shown) and to correlate with serum IL-8 in our cohort (Table 2). These findings are in line with the current concept that advanced fibrotic disorders are generally characterized by strong Th2-biased immune responses [43].

Although our data demonstrate an association between IL-8 expression, macrophage infiltration and disease progression in patients with liver cirrhosis, the direct functional role of IL-8 in human liver disease is difficult to dissect. Functional experimental approaches with animal models are limited, because mice do not bear an IL-8 encoding gene, but only express the gene *gro*, whose gene product is the chemokine CXCL1/KC. Murine CXCL1 shows only 68% sequence identity with the human CXCL1. These differences between species are certainly a main reason why it is difficult to further dissect the role of this ELR^{+} chemokine in liver inflammation [44]. However, *in vitro* experiments characterized $CXCR1^{+}$ macrophages as polarized towards the alternatively activated M2 macrophage phenotype [38], which is believed to act pro-fibrogenic in hepatic fibrosis [45]. Interestingly, IL-8 secreted by injured hepatocytes was shown to activate collagen-producing hepatic stellate cells *in vitro* [27]. Our study expands the profibrogenic potential of IL-8 by showing that the IL-8 signal is also amplified by 'non-classical', fibrosis-associated $CD16^{+}$ monocytes/macrophages [4] and that IL-8 is in chronically inflamed liver directly associated with the number of hepatic macrophages, rather than hepatic neutrophils. Thus, our data support that IL-8 contributes to establish a profibrogenic microenvironment in chronic liver diseases and propose a novel role of IL-8 for the recruitment and activation of hepatic macrophages in human liver cirrhosis.

Acknowledgments

The authors thank Aline Müller and Silke Ensslen for excellent technical assistance.

Author Contributions

Conceived and designed the experiments: HWZ CT FT. Performed the experiments: HWZ SS NG. Analyzed the data: HWZ TL CT FT. Contributed reagents/materials/analysis tools: NG JN. Wrote the paper: HWZ CT.

References

1. Schuppan D, Afdhal NH (2008) Liver cirrhosis. Lancet 371: 838–851.
2. Iredale JP (2007) Models of liver fibrosis: exploring the dynamic nature of inflammation and repair in a solid organ. J Clin Invest 117: 539–548.
3. Karlmark KR, Wasmuth HE, Trautwein C, Tacke F (2008) Chemokine-directed immune cell infiltration in acute and chronic liver disease. Expert Rev Gastroenterol Hepatol 2: 233–242.
4. Zimmermann HW, Seidler S, Nattermann J, Gassler N, Hellerbrand C, et al. (2010) Functional contribution of elevated circulating and hepatic non-classical CD14CD16 monocytes to inflammation and human liver fibrosis. PLoS One 5: e11049.
5. Karlmark KR, Weiskirchen R, Zimmermann HW, Gassler N, Ginhoux F, et al. (2009) Hepatic recruitment of the inflammatory Gr1+ monocyte subset upon liver injury promotes hepatic fibrosis. Hepatology 50: 261–274.
6. Marra F, Aleffi S, Galastri S, Provenzano A (2009) Mononuclear cells in liver fibrosis. Semin Immunopathol 31: 345–358.
7. Bautista AP (2002) Neutrophilic infiltration in alcoholic hepatitis. Alcohol 27: 17–21.
8. French SW (2002) Alcoholic hepatitis: inflammatory cell-mediated hepatocellular injury. Alcohol 27: 43–46.
9. Jaeschke H (2006) Mechanisms of Liver Injury. II. Mechanisms of neutrophil-induced liver cell injury during hepatic ischemia-reperfusion and other acute inflammatory conditions. Am J Physiol Gastrointest Liver Physiol 290: G1083–1088.
10. Jaeschke H (2002) Neutrophil-mediated tissue injury in alcoholic hepatitis. Alcohol 27: 23–27.
11. Tritto G, Bechlis Z, Stadlbauer V, Davies N, Frances R, et al. (2011) Evidence of Neutrophil Functional Defect Despite Inflammation in Stable Cirrhosis. J Hepatol, in press.
12. Kirsch R, Woodburne VE, Shephard EG, Kirsch RE (2000) Patients with stable uncomplicated cirrhosis have normal neutrophil function. J Gastroenterol Hepatol 15: 1298–1306.

13. Shawcross DL, Wright GA, Stadlbauer V, Hodges SJ, Davies NA, et al. (2008) Ammonia impairs neutrophil phagocytic function in liver disease. Hepatology 48: 1202–1212.
14. Neugebauer H, Hartmann P, Krenn S, Gluck T, Scholmerich J, et al. (2008) Bacterial translocation increases phagocytic activity of polymorphonuclear leucocytes in portal hypertension: priming independent of liver cirrhosis. Liver Int 28: 1149–1157.
15. Jaeschke H, Hasegawa T (2006) Role of neutrophils in acute inflammatory liver injury. Liver Int 26: 912–919.
16. Baggiolini M, Walz A, Kunkel SL (1989) Neutrophil-activating peptide-1/interleukin 8, a novel cytokine that activates neutrophils. J Clin Invest 84: 1045–1049.
17. Matsushima K, Oppenheim JJ (1989) Interleukin 8 and MCAF: novel inflammatory cytokines inducible by IL 1 and TNF. Cytokine 1: 2–13.
18. Kaplanski G, Farnarier C, Kaplanski S, Porat R, Shapiro L, et al. (1994) Interleukin-1 induces interleukin-8 secretion from endothelial cells by a juxtacrine mechanism. Blood 84: 4242–4248.
19. Hashimoto S, Yoda M, Yamada M, Yanai N, Kawashima T, et al. (1996) Macrophage colony-stimulating factor induces interleukin-8 production in human monocytes. Exp Hematol 24: 123–128.
20. Murphy PM (1997) Neutrophil receptors for interleukin-8 and related CXC chemokines. Semin Hematol 34: 311–318.
21. Ahuja SK, Murphy PM (1996) The CXC chemokines growth-regulated oncogene (GRO) alpha, GRObeta, GROgamma, neutrophil-activating peptide-2, and epithelial cell-derived neutrophil-activating peptide-78 are potent agonists for the type B, but not the type A, human interleukin-8 receptor. J Biol Chem 271: 20545–20550.
22. Morohashi H, Miyawaki T, Nomura H, Kuno K, Murakami S, et al. (1995) Expression of both types of human interleukin-8 receptors on mature neutrophils, monocytes, and natural killer cells. J Leukoc Biol 57: 180–187.
23. Sallusto F, Baggiolini M (2008) Chemokines and leukocyte traffic. Nat Immunol 9: 949–952.
24. Huang YS, Chan CY, Wu JC, Pai CH, Chao Y, et al. (1996) Serum levels of interleukin-8 in alcoholic liver disease: relationship with disease stage, biochemical parameters and survival. J Hepatol 24: 377–384.
25. Hill DB, Marsano LS, McClain CJ (1993) Increased plasma interleukin-8 concentrations in alcoholic hepatitis. Hepatology 18: 576–580.
26. Polyak SJ, Khabar KS, Rezeiq M, Gretch DR (2001) Elevated levels of interleukin-8 in serum are associated with hepatitis C virus infection and resistance to interferon therapy. J Virol 75: 6209–6211.
27. Clement S, Pascarella S, Conzelmann S, Gonelle-Gispert C, Guilloux K, et al. (2010) The hepatitis C virus core protein indirectly induces alpha-smooth muscle actin expression in hepatic stellate cells via interleukin-8. J Hepatol 52: 635–643.
28. Schauer IG, Ressler SJ, Tuxhorn JA, Dang TD, Rowley DR (2008) Elevated epithelial expression of interleukin-8 correlates with myofibroblast reactive stroma in benign prostatic hyperplasia. Urology 72: 205–213.
29. Motoo Y, Xie MJ, Mouri H, Sawabu N (2004) Expression of interleukin-8 in human obstructive pancreatitis. JOP 5: 138–144.
30. Carre PC, Mortenson RL, King TE, Jr., Noble PW, Sable CL, et al. (1991) Increased expression of the interleukin-8 gene by alveolar macrophages in idiopathic pulmonary fibrosis. A potential mechanism for the recruitment and activation of neutrophils in lung fibrosis. J Clin Invest 88: 1802–1810.
31. Seidler S, Zimmermann HW, Bartneck M, Trautwein C, Tacke F (2010) Age-dependent alterations of monocyte subsets and monocyte-related chemokine pathways in healthy adults. BMC Immunol 11: 30.
32. Ingersoll MA, Spanbroek R, Lottaz C, Gautier EL, Frankenberger M, et al. (2010) Comparison of gene expression profiles between human and mouse monocyte subsets. Blood 115: e10–19.
33. Karlmark KR, Zimmermann HW, Roderburg C, Gassler N, Wasmuth HE, et al. (2010) The fractalkine receptor CX3CR1 protects against liver fibrosis by controlling differentiation and survival of infiltrating hepatic monocytes. Hepatology 52: 1769–1782.
34. Tacke F, Zimmermann HW, Trautwein C, Schnabl B (2011) CXCL5 plasma levels decrease in patients with chronic liver disease. J Gastroenterol Hepatol 26: 523–529.
35. Isse K, Harada K, Nakanuma Y (2007) IL-8 expression by biliary epithelial cells is associated with neutrophilic infiltration and reactive bile ductules. Liver Int 27: 672–680.
36. Afford SC, Fisher NC, Neil DA, Fear J, Brun P, et al. (1998) Distinct patterns of chemokine expression are associated with leukocyte recruitment in alcoholic hepatitis and alcoholic cirrhosis. J Pathol 186: 82–89.
37. Kobayashi Y (2008) The role of chemokines in neutrophil biology. Front Biosci 13: 2400–2407.
38. Bonecchi R, Facchetti F, Dusi S, Luini W, Lissandrini D, et al. (2000) Induction of functional IL-8 receptors by IL-4 and IL-13 in human monocytes. J Immunol 164: 3862–3869.
39. Tacke F, Zimmermann HW, Berres ML, Trautwein C, Wasmuth HE (2011) Serum chemokine receptor CXCR3 ligands are associated with progression, organ dysfunction and complications of chronic liver diseases. Liver Int, in press.
40. Emadi S, Clay D, Desterke C, Guerton B, Maquarre E, et al. (2005) IL-8 and its CXCR1 and CXCR2 receptors participate in the control of megakaryocytic proliferation, differentiation, and ploidy in myeloid metaplasia with myelofibrosis. Blood 105: 464–473.
41. Nolan JP (2010) The role of intestinal endotoxin in liver injury: a long and evolving history. Hepatology 52: 1829–1835.
42. Dominguez M, Miquel R, Colmenero J, Moreno M, Garcia-Pagan JC, et al. (2009) Hepatic expression of CXC chemokines predicts portal hypertension and survival in patients with alcoholic hepatitis. Gastroenterology 136: 1639–1650.
43. Hammerich L, Heymann F, Tacke F (2011) Role of IL-17 and Th17 cells in liver diseases. Clin Dev Immunol 2011: 345803.
44. Wasmuth HE, Tacke F, Trautwein C (2010) Chemokines in liver inflammation and fibrosis. Semin Liver Dis 30: 215–225.
45. Heymann F, Trautwein C, Tacke F (2009) Monocytes and macrophages as cellular targets in liver fibrosis. Inflamm Allergy Drug Targets 8: 307–318.

A Boswellic Acid-Containing Extract Ameliorates Schistosomiasis Liver Granuloma and Fibrosis through Regulating NF-κB Signaling in Mice

Miao Liu[1,2]☯, Qingsi Wu[1,2]☯, Peng Chen[3], Berthold Büchele[4], Maohong Bian[5], Shengjian Dong[6], Dake Huang[1,2], Cuiping Ren[1,2], Yuxia Zhang[1], Xin Hou[1,2], Thomas Simmet[4]*, Jijia Shen[1,2]*

1 Department of Microbiology and Parasitology, Anhui Medical University, Hefei, Anhui, People's Republic of China, **2** Anhui Provincial Laboratory of Microbiology and Parasitology, Anhui Medical University, Hefei, Anhui, People's Republic of China, **3** College of Clinical Medical Sciences, Anhui Medical University, Hefei, Anhui, People's Republic of China, **4** Institute of Pharmacology of Natural Products & Clinical Pharmacology, Ulm University, Ulm, Germany, **5** Department of Blood Transfusion, The First Affiliated Hospital, Anhui Medical University, Hefei, Anhui, People's Republic of China, **6** Department of Clinical Laboratory, Hefei Second People's Hospital, Hefei, Anhui, People's Republic of China

Abstract

Boswellic acid (BA)-containing extracts such as BSE have anti-inflammatory and immunomodulatory activity. In chronic schistosomiasis, the hepatic granuloma and fibrosis induced by egg deposition in the liver is the most serious pathological manifestations. However, little is known regarding the role of BAs in *Schistosoma japonicum* (*S. japonicum*) egg-induced liver granuloma and fibrosis. In order to investigate the effect of a water-soluble complex preparation of BSE, BSE-CD, on *S. japonicum* egg-induced liver pathology, liver granuloma and fibrosis were induced by infecting C57BL/6 mice with 18–22 cercariae of *S. japonicum. S. japonicum* cercariae infected mice were injected with BSE-CD at the onset of egg granuloma formation (early phase BSE-CD treatment after 4 weeks infection) or after the formation of liver fibrosis (late phase BSE-CD treatment after 7 weeks infection). Our data show that treatment of infected mice with BSE-CD significantly reduced both the extent of hepatic granuloma and fibrosis. Consistent with an inhibition of NF-κB signaling as evidenced by reduced IκB kinase (IKK) activation, the mRNA expression of VEGF (vascular endothelial growth factor, VEGF), TNF-α (tumor necrosis factor-alpha TNF-α) and MCP-1 (monocyte chemotactic protein 1, MCP-1) was decreased. Moreover, immunohistochemical analysis (IHC) revealed that the content of α-SMA in liver tissue of BSE-CD treated mice was dramatically decreased. Our findings suggest that BSE-CD treatment attenuates *S. japonicum* egg-induced hepatic granulomas and fibrosis, at least partly due to reduced NF-κB signaling and the subsequently decreased expression of VEGF, TNF-α, and MCP-1. Suppression of the activation of hepatic stellate cells (HSC) may also be involved in the therapeutic efficacy of BSE-CD.

Editor: Laurent Rénia, Agency for Science, Technology and Research - Singapore Immunology Network, Singapore

Funding: This work was supported by Natural Science Foundation of China (http://www.nsfc.gov.cn) (grant numbers 30901251 and 30972569). The funders had no role in study design, data collection and analysis, decision to publish, or preparation of the manuscript.

Competing Interests: The authors have declared that no competing interests exist.

* E-mail: thomas.simmet@uni-ulm.de (TS); shenjijia@hotmail.com (JS)

☯ These authors contributed equally to this work.

Introduction

Schistosomiasis is an important disease among the neglected tropical diseases. It is caused by several species of the genus schistosoma and remains a serious public health problem that affects more than 200 million people in 74 countries [1–2]. The three important species affecting humans are *Schistosoma haematobium*, *Schistosoma japonicum* and *Schistosoma mansoni*. *S. japonicum* is mainly prevalent in China. By the end of 2012, the total number of schistosomiasis japonica cases were estimated to be 240597, the total number of advanced schistosomiasis cases were estimated to be 30396. Schistosomiasis mainly was endemic in 7 provinces in the south of China, including Hubei, Hunan, Jiangxi, Anhui, Jiangsu, Yunnan, Guangxi, and Sichuan [3]. The total infection rate in fishermen was 40.4% in two fisherman villages in Yueyang County of Hunan Province, 58.6% schistosomiasis had hepatic fibrosis [4]. 66.2% schistosomiasis had hepatic fibrosis by Type-B ultrasonic examining the status of hepatic fibrosis from 447 chronic schistosomiasis patients in Tongling County of Anhui Province [5]. In schistosomiasis, the adult worms grow inside the mesenteric and portal vein system of the human body where they are laying eggs. The eggs become trapped mainly in the liver and gut, where they induce a vigorous granulomatous response. Subsequently, fibrosis and portal hypertension may develop, which are responsible for morbidity and the potentially fatal outcome in infected individuals. Thus, much of the clinical manifestation of schistosomiasis is ascribed to the egg-induced granulomatous inflammatory response and the associated fibrosis [6]. The latter is a serious consequence of *S. japonicum* infection that involves remodeling of the extracellular matrix (ECM) and excessive deposition of collagen, primarily by hepatic stellate cells (HSCs) [7]. Effective medical interventions to control and treat granuloma and fibrosis in schistosomiasis are lacking so far.

NF-κB is an important transcription factor involved in the expression of a variety of inflammatory genes in response to pathogens and cytokines [8]. It has been shown that activation of the NF-κB signaling pathway is closely associated with the development of granuloma and hepatic fibrosis [9–10]. Both Th1 and Th2 cytokines determine the hepatic granuloma size [11–12]. Particularly chemokines, such as MCP-1, contribute to the formation of hepatic granuloma in schistosomiasis. Accordingly, injection of anti-MCP-1 or anti-MCP-1α antibodies can inhibit granuloma formation [13]. Besides, VEGF is an important signaling protein involved in both vasculogenesis and angiogenesis. To that effect, previous studies have demonstrated that VEGF also plays an important role in promoting granuloma formation and fibrosis in experimental schistosomiasis [14–15].

Extracts of the oleogum resin from *Boswellia serrata* (BSE) containing a mixture of boswellic acids (BAs) have been confirmed to regulate inflammation and immune responses [16–17]. Likewise, recent studies have demonstrated that boswellic acid extracts attenuate pulmonary fibrosis and colonic fibrosis in rats [18–19]. Thus, these studies suggest that BSE might be valuable for the treatment of fibrosis associated with diverse clinical diseases. We have previously shown that water-soluble BSE-CD could attenuate *S. japonicum* egg-induced hepatic granuloma [20]. This prompted us to address in greater detail the role and mechanism of boswellic acids in *S. japonicum* egg-induced liver granuloma and the subsequent development of hepatic fibrosis.

The aim of our present work was to investigate whether the BA-containing extract (BSE) administered as a special cyclodextrin complex (CD), could attenuate *S. japonicum* egg-induced liver granuloma and fibrosis by a mechanism involving the inhibition of the NF-κB signaling pathway and the expression of selected NF-κB-dependent genes.

Materials and Methods

Ethics Statement

All mice were maintained in a specific pathogen-free microenvironment, and received care in compliance with the guidelines outlined in the *Guide for the Care and Use of Laboratory Animals*. All work was conducted with the approval of the Anhui Experimental Animal Training Base. The permit license number is LLSC2012-001.

Parasites and Animals

Oncomelania hupensis snails, infected with the Chinese strain of *S. japonicum* were provided by the Jiangxi Provincial Institute of Parasitic Diseases. Six weeks old female C57BL/6 mice, weighing 18–20 g, were purchased from the Experimental Animal Center of Chinese Science Academy. They were housed in a specific pathogen-free microenvironment in the animal facility, and received care in compliance with the guidelines for the Care and Use of Laboratory Animals. All work was approved by the Anhui Experimental Animal Training Base.

Infection of Mice with *S. japonicum*

Cercariae were shed in a beaker after exposing thirty infected *Oncomelania* to sunlight for 4 h (25–28°C). Mice were infected percutaneously with 20±2 *S. japonicum* cercariae.

Treatment of Mice with BSE-CD

The German drug authorities (BfArM) had previously approved BSE for testing in clinical studies. The extract composition of major BA derivatives is as follows: 1. α-boswellic acid (138 mg/g), 2. acetyl-α-boswellic acid (34 mg/g), 3. β-boswellic acid (192 mg/g), 4. acetyl-β-boswellic acid (100 mg/g), 5. 9,11-dehydro-α-boswellic acid (2 mg/g), 6. acetyl-9,11-dehydro-α-boswellic acid (0.6 mg/g), 7. 9,11-dehydro-β-boswellic acid (8 mg/g, 8. acetyl-9,11-dehydro-β-boswellic acid (6 mg/g), 9. lupeolic acid (26 mg/g), 10. acetyl-lupeolic acid (12 mg/g), 11. 11-keto-β-boswellic acid (66 mg/g), 12. acetyl-11-keto-β-boswellic acid (38 mg/g).

To allow the application of lipophilic BAs in aqueous solutions, BSE was complexed with cyclodextrin (CD) yielding BSE-CD ready for *in vivo* applications. For early phase BSE-CD treatment, the animals were divided into 5 groups: BSE-CD (280 mg/kg), BSE-CD (140 mg/kg), cyclodextrin (280 mg/kg), infected mice and normal mice, every group had 8 mice. Mice were injected intraperitoneally with BSE-CD (280 mg/kg) or BSE-CD (140 mg/kg) every day for 21 days of successive administration starting at 4 weeks after infection. In analogy, control mice were given intraperitoneally injections of cyclodextrin (280 mg/kg) for 21 days of successive administration starting at 4 weeks after infection. Another group of infected mice did not receive any treatment. Mice were sacrificed 24 h after the last administration. For late phase BSE-CD treatment, the animals were divided into 5 groups: BSE-CD (280 mg/kg), BSE-CD (140 mg/kg), cyclodextrin (280 mg/kg), infected mice and normal mice, every group had 8 mice. Mice were orally administered praziquantel on week 6 to eliminate the adult worms followed by injection with BSE-CD or cyclodextrin control from week 7 until week 10.

Histology and Immunohistochemistry of Liver Sections

Livers were excised from sacrificed mice, instantly fixed in 10% formalin in PBS and embedded in paraffin. Then tissue sections (4 μm) were stained with hematoxylin and eosin (H&E) or with Masson trichrome to examine the size of the granulomas and the extent of hepatic fibrosis, respectively. Immunostaining for phosphor-IκB kinase (IKK) was performed using a monoclonal phosphor-IKK primary Ab (Cell Signaling Technology, Beverly, MA, USA); immunostaining for α-smooth muscle actin (α-SMA) was performed using polyclonal α-SMA primary antibody (Bioss Inc., Bejing, China). Immunohistochemical analysis was performed with the Powervision Two-Step detection system (Zhongshan Biotechnology Co., Beijing, China). Six to ten microphotographs per mouse liver were recorded using an inverted microscope (Nikon 80I, Japan). Quantitative and qualitative changes were analyzed by means of morphometric software (Image-Pro Plus software). At least three non-continuous tissue sections were measured, and the mean values obtained from eight mice were used for statistical analysis.

Quantitative PCR

Total RNA of fresh liver tissue was isolated with Trizol Reagent (Invitrogen, Carlsbad, CA, USA) and transcribed into cDNA. Quantitaive PCR was performed using an ABI-Prism StepOne Plus Sequence Detector Systems (Applied Biosystems) and SYBR Premix Ex Taq (Takara Dalian, China). The primers used in this experiment are listed in Table S1. For normalization, we used the housekeeping gene encoding β-actin. Gene expression values were then calculated based on the ΔΔCt method [21]. The mean of the respective cytokines in uninfected mice was used as a calibrator. The relative quantity of target cytokine mRNA was expressed as $2^{-\Delta\Delta Ct}$.

Electrophoretic Mobility Shift Assay (EMSA)

For electrophoretic mobility shift assays (EMSA), we isolated nuclear proteins from the liver samples according to the manufacturer's instruction; protein concentrations were determined using a BCA assay kit (Viagene Biotech, Ningbo, China).

The binding of NF-κB to consensus oligonucleotides was analyzed using an EMSA kit (Viagene Biotech, Ningbo, China) according to the manufacturer's instruction. The sequences of the oligonucleotides used for the EMSA are 5′-AGTTGAGGGGACTTTCC-CAGGC-3′ served as the probe.

Statistical Analysis

The results were analyzed by the Student's *t*-test or analysis of variance where appropriate. All data were shown as mean ± standard error of the mean (SEM). *P* value <0.05 was considered to be statistically significant.

Results

Early Phase BSE-CD Treatment Suppresses *S. japonicum* Egg-induced Liver Granuloma Formation

To investigate the effect of BSE-CD on *S. japonicum* egg-induced liver granuloma, mice were intraperitoneally injected with BSE-CD or CD control once a day for a total of 21 days commencing 4 weeks after infection. Then mice were sacrificed, To investigate whether the above differences in liver granuloma size are due to dissimilar worm pairs, total worms, and total parasite eggs in the livers, we measured worm pairs, total worms, and total parasite eggs in the livers. Worm pairs, total worms, and total parasite eggs in the livers were similar between BSE-CD treatment groups and the control groups (Table S2)), liver tissues were fixed and stained with H&E. Strikingly, compared with control mice, early liver granulomas were attenuated in the group treated with 280 mg/kg BSE-CD. Likewise, in this group, H&E staining also showed a regression of the granulomatous inflammatory reaction compared with control mice (Fig. 1).

BSE-CD Treatment Markedly Suppresses the NF-κB Signaling Pathway

IκBα acts as endogenous NF-κB inhibitor by keeping the proteins in the cytosolic localization. After IκBα is targeted for degradation by phosphorylation activated IKK, NF-κB translocates into the cell nucleus where it activates the expression of target genes. To address NF-κB signaling, we analyzed the phosphorylation of IKK as parameter of NF-κB activity. Indeed, our results show that phospho-IKK staining intensities in hepatic granuloma from BSE-CD -treated animals were clearly reduced in comparison to control mice (Fig. 2). We also investigated the effects of BSE-CD on NF-κB activation using an EMSA method. Fig. 2 shows that BSE-CD (280 mg/kg) suppressed the constitutive activation of NF-κB in the liver tissue.

Early Phase BSE-CD Treatment Markedly Decreases MCP-1, TNF-α and VEGF mRNA Levels

To explore the molecular mechanism underlying the anti-granuloma effect mediated by early phase BSE-CD treatment, we analyzed some gene mRNA levels in the liver of BSE-CD-treated mice compared with control mice. Our data show that MCP-1, TNF-α and VEGF mRNA expression as determined by real time PCR were dose-dependently decreased in the liver of BSE-CD (280 mg/kg)-treated mice (*P*<0.05). No significant differences in the expression of IL-1, IL-6, IL-13 and TGF-β were detected in the livers of the four groups (Fig. 3).

Late Phase *BSE-CD* Treatment Reverses *S. japonicum* Egg-induced Liver Fibrosis

To investigate the effect of BSE-CD on *S. japonicum* egg-induced liver fibrosis, we assayed the effect of late phase BSE-CD treatment on pre-existent fibrosis, *i.e.* after fibrosis had already developed, We eliminated all worms in infected mice with praziquantel on week 6, and subsequently treated the mice with BSE-CD or placebo every day at 7 weeks (21 days of successive administration). Examination by Masson staining showed a significant decrease in the extent of fibrosis in the liver sections of BSE-CD (280 mg/kg)-treated mice compared with control mice (*P*<0.05) (Fig. 4A). The results also showed that more fibrous septa were formed in the model mice, and more collagen accumulated and deposited in the sinusoids and liver lobules. However, less fibrous septa and collagen were found in BSE-CD-treated mice (Fig. 4A). Furthermore, a significant decrease of α-SMA positive areas was also observed in BSE-CD (280 mg/kg)-treated mice compared with control mice (*P*<0.05) (Fig. 4B).

Late Phase BSE-CD Treatment Markedly Decreases MCP-1, TNF-α and VEGF mRNA Levels

To explore the molecular mechanism underlying the anti-fibrotic effect mediated by the late phase BSE-CD treatment, we analyzed some gene mRNA levels in the liver of BSE-CD-treated mice compared with control mice. We found that the expression of MCP-1, TNF-α, and VEGF was decreased in liver tissue of BSE-CD (280 mg/kg)-treated mice as detected by real time PCR assay (*P*<0.05), whereas no difference was found regarding the expression of IL-1, IL-6, IL-13 and TGF-β in the livers of the four groups of mice (Fig. 5).

Discussion

Although BSE is a contemporary phytomedicine, BA-containig remedies have already been used in traditional medicine for the treatment of various inflammatory diseases. The fact, that treatment with BSE and other BA-containing phytomedicines cause only minor side effects makes such preparations particularly appealing therapeutics [16]. The anti-inflammatory mechanism of BA-containing preparations such as BSE has been partly ascribed to their suppressive activity on lipid mediator biosynthesis encompassing leukotrienes and PGE_2 [22–24]. More importantly, several BAs have been shown to interfere with NF-κB signaling leading to inhibition of proinflammatory NF-κB activation [25–28]. Similarly, Kumar confirmed acyl derivatives of BAs can inhibit NF-κB and STATs pathway [29]. Latella have demonstrated the extracts from *Boswellia serrata* and *Scutellaria baicalensis* prevented the development of colonic fibrosis in rats [18]. Ali found that a BA extract could attenuate pulmonary fibrosis induced by bleomycin and oxidative stress from gamma irradiation in rats [19]. We have confirmed that BSE-CD could attenuate *S. japonicum* egg-induced hepatic granuloma, which may be partly dependent on the down-regulation of some biochemical mediators [20]. Here, we wanted to study in greater detail the role of BAs in *S. japonicum* egg-induced liver granuloma and fibrosis. We found that early BSE-CD treatment significantly attenuated *S. japonicum* egg-induced granuloma and significantly improved hepatic gross appearance (Fig. 1). We also observed that late BSE-CD treatment significantly attenuated *S. japonicum* egg-induced fibrosis (Fig. 4).

In resting cells, the transcription factor NF-κB is bound to inhibitor of nuclear factor κB (IκB) proteins, keeping the transcription factor in a cytosolic localization. Upon stimulation by many factors, IκB kinases (IKK) become activated and mediate phosphorylation and degradation of the inhibitor. Subsequently, free NF-κB is translocating into the nucleus where it activates target gene expression [8]. In line with previous findings [25–29], our data show that phospho-IKK staining intensities in hepatic granuloma from BSE-CD (280 mg/kg) treated animals were

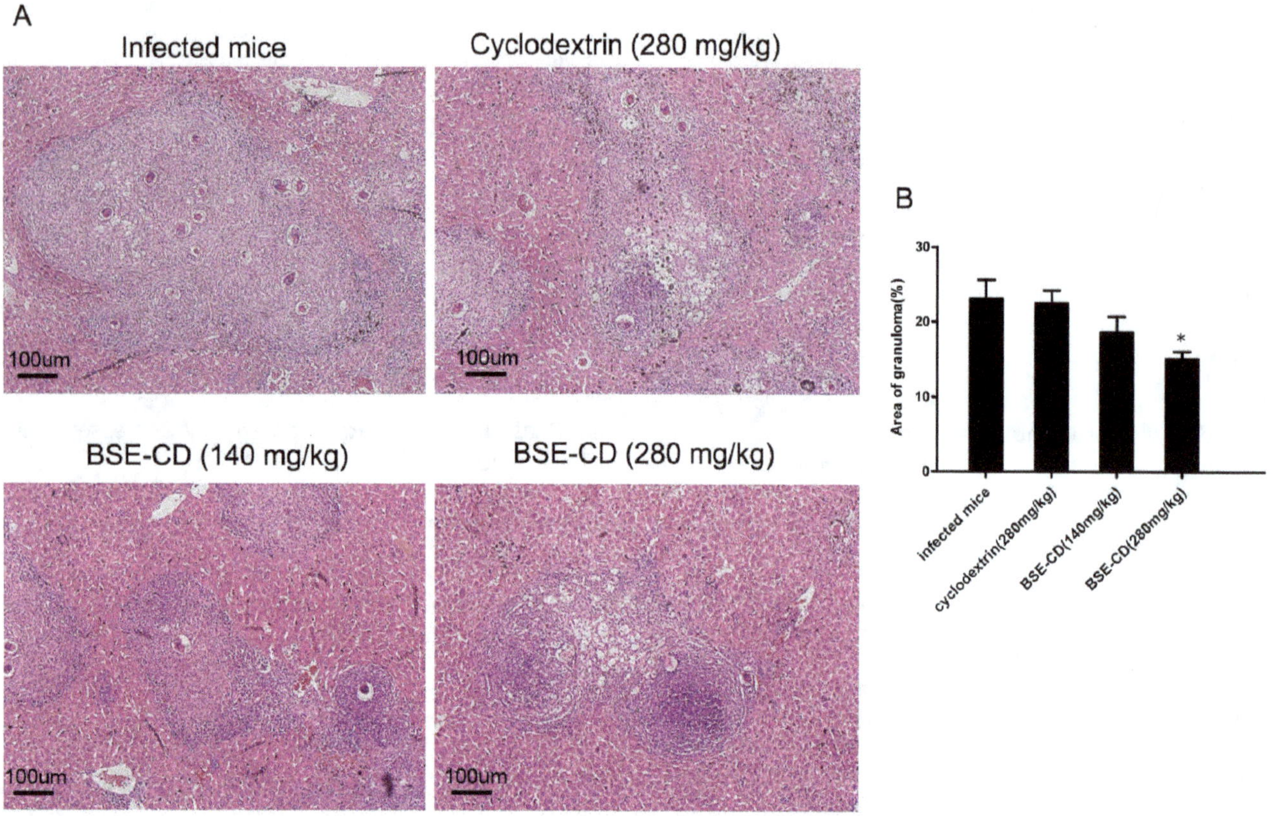

Figure 1. Effect of early phase BSE-CD treatment on hepatic granulomatous inflammation in mice infected with *S. japonicum*. Mice were infected with 20±2 cercariae, Treatment with BSE-CD or placebo from week 5 to week 7. Mice were killed, and liver tissues were fixed by formalin and stained with H&E. (A) Liver tissues stained with H&E. (B) Hepatic egg granuloma size was measured by computer-assisted histomorphometric analysis. All data are expressed as mean ± SEM (n = 8 for each group). **P*<0.05 *versus* corresponding infected mice or the cyclodextrin (280 mg/kg) group.

clearly reduced in comparison to control mice (P<0.05). Besides EMSA data confirmed that *in vivo* treatment with BSE-CD (280 mg/kg) suppressed NF-κB signal transduction in the liver tissue (P<0.05) (Fig. 2).

The NF-κB signaling pathway modulates hepatic fibrogenesis predominantly by regulating stellate cell survival and hepatocyte injury, the primary effects of fibrogenic and inflammatory signals eliciting hepatic inflammation. Indeed, the activation of NF-κB seems to play a key role in the pathogenesis of liver fibrosis by regulating hepatocyte, HSC and Kupffer cell functions [10,30–31]. Consistently, multiple studies have demonstrated inhibiton of hepatic fibrosis by targeting NF-κB signaling [32–33]. In line with those findings, BSE-CD could also significantly reduce the hepatic granuloma and fibrosis size in our study, which could at least be partly due to inhibiting the NF-κB signaling pathway.

The process of fibrosis formation from granular tissue in the liver is dependent on activation of stellate cells [34]. Activated HSCs are considered to be effector cells of liver fibrosis playing an important role in the granulomatous, fibrotic process induced by *S. japonicum* eggs [35]. Our data show that BSE-CD could markedly reduce HSC activation (Fig. 4), which is expected to contribute to the suppression of hepatic fibrosis formation.

Vascular endothelial growth factor (VEGF) contributes to the regulation of vasculogenesis, and induces angiogenesis and endothelial cell proliferation [36]. Some studies have linked VEGF with harmful effects in the state of hepatic granuloma and fibrosis and cirrhosis in patients and experimental animal models [37–38]. Consistently, application of an angiogenic inhibitorin an experimental murine model of *S. mansoni* resulted in reduced injury characterized by attenuated hepatic granuloma formation and fibrosis [15]. MCP-1can trigger migration of monocytes into the hepatic granuloma. To that effect, the expression profile of MCP-1 has close correlation with granuloma diameter. It has been reported that MCP-1 might play a key role in initiating and maintaining the immune response to tissue egg deposition, injection of anti-MCP-1 antibodies could inhibit granuloma formation [13]. TNF-α is a cytokine taking part in many processes, including inflammation, proliferation and programmed cell death. Studies *in vitro* and in experimental models *in vivo* have demonstrated that TNF-α plays a role in granuloma formation and hepatic fibrosis [39]. In fact, TNF-α seems to play a central role in promoting periportal fibrosis during *S. mansoni* infection and was found to be elevated in peripheral blood eosinophils from chronic Schistosoma mansoni-infected patients [40].

Multiple studies have demonstrated that BA treatment significantly decreases VEGF [25,28,41–42], MCP-1 [25,28] and TNF-α [28,40,43] in different animal model such as in LPS-challenged ApoE mice [25,28], in a transgenic model of psoriasis [44], in an orthotopic nude mouse model of PaCa [41] and in a murine sponge model [43]. Our results show that the early and late treatment of mice with *S. japonicum* infection by BSE-CD also significantly reduces VEGF, TNF-α and MCP-1 levels; the genes of those proteins were reported to be under the control of NF-κB (Fig. 3, Fig. 5). The attenuating effect of BSE-CD on liver

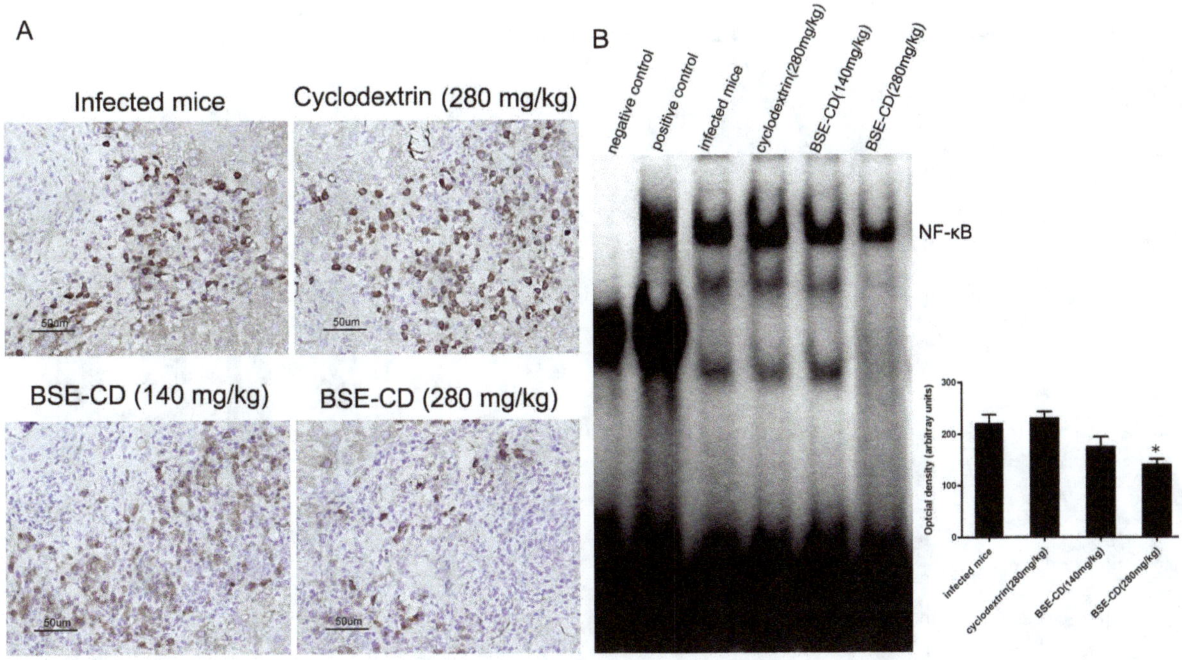

Figure 2. Effects of BSE-CD treatment on the NF-κB pathway activation in the liver tissue of mice infected *with S. japonicum.* Mice were treated as described in Fig. 1. (A) Sections of the liver tissue were analyzed immunohistochemically for the phosphorylated form of IKK. (B) The activation of NF-κB was measured by EMSA. All data are expressed as mean ± SEM (n = 8 for each group). **P*<0.05 versus corresponding infected mice or the cyclodextrin (280 mg/kg) group.

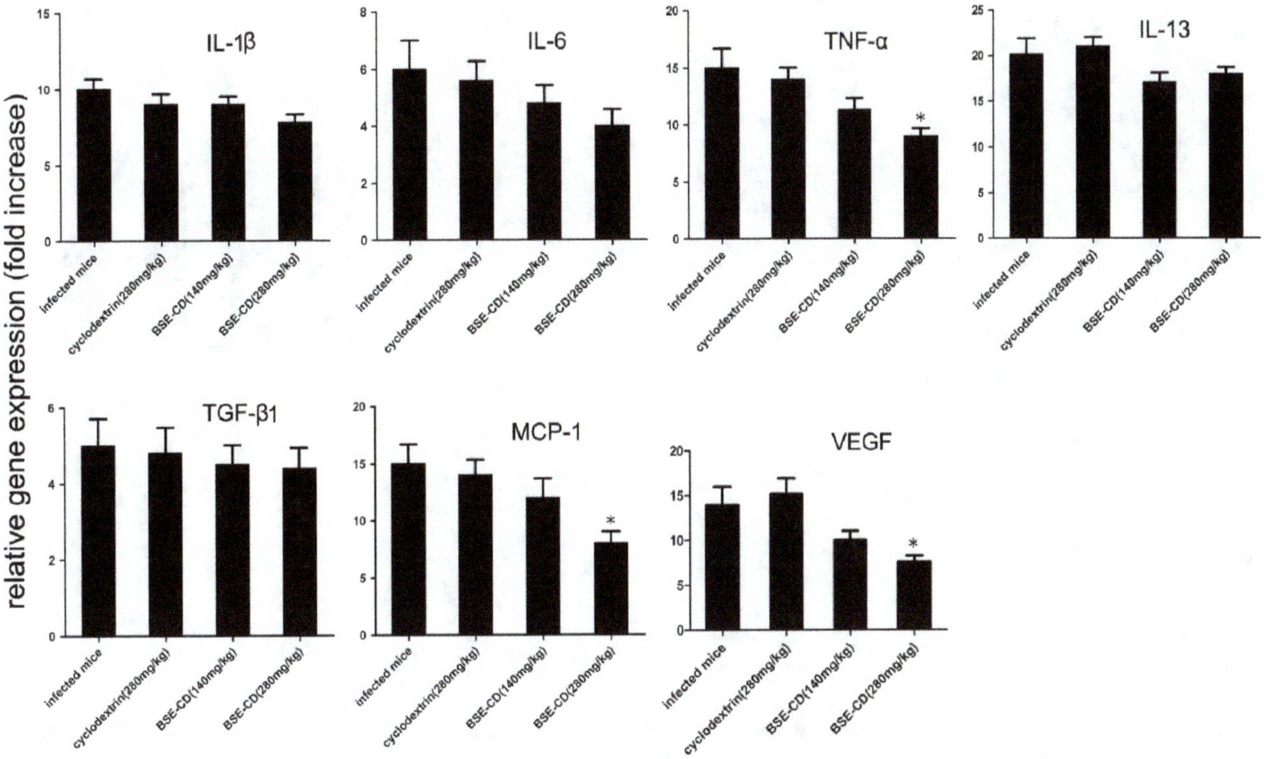

Figure 3. Effect of early phase BSE-CD treatment on cytokine mRNA expression in the liver of mice infected with *S. japonicum.* Mice were treated as described in Fig. 1. The mRNA levels were expressed relative to the levels in uninfected controls following normalization with β-actin. All data are expressed as mean ± SEM (n = 8 for each group). **P*<0.05 versus corresponding infected mice or the cyclodextrin (280 mg/kg) group.

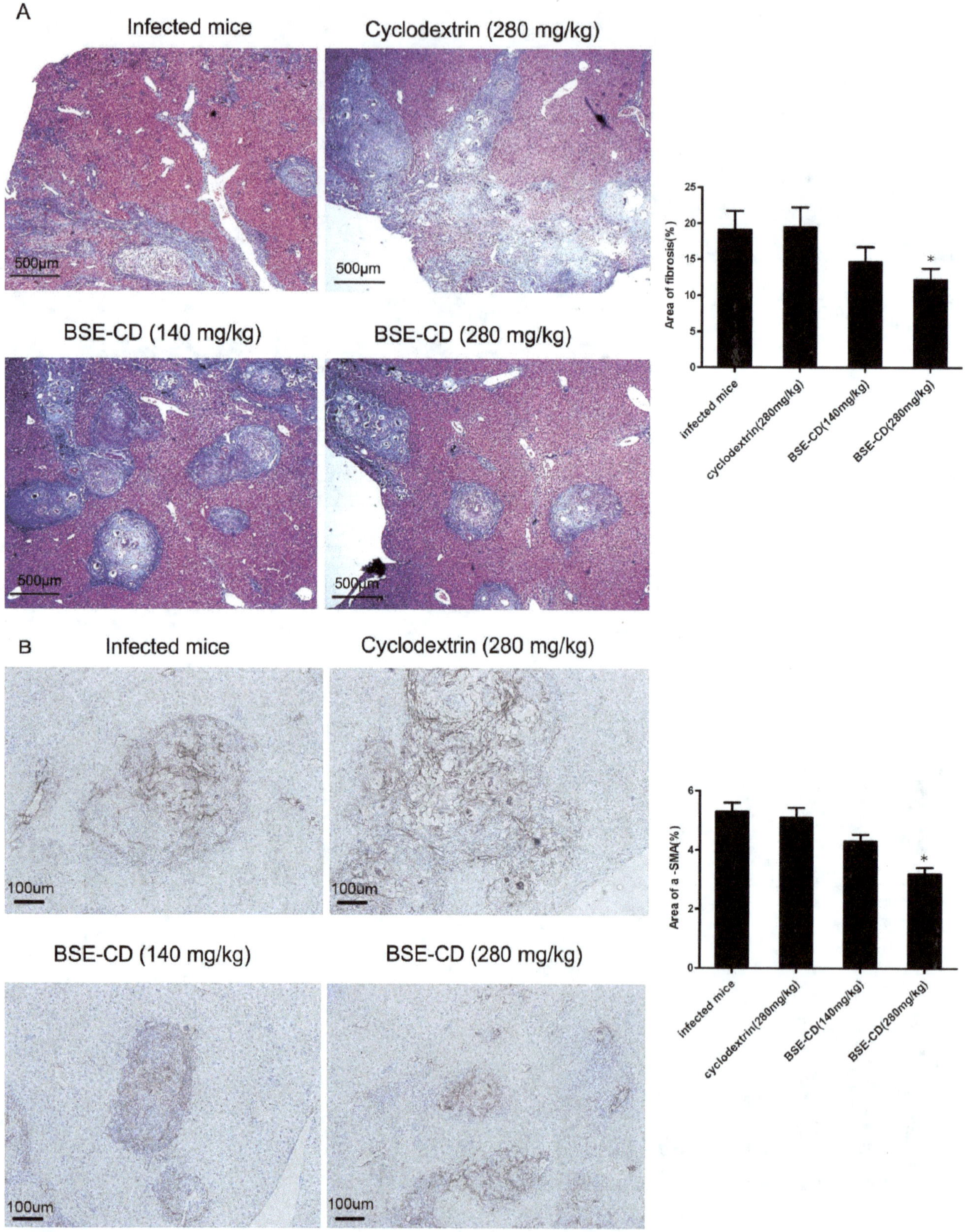

Figure 4. Effect of late phase BSE-CD treatment on hepatic fibrosis of liver tissue from mice that had been infected with *S. japonicum.* Mice were infected with 20±2 cercariae, Treatment with BSE-CD or placebo from week 7 until week 11. (A) Mice were killed, and liver tissues were fixed in formalin and stained with Masson trichrome or (B) anti-SMA antibody. Collagen deposition and the α-SMA positive areas were quantified as shown on the right hand panel, respectively. All data are expressed as mean ± SEM (n = 8 for each group). **P*<0.05 versus corresponding infected mice or the cyclodextrin (280 mg/kg) group.

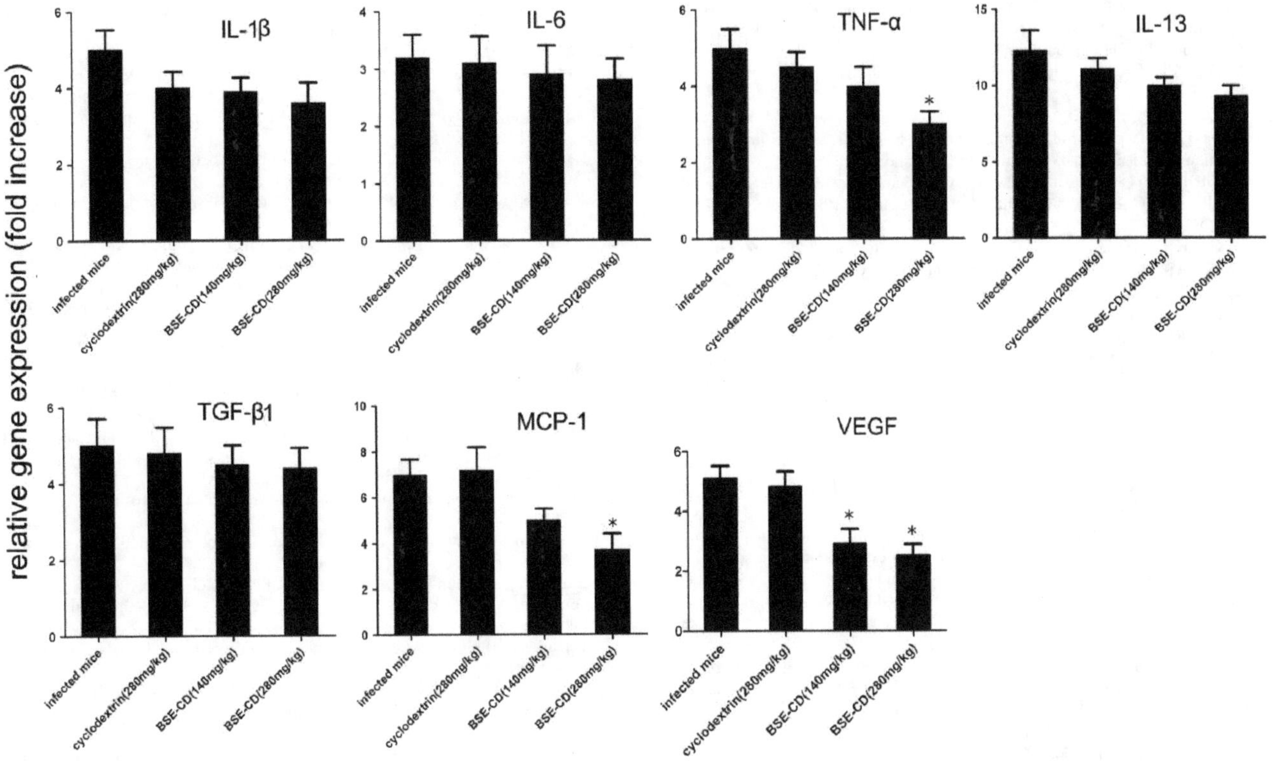

Figure 5. Effect of late phase BSE-CD treatment on cytokine mRNA expression in the liver tissue of mice. Mice were treated as described in Fig. 4. The mRNA levels were expressed relative to the levels in uninfected controls following normalization with β-actin. All data are expressed as mean ± SEM (n = 8 for each group). $^{*}P<0.05$ versus corresponding infected mice or the cyclodextrin (280 mg/kg) group.

granuloma and fibrosis was accompanied by decreased MCP-1, TNF-α, and VEGF levels expression, which may contribute to the inhibition of macrophage recruitment, and to the reduction of peri-ovular inflammatory responses and vasculogenesis.

Both IL-13 and TGF-β1 are involved in the activation of "resting" HSCs and they are known to play an important role in promoting hepatic fibrosis in schistosomiasis [35,45]. There have been reports that BSE treatment could downregulate the expression of transforming growth factor (TGF-β 1) in vivo [19]. However, we found BSE treatment had little effect on TGF-β 1 and IL-13 mRNA expression in the liver tissue (Fig. 3, Fig. 5). Thus, BSE-CD treatment attenuates *S. japonicum* egg-induced hepatic fibrosis independent from a decreased expression of IL-13 and TGF-β1. We also observed that the expression level of IL-1β and IL-6 tended to decrease in the BSE-CD-treatment groups. However, there was no significant difference in the expression of IL-1β and IL-6 between the four group mice (Fig. 3, Fig. 5).

In conclusion, our data show that BSE-CD treatment can attenuate *S. japonicum* egg-induced hepatic granulomas and fibrosis, which might be partly due to the suppression of the NF-κB pathway and a decreased expression of VEGF, TNF-α and MCP-1. Suppression of HSC activation may also play a role in the therapeutic effect of BSE-CD. This study explores BSE-CD in treatment of *S. japonicum* egg-induced hepatic granuloma and fibrosis as well as its mechanism. Our findings may provide the theoretical and practical basis for a novel treatment of schistosomal hepatic granuloma and fibrosis.

Supporting Information

Table S1 Sequences of primers used in this study.

Table S2 Parasitological measurements in infected mice treated with BSE-CD or cyclodextrin in early phase. Mice were treated as described in Fig. 1, and then we measured worm pairs, total worms, and total parasite eggs in the livers. Worm pairs, total worms, and total parasite eggs in the livers were similar between BSE-CD treatment groups and the control groups($P>0.05$). All data are expressed as mean ± SEM (n = 8 for each group).

Author Contributions

Conceived and designed the experiments: JS ML TS. Performed the experiments: ML QW PC MB SD CR. Analyzed the data: ML QW YZ XH. Contributed reagents/materials/analysis tools: TS BB DH CR. Wrote the paper: JS ML TS.

References

1. Molyneux DH, Malecela MN (2011) Neglected tropical diseases and the millennium development goals: why the "other diseases" matter: reality versus rhetoric. Parasit Vectors 4: 234.
2. Steinmann P, Keiser J, Bos R, Tanner M, Utzinger J (2006) Schistosomiasis and water resources development: systematic review, meta-analysis, and estimates of people at risk. Lancet Infect Dis 6: 411–425.
3. Li SZ, Zheng H, Gao J, Zhang LJ, Zhu R, et al. (2013) Endemic status of schistosomiasis in People's Republic of China in 2012. Zhongguo xue xi chong bing fang zhi za zhi 25: 557–563.
4. Yu XL, Zhou J, He YK, Huang MZ, Li YS, et al. (2013) Influence factors of schistosoma japonum infection among fishermen in eastern dongting lake region. Zhongguo xue xi chong bing fang zhi za zhi. 31: 307–309.

5. Wang XH, Zhang Y, Tan YQ (2008) Image analysis of ultrasonography on the liver and spleen of chronic schistosomiasis patients: a report of 447 cases Zhongguo xue xi chong bing fang zhi za zhi 28: 314.
6. Andrade ZA (2008) Schistosomiasis and hepatic fibrosis regression. Acta Trop 108: 79–82.
7. Mohamed-Ali Q, Elwali N, Abdelhameed A, Mergani A, Rahoud S, et al. (1999) Susceptibility to periportal (Symmers) fibrosis in human Schistosoma mansoni infections: evidence that intensity and duration of infection, gender, and inherited factors are critical in disease progression. J Infect Dis 180: 1298–1306.
8. Hayden MS, Ghosh S (2008) Shared principles in NF-κB signaling. Cell 132: 344–362.
9. Friedman SL, Rockey DC, Bissell DM (2007) Hepatic fibrosis 2006: report of the Third AASLD Single Topic Conference. Hepatology 45: 242–249.
10. Luedde T, Schwabe RF (2011) NF-κB in the liver–linking injury, fibrosis and hepatocellular carcinoma. Nat Rev Gastroenterol Hepatol 8: 108–118.
11. Caldas IR, Campi-azevedo AC, Oliveira LF, Silveira AM, Oliveira RC, et al. (2008) Human schistosomiasis mansoni: immune responses during acute and chronic phases of the infection. Acta Trop 108: 109–117.
12. Herbert DR, Orekov T, Perkins C, Finkelman FD (2008) IL-10 and TGF-βredundantly protect against severe liver injury and mortality during acute schistosomiasis. J Immunol 181: 7214–7220.
13. Souza PR, Souza AL, Negrão-correa D, Teixeira AL, Teixeira MM (2008) The role of chemokines in controlling granulomatous inflammation in Schistosoma mansoni infection. Acta Trop 108: 135–138.
14. Abdel fattah NS, Ahmed NS (2012) Evidence of intra-hepatic vascular proliferation remodeling early after cure in experimental schistosomiasis mansoni: an immunohistochemical descriptive study. Exp Parasitol 130: 58–62.
15. Shariati F, Pérez-arellano JL, Carranza C, López-abán J, Vicente B, et al. (2011) Evaluation of the role of angiogenic factors in the pathogenesis of schistosomiasis. Exp Parasitol 128: 44–49.
16. Abdel-tawab M, Werz O, Schubert-Zsilavecz M (2011) Boswellia serrata: an overall assessment of in vitro, preclinical, pharmacokinetic and clinical data. Clin Pharmacokinet 50: 349–369.
17. Ammon HP (2010) Modulation of the immune system by Boswellia serrata extracts and boswellic acids. Phytomedicine 17: 862–867.
18. Latella G, Sferra R, Vetuschi A, Zanninelli G, D'angelo A, et al. (2008) Prevention of colonic fibrosis by Boswellia and Scutellaria extracts in rats with colitis induced by 2,4,5-trinitrobenzene sulphonic acid. Eur J Clin Invest 38: 410–420.
19. Ali EN, Mansour SZ (2011) Boswellic acids extract attenuates pulmonary fibrosis induced by bleomycin and oxidative stress from gamma irradiation in rats. Chin Med 6: 36.
20. Liu M, Chen P, Büchele B, Dong S, Huang D, et al. (2013) A boswellic acid-containing extract attenuates hepatic granuloma in C57BL/6 mice infected with Schistosoma japonicum. Parasitol Res 112: 1105–1111.
21. Hou X, Zhou R, Wei H, Sun R, Tian Z (2009) NKG2D-retinoic acid early inducible-1 recognition between natural killer cells and Kupffer cells in a novel murine natural killer cell-dependent fulminant hepatitis. Hepatology 49: 940–949.
22. Safayhi H, Sailer ER, Ammon HP (1995) Mechanism of 5-lipoxygenase inhibition by acetyl-11-keto-β-boswellic acid. Mol Pharmacol 47: 1212–1216.
23. Sailer ER, Subramanian LR, Rall B, Hoernlein RF, Ammon HP, et al. (1996) Acetyl-11-keto-β-boswellic acid (AKBA): structure requirements for binding and 5-lipoxygenase inhibitory activity. Br J Pharmacol 117: 615–618.
24. Siemoneit U, Koeberle A, Rossi A, Dehm F, Verhoff M, et al. (2011) Inhibition of microsomal prostaglandin E_2 synthase-1 as a molecular basis for the anti-inflammatory actions of boswellic acids from frankincense. Br J Pharmacol 162: 147–162.
25. Kiela PR, Midura AJ, Kuscuoglu N, Jolad SD, Sólyom AM, et al. (2005) Effects of Boswellia serrata in mouse models of chemically induced colitis. Am J Physiol Gastrointest Liver Physiol 288: G798-G808.
26. Syrovets T, Gschwend JE, Büchele B, Laumonnier Y, Zugmaier W, et al. (2005) Inhibition of IκB kinase activity by acetyl-boswellic acids promotes apoptosis in androgen-independent PC-3 prostate cancer cells in vitro and in vivo. J Biol Chem 280: 6170–6180.
27. Cuaz-pérolin C, Billiet L, Baugé E, Copin C, Scott-algara D, et al. (2008) Antiinflammatory and antiatherogenic effects of the NF-κB inhibitor acetyl-11-keto-β-boswellic acid in LPS-challenged ApoE−/− mice. Arterioscler Thromb Vasc Biol 28: 272–277.
28. Syrovets T, Büchele B, Krauβ C, Laumonnier Y, Simmet T (2005) Acetyl-boswellic acids inhibit lipopolysaccharide-mediated TNF-α induction in monocytes by direct interaction with IκB kinases. J Immunol 174: 498–506.
29. Kumar A, Shah BA, Singh S, Hamid A, Singh SK, et al. (2012) Acyl derivatives of boswellic acids as inhibitors of NF-κB and STATs. Bioorg Med Chem Lett 22: 431–435.
30. Bataller R, Brenner DA (2012) Liver fibrosis. J Clin Invest 115: 209–218.
31. Friedman SL (2004) Mechanisms of disease: Mechanisms of hepatic fibrosis and therapeutic implications. Nat Clin Pract Gastroenterol Hepatol 1: 98–105.
32. Mann DA, Smart DE (2002) Transcriptional regulation of hepatic stellate cell activation. Gut 50: 891–896.
33. Anan A, Baskin-bey ES, Bronk SF, Werneburg NW, Shah VH, et al. (2006) Proteasome inhibition induces hepatic stellate cell apoptosis. Hepatology 43: 335–344.
34. Friedman SL (2008) Hepatic stellate cells: protean, multifunctional, and enigmatic cells of the liver. Physiol Rev 88: 125–172.
35. Bartley PB, Ramm GA, Jones MK, Ruddell RG, Li Y, et al. (2006) A contributory role for activated hepatic stellate cells in the dynamics of Schistosoma japonicum egg-induced fibrosis. Int J Parasitol 36: 993–1001.
36. Ferrara N (1999) Molecular and biological properties of vascular endothelial growth factor. J Mol Med 77: 527–543.
37. Giatromanolaki A, Kotsiou S, Koukourakis MI, Sivridis E (2007) Angiogenic factor expression in hepatic cirrhosis. Mediators Inflamm: 67187.
38. Makhlouf MM, Awad A, Zakhari MM, Fouad M, Saleh WA (2002) Vascular endothelial growth factor level in chronic liver diseases. J Egypt Soc Parasitol 32: 907–921.
39. Fallon PG, Dunne DW (1999) Tolerization of mice to Schistosoma mansoni egg antigens causes elevated type 1 and diminished type 2 cytokine responses and increased mortality in acute infection. J Immunol 162: 4122–4132.
40. Silveira-lemos D, Teixeira-carvalho A, Martins-filho OA, Alves oliveira LF, Costa-silva MF, et al. (2008) Eosinophil activation status, cytokines and liver fibrosis in Schistosoma mansoni infected patients. Acta Trop 108: 150–159.
41. Park B, Prasad S, Yadav V, Sung B, Aggarwal BB (2011) Boswellic acid suppresses growth and metastasis of human pancreatic tumors in an orthotopic nude mouse model through modulation of multiple targets. PLoS One 6: e26943.
42. Shehata AM, Quintanilla-fend L, Bettio S, Singh CB, Ammon HP (2011) Prevention of multiple low-dose streptozotocin (MLD-STZ) diabetes in mice by an extract from gum resin of Boswellia serrata (BE). Phytomedicine 18: 1037–1044.
43. Saraswati S, Pandey M, Mathur R, Agrawal SS (2011) Boswellic acid inhibits inflammatory angiogenesis in a murine sponge model. Microvasc Res 82: 263–268.
44. Wang H, Syrovets T, Kess D, Büchele B, Hainzl H, et al. (2006) Targeting NF-κB with a natural triterpenoid alleviates skin inflammation in a mouse model of psoriasis. J Immunol 183: 4755–4763.
45. Weng HL, Liu Y, Chen JL, Huang T, Xu LJ, et al. (2009) The etiology of liver damage imparts cytokines transforming growth factor β1 or interleukin-13 as driving forces in fibrogenesis. Hepatology 50: 230–243.

HGF and Direct Mesenchymal Stem Cells Contact Synergize to Inhibit Hepatic Stellate Cells Activation through TLR4/NF-kB Pathway

Pei-pei Wang[1,4 9], Dong-ying Xie[1,4 9], Xu-Jing Liang[2], Liang Peng[1], Geng-lin Zhang[1], Yi-nong Ye[3], Chan Xie[1,4]*, Zhi-liang Gao[1,4]*

1 Department of Infectious Diseases, the Third Affiliated Hospital of Sun Yat-Sen University, Guangzhou, Guangdong Province, China, **2** Department of Infectious Disease, the First Affiliated Hospital, Jinan University, Guangzhou, Guangdong, China, **3** Department of Infectious Diseases, the First Peoples Hospital of Foshan City, Foshan, Guangdong Province, China, **4** Key Laboratory of Tropical Disease Control, Ministry of Education, Sun Yat-sen University, Guangzhou, Guangdong Province, China

Abstract

Aims: Bone marrow-derived mesenchymal stem cells (BMSCs) can reduce liver fibrosis. Apart from the paracrine mechanism by which the antifibrotic effects of BMSCs inhibit activated hepatic stellate cells (HSCs), the effects of direct interplay and juxtacrine signaling between the two cell types are poorly understood. The purpose of this study was to explore the underlying mechanisms by which BMSCs modulate the function of activated HSCs.

Methods: We used BMSCs directly and indirectly co-culture system with HSCs to evaluate the anti-fibrosis effect of BMSCs. Cell proliferation and activation were examined in the presence of BMSCs and HGF. c-met was knockdown in HSCs to evaluate the effect of HGF secreted by BMSCs. The TLR4 and Myeloid differentiation primary response gene 88(MyD88) mRNA levels and the NF-kB pathway activation were determined by real-time PCR and western blotting analyses. The effect of BMSCs on HSCs activation was investigated in vitro in either MyD88 silencing or overexpression in HSCs. Liver fibrosis in rats fed CCl_4 with and without BMSCs supplementation was compared. Histopathological examinations and serum biochemical tests were compared between the two groups.

Results: BMSCs remarkably inhibited the proliferation and activation of HSCs by interfering with LPS-TLR4 pathway through a cell–cell contact mode that was partially mediated by HGF secretion. The NF-kB pathway is involved in HSCs activation inhibition by BMSCs. MyD88 over expression reduced the BMSC inhibition of NF-kB luciferase activation. BMSCs protected liver fibrosis in vivo.

Conclusion: BMSCs modulate HSCs in vitro via TLR4/MyD88/NF-kB signaling pathway through cell–cell contact and secreting HGF. BMSCs have therapeutic effects on cirrhosis rats. Our results provide new insights into the treatment of hepatic fibrosis with BMSCs.

Editor: Yao Liang Tang, University of Cincinnati, United States of America

Funding: Grant Support: The Natural Science Foundation of China (No. 81101864/H1617), Baiyang liver cirrhosis grand (No. 2010-004), the Fundamental Research Funds for the Central Universities (09 ykzs07,10 ykzs04). The funders had no role in study design, data collection and analysis, decision to publish, or preparation of the manuscript.

Competing Interests: The authors have declared that no competing interests exist.

* E-mail: happyxiechan@gmail.com (CX); gaozl@yahoo.com.cn (ZG)

9 These authors contributed equally to this work.

Introduction

Liver fibrosis is the excessive deposition of extracellular matrix and scar formation surrounding damaged liver and this can be effectively reversed [1,2]. Activated hepatic stellate cells are generated in the extracellular matrix (ECM) of the principal cells during the process of liver fibrosis. ECM production is the primary reason for the excessive fibrosis formation, which eventually leads to cirrhosis. Acquired fibrosis may result from the action of a number of pathogenic factors, toxic exposures, chronic viral hepatitis or the presence of non-alcoholic fatty liver disease. These etiological factors may work separately or in combination with each other to produce cumulative effects [3]. A large number of in vivo experimental and clinical studies have shown that endotoxin levels in patients with liver cirrhosis are significantly increased, and LPS (an endotoxin) can directly activate HSC in vivo. TLR4 is the primary LPS receptor, and TLR4 polymorphisms are closely related to liver fibrosis. Thus, the LPS-TLR4 pathway plays an important role in fibrosis [4]. TLR4 signals through adaptor proteins, including MyD88, to activate down-stream effectors that include NF-kB, mitogen-activated protein kinase (MAPK), and phosphatidylinositol 3-kinase (PI3K). Collectively, these pathways regulate the expression of pro-inflammatory cytokines and genes that control cell survival and apoptosis.

BMSCs are pluripotent stem cells with the potential to differentiate into liver cells. Recent studies have also shown that BMSCs play a substantial role in liver fibrosis treatment without allograft rejection. Studies from animal models have shown that BMSCs infusion ameliorates liver fibrosis and reverses fulminant hepatic failure. A number of clinical trials also proved that BMSCs can effectively alleviate end-stage liver disease and improve symptoms and liver function, indicating the effectiveness and safety of BMSCs in clinical implantation [5–7]. However, it has also been reported that BMSCs have the potential to promote fibrosis [8,9]. Therefore, for therapeutic applications, it will be important to understand the potency and possible repair mechanisms of BMSCs to help us understand the nature of hepatic fibrosis.

Since both the LPS-TLR4 pathway and BMSCs are involved in liver fibrosis, we hypothesized that BMSCs may interfere LPS-TLR4 pathway and inhibit NF-kB activation during fibrosis. To test this hypothesis, we examined the expression of TLR4 in HSCs stimulated with different doses of LPS and investigated the regulatory role of BMSCs in MyD88-mediated LPS-stimulated TLR4 expression.

Materials and Methods

Ethics Statement

Normal liver and bone marrow samples. Normal liver samples were collected from patients undergoing resection of hepatic hemangiomas at the Department of Hepatobiliary Surgery, the third affiliated hospital of Sun Yat-sen University. Bone marrow suspension cells (10 ml) were obtained from healthy donors in the department of infectious diseases, the third affiliated hospital of Sun Yat-Sen university. All samples were obtained with written, informed consent in accordance with the Sun Yat-sen University Ethical Committee requirements.

Bone Marrow Separation for Primary Human BMSCs Cultures

BMSCs isolation and culture were described in our previously study [10]. Prior to experimental use, the third generation BMSCs were determined to be CD44, CD90 positive and lack expression of CD45 and CD34 by flowcytometry analysis.

Human HSCs Isolation and Cell Line Culture

HSCs were isolated by a 2-step collagenase perfusion from surgical specimens of two normal human livers as described previously [11]. All tissues were obtained by qualified medical staff, with donor consent and the approval of the Sun Yat-sen University Ethical Committee requirements. Cell viability was determined using trypan blue exclusion staining. Hepatic stellate cell line LX2 was obtained from the Cancer Center of Sun Yat-sen University. Isolated HSCs and LX2 were seeded on uncoated plastic tissue culture dishes and cultured in Dulbecco's modified Eagle medium (DMEM, Invitrogen, Carlsbad, CA, USA) supplemented with 10% fetal bovine serum (FBS, HyClone, Logan, UT, USA), 2 mM L-glutamine, 100 units/ml penicillin and 100 ug/ml streptomycin, cultured at 37°C in a humidified atmosphere containing 5% CO_2.

Physical Contact Co-culture System and Insert Co-culture System

The GFP-labeled LX2 cells were mixed and co-cultured with BMSCs in supplemented DMEM containing 10% FBS at a density of 1:1 for LX2 and BMSCs. Since there is no barrier between the two populations, effects are produced from both the exchange of soluble factors and from physical contact. As a comparison to the physical contact co-culture system, LX2 cells and BMSCs were also co-cultured in a bicompartmental system by using 6.5 mm Transwell® with 1.0 μm Pore Polycarbonate Membrane Insert, which were purchased from Corning (Corning, NY, USA). In this case, two types of cells shared the culture medium but were not in physical contact. Cells were seeded in DMEM and incubated overnight. Immediately prior to treatment the medium was changed for fresh DMEM. A total of 2×10^5 LX2/ml and equivalent volumes of BMSCs releasate and pellet fractions were added. Where indicated, cells were treated with 5 or 50 ng/ml of recombinant HGF (R&D Systems).

In Vivo Transplantation of BMSCs

Fourty SD rats in six weeks were purchased from the Institute of Materia Medica (Chinese Academy of Sciences, Beijing, China). This study was carried out in strict accordance with the recommendations in the Guide for the Care and Use of Laboratory Animals of the National Institutes of Health. The protocol was approved by the Committee on the Ethics of Animal Experiments of Sun Yat-Sen University. To induce liver cirrhosis, 6.0 ml/kg body weight of carbon tetrachloride (CCl4) mixed with olive oil (1:1 ratio) was injected intraperitonealy into rats twice a week up to 7 weeks. Five rats were random sacrificed to evaluate if the model was successful. Then the rest rats were divided into two group: BMSC treatment group (25 rats) and control group (10 rats): 1×10^6 BMSC in 100 ul PBS or 100 ul PBS as a control were injected into tail vein of rats. Three rats were sacrificed at each predetermined time interval (12 h, 24 h, 48 h, 72 h, 144 h) after BMSC post-transplantation to track the BMSC location. CCl4(3 ml/kg) was injected for another two weeks after cell transplantation to maintain persistent liver damage and all the left rats were sacrificed after 3 weeks BMSC post-transplantation. Liver tissue was collected after perfusing with 4% paraformaldehyde solution and preserved in formalin buffer solution for histopathological studies. For protein and total RNA isolation, liver tissue was snap-frozen in liquid nitrogen and then stored at −80°C.

Hematoxylin and Eosin (HE) and Masson Staining

The rat livers were fixed in formalin for 48 h, paraffin embedded and sectioned into 4-μm thick slices for HE staining or Masson staining. After sealing the slides containing the tissue slices with neutral gum, the stained tissue slices were microscopically examined at 200 × magnification. Subsequently, color images in five randomly chosen microscopic fields of each slice were captured and analyzed by a medical image software program (Image-Pro Plus, Media Cybernetics, USA) to semi-quantitatively determine the areal density (AD) i.e. collagen fiber area over liver area.

Scheuer Scoring System

A semiquantitative histological score was applied based on the histological classification and quantitation of the Scheuer scoring system using a scale of 0–3 for the inflammatory activity (0, absent; 0.5, minimal; 1, mild; 2, moderate; 3, severe), and 0–4 for the evaluation of fibrosis (0, absent; 1, mild; 2, moderate without septa; 3, moderate with septa; 4, cirrhosis) [12].

Serum Assay

Blood was taken from the abdominal aorta, and the following indicators were analyzed: total protein (TP), albumin (ALB), alanine aminotransferase (ALT), and aspartate aminotransferase (AST).

Other experimental procedures are available in Materials and Methods S1.

Statistical Analysis

Data are reported as mean values ± SD. The statistical significance of differences between mean values was determined by Student's t test. A *P* value of less than 0.05 was considered significant. Statistical calculations were performed using SPSSv16 software (SPSS Inc., Chicago, Illinois, USA).

Results

Bone Marrow-derived Cells Expressed Characteristic Surface Markers of BMSCs

BMSCs obtained by bone marrow aspiration and expanded in vitro appeared similar to fibroblasts, with a characteristic spindle-shaped fusiform morphology (Figure 1A). LX2 and primary HSCs were also fibroblasts alike (Figure 1A and 1B). In cultured cells of the 3rd generation analyzed by flow cytometry, more than 97% of the cells expressed CD44 (97.2±1.35%, Fig. 1B) and CD90 (98.0±1.20%, Figure 1C), a surface marker characteristic of BMSCs. The absence of contaminating hematopoietic cells in the BMSCs population was verified by the lack of surface antigens defining hematopoietic progenitor cells (CD34, 1.1±0.03%) or leukocytes (CD45, 0.68±0.05%). Thus, the bone marrow cells after the 3rd passage were of high purity, and expressed CD44^{+}, CD90^{+}, CD34^{-} and CD45^{-}, which are markers for BMSCs.

LPS induced Activation of LX2 Cells and Upregulation of TLR4

We first evaluated the effect of LPS stimulate hepatic stellate cells in vitro. LX2 cells were cultured with different concentrations of LPS (0, 50, 100, 125 ng/ml) to evaluate if there is a dose depended effect. IL-8 and TGF-β which was secreted by activated hepatic stellate cells were measured by ELISA. Results showed quiescent LX2 cells only secreted small amounts of IL-8 (0.33±0.04 pg/ml) and TGF-β (0.31±0.05 pg/ml) (Figure 2A). However, the secretion of IL-8 and TGF-β of LX2 was significantly increased when LPS added. Results of ELISA showed that IL-8 and TGF-β secretion from LPS-activated LX2 cells was 0.88±0.03 pg/ml and 0.74±0.05 pg/ml respectively after 100 ng/ml LPS stimulation (Figure 2A). Furthermore, the expression IL-8 and TGF-β was increased in parallel to increasing concentrations of LPS. When the LPS concentration reached 100 ng/ml, IL-8 and TGF-β expression levels reached up to three times that of the untreated cells. However, as the LPS concentration was increased to 125 ng/ml, a significant amount of cell died. As such, 100 ng/ml LPS were used in all subsequent experiments. Then the expression of TLR4 in two human primary HSCs cell lines and LX2 cells were assessed by RT-PCR. In quiescent LX2 cells and primary HSCs cells (no LPS stimulation), only low levels of TLR4 mRNA were detected. However, TLR4 was substantially up-regulated in LPS-activated primary HSCs cells and LX2 cells for more than 2 times in vitro (Figure 2B). These results suggested that LPS can stimulate HSC activation and TLR4 gene expression.

BMSCs Inhibit the Activation of LX2 Cells by Interfering with LPS-TLR4 Pathway

Since BMSCs had benefit to liver fibrosis patients, we test if BMSCs also had the effect to inhibit the activation of LX2 in vitro. We co-cultured LX2 with BMSCs separated by transwell to test if BMSC had the same effect on LPS induced LX2 activation. RT-PCR analysis indicated that LX2 and BMSCs without LPS stimulation only expressed small amount of TLR4, a-SMA, and Col-1. However, after LPS stimulation, the levels of TLR4, a-SMA, and Col-1 expression from LX2 cells were significantly increased for more than two times (Figure 2C), while addition of BMSCs significantly reduced the effect. Furthermore, the results of western blot analysis indicated that LX2 cells without LPS stimulation express only small amounts of a-SMA, Col-1, and TLR4, and addition of LPS stimulated increased expression of these proteins, which are known markers of HSCs activation. However, when BMSCs or the TLR4 inhibitor was added, the expression of these proteins from LX2 cells was decreased significantly (Figure 2D). These data suggest that protection of LPS induced LX2 activation by BMSCs was associated with TLR4.

BMSC Promote Activation of the HGF Pathway in LX2 Activation

To gain better insight into the signaling pathways involved in BMSCs-to-LX2 cell communication, we detected the effect of BMSCs-secreted cytokines on protection of LPS induced LX2 activation. Of the many cytokines, we tested HGF, IL-8, IL-2, IL-6, and TNF-a for their ability to effect Col-1 and a-SMA expression of LX2. The RT-PCR showed only HGF decreased Col-1 and a-SMA mRNA expression in LX2 cells for more than two times (Figure S1A). Considering that a prolonged exposure to HGF protects fibrosis in LX2, we investigated whether BMSC-derived HGF could inhibit fibrosis in LX2 cells. As shown in Figure S1B-1E, the mRNA and protein level of Col-1 and a-SMA in LPS stimulated LX2 cells decreased by approximately 1.5- to 2-fold within 6 to 24 hours after HGF treatment and increasing dose of HGF from 20 to 50 ng/ml, demonstrating that effect of HGF on LX2 cells. We next investigated whether HGF protection of LX2 cell is dependent on TLR4 signaling. Interestingly, When LX2 cells were treated with different cytokines for 6 h, we found only HGF induced decrease in TLR4 mRNA expression (Figure 3A). We also combined HGF with other cytokines to evaluate the co-effect on LX2. Western blot showed that quiescent LX2 cells (without LPS stimulation) only expressed a small amount of TLR4. While after LPS stimulation, TLR4 expression increased obviously. Then we used IL-8, HGF, IL-2, IL-6, and TNF-a stimulated LX2 along, and found only HGF deduced TLR4 expression. Besides of these, we combined two or three cytokines together and stimulate LX2, and the results of western blot showed that only when the combination included HGF, there was an effect of TLR4 down-regulation. The combination without HGF demonstrated no effect. Furthermore, no synergistic effect was found when HGF was used together with other cytokines (Figure 3B).

Then we knockdown the HGF receptor, c-met, of LX2 cell and investigate if LX2 activation inhibited by BMSCs was through HGF. As Figure 3C indicated, two c-met siRNA knockdown c-met protein in LX2 cell. When using BMSCs treating LX2/c-met-RNAi, we found that LPS induced LX2 activation could not be suppressed (Figure 3D). The results conferred BMSCs protected LX2 cells from LPS through secreating HGF.

HGF and Direct BMSC-LX2 Cell Contact Synergize to Inhibit LX2 Activation Gene Expression

It is believed that effective treatments aimed at suppressing the activation and proliferation of LX2 would reduce the deleterious

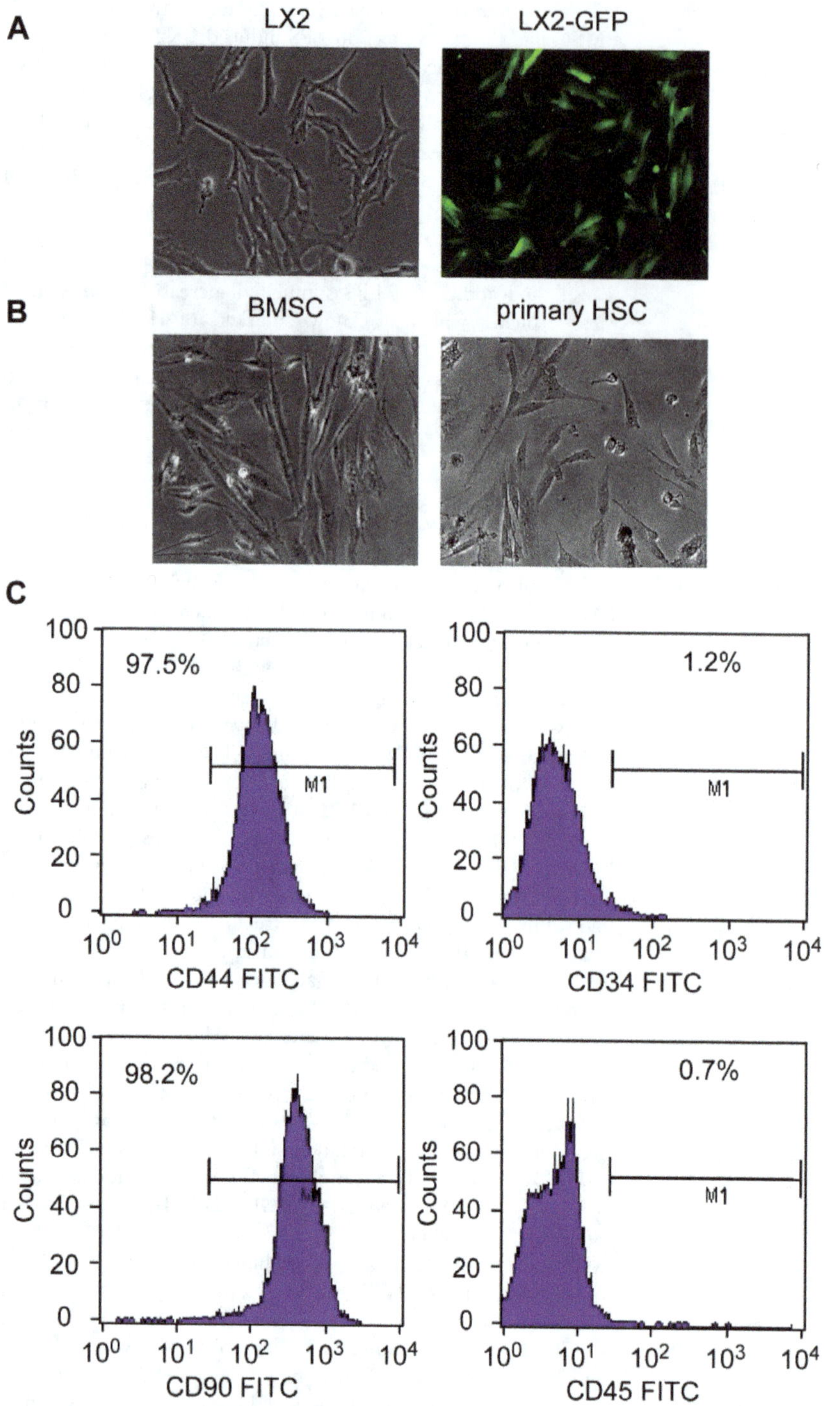

Figure 1. Primary Cells morphology and molecular expression. (A) HSC cell line LX2 (left) and GFP labeled LX2 (right). (B) BMSCs were separated from bone marrow and purified by removing the non-adherent cells at least three times. The 3rd generation BMSCs (medium) were fusiform and fibroblast-like (100×). Primary human HSC (right). (C) FCM analysis showed that the 3rd generation BMSCs expressed CD44 and CD90 but not CD45 or CD34.

effects of LX2 on the progression of fibrosis. The proliferation of GFP labeled cells leads to a progressive reduction in mean fluorescence intensity (MFI). We therefore calculated the in vitro growth rate of LX2 by MFI after interaction with BMSCs. Flow cytometry analyses suggested that the MFI of GFP gradually decreased with incubation time during LX2 growth and that direct co-cultured LX2 exhibited relatively slow proliferation rates compared to monocultured cells (Figure 4A).

When GFP-labeled LX2 cells and BMSCs were co-cultured with direct cell-cell contact, the fluorescence labeled LX2 cells was inherited by daughter cells after cell division, but was not transferred to adjacent BMSCs in the co-culture population. Fluorescence-activated cell sorting was then performed to separate

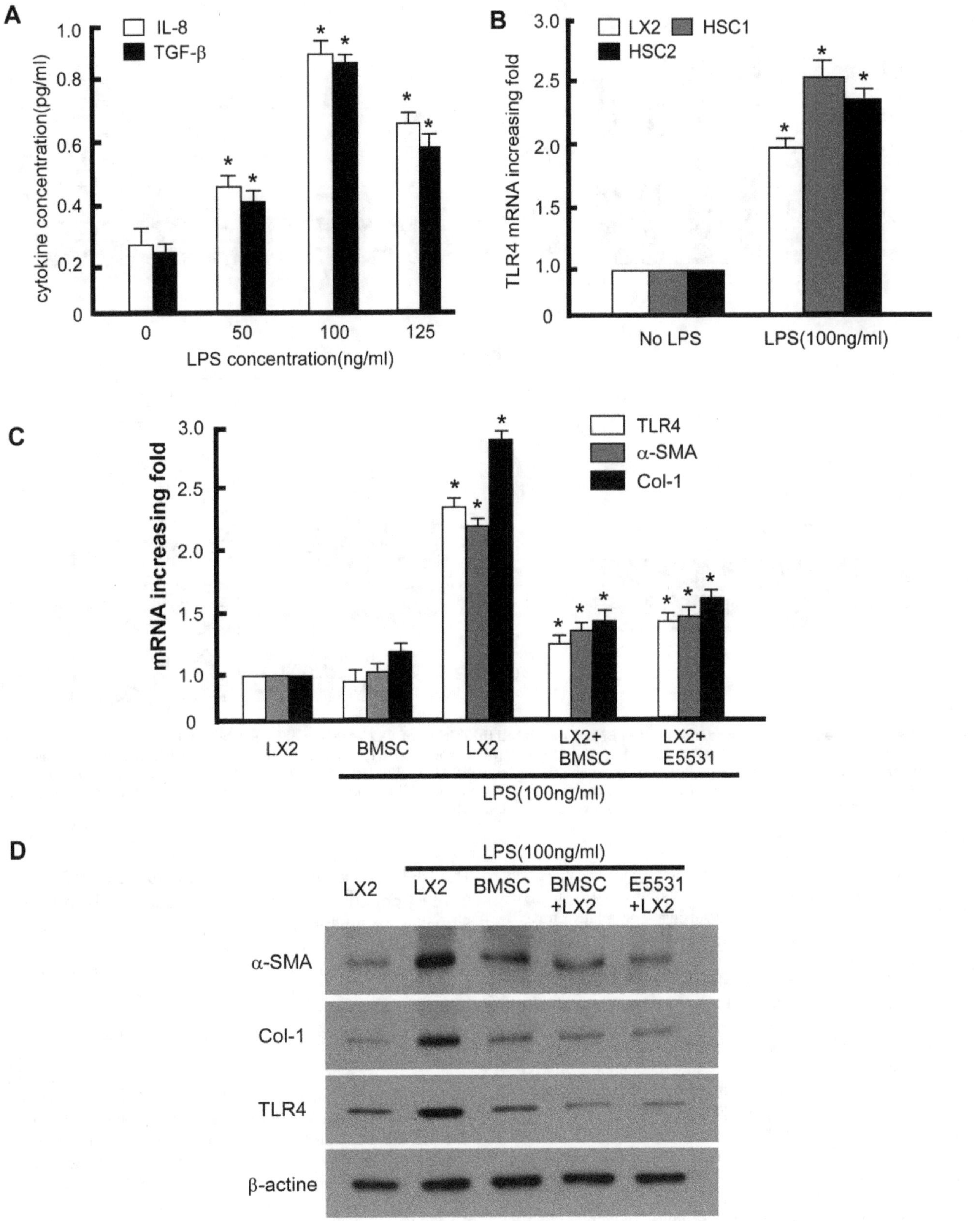

Figure 2. BMSC inhibited LPS induced activation of LX2 and upregulation of TLR4. (A) The effect of different dose of LPS on LX2 cells activation as the IL-8 and TGF-β secretion. All data are shown as mean ± SD from three independent experiments. * $P<0.05$. (B) Relative mRNA expression of TLR4 in LX2 cells and two HSCs in response to LPS. Data are depicted relative to expression in cells without LPS, which are assigned a value of 1. (C) RT-PCR analysis of the HSC activation marker α-SMA, Col-1 and TLR4 in the indicated treatments. (D) Western blot analysis of the HSC activation marker α-SMA, Col-1 and TLR4 in the indicated treatments. Expression levels were normalized with GAPDH.

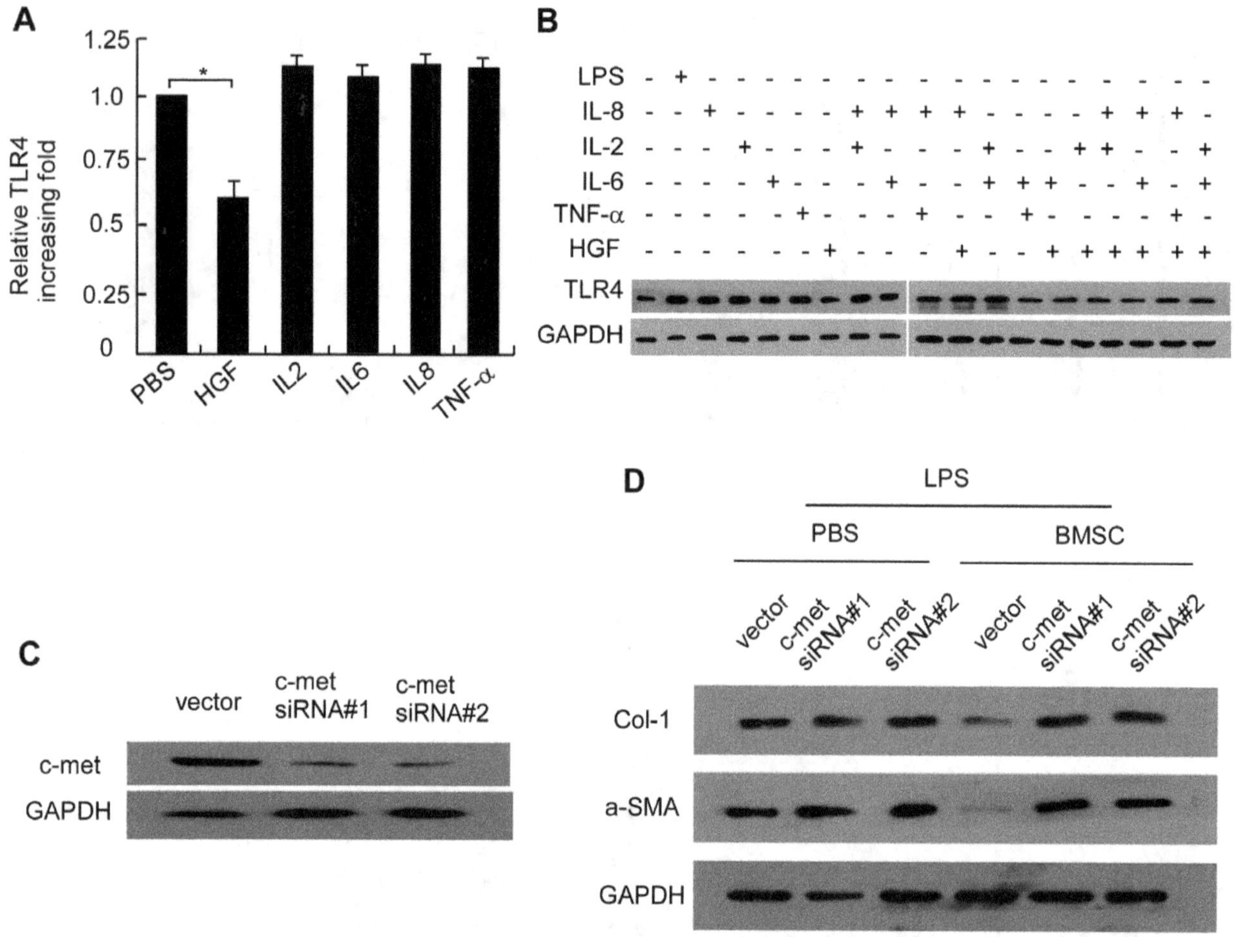

Figure 3. HGF is the major cytokine involved in BMSC-mediated inhibition of LX2 activation. (A) Relative mRNA expression of Col-1 and α-SMA in LX2 with different cytokine stimulation. Data are depicted relative to expression in LX2 cells cultured with PBS, which are assigned a value of 1. All data are shown as mean ± SD from three independent experiments. * $P<0.05$. (B) Western blot analysis for TLR4 expression under different combination of cytokine. GAPDH was used as a loading control for all Western blots (C) Knockdown of c-met in two specific shRNA-transduced LX2 cell lines. (D) Western blot analysis for Col-1 and α-SMA expression in LX2 with c-met knockdown.

fluorescence-positive cells (LX2) and fluorescence-negative cells (BMSCs). Co-cultured cells (3×10^6) were sorted and $0.9-1.2\times10^6$ of each type was obtained after cell sorting. The relative mRNA expression levels of a-SMA, Col-1, TLR4, MyD88 in LX2 co-culture with physical contact, and in the insert co-culture system (no physical contact) versus LX2 alone with HGF are significant deduced compared to PBS control group (Figure 4B). In the LX2 co-culture with physical contact with BMSCs group, the gene relative expression levels were much lower than the groups which were in the insert co-culture system and LX2 alone with HGF. Results for time and dose-depend effect of the three kinds of treatments on LX2 cells using RT-PCR are also shown (Figure 4C and 4D). Genes that were down-regulated at least one half are identified in the BMSCs physical contact co-culture and HGF. The patterns of gene expression for cells exposed to contact co-culture are different from co-culture that only permitted soluble interactions only (i.e. the insert co-culture system). WB also showed the same Synergize effect of HGF and direct BMSC-LX2 cell contact (Figure 4E and 4F). Taken together, these results show that BMSC-derived HGF is necessary to deduce the expression of several fibro-activation genes in vitro but that, in addition, BMSCs provide other signals through physical contacting which synergize with HGF signaling.

The NF-kB Signaling Pathway is Inhibited by BMSCs in a Contact-dependent Manner and Cooperates with HGF Signaling to Inhibit LX2 Activation

We next sought to define the molecular pathway induced upon BMSCs contact that cooperate with HGF to inhibit fibro-activation gene expression. Using a set of luciferase reporter assays for several pathways, we screened for their activation in LPS treated LX2 cells in response to interaction with BMSCs or HGF (Figure 5A). Interestingly, co-incubation with BMSCs or HGF addition decreased activation of the NF-kB pathways in LX2 cells (Figure 5A). Activation of the NF-kB pathway was decreased when cells were incubated with either BMSCs or the pellet fraction from BMSCs. RT-PCR further proved the NF-kB downstream genes including cyclinD1, c-Myc, Mmp9, CXCR4, Cox2 and VEGF, were inhibited by BMSCs, HGF or HGF+BMSC (Figure 5B). NF-kB is composed of the p50 and p65 subunits, and in resting cells the NF-kB complex is sequestered in the cytosol by an inhibitory subunit, IkB. Once stimulated, IkB is phosphorylated and degraded, which allows NF-kB to translocate to the nucleus and induce the expression of its target genes. So we did p65 staining to evaluate the effect of BMSCs on NF-kB signaling. As indicated in Figure 5C, LPS-treated LX2 cells demonstrated primarily nuclear NF-kB staining, whereas exposure to BMSC or HGF for 1 h

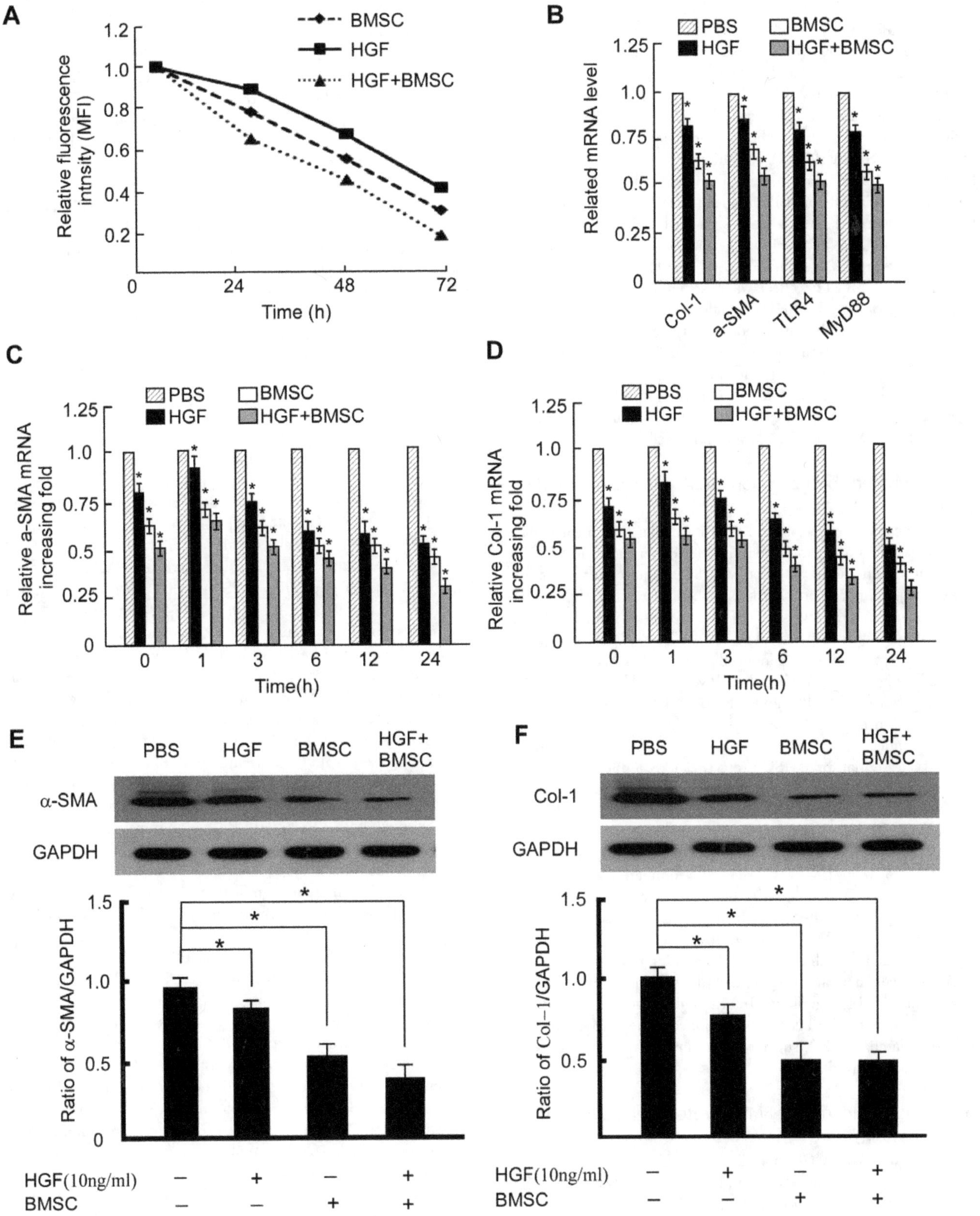

Figure 4. HGF and direct BMSC-LX2 cell contact synergize to inhibit LX2 activation gene expression. (A) MFI of GFP at the indicated times during HSC culture. (B) Relative mRNA expression of Col-1, a-SMA, MyD88 and TLR4 in LX2 with the indicated treatments. Data are depicted relative to expression in LX2 cells with PBS stimulation, which are assigned a value of 1. All data are shown as mean ± SD from three independent experiments. * $P<0.05$. (C) Real-time PCR show that expression of α-SMA and Col-1(D) in LX2 cells with indicated treatments in different time point. Expression levels were normalized with GAPDH. Western blot analysis of a-SMA (E) and Col-1(F) in LX2 cells with the indicated treatments.

resulted in a rapid translocation of NF-kB to the cytoplasm. The effect was enforced by co-cultured with BMSCs directly with HGF addition. Additionally, when we examined the cellular localization of NF-kB expression within the cell, we noted a decrease in nuclear NF-kB expression in BMSC or HGF treated cells, and the effect was also enforced by co-cultured with BMSCs directly with HGF addition (Figure 5D). WB further proved the protection of BMSCs or HGF in LPS induced LX2 activation through inhibited TLR4/ M yD88/NF-kB signaling (Figure 5E). To determine if BMSC had the protection ability in LPS induced NF-κB DNA binding in LX2, we performed EMSA analysis on nuclear lysates from LX2. As showed in Figure 5F, nuclear NF-κB constitutively bound DNA in LPS-stimulated LX2. While BMSCs and HGF repressed DNA binding of NF-kB. The effect was also enforced by co-cultured with BMSCs directly with HGF addition. When we knockdown c-met in LX2 cells, the protection ability of BMSCs, HGF or director BMSCs co-culture on LX2 cell were significantly impaired (Figure 5G). These data proved the ability of BMSCs to prime LX2 cells activation depends on the synergistic interaction between the NF-kB and HGF signaling pathways, which is triggered by direct BMSC-tumor cell contact.

BMSC Inhibited the Activation of LX2 Cells Depended on MyD88

TLR4 acts as a receptor for LPS and mediates its intracellular actions via the adapter molecule MyD88. Experiments in MyD88 knockout mice demonstrated that MyD88 is required for induction of liver injury in response to hypoxia and LPS [14,15]. So we further examining the levels of MyD88 and NF-kB in LPS induced activated LX2 cells response to BMSCs. The MyD88 and NF-kB was highly expressed in LPS induced activated LX2 cells based on RT-PCR (Figure 4B). While when BMSCs or HGF was added, the expression of MyD88 and NF-kB of LX2 was significantly decreased. Since MyD88 was important in LPS-TLR4 pathway and responded to BMSCs treating, we further investigate if MyD88 is essential for BMSC protecting LPS induced activation of LX2. We established MyD88-overexpressing or -silenced LX2 stable cell line (Figure 6A). Inhibition of LPS-induced LX2 activation by BMSCs was significantly decreased when MyD88 was overexpressed (LX2/MyD88 cells) (Figure 6B). When MyD88 was knockdown in LX2 cells, the LPS stimulated activation of LX2 was inhibited as treated by BMSCs alone (Figure 6B). The luciferase activity of NF-kB in activated LX2 was also blocked by BMSCs or when MyD88 knockdown, while overexpressing MyD88 rescued the inhibited effect, suggesting that these markers of stellate cell activation were directly regulated by MyD88-dependent TLR4 signaling. Interestingly, the LPS induced luciferase activity of LX2 was inhibited when MyD88 was down-regulated in LX2, suggesting the involvement of TLR4 in this process (Figure 6C and 6D).

In Vivo Determination of BMSC-protected HSC Activation and Liver Fibrosis

After 8 weeks of CCl_4 injection, liver fibrosis was observed (Figure 7A) and proved by HE and Masson-stained sections. The Scheuer score in control group was 9±1.25 compared 3±0.37 in BMSCs transplantation group ($P<0.05$) (Figure 7B). So BMSCs transplantation had 2-fold decrease of fibrotic area and ameliorated the formation of liver fibrosis (Figure 7B). Rats with fibrosis treated with PBS alone had 4-fold increase of serum ALT (533.6±45.1 U/dl) (Figure 7C) and 2.5-fold increase of serum AST (489.7±42.8 U/dl) (Figure 7D) activity relative to those with BMSCs group (ALT 136.1±38.6 U/dl, $P<0.05$ and AST 152.3±10.3 U/dl, $P<0.01$), respectively. The TP of the rats treated with PBS alone was 38.2±7.1 umol/L, and 50.1±7.8 umol/L for the rats treated with BMSCs (Figure 7E). ALB level of the rats treated with BMSCs was 28.7±3.4 umol/L compared to18.5±3.8 umol/L in PBS treated rats (Figure 7F). The results suggested that BMSCs transplantation ameliorates the CCl4-induced deterioration of liver function. Meanwhile, GFAP-labeled BMSCs were strongly and diffusely present near the expanding septa and in the perisinusoidal spaces of sidual hepatic parenchyma when frozen tissue sections from these livers since 24 h after BMSCs injection and proliferated at 144 h were observed under fluorescence microscopy (Figure 7G); however, no fluorescent cells were observed in sections from the untreated cirrhotic rats and few BMSCs were stayed at lung and spleen. These results suggest that BMSC labeled with GFP in vitro are able to survive in the livers of cirrhotic rats without effect other organs. Thus, BMSCs transplantation relived liver fibrosis safe and effect.

Discussion

In this study, we found that BMSCs inhibited LX2 cell activation in vitro and relieved liver fibrosis in vivo. Furthermore, we showed that the anti-fibrotic effect of BMSCs was through induction of HGF and cell-to-cell contact. C-met knockdown or MyD88 over expression reversed the BMSCs inhibition of NF-kB luciferase activation. These data suggested that BMSCs plays an important role in protecting LPS induced LX2 activation via inhibition of the LPS-TLR4-MyD88-NF-kB pathway and may represent a novel therapeutic way for the disease.

After liver injury, LPS levels increase in the portal and systemic circulation, owing to changes in the intestinal mucosal permeability and increased bacterial translocation. Animal studies have shown that LPS can increase hepatic fibrosis [13,14]. Patients with liver cirrhosis of Child-Pugh A class, B class, and C class, followed by LPS increased [15]. TLR4 is an important member of the TLR family and a receptor for LPS, has been found in the portal vein of chronic hepatitis patients and expressed in HSCs and KC cells too [16]. Although both LPS and TLR4 has an important role in liver cirrhosis, the mechanism is still unclear. A recent report documents the discovery of a single nucleotide polymorphism (T399I) in TLR4 that can significantly reduce the risk of hepatic fibrosis [17]. As such, therapeutic targeting of this pathway may block the formation of fibrosis and has important research value. Our experiments also indicated that LPS activated LX2 cell, which significantly increased TLR4 as well as collagen synthesis. TLR activation can stimulate two main pathways. One is dependent upon the adapter protein MyD88 (MyD88-dependent pathway) and the other is not (MyD88-independent pathway). The differential responses mediated by distinct TLR ligands and had different effect. Our results showed the protection of BMSCs on LX2 was MyD88 depended and found that at least part of the effects of BMSCs may have resulted from the suppression of NF-kB activation, which would normally occur in response to MyD88-dependent ligand-induced stimulation of TLRs. In the present study, the MyD88-overexpressing LX2 cells demonstrated increased NF-kB activity even when co-cultured with BMSCs and MyD88-knocdown decreased NF-kB activity of LX2 even without BMSCs protection. These findings confirmed the critical role of TLR4-MyD88 signaling in regulation of LX2 cell activation and identified novel biologic pathways affecting the risk of hepatic fibrosis progression. In our experiments, LX2 cell activation was inhibited when these cells were co-cultured with BMSCs, and

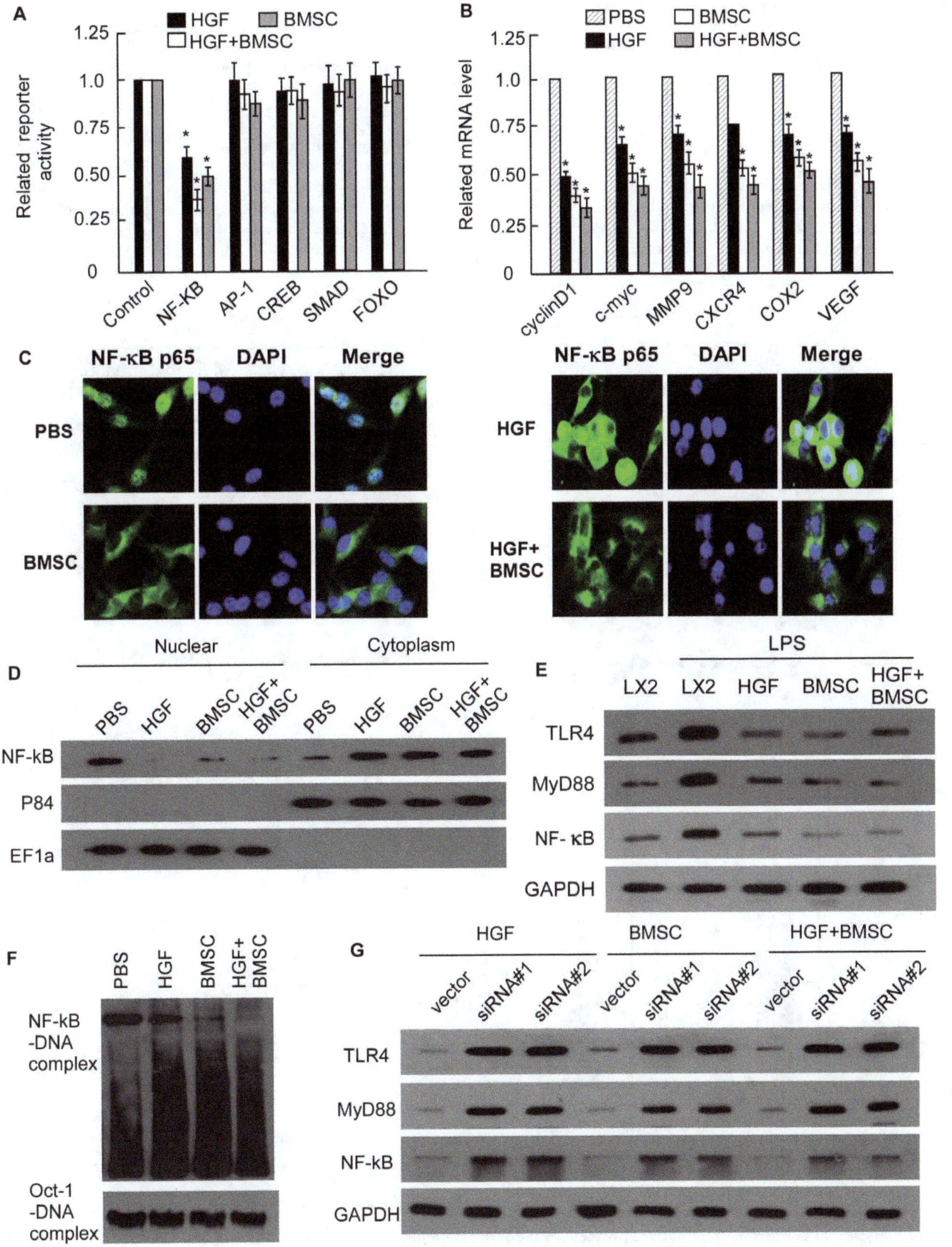

Figure 5. NF-kB signaling pathway is activated by BMSC in a contact-dependent manner and cooperates with HGF signaling to inhibit LX2 activation. (A) Relative luciferase activity in the LPS stimulated LX2 cell with BMSC in a Contact-Dependent Manner (BMSC), BMSC in a contact-dependent manner with HGF addition (BMSC+HGF) and HGF stimulation alone (HGF). (B) Real-time PCR show the expression of cyclinD1, c-

Myc, Mmp9, CXCR4, Cox2 and VEGF in LX2 cells with indicated treatments. Expression levels were normalized with GAPDH. (C) Doubling staining with anti-p65 antibody and DAPI was performed, and the NF-kB localization was identified in LX2 cells with indicated treatments (400×). (D) Cytoplasmic and nuclear levels of NF-kB in LX2 cells with indicated treatments were analyzed by WB. (E) WB analysis of TLR4, MyD88 and NF-kB in LX2 cells with the indicated treatments. (F) NF-κB DNA binding activity was analyzed by EMSA Shown is a representative blot from three independent experiments. (G) MWB analysis of TLR4, MyD88 and NF-kB in LX2 cells with c-met knockdown.

BMSCs inhibit LX2 activation through inhibiting the LPS-TLR4-MyD88 pathway.

Animal experiments have shown that BMSCs can effectively relieve fibrosis, improve liver function, and effect the remodeling of fibrous tissue, which may be related to the integration of bone marrow cells and the expression of matrix metalloproteinase 9 [18–22]. In addition, transplantation of BMSCs can result in a large increase in the number of liver and bile duct cells, subsequently improving liver function. We have previously reported good results with autologous transplantation of BMSCs through the hepatic artery for treatment of patients with liver failure [23]. To evaluate the function of BMSCs on HSCs, we

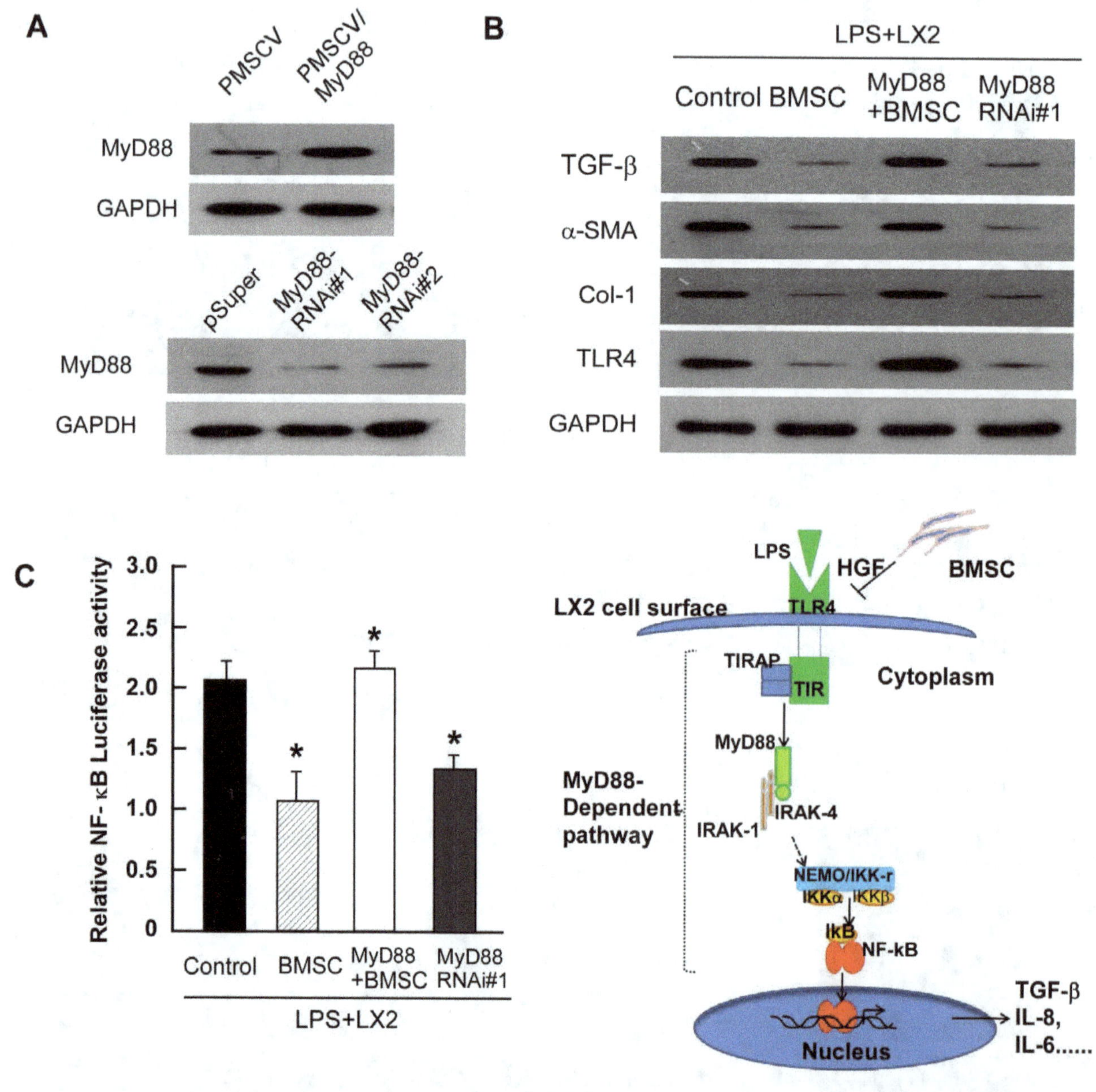

Figure 6. MyD88 was necessary for BMSCs to protect LPS induced activation of LX2. (A) Western blotting analysis of MyD88 expression in indicated cells. GAPDH was used as a loading control. (B) TGF-β, a-SMA, Col-1 and TLR4 was analysis by western blotting on LPS stimulated LX2 cell under BMSC treatment, MyD88 overexpress (MyD88) and MyD88 RNAi#1. (C) Relative NF-kB luciferase activity in the LPS stimulated LX2 cell with BMSC treated and MyD88 overexpress and MyD88 shRNA. (D) Proposed scheme for BMSC inhibition in LPS-stimulated signaling in the activation of LX2.

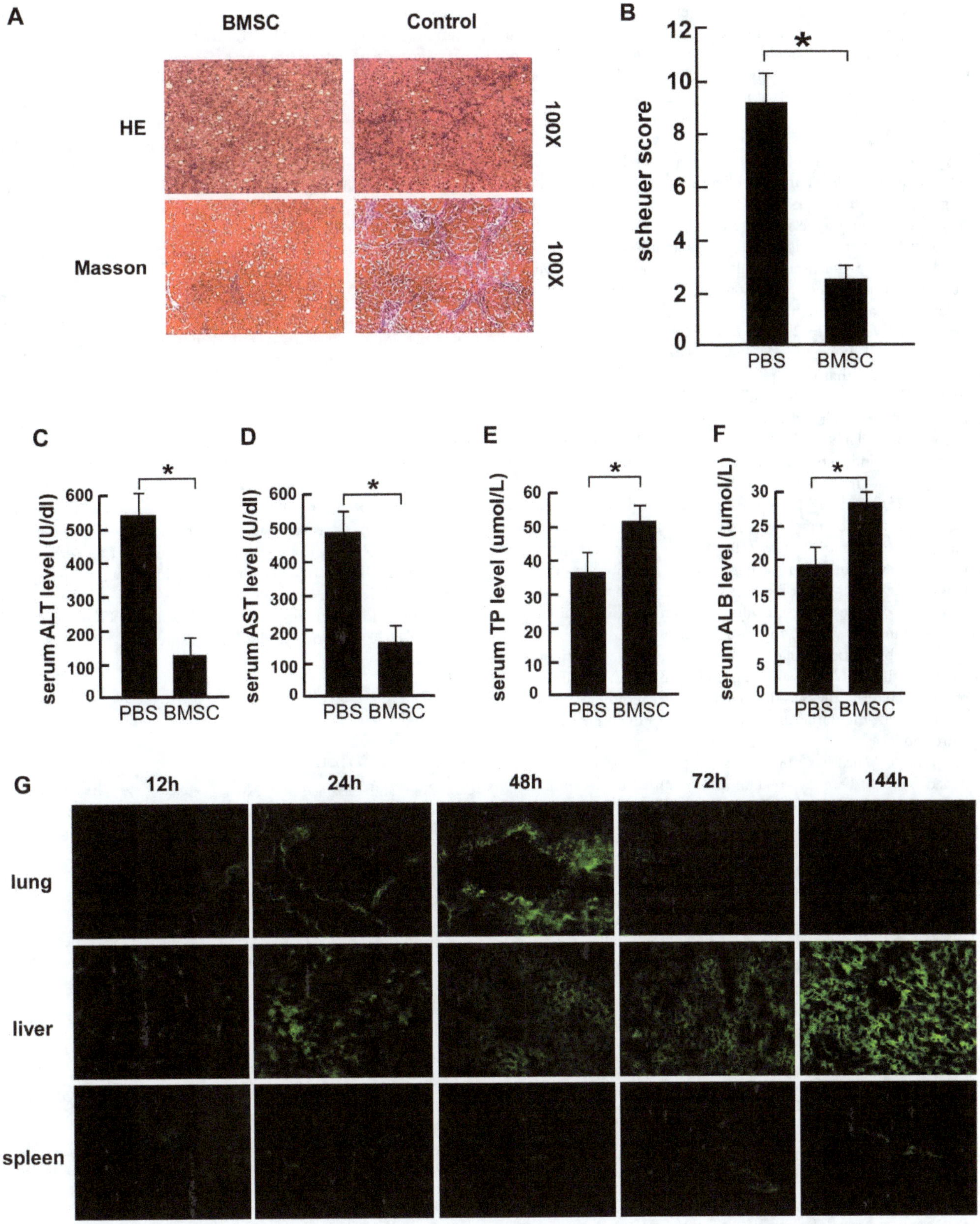

Figure 7. BMSCs transplantation reduced CCl4-induced hepatic fibrosis. (A) Hematoxylin and eosin (up panel) and Micrographs of Masson's trichrome staining (down panel) of liver paraffin sections from control group and BMSCs group (100X). (B) Scheuer score was quantified. Each value is the mean±SEM of determinations in 10 rats of each group. *$P<0.05$ compared with PBS control group. Rats serum ALT (C), AST (D), TP (E) and ALB (F) level in each group. (G) Tracking GFP-labeled BMSCs in lung, liver and spleen frozen sections (12 to 144 h following transplantation) using fluorescence microscopy (100×).

further conclude from in vivo experiments that BMSCs confer their liver protective effects. This suggests that BMSCs can evoke endogenous repair mechanisms in liver. Indeed, BMSCs are capable of producing a variety of cytokines and hematopoietic growth factors [24–26]. Among the great number of growth factors liver protective effects have been most attributed to HGF. HGF is a potent growth factor involved in liver regeneration that has various effects on epithelial and nonepithelial cells. HGF is a polypeptide originally characterized as a highly potent hepatocyte mitogen [27,28]. HGF also suppresses the onset of severe hepatic injury and maintains the integrity of hepatocytes in the livers of mice with cholestasis induced by alphanaphthylisothiocyanate [29–31]. Using a transwell co-culture assay, our study suggested that BMSCs protected activation of HSCs. This effect was mediated in part through paracrine signaling by HGF secreted by BMSCs. When we knockdown HGF receptor c-met, the protection of BMSCs and HGF decreased. Our results could therefore indicate that HGF production is upregulated in BMSCs-CM compared to DMEM, inhibiting NF-kB pathway which is important in LPS induced LX2 activation.

Importantly, labeled LX2 and BMSCs directly co-culture inhibited LPS induced LX2 activation much more effect. These results present the possibility of direct interactions between activated HSCs and BMSCs through direct cell-to-cell contact, although we and others have previously investigated paracrine regulation between these two cells. In this study, we therefore propose a new potential mechanism of the anti-fibrotic effect of BMSCs. The present data indicate that BMSCs in direct cell-cell contact not only result in growth inhibition in HSCs compared with the transwell system, but also suppress HSCs activation in vitro. This observation provides evidence that cell–cell adhesion is involved in the HSCs growth inhibition by BMSCs. In particular, directly co-cultured BMSCs displayed stronger inhibitory activities compared with the paracrine blockade effect in two-chamber co-culture models.

In summary, BMSCs are able to protect against liver fibrosis induced by LPS. Directly co-culture, in contrast to the indirectly co-culture of BMSCs, provides the most effective treatment to prevent LX2 activation. These results are due to the fact that BMSCs can secret HGF, which, in turn, can modulate the host immune response and homeostasis between TLR4 and NF-kB pathway. The results of this study provide several new insights into reversing hepatic fibrosis through the anti-fibrotic effects of treated BMSCs targeting HSCs in vitro. The direct co-culture system we have established was applied to explore the effect of direct interplay between BMSCs and HSCs involving paracrine signaling as well as cell–cell adhesion and juxtacrine signaling. Regardless of the mechanism, our study is the first to demonstrate that induction of the TLR4-MyD88-NF-kB signaling pathway can dramatically repress proliferation of HSCs co-cultured with BMSCs in vitro. But the in vivo effect of BMSCs inhibited HSC activation through TLR4-MyD88-NF-kB pathway is still unclear. Therefore, more studies needed to clarify the mechanism and make BMSCs more effectively to reduce liver inflammation and reduce scar formation, thus inhibiting liver fibrosis and improving the quality of life of patients and prolonging their survival time.

Supporting Information

Figure S1 (A) Relative mRNA expression of TLR4 in LX2 with different cytokine stimulation. Data are depicted relative to expression in LX2 cells cultured with PBS, which are assigned a value of 1. (B) Real-time PCR show that HGF induces Col-1 and a-SMA mRNA expression in a dosage-dependent manner. (C) Real-time PCR show that expression of Col-1 and α-SMA in LX2 cells with HGF (50 ng/ml) stimulation in different time point. Expression levels were normalized with GAPDH. (D, E) Western blot analysis for a dosage and time -dependent (HGF 50 ng/ml) effects of HGF on Col-1 and a-SMA expression.

Materials and Methods S1

Author Contributions

Conceived and designed the experiments: CX ZG. Performed the experiments: DX PW. Analyzed the data: LP. Contributed reagents/materials/analysis tools: YY GZ XL. Wrote the paper: CX. No.

References

1. Schiff ER, Lee SS, Chao YC, Kew Yoon S, Bessone F, et al (2003) Long-term treatment with entecavir induces reversal of advanced fibrosis or cirrhosis in patients with chronic hepatitis B. Clin Gastroenterol Hepatol 9: 274–276.
2. Chang TT, Liaw YF, Wu SS, Schiff E, Han KH, et al (2010) Long-term entecavir therapy results in the reversal of fibrosis/cirrhosis and continued histological improvement in patients with chronic hepatitis B. Hepatology 52: 886–893.
3. Baranova A, Lal P, Birerdinc A, Younossi ZM (2011) Non-Invasive markers for hepatic fibrosis. BMC Gastraenterology 11: 1–15.
4. Soares J-B, Pimentel-Nunes P, Roncon-Albuquerque R Jr, Leite-Moreira A (2010) The role of lipopolysaccharide/toll-like receptor 4 signaling in chronic liver diseases. Hepatol Int 4: 659–672.
5. Gaia S, Smedile A, Omedè P, Olivero A, Sanavio F, et al. (2006) Feasibility and safety of G-CSF administration to induce bone marrow-derived cells mobilization in patients with end stage liver disease. J Hepatol 45: 13–19.
6. Terai S, Ishikawa T, Omori K, Aoyama K, Marumoto Y, et al. (2006) Improved liver function in patients with liver cirrhosis after autologous bone marrow cell infusion therapy. Stem Cells 24: 2292–2298.
7. Gordon MY, Levicar N, Pai M, Bachellier P, Dimarakis I, et al. (2006) Characterisation and clinical application of human CD34+stem/progenitor cell populations mobilized into the blood by granulocyte colony-stimulating factor. Stem Cells 24: 1822–1830.
8. Baertschiger RM, Serre-Beinier V, Morel P, Bosco D, Peyrou M, et al. (2009) Fibrogenic Potential of Human Multipotent Mesenchymal Stromal Cells in Injured Liver. PLoS One 17: e6657.
9. Sakaida I, Terai S, Nishina H, Okita K (2005) Developmentof cell therapy using autologous bone marrow cells for liver cirrhosis. Med Mol Morphol 38: 197–202.
10. Xie C, Zheng YB, Zhu HP, Peng L, Gao ZL (2009) Human Bone Marrow Mesenchymal Stem Cells are resistant to HBV Infection during differentiation towards Hepatocytes in vivo and vitro. Cell Biology Int 33: 493–500.
11. Schwabe RF, Schnabl B, Kweon YO, Brenner DA (2001) CD40 activates NF-kB and c-Jun N-terminal kinase and enhances chemokine secretion on acti-vated human hepatic stellate cells. J Immunol 166: 6812–6819.
12. Desmet VJ, Gerber M, Hoofnagle JH, Manns M, Scheuer PJ(1994) Classification of chronic hepatitis: diagnosis, grading and staging. Hepatology 19:1513–1520.
13. Wiest R, Garcia-Tsao G (2005) Bacterial translocation (BT) in cirrhosis. Hepatology 41: 422–433.
14. Nolan JP, Leibowitz AI (1978) Endotoxin and the liver. III. Modification of acute carbon tetrachloride injury by polymyxin b – an antiendotoxin. Gastroenterology 75: 445–449.
15. Grinko I, Geerts A, Wisse E (1995) Experimental biliary fibrosis correlates with increased numbers of fat-storing and Kupffer cells, and portal endotoxemia. J Hepatol 23: 449–458.
16. Lin RS, Lee FY, Lee SD, Tsai YT, Lin HC, et al. (1995) Endotoxemia in patients with chronic liver diseases: relationship to severity of liver diseases, presence of esophageal varices, and hyperdynamic circulation. J Hepatol 22: 165–172.
17. Brun P, Castagliuolo I, Pinzani M, Palù G, Martines D (2005) Exposure to bacterial cell wall products triggers an inflammatory phenotype in hepatic stellate cells. Am J Physiol Gastrointest Liver Physiol 289: 571–578.
18. Guo J, Loke J, Zheng F, Hong F, Yea S, et al. (2009) Functional linkage of cirrhosis-predictive single nucleotide polymorphisms of Toll-like receptor 4 to hepatic stellate cell responses. Hepatology 49: 960–968.

19. Jiang Y, Jahagirdar BN, Reinhardt RL, Schwartz RE, Keene CD, et al. (2002) Pluripotency of mesenchymal stem cells derived from adut marrow. Nature 418: 41–49.
20. Sakaida I, Terai S, Yamamoto N, Aoyama K, Ishikawa T, et al. (2004) Transplantation of bone marrow cells reduces CCL4-induced liver fibrosis in mice. Hepatology 40: 1304–1311.
21. Oyagi S, Hirose M, Kojima M, Okuyama M, Kawase M, et al. (2006) Therapeutic effect of transplanting HGF-treated bone marrow mesenchymal cells into CCl4- injured rats. J Hepatol 44: 742–748.
22. Payne C, Samuel K, Pryde A (2007) The impact of bone marrow stem cells on liver fibrosis in critically determined by their route of cell trafficking. Hepatology 46: 710A.
23. Sakaida I, Terai S, Nishina H, Okita K (2005) Developmentof cell therapy using autologous bone marrow cells for liver cirrhosis. Med Mol Morphol 38: 197–202.
24. Peng L, Xie DY, Lin BL, Liu J, Zhu HP, et al. (2011) Autologous bone mesenchymal stem cell transplantation in liver failure patients caused by hepatitis B: short-term and long-term outcomes. Hepatology 54: 820–828.
25. Chen X, Katakowski M, Li Y, Lu D, Wang L, et al. (2002) Human bone marrow stromal cell cultures conditioned by traumatic brain tissue extracts: growth factor production. J Neurosci Res 69: 687–691.
26. Haynesworth SE, Baber MA, Caplan AI (1996) Cytokine expression by human marrow-derived mesenchymal progenitor cells in vitro: effects of dexamethasone and IL-1 alpha. J Cell Physiol 166: 585–592.
27. Liu Y, Dulchavsky DS, Gao X, Kwon D, Chopp M, et al. (2006) Wound repair by bone marrow stromal cells through growth factor production. J Surg Res 136: 336–341.
28. Gohda E, Tsubouchi H, Nakayama H, Hirono S, Sakiyama O, et al. (1988) Purification and partial characterization of hepatocyte growth factor from plasma of a patient with fulminant hepatic failure. J Clin Invest 81: 414–419.
29. Nakamura T, Nishizawa T, Hagiya M, Seki T, Shimonishi M, et al. (1989) Molecular cloning and expression of human hepatocyte growth factor. Nature 342: 440–443.
30. Ishiki Y, Ohnishi H, Muto Y, Matsumoto K, Nakamura T (1992) Direct evidence that hepatocyte growth factor is a hepatotrophic factor for liver regeneration and has a potent antihepatitis effect in vivo. Hepatology 16: 1227–1235.
31. Roos F, Terrell TG, Godowski PJ, Chamow SM, Schwall RH (1992) Reduction of alpha-naphthylisothiocyanate-induced hepatotoxicity by recombinant human hepatocyte growth factor. Endocrinology 131: 2540–2544.

13

Hedgehog Signaling Antagonist Promotes Regression of Both Liver Fibrosis and Hepatocellular Carcinoma in a Murine Model of Primary Liver Cancer

George M. Philips[1]*, Isaac S. Chan[1,2]*, Marzena Swiderska[1], Vanessa T. Schroder[3], Cynthia Guy[4], Gamze F. Karaca[1], Cynthia Moylan[1], Talaignair Venkatraman[5], Sebastian Feuerlein[5], Wing-Kin Syn[1], Youngmi Jung[1,6], Rafal P. Witek[1], Steve Choi[1], Gregory A. Michelotti[1], Fatima Rangwala[7], Elmar Merkle[5], Christopher Lascola[5], Anna Mae Diehl[1]*

1 Division of Gastroenterology, Department of Medicine, Duke University Medical Center, Durham, North Carolina, United States of America, **2** Department of Genetics, The University of North Carolina School of Medicine, Chapel Hill, North Carolina, United States of America, **3** Department of Surgery, Duke University Medical Center, Durham, North Carolina, United States of America, **4** Department of Pathology, Duke University Medical Center, Durham, North Carolina, United States of America, **5** Department of Radiology, Duke University, Durham, North Carolina, United States of America, **6** Department of Biological Science, Pusan National University, Pusan, Korea, **7** Divisions of Cell Therapy, Hematology and Medical Oncology, Duke University Medical Center, Durham, North Carolina, United States of America

Abstract

Objective: Chronic fibrosing liver injury is a major risk factor for hepatocarcinogenesis in humans. Mice with targeted deletion of Mdr2 (the murine ortholog of MDR3) develop chronic fibrosing liver injury. Hepatocellular carcinoma (HCC) emerges spontaneously in such mice by 50–60 weeks of age, providing a model of fibrosis-associated hepatocarcinogenesis. We used Mdr2$^{-/-}$ mice to investigate the hypothesis that activation of the hedgehog (Hh) signaling pathway promotes development of both liver fibrosis and HCC.

Methods: Hepatic injury and fibrosis, Hh pathway activation, and liver progenitor populations were compared in Mdr2$^{-/-}$ mice and age-matched wild type controls. A dose finding experiment with the Hh signaling antagonist GDC-0449 was performed to optimize Hh pathway inhibition. Mice were then treated with GDC-0449 or vehicle for 9 days, and effects on liver fibrosis and tumor burden were assessed by immunohistochemistry, qRT-PCR, Western blot, and magnetic resonance imaging.

Results: Unlike controls, Mdr2$^{-/-}$ mice consistently expressed Hh ligands and progressively accumulated Hh-responsive liver myofibroblasts and progenitors with age. Treatment of aged Mdr2-deficient mice with GDC-0449 significantly inhibited hepatic Hh activity, decreased liver myofibroblasts and progenitors, reduced liver fibrosis, promoted regression of intra-hepatic HCCs, and decreased the number of metastatic HCC without increasing mortality.

Conclusions: Hh pathway activation promotes liver fibrosis and hepatocarcinogenesis, and inhibiting Hh signaling safely reverses both processes even when fibrosis and HCC are advanced.

Editor: Pranela Rameshwar, University of Medicine and Dentistry of New Jersey, United States of America

Funding: This work was supported, in part, by National Institutes of Health (NIH) RO1 DK077794, NIH RO1 AA010154, NIH T32 DK007568, and NIH T32 CA071341. A portion of the imaging was performed at the Duke Center for In Vivo Microscopy, supported, in part, by National Center for Research Resources National Biomedical Technology Research Center (P41 RR005959) and National Cancer Institute Small Animal Imaging Resource Program (U24 CA092656). The funders had no role in study design, data collection and analysis, decision to publish, or preparation of the manuscript.

Competing Interests: The authors have declared that no competing interests exist.

* E-mail: annamae.diehl@duke.edu

These two authors contributed equally to the work.

Introduction

Hepatocellular carcinoma (HCC) is an insidious cancer that accounts for up to 1 million deaths a year and is the third leading cause of cancer deaths worldwide [1]. Cirrhosis, a consequence of progressive liver injury and fibrosis, is the single largest risk factor for HCC [2]. An altered wound healing response to chronic liver injury, with resultant dysregulated activation of myofibroblasts and progenitor cell populations, has been implicated in cirrhosis pathogenesis and eventual carcinogenesis [3].

Loss-of-function mutations in the hepatocyte canalicular phospholipid flippase MDR3 (ABCB4) have been associated with a wide range of human biliary diseases including progressive familial intrahepatic cholestasis type 3 (PFIC3), cholestasis of pregnancy, drug induced cholestasis and an adult biliary cirrhosis with features similar to primary sclerosing cholangitis (PSC) [4,5,6,7]. Mice with a targeted deletion of Mdr2 (the murine ortholog of MDR3) lack the liver-specific P-glycoprotein that transports phosphatidylcholine (PC) across the canalicular membrane. The absence of phospholipids in bile results in progressive sclerosing cholangitis with accompanying portal inflammation, ductular proliferation and portal fibrosis. Liver injury manifests shortly after birth and hepatocellular carcinomas emerge spontaneously between 50 to 60 weeks of age [8,9,10,11,12,13,14]. Unlike xenograft models that are widely utilized to examine mechanisms of- and treatments for- HCC, Mdr2$^{-/-}$ mice provide a model that parallels the natural evolution of HCC on a background of chronic inflammation, liver injury and fibrosis [15].

Gene expression analyses in Mdr2-deficient mice and heterozygote controls have demonstrated robust and sustained induction of multiple adaptive mechanisms that control cellular responses related to oxidative stress, inflammation, lipid metabolism, and proliferation, prompting speculation that these processes contribute to hepatocarcinogenesis [16]. Although not formally assessed by earlier studies of Mdr2-deficient mice, another pathway that might play a role in fibrosis-associated hepatocarcinogenesis is Hedgehog (Hh), because Hh signaling has been implicated in both fibrogenic repair of liver injury and HCC.

The Hh pathway is an evolutionarily conserved signaling pathway that is activated when Hh ligands (Sonic hedgehog and Indian hedgehog) bind to Patched (Ptc), a transmembrane receptor that is expressed on the surface of Hh-responsive cells. Upon ligand binding, Ptc is inactivated, relieving its repression of Smoothened (Smo), a trans-membrane protein that mediates Hh signaling inside the cell. Smo activation culminates in the nuclear localization of Gli-family transcription factors, Gli1, Gli2, and Gli3, which, in turn, regulate downstream gene expression. The pathway is quiescent in normal liver [17,18], but becomes re-activated as a repair mechanism in chronic liver injury [19,20, 21,22,23]. Hh ligands promote the growth and viability of myofibroblasts, the accumulation of which leads to abnormal liver repair, fibrosis and eventual cirrhosis [24,25]. Hh ligands also serve as viability and proliferative factors for liver epithelial progenitors, and expansion of this compartment has been linked to the formation and maintenance of hepatocellular carcinomas [26]. The possibility that Hh pathway activation contributes to hepatocarcinogenesis is supported by the fact that Sonic hedgehog (Shh) ligand expression is noted in approximately 60% of human HCCs, and expression of the Hh-regulated genes, Gli1 and Ptc, occurs in 50% of human tumors [27,28,29,30].

Based on these observations, we postulated that Hh pathway activation contributes to the pathogenesis of both liver fibrosis and fibrosis-associated HCC. To test this hypothesis, we treated aged Mdr2-deficient mice with the Hh pathway inhibitor, GDC-0449, a small-molecule inhibitor that binds to Smoothened (SMO). This agent was selected because of its human safety profile in phase 1 trials, as well as its effectiveness in solid organ tumors like basal cell carcinoma (BCC) and medulloblastoma [31,32,33]. Our aims were to determine whether or not mice with advanced liver disease and HCCs would tolerate Hh pathway inhibition and experience improvements in liver fibrosis and/or tumor burden.

Methods

Mice

Mdr2$^{-/-}$ mice were a gift from Dr. Detlef Schuppan (Beth Israel Deaconess Medical Center, Boston, MA). Age matched FVB/NJ wild type mice were obtained from Jackson Laboratory (Bar Harbor, ME). All mice were housed with a 12-h light-dark cycle and given water and standard chow *ad libitum*. At ages, 2, 4, 12, 36 52 and 62-weeks, mice were sacrificed under general anesthesia. Liver weight and body weight were recorded, serum and liver tissue were collected. Animal studies were approved by the Institutional Animal Care and Use Committee as governed by the National Institute of Health's "Guide for the Care and Use of Laboratory Animals", Duke University Animal Welfare Assurance Number A3195-01.

Serum AST/ALT determination

Serum aspartate aminotransferase (AST) and alanine aminotransferase (ALT) were measured using kits commercially available from Biotron Diagnostics (66-D and 68-D respectively; Hemet, CA) according to the manufacturers' instructions.

Western Blot

Total protein was extracted from snap frozen whole liver tissue in RIPA buffer. Samples were pooled by age (2–4 samples per age group) except as noted. Western blot analysis was performed as previously described. Membranes were probed with the following primary antibodies: Sonic hedgehog (sc-9024; Santa Cruz Biotechnology, Santa Cruz, CA), Indian hedgehog (ab39634; Abcam), β-actin (sc-47778, Santa Cruz Biotechnology), Gli2 (18-732-292462, Genway, San Diego, CA). All antibodies were diluted 1:1000 and were incubated at 4°C overnight. Western blot images were acquired using a FluorChem HD2 digital darkroom system (Cell Biosciences, Santa Clara, California).

Immunohistochemistry

4 μm formalin-fixed, paraffin-embedded samples were dewaxed and rehydrated. To evaluate tissue architecture, slides were stained with hematoxylin and eosin (H&E) and Sirius red per standard protocol. For immunohistochemistry, slides were incubated in 3% hydrogen peroxide/methanol. Antigen retrieval was performed by heating in 10 mM sodium citrate buffer or 0.25% pepsin (K19; Invitrogen, Carlsbad, CA) for 10 minutes. Sections were blocked (Dako Envision, Carpinteria, CA) and incubated with primary antibodies overnight at 4°C: glioblastoma-2 (Gli-2; 18-732-292462; 1:2000; Genway, San Diego, CA); cytokeratin 19 (Troma-III; Hybridoma Bank, Iowa City, IA; 1:500); α-fetoprotein (AFP) (Dako, 1:1000); Indian hedgehog (Abcam; 1:750, Cambridge, MA); Polymer-HRP anti-rabbit (K4003; Dako) or anti-mouse (K40011; Dako) or MACH3 mouse AP polymer kit (MP530, Biocare Medical, Concord, California, USA) were used as secondary antibodies. 3,3′-Diaminobenzidine (DAB) Substrate Chromogen System (K3466; Dako) and/or Ferangi Blue (Biocare) was employed in the detection procedure. Omitting primary antibodies from the reactions eliminated staining which demonstrated staining specificity. Images were acquired on an Olympus IX71 (Tokyo, Japan) inverted microscope using the DP2-BSW (Olympus) image acquisition software system.

Quantitative Real-Time Reverse Transcription PCR

RNA was isolated from whole liver, as well as from resected tumor specimens had standard TriZol extraction as has been previously described [24]. A table of primers has been included in the Supplementary Materials.

Morphometry

Formalin-fixed liver and tumor sections were stained for CD44 and osteopontin as described above, and were quantified by morphometric analysis with MetaView software (Universal Imaging, Downington, PA). A minimum of 5 randomly selected 10× or 20× fields/section were evaluated for each mouse.

Quantitative Immunohistochemical Analysis

Formalin-fixed liver and tumor sections were costained for Gli2 and CK19. A minimum of 5 ductular regions, 20× fields per section, were evaluated for each mouse by counting the number of cells co-labelled.

Hepatic hydroxyproline assay

The hydroxyproline content in whole liver specimens was quantified colorimetrically as previously reported [34].

GDC-0449 treatment

In the initial, dose-finding cohort of animals, 16 Mdr2$^{-/-}$ mice (age 57–68 weeks) were assigned to treatment with vehicle control (DMSO, n = 5), 20 mg/kg GDC-0449 (n = 5), or 40 mg/kg GDC-0449 (n = 6). Male-female ratios were balanced between the groups. GDC-0449 (Selleck Chemicals, Houston, TX) was freshly constituted daily in DMSO. All mice were given a daily intraperitoneal injection for 9 days. On day 10, animals were sacrificed. Samples were collected as above. A second cohort of 20 Mdr2$^{-/-}$ mice (age 51–59 weeks of age) were subjected to whole body magnetic resonance imaging to assess tumor burden and then pairs of mice with comparable tumor burdens were assigned to treatment with either DMSO (control, n = 10) or 40 mg/kg GDC-0449 (n = 10). Drugs were delivered as described above; MRI scanning was repeated after the 9th day of treatment; mice were sacrificed for necropsy and tissue harvest.

Pathology

H&E and sirius red staining of liver sections was evaluated by a board-certified pathologist. Representative sections of tumor and non-tumor tissue were examined. Tumor tissue was defined as grossly visible nodules that were at least 10 mm in size and resectable.

Abdominal magnetic resonance imaging

Animals were assigned a blinding code, which was maintained during magnetic resonance (MR) data acquisition and analysis. MR mouse liver imaging was performed on a 7T Bruker Biospec 70/30 horizontal bore system (Billerica, MA). Animals were lightly anesthetized under isofluorane with continuous monitoring and maintenance of physiological parameters throughout the imaging session (~60 min for each animal). Axial and coronal 2D T2-weighted fast spin echo images (TURBO-RARE, TE/TR = 11/4200 ms with 1 mm slice thick, matrix = 256×256 and FOV of 2.4 cm×2.4 cm, 5 averages, 0.0 mm interslice gap) images were first obtained for screening purposes and supplemental anatomic information. For directed tumor volumetric analysis, 64 contiguous 500 μM thick 3D FSE proton density images biased towards T1 weighting (TURBO-RARE, TE/TR = 9/1500 ms, matrix = 256×256×64 and FOV 2.2 cm×2.2 cm×2.2 cm, 25 minutes duration) were acquired. All imaging sequences were performed using respiratory gating.

Volumetric analysis from MR data sets was performed in Osirix software, an open source image processing application developed and maintained by Pixmeo (Geneva, SUI). Liver tumors were manually segmented in each animal by a board-certified radiologist (blinded to treatment) post-treatment. Selected areas were reviewed for consistency on coronal and sagittal representations, and cross-correlated with axial 2D FSE images. For volumetry, two separate volume measurements were obtained for each lesion, with the average volume then taken. Interrater reliability (kappa value) was = 0.97. T1 and T2-weighted scanning sequences were performed.

Statistical analyses

Results expressed as mean±SD. Significance established using the Student's t-test. Differences were considered significant when $p<0.05$.

Results

Progressive accumulation of Hh-responsive cells in Mdr2$^{-/-}$ mice

Various forms of acute and chronic liver injury induce hepatic expression of Hh ligands and activation of Hh responsive cells. Serum levels of AST and ALT were consistently higher in Mdr2$^{-/-}$ mice than age-matched controls (**Figure S1**), confirming that the knockout mice had chronic liver injury. Thus, we surveyed livers from Mdr2$^{-/-}$ mice for Hh pathway activation. Compared to liver protein lysates from wild type controls, lysates from Mdr2$^{-/-}$ mice demonstrated an increase in Sonic hedgehog (Shh) and Indian hedgehog (Ihh) by Western blot analysis. This was apparent at the first time point examined (2 weeks after birth) and maintained throughout the lifespan of the animals (up to 64 weeks of age) (**Figure 1A**). Immunohistochemistry for the Hh-regulated transcription factor, Gli2, demonstrated progressive, age-related accumulation of cells with nuclear Gli2 staining in Mdr2$^{-/-}$ mice. Such Gli2-positive cells included stromal cells, as well as hepatocytic and ductular cells (**Figure 1B–C**). Together, these data suggest that the Hh pathway is activated in chronically injured livers of Mdr2-deficient mice, resulting in progressive expansion of various Hh-responsive cell populations.

Treatment of Mdr2$^{-/-}$ mice with the Smoothened inhibitor, GDC-0449, is safe and decreases Hedgehog pathway signaling

To determine the appropriate dose of GDC-0449, a pilot study was done with 16 aged (57–68 week old) Mdr2$^{-/-}$ mice. Animals were given a daily intraperitoneal injection of 20 mg/kg GDC-0449 (n = 5), 40 mg/kg GDC-0449 (n = 6), or DMSO vehicle control (n = 5) for 9 days and then sacrificed. There was no statistical difference in mortality between the control and high dose (40 mg/kg) GDC-0449 groups. At sacrifice, liver/body weight ratios of mice in the three groups were also similar, suggesting that a relatively short course of systemic treatment with GDC-0449 at 40 mg/kg is well tolerated by mice with advanced liver disease and HCC (**Figures S2A–B**). Western blot analysis of liver lysates from this cohort of animals demonstrated that GDC-0449 treatment caused a decrease in Shh ligand levels at the higher dose, and Gli2 expression attenuation at both doses (**Figure S2C**).

Hedgehog signaling inhibition with GDC-0449 abrogates effects of Hh signaling on target gene expression

Based on the data acquired in our dose-finding study, a second cohort of Mdr2$^{-/-}$ mice (51–59 weeks of age) were assigned to treatment with vehicle (DMSO; n = 10) or 40 mg/kg GDC-0449 (n = 10) via daily i.p injection for 9 days. Overall survival between the two groups in the second cohort was equal, with no deaths in the DMSO treatment group and 1 death in the GDC-0449 treatment group secondary to iatrogenic injury. Both the liver parenchyma and tumors of treated mice showed decreased expression of the Hh pathway target Gli2 (**Figures 2A–B**). Real-time PCR analysis of resected tumors revealed that GDC-0449 treatment released the inhibitory effects of Hh signaling on PPARã, causing a significant increase in its gene expression (**Figure 2C**). Treatment with GDC-0449 also caused a significant decrease in expression of Gli1, another Hh target gene (**Figure 2D**).

Hedgehog signaling inhibition with GDC-0449 reduces liver fibrosis

Mdr2$^{-/-}$ mice demonstrated progressive age-related increases in hepatic expression of alpha-smooth muscle actin (α-sma), a marker of myofibroblastic hepatic stellate cells (**Figure 3A, top panel**). This was accompanied by enhanced expression of pro-fibrogenic factors, such as transforming growth factor TGF-β and platelet derived growth factor PDGF-β (**Figures S3A–B**), and progressive fibrosis, as evidenced by Sirius red staining (**Figure 3A, bottom panel**) and quantification of the hepatic hydroxyproline content

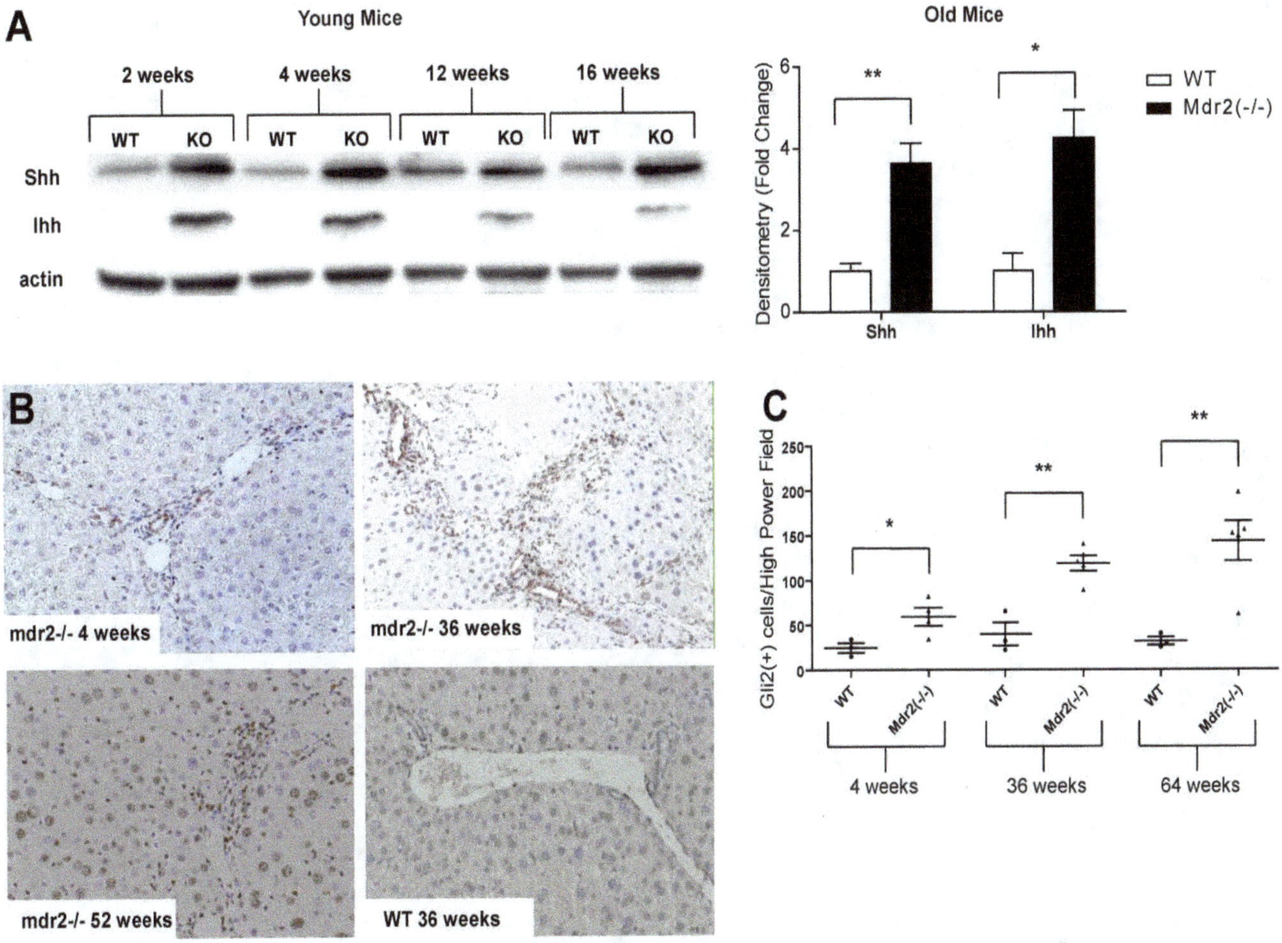

Figure 1. Increased hepatic Hedgehog (Hh) pathway activity in Mdr2$^{-/-}$ mice. A. Western blot analysis for Sonic Hedgehog (SHh) and Indian Hedgehog (IHh) in whole liver extracts pooled from young Mdr2$^{-/-}$ mice (2–16 weeks old), old (36–64 weeks old) Mdr2$^{-/-}$ mice and age-matched controls (n = 3–5 mice/group/time point). A representative Western blot demonstrating results from young mice is shown. Mean±SEM data from older mice are graphed. **B.** Representative liver sections stained to demonstrate Gli2 from young (4 wk old), middle aged (36 wk old) and old (52 wk old) Mdr2$^{-/-}$ mice. Little Gli2 expression was noted in wildtype mice at any age, so results from a representative 36 wk old wild type mouse is shown. (10×) **C.** Quantitative Gli2 immunohistochemical data. The number of nuclear Gli2(+) cells was counted in at least 5 high power fields (HPF) per liver section in Mdr2$^{-/-}$ mice and wild type controls at 4, 36 and 64 weeks of age (n = 3–4 mice/group/time point) and mean±SEM are graphed. $^*p<0.05$, $^{**}p<0.01$ in Mdr2$^{-/-}$ groups vs. respective controls.

(**Figure 3B**). Treatment with GDC-0449 decreased α-sma-expressing myofibroblastic cells, hepatic expression of TGF-β and PDGF-β, Sirius red staining, and hydroxyproline content, demonstrating that Hh pathway inhibition reduced liver fibrosis (**Figures 3C–D and Figures S3C–D**).

Hedgehog signaling inhibition with GDC-0449 decreases accumulation of liver progenitor cells

In response to injury, progenitor populations in the liver proliferate. Hence, immunohistochemical analysis for progenitor markers, such as cytokeratin-19 (CK-19) and α-fetoprotein (AFP), showed age-related increases in Mdr2$^{-/-}$ mice (**Figure 4A**). Co-staining for CK19 and Gli2 confirmed that the progenitor population was Hh responsive (**Figure 4B**). Upon treatment with GDC-0449, progenitor markers decreased (**Figure 4C**), indicating that Hh signaling was required to maintain progenitor populations during tumorigenesis, and that Hh inhibition was sufficient to shrink the size of progenitor populations even in mice with advanced HCC.

Decreasing Hedgehog signaling reduces expression of osteopontin and prevents accumulation of osteopontin-responsive (CD44-positive) cells

Stem/progenitor cell populations for many types of cancer, including HCC, are thought to be enriched with cells that express CD44, a receptor for the stem cell growth factor, osteopontin [35,36]. Osteopontin expression is regulated by Hh signaling [37]. Therefore, we examined the effects of GDC-0449 on osteopontin and its receptor, CD44. Immunohistochemistry and quantitative morphometry demonstrated that inhibition of the Hh pathway with GDC-0449 significantly decreased osteopontin staining within primary liver tumors (**Figure 5A**). Similar treatment-related decreases in CD44+ tumor cells were also noted (**Figure 5B**). Gene expression analysis showed that expression of both osteopontin and CD44 mRNAs also tended to decrease in GDC-0449-treated mice (**Figure 5C**). Together, these results suggest that Hh signaling may regulate putative liver cancer stem/progenitor cells by modulating availability of osteopontin.

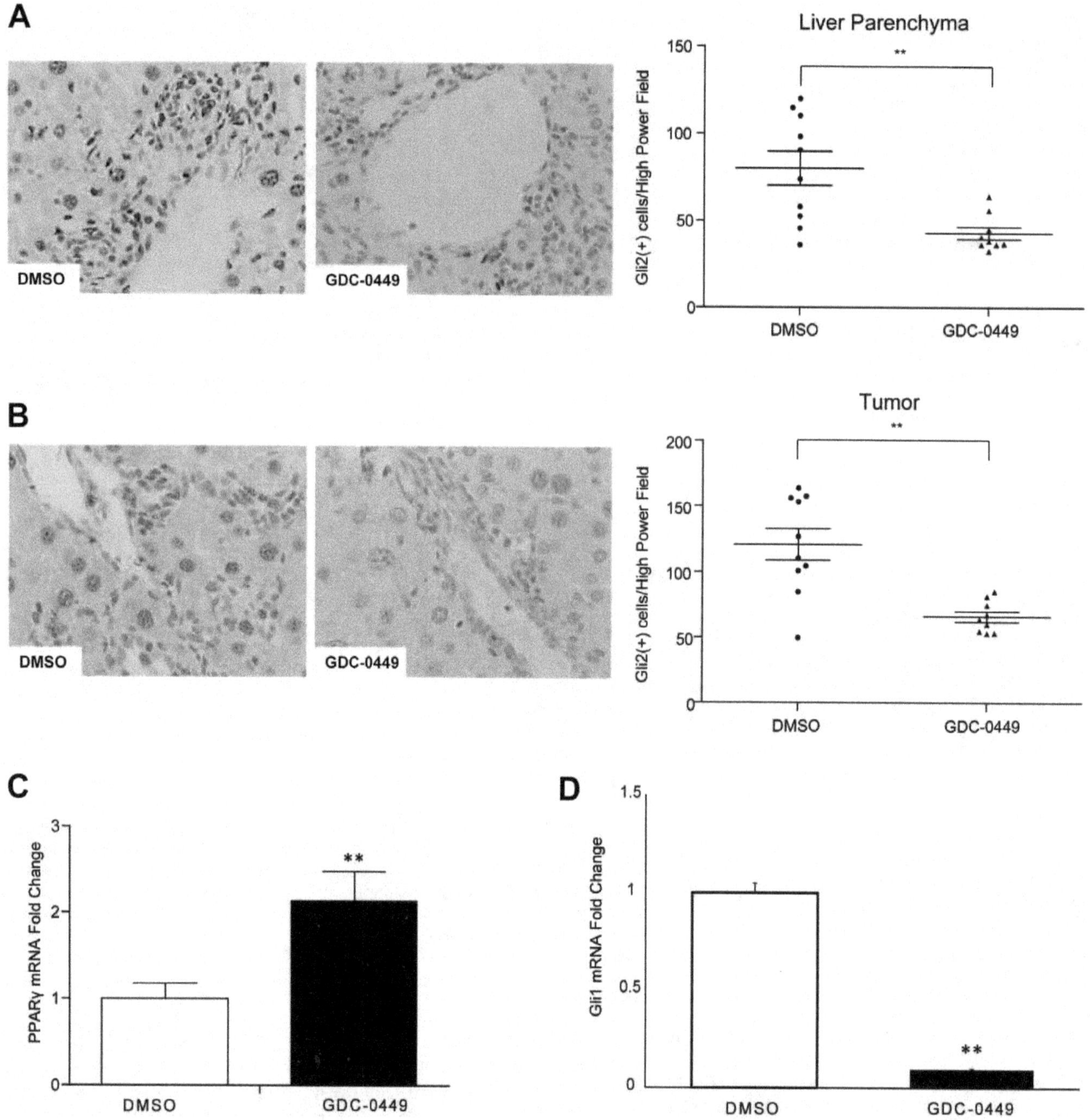

Figure 2. Hedgehog (Hh) inhibitor, GDC-0449, abrogates effects of Hh signaling within liver parenchyma and HCC nodules. A. Liver sections stained for Gli2 from representative DMSO- and GDC-0449- treated mice (40×). Quantitative Gli2 immunohistochemistry data in non-tumor livers of mice treated with DMSO or GDC-0449 (n = 9–10/group) are graphed as mean±SEM (*$^{**}p<0.01$*. The number of ductular cells with Gli2 positive staining were counted in each portal tract/section under 40× magnification. **B.** Tumor sections from the same mice were also stained to demonstrate Gli2. Results from representative DMSO- and GDC-0449-treated mice are displayed. Quantitative Gli2 immunohistochemistry data were generated by counting nuclear Gli2 positive ductular and hepatocytic cells in tumor sections under 40× magnification. Results are graphed as mean±SEM Gli2-positive cells/40× high power field (**p<0.01) **C–D** Quantitative reverse transcription-PCR (qRT-PCR) analysis of whole liver RNA from DMSO-(open bar) and GDC-0449 (black bar) treated mice. **C.** PPAR-γ, a gene that is normally repressed by Hh signaling. **D.** Gli1, a gene that is induced by Hh signaling. Mean±SEM are graphed (**p<0.01).

MRI and histological evidence of liver tumor involution following GDC-0449 treatment

To evaluate the potential impact of changes in matrix and progenitor cells on HCC, pre- and post-treatment tumor volumes were analyzed using magnetic resonance imaging (**Figures 6A–B**). An analysis of tumors in mice without overt metastasis demonstrated that tumor volumes decreased in mice that received a 9 day course of GDC-0449-treatment, while vehicle-treated animals evidenced persistent tumor growth (**Figure 6C**; −6.7%+/−11.7% vs 22.7% +/−9.1%, p = 0.03). This data correlated with

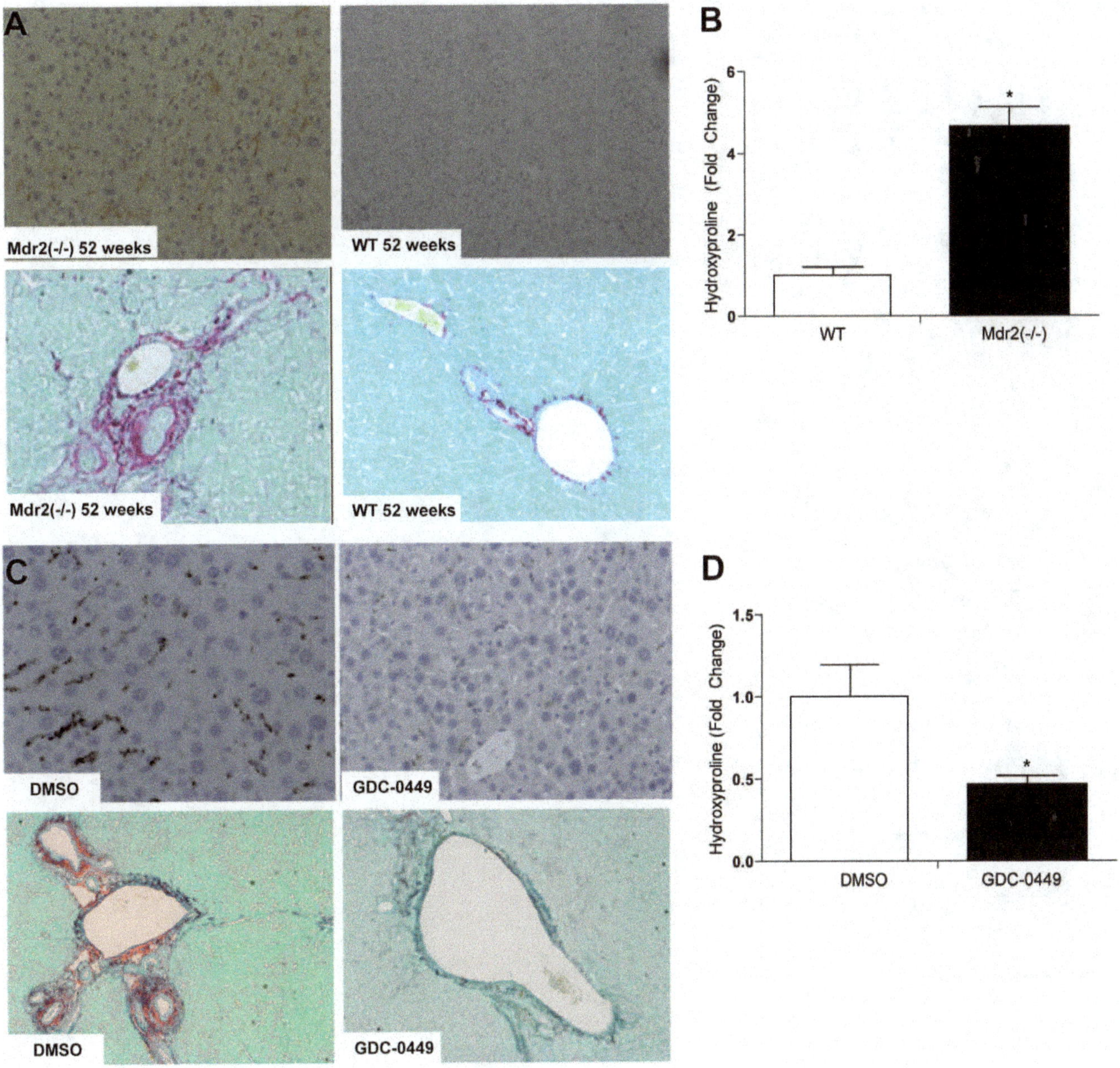

Figure 3. GDC-0449 treatment reduces fibrosis in Mdr2$^{-/-}$ mice. A. Immunohistochemical staining for α-SMA (top panel) and Sirius red (bottom panel) in sections of non-tumor liver from representative age-matched Mdr2$^{-/-}$ and wildtype mice (10×). **B.** Pooled Hepatic hydroxyproline content of 2–*52 wk-old* wildtype (WT) and age-matched Mdr2$^{-/-}$ mice (n = 3–5/group). Results in Mdr2$^{-/-}$ mice were normalized to that of age-matched WT mice and graphed as fold change. Data are displayed as mean +/− SD (*p<0.05) **C.** Non-tumor liver sections stained for α-SMA (top panel, 20×) and Sirius red (bottom panel, 10×) in representative DMSO- and GDC- treated Mdr2$^{-/-}$ mice. **D.** Heptic hydroxyproline content of DMSO- and GDC- treated mice (n = 9/group). Results in GDC-0449-treated mice were normalized to that of DMSO vehicle-treated mice and graphed as fold change. Data are displayed as Mean +/− SEM (*p<0.05).

necropsy findings: Only 56% of GDC-0449-treated mice had visible liver tumor nodules, compared to 80% of the DMSO mice (**Table 1**). Furthermore, both MRI and necropsies showed a decreased number of metastasis in GDC-0449-treated mice compared to vehicle-treated controls (**Table 1**). Histological analysis of H&E-stained liver sections was also performed on all animals from both cohorts. If tumor nodules were not grossly visible or greater than 10 mm in size, the samples were excluded from analysis. Microscopic tumor nodules in GDC-0449 treated animals demonstrated increased rates of hemorrhagic infarct (20% vs 0%; **Figure 6D, top panel**), microvesicular steatosis (40% vs 0%, **Figure 6D, middle panel**), acidophilic necrosis and degenerative cytoplasmic changes (70% vs 40%, **Figure 6D, bottom panel**) in comparison to tumors from vehicle treated animals. Thus, findings on MRI, necropsy, and liver histology were consistent and demonstrated that Hh pathway inhibition caused significant regression of primary and metastatic HCC.

Discussion

We studied Mdr2$^{-/-}$ mice to determine whether or not activation of the Hh pathway contributes to hepatocarcinogenesis

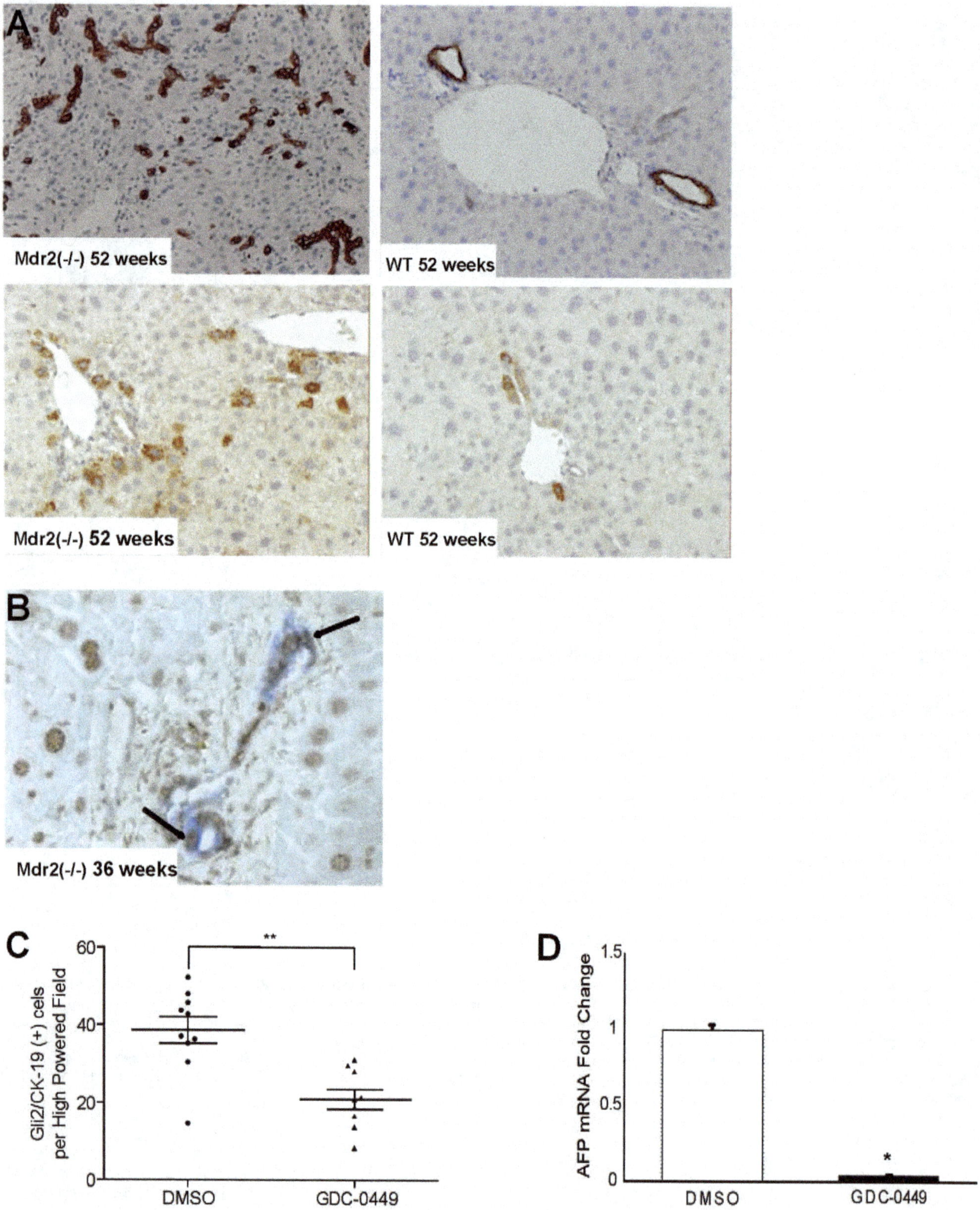

Figure 4. Effects of Mdr2 deficiency and Hedgehog (Hh) inhibition on hepatic progenitor populations. A. Immunohistochemical staining of liver sections from representative, age-matched Mdr2$^{-/-}$ and wildtype mice for progenitor markers, cytokeratin-19 (CK-19) (top panels) and α -fetoprotein (AFP) (bottom panels) (20×). **B.** Representative micrograph of a portal triad in liver of an Mdr2$^{-/-}$ mouse, demonstrating co-localization of CK-19 (blue) and Gli2 (brown) in the ductular compartment (40×). **C.** Quantitative Gli2 and CK19 immunohistochemistry in DMSO- and GDC-0449-treated Mdr2$^{-/-}$ mice (n=9–10/group). The number of Gli2 and CK19 double-positive ductular-appearing cells were counted within tumors under 20× magnification. Mean±SEM double(+) cells t per high power field (HPF) are graphed (* $p<0.05$) **D.** QRT-PCR analysis of AFP in tumor RNA from mice treated with DMSO (open bar) or GDC-0449 (closed bar) Results in the GDC-0449-treated mice were normalized to that of the mice treated with DMSO vehicle and graphed as Mean±SEM (*$p<0.05$).

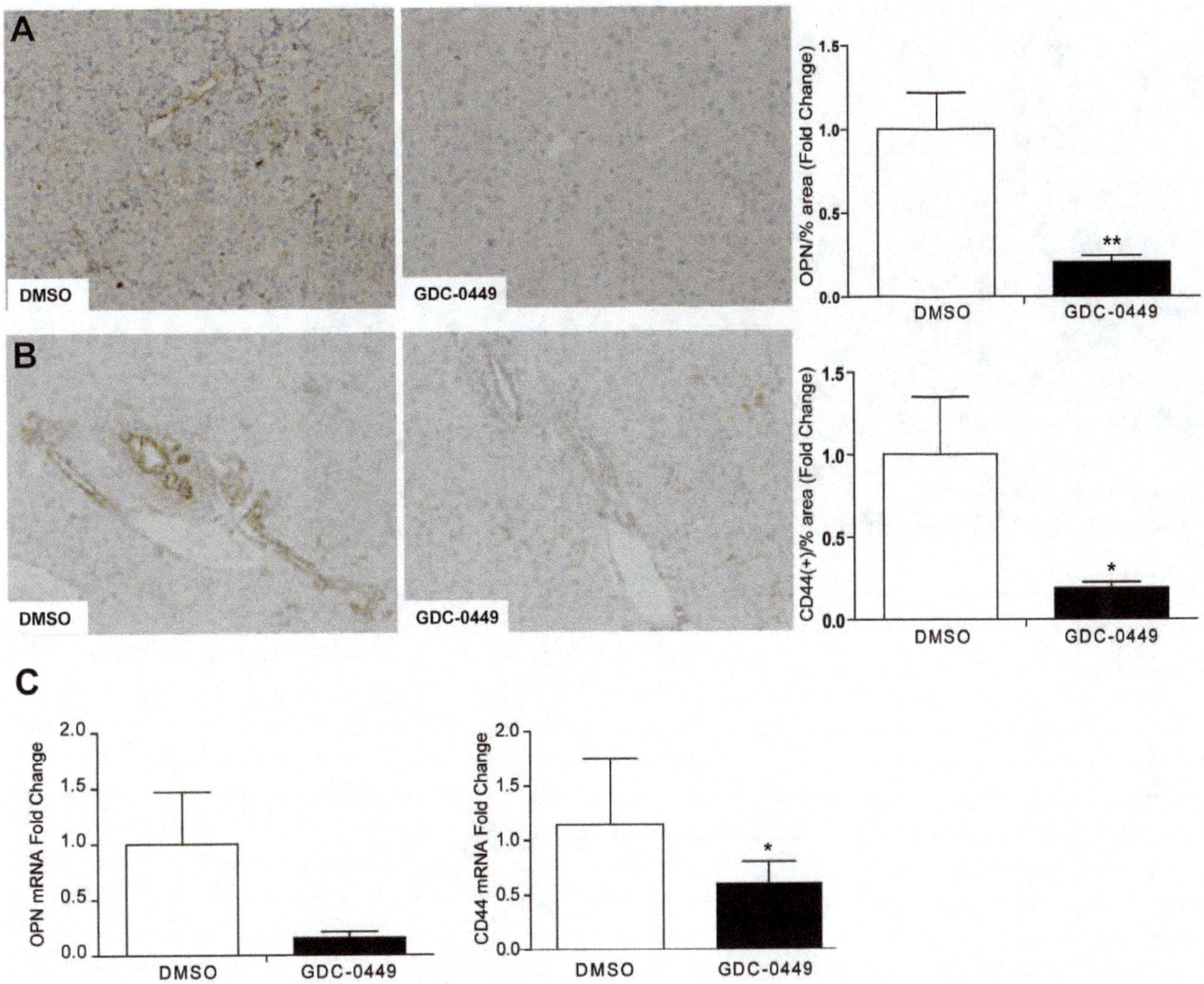

Figure 5. Inhibition of Hh signaling decreases osteopontin and osteopontin-responsive (CD44) positive cells in tumors and peri-tumoral tissues of aged Mdr2$^{-/-}$ mice. A. Tumor sections from representative DMSO- and GDC-0449 treated Mdr2$^{-/-}$ mice were stained to demonstrate osteopontin (OPN) Representative sections are displayed (*Right panel*). OPN staining was quantified by morphometric analysis of at least 5 HPF per tumor section using 20× magnification (n = 5 mice/group). Results in the GDC-0449-treated group were normalized to that of the group treated with DMSO vehicle and graphed as fold change. Data are displayed as Mean±SEM (**p<0.01). **B.** Immunohistochemical staining for the osteopontin receptor, CD44, in peri-tumoral tissues of representative DMSO- and GDC-0449- treated Mdr2$^{-/-}$ mice. (*Right panel*) CD44 staining was quantified by morphometric analysis as described in A. Results in GDC-0449-treated mice were normalized to those of vehicle-treated controls and graphed as Mean±SEM (**p<0.01). **C.** QRT-PCR analysis of liver tumor RNA from DMSO- (open bar) and GDC-0449- (closed bar) treated Mdr2$^{-/-}$ mice for OPN (left) and CD44 (right). After normalization to results in the DMSO-treated group, Mean±SEM were graphed (*p<0.05).

during chronic fibrosing liver injury. Mdr2-deficient mice lack a phospholipid flippase that is required for normal bile formation, and consequently exhibit liver injury and ductular proliferation from a young age. All afflicted mice eventually develop significant liver fibrosis and metastatic HCC. Our results demonstrate that this pathology is accompanied by progressive activation of the Hh pathway. Introduction of a specific inhibitor of the key Hh signaling intermediate, Smoothened, reduced pathway activity and proved that sustained Hh signaling was required to maintain the expanded populations of liver myofibroblasts and progenitors that had accumulated in the damaged livers. Moreover, treating aged Mdr2-deficient mice (which already had advanced liver fibrosis and HCC) with the Hh pathway inhibitor significantly reduced liver fibrosis and tumor burden, demonstrating for the first time that inhibiting Hh signaling has clinically-relevant, therapeutic value for both liver fibrosis and HCC. Even more exciting is evidence that the prohibitive effect on hepatic tumor growth *in vivo* pertains to both intra-hepatic HCC and distant metastasis.

In addition, our results provide insight into some of the underlying mechanisms involved. Hepatic production of Hh ligands was increased in mice that developed progressive liver fibrosis and invasive HCC. These mice also demonstrated consistently higher serum aminotransferase levels, in keeping with other evidence that Mdr2 deficiency provokes chronic hepatocyte injury [38,39]. Various stressors that reduce hepatocyte viability have been shown to induce production and release of Hh ligands by wounded hepatocytes [40,41]. Thus, hepatocyte injury is likely one of the factors that increases Hh ligand generation in mdr2-deficient livers. Myofibroblastic cells and ductular-type progenitors that progressively accumulate in chronically injured livers also produce Hh ligands, as well as other factors, such as PDGF-β, that

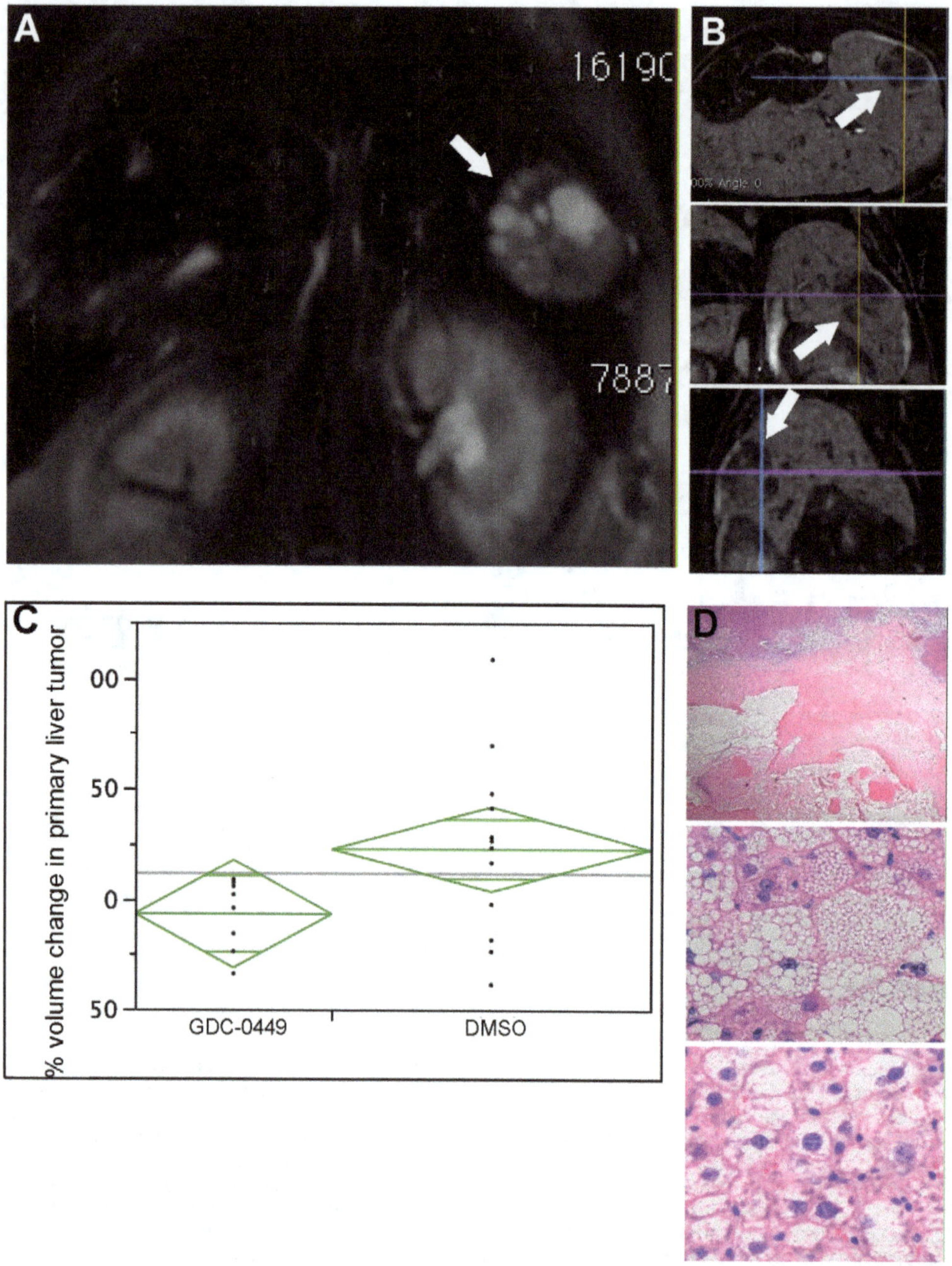

Figure 6. Hh pathway inhibition decreases in liver tumor volume by magnetic resonance imaging (MRI) and induces histologic features of tumor involution. A. Representative cross-sectional image of intrahepatic tumor as identified by contrast-enhanced MRI following GDC-0449 treatment. **B.** Representative MRI images of sagittal, coronal, and oblique perspectives used for volumetric analysis. **C.** Change in tumor volume were quantified by computerize generated volumetric measurements and graphed as Mean±SD (*$p<0.05$). **D.** Micrographs of representative histologic changes induced by, GDC-0449, treatment. Top panel shows tumor necrosis; middle panel demonstrates fatty degeneration; bottom panel show vacuolated tumor cells with pyknotic nuclei.

stimulate autocrine-paracrine synthesis of Hh ligands [20,42]. Relative to age/gender matched healthy control mice, aged mdr2-deficient mice with ductular reactions and liver fibrosis demonstrated higher hepatic mRNA levels of PDGF-β, suggesting a mechanism by which the fibrogenic repair response itself might perpetuate excessive hepatic accumulation of Hh ligands. The latter concept is supported by evidence that inhibiting Hh signaling with GDC-0449 reduced accumulation of myofibroblasts and ductular-type progenitors, decreased expression of PDGF-β, and suppressed hepatic expression Hh ligands in mice that remained at risk for hepatocyte injury due to genetic deficiency of Mdr2.

Chronic over-production of Hh ligands has important pathobiological implications because mice that generated increased Hh ligands also demonstrated excessive activation of the Hh pathway in their livers. This was evidenced by larger numbers of cells with nuclear staining for the Hh-regulated transcription factor, Gli2, and enhanced expression of various Hh-target genes, including Gli1 and osteopontin. In such animals, we showed that treatment with a highly specific antagonist of Smoothened was able to

Table 1. Effect of GDC-0449 treatment on intrahepatic HCC and HCC metastases.

	Surgical Resection		MRI Imaging	
	Vehicle	Treatment	Vehicle	Treatment
Intrahepatic Tumor Nodules	80%	56%	78%	50%
Metastases	20%	0%	50%	20%

suppress all of these responses, consistent with published evidence that activation of Smoothened in Hh-responsive cells promotes nuclear localization of Gli2, and consequent induction of Gli1 and osteopontin transcription [43,44]. Osteopontin, in turn, has been shown to promote myofibroblast accumulation and liver fibrosis in mice [37,45]. It also acts via its receptor, CD44, to enhance the viability and growth of certain types of liver progenitors, including liver cancer stem/progenitor cells [35,36,46,47]. Hence, the Hh pathway might be modulating both liver fibrosis and HCC outgrowth by regulating the autocrine/paracrine availability of osteopontin.

Myofibroblasts and ductular progenitor cells are also important sources of other pro-fibrogenic factors (e.g., PDGF-β and TGF-β) that are capable of activating Gli2 via mechanisms that do not require Smoothened [48,49,50]. We observed increased hepatic expression of both PDGF-β and TGF-β in Mdr2-deficient mice. This suggests that Smoothened-independent mechanisms that re-enforce the effects of the canonical Hh pathway may evolve during fibrogenic repair. In mdr2-deficient mice, however, GDC-0449 significantly reduced expression of TGF-β and tended to suppress expression of PDGFβ, demonstrating that canonical Hh signaling with resultant Smoothened activation is ultimately required to fully engage noncanonical pathways that rely on interaction of TGF-β and PDGF-β with their respective receptors to activate Gli2 in injured, fibrotic livers.

Finally, the fact that liver fibrosis/cirrhosis is a major risk factor for the development of HCC should not be misconstrued to imply that fibrosis *per se* causes cancer. It is conceivable that fibrosis and HCC each result from some adaptive response that occurs during chronic liver injury. Our results demonstrate that injury-related activation of the Hh pathway typifies an adaptive response that is both pro-fibrogenic and pro-carcinogenic. This discovery, in turn, provides novel evidence that helps to explain why fibrosis and HCC often develop in the same livers. As such, it has immediate clinical relevance to the many cirrhotic patients with HCC. Additional research will be required, however to delineate the precise down-stream mechanism(s) involved and to determine which (if any) of those subsequent fibrogenic and carcinogenic processes are inter-dependent, and which are totally independent of each other.

Proof that inhibition of Hh signaling substantially reduced the hepatic content of myofibroblasts and progenitors suggests that these cell types promote and/or maintain the outgrowth of malignant hepatocytes. This finding, in turn, provides a starting point for further research. Indeed, others have reported that Smoothened antagonists lead to the involution of pancreatic cancers by influencing tumor angiogenesis [51]. Myofibroblasts are known to be an important source of vascular growth factors, such as VEGF [52,53,54], and we found increased hepatic expression of VEGF and its receptor, VEGFR1, in the diseased livers of Mdr2-deficient mice compared to the healthy livers of age/gender-matched controls (data not shown). Hence, it is possible that myofibroblast depletion exerted a negative impact on the hepatic vasculature that ultimately resulted in HCC involution. This concept is supported by evidence that GDC-0449 tended to suppress hepatic expression of VEGF/VEGFR1 (data not shown) and increased necrosis in the HCC of GDC-0449-treated mice. Hh signaling is also known to maintain various progenitor populations [55,56,57]. Previously, we reported that Hh ligands function as autocrine and paracrine survival signals for liver progenitors and showed that liver myofibroblasts are an important paracrine source of Hh ligands that serve this purpose [40,42,58,59,60]. Liver progenitors, in turn, generate Hh ligands that provide paracrine signals that re-enforce the growth of liver myofibroblasts [61,62]. Given this background, it is not surprising that blocking Hh signaling with a Smoothened antagonist resulted in the mutual depletion of both cell types. To our knowledge, however, by demonstrating marked treatment-related decreases in CD44, cytokeratin-19, and α-fetoprotein within HCC tumors, the current data provide the first evidence that Smoothened antagonists reduce populations of cells that exhibit features of tumor stem/progenitor cells. Further investigation is required to ascertain how aberrant Hedgehog signaling promotes these cancer stem cell compartments.

In conclusion, our findings in the Mdr2$^{-/-}$ mouse model of progressive liver fibrosis and spontaneous hepatocarcinogenesis demonstrate that increased production of Hh ligands and progressive accumulation of Hh-responsive cell types, such as myofibroblasts and liver progenitor cells, precede the emergence of HCC, and persist after the development of HCC. Despite advanced liver fibrosis and HCC, a short course of treatment with a highly-specific and clinically available Hh signaling inhibitor is well-tolerated and demonstrates appreciable anti-tumor effects. Thus, Hh pathway inhibition with GDC-0449 merits evaluation as a potential treatment for HCC arising in cirrhotic patients, providing a novel treatment option for an emerging disease with a poor prognosis and limited therapeutics.

Supporting Information

Figure S1 Evidence of ongoing liver injury in Mdr2$^{-/-}$ mice. AST and ALT measurements from Mdr2$^{-/-}$ mice and their age-matched wild type counterparts at various time points. Each data point represents n = 2–7 animals and Mean±SD is graphed. (*$p<0.05$ vs the age-matched wild-type control).

Figure S2 Systemic treatment of GDC-0449 treatment is well tolerated in Mdr2$^{-/-}$ mice with advanced liver disease and HCC. A. Daily body weight measurements were obtained for all animals in each of the three treatment groups and graphed over time. Data expressed as Mean±SD. **B.** Liver to body weight ratios of animals in each of the three treatment groups. Data expressed as Mean±SD. **C.** Western blot analysis for Shh, Gli1, Gli2 and actin (loading control) in whole liver extracts from Mdr2−/− mice treated with vehicle, 20 mg/kg GDC-0449, and 40 mg/kg GDC-0449. Liver extracts from each treated mouse were loaded individually.

Figure S3 Increased hepatic expression of TGFβ and PDGFβ in Mdr2$^{-/-}$ mice is reversed by GDC-0449 treatment. Whole liver RNA was isolated from Mdr2$^{-/-}$ mice and age/gender-matched wild type controls (WT) (n = 3 mice/group) and QRT PCR was done to compare expression of (**A**) TGFβ and (**B**) PDGFβ. Similar approaches were used to assess the effects of a 9 day course of treatment with either the Hh pathway inhibitor GDC-0449 or vehicle (DMSO) on expression of (**C**) TGFβ and (**D**) PDGFβ in Mdr2$^{-/-}$ mice (n = 5 mice/group). Gene expression was normalized to expression of S9 in the same samples; mean +/− SEM values were calculated; values in the experimental groups were graphed relative those in the respective controls. P values are shown.

Table S1

Author Contributions

Conceived and designed the experiments: GMP ISC VTS FR CL AMD. Performed the experiments: GMP ISC MS VTS CG GFK CM W-KS YJ RPW SC FR EM CL AMD. Analyzed the data: GMP ISC MS VTS CG TV SF W-KS SC GAM EM CL AMD. Contributed reagents/materials/analysis tools: EM CL AMD. Wrote the paper: GMP ISC FR GAM SC AMD.

References

1. Rahbari NN, Mehrabi A, Mollberg NM, Muller SA, Koch M, et al. (2011) Hepatocellular carcinoma: current management and perspectives for the future. Ann Surg 253: 453–469.
2. Luedde T, Schwabe RF (2011) NF-kappaB in the liver–linking injury, fibrosis and hepatocellular carcinoma. Nat Rev Gastroenterol Hepatol 8: 108–118.
3. Schuppan D, Afdhal NH (2008) Liver cirrhosis. Lancet 371: 838–851.
4. Gonzales E, Davit-Spraul A, Baussan C, Buffet C, Maurice M, et al. (2009) Liver diseases related to MDR3 (ABCB4) gene deficiency. Front Biosci 14: 4242–4256.
5. Jacquemin E (2001) Role of multidrug resistance 3 deficiency in pediatric and adult liver disease: one gene for three diseases. Semin Liver Dis 21: 551–562.
6. Trauner M, Fickert P, Halilbasic E, Moustafa T (2008) Lessons from the toxic bile concept for the pathogenesis and treatment of cholestatic liver diseases. Wien Med Wochenschr 158: 542–548.
7. Trauner M, Fickert P, Wagner M (2007) MDR3 (ABCB4) defects: a paradigm for the genetics of adult cholestatic syndromes. Semin Liver Dis 27: 77–98.
8. Baghdasaryan A, Fickert P, Fuchsbichler A, Silbert D, Gumhold J, et al. (2008) Role of hepatic phospholipids in development of liver injury in Mdr2 (Abcb4) knockout mice. Liver Int 28: 948–958.
9. De Vree JM, Ottenhoff R, Bosma PJ, Smith AJ, Aten J, et al. (2000) Correction of liver disease by hepatocyte transplantation in a mouse model of progressive familial intrahepatic cholestasis. Gastroenterology 119: 1720–1730.
10. Fickert P, Fuchsbichler A, Wagner M, Zollner G, Kaser A, et al. (2004) Regurgitation of bile acids from leaky bile ducts causes sclerosing cholangitis in Mdr2 (Abcb4) knockout mice. Gastroenterology 127: 261–274.
11. Fickert P, Zollner G, Fuchsbichler A, Stumptner C, Weiglein AH, et al. (2002) Ursodeoxycholic acid aggravates bile infarcts in bile duct-ligated and Mdr2 knockout mice via disruption of cholangioles. Gastroenterology 123: 1238–1251.
12. Frijters CM, Ottenhoff R, Van Wijland MJ, Van Nieuwkerk C, Groen AK, et al. (1996) Influence of bile salts on hepatic mdr2 P-glycoprotein expression. Adv Enzyme Regul 36: 351–363.
13. Popov Y, Patsenker E, Fickert P, Trauner M, Schuppan D (2005) Mdr2 (Abcb4)−/− mice spontaneously develop severe biliary fibrosis via massive dysregulation of pro- and antifibrogenic genes. J Hepatol 43: 1045–1054.
14. Van Nieuwkerk CM, Elferink RP, Groen AK, Ottenhoff R, Tytgat GN, et al. (1996) Effects of Ursodeoxycholate and cholate feeding on liver disease in FVB mice with a disrupted mdr2 P-glycoprotein gene. Gastroenterology 111: 165–171.
15. Katzenellenbogen M, Mizrahi L, Pappo O, Klopstock N, Olam D, et al. (2007) Molecular mechanisms of liver carcinogenesis in the mdr2-knockout mice. Mol Cancer Res 5: 1159–1170.
16. Katzenellenbogen M, Pappo O, Barash H, Klopstock N, Mizrahi L, et al. (2006) Multiple adaptive mechanisms to chronic liver disease revealed at early stages of liver carcinogenesis in the Mdr2-knockout mice. Cancer Res 66: 4001–4010.
17. Ramalho-Santos M, Melton DA, McMahon AP (2000) Hedgehog signals regulate multiple aspects of gastrointestinal development. Development 127: 2763–2772.
18. Berman DM, Karhadkar SS, Maitra A, Montes De Oca R, Gerstenblith MR, et al. (2003) Widespread requirement for Hedgehog ligand stimulation in growth of digestive tract tumours. Nature 425: 846–851.
19. Omenetti A, Diehl AM (2008) The adventures of sonic hedgehog in development and repair. II. Sonic hedgehog and liver development, inflammation, and cancer. Am J Physiol Gastrointest Liver Physiol 294: G595–598.
20. Omenetti A, Popov Y, Jung Y, Choi SS, Witek RP, et al. (2008) The hedgehog pathway regulates remodelling responses to biliary obstruction in rats. Gut 57: 1275–1282.
21. Omenetti A, Porrello A, Jung Y, Yang L, Popov Y, et al. (2008) Hedgehog signaling regulates epithelial-mesenchymal transition during biliary fibrosis in rodents and humans. J Clin Invest 118: 3331–3342.
22. Omenetti A, Yang L, Li YX, McCall SJ, Jung Y, et al. (2007) Hedgehog-mediated mesenchymal-epithelial interactions modulate hepatic response to bile duct ligation. Lab Invest 87: 499–514.
23. Syn WK, Jung Y, Omenetti A, Abdelmalek M, Guy CD, et al. (2009) Hedgehog-mediated epithelial-to-mesenchymal transition and fibrogenic repair in nonalcoholic fatty liver disease. Gastroenterology 137: 1478–1488 e1478.
24. Choi SS, Omenetti A, Witek RP, Moylan CA, Syn WK, et al. (2009) Hedgehog pathway activation and epithelial-to-mesenchymal transitions during myofibroblastic transformation of rat hepatic cells in culture and cirrhosis. Am J Physiol Gastrointest Liver Physiol 297: G1093–1106.
25. Sicklick JK, Li YX, Choi SS, Qi Y, Chen W, et al. (2005) Role for hedgehog signaling in hepatic stellate cell activation and viability. Lab Invest 85: 1368–1380.
26. Huang S, He J, Zhang X, Bian Y, Yang L, et al. (2006) Activation of the hedgehog pathway in human hepatocellular carcinomas. Carcinogenesis 27: 1334–1340.
27. Sicklick JK, Li YX, Jayaraman A, Kannangai R, Qi Y, et al. (2006) Dysregulation of the Hedgehog pathway in human hepatocarcinogenesis. Carcinogenesis 27: 748–757.
28. Patil MA, Zhang J, Ho C, Cheung ST, Fan ST, et al. (2006) Hedgehog signaling in human hepatocellular carcinoma. Cancer Biol Ther 5: 111–117.
29. Chen W, Tang T, Eastham-Anderson J, Dunlap D, Alicke B, et al. (2011) Canonical hedgehog signaling augments tumor angiogenesis by induction of VEGF-A in stromal perivascular cells. Proc Natl Acad Sci U S A 108: 9589–9594.
30. Pereira Tde A, Witek RP, Syn WK, Choi SS, Bradrick S, et al. (2010) Viral factors induce Hedgehog pathway activation in humans with viral hepatitis, cirrhosis, and hepatocellular carcinoma. Lab Invest 90: 1690–1703.
31. Lorusso PM, Rudin CM, Reddy JC, Tibes R, Weiss GJ, et al. (2011) Phase I Trial of Hedgehog Pathway Inhibitor Vismodegib (GDC-0449) in Patients with Refractory, Locally Advanced or Metastatic Solid Tumors. Clin Cancer Res 17: 2502–2511.
32. Von Hoff DD, LoRusso PM, Rudin CM, Reddy JC, Yauch RL, et al. (2009) Inhibition of the hedgehog pathway in advanced basal-cell carcinoma. N Engl J Med 361: 1164–1172.
33. Rudin CM, Hann CL, Laterra J, Yauch RL, Callahan CA, et al. (2009) Treatment of medulloblastoma with hedgehog pathway inhibitor GDC-0449. N Engl J Med 361: 1173–1178.
34. Witek RP, Stone WC, Karaca FG, Syn WK, Pereira TA, et al. (2009) Pan-caspase inhibitor VX-166 reduces fibrosis in an animal model of nonalcoholic steatohepatitis. Hepatology 50: 1421–1430.
35. Orian-Rousseau V (2010) CD44, a therapeutic target for metastasising tumours. Eur J Cancer 46: 1271–1277.
36. Yang GH, Fan J, Xu Y, Qiu SJ, Yang XR, et al. (2008) Osteopontin combined with CD44, a novel prognostic biomarker for patients with hepatocellular carcinoma undergoing curative resection. Oncologist 13: 1155–1165.
37. Syn WK, Choi SS, Liaskou E, Karaca GF, Agboola KM, et al. (2011) Osteopontin is induced by hedgehog pathway activation and promotes fibrosis progression in nonalcoholic steatohepatitis. Hepatology 53: 106–115.
38. Mauad TH, van Nieuwkerk CM, Dingemans KP, Smit JJ, Schinkel AH, et al. (1994) Mice with homozygous disruption of the mdr2 P-glycoprotein gene. A novel animal model for studies of nonsuppurative inflammatory cholangitis and hepatocarcinogenesis. Am J Pathol 145: 1237–1245.
39. Smit JJ, Schinkel AH, Oude Elferink RP, Groen AK, Wagenaar E, et al. (1993) Homozygous disruption of the murine mdr2 P-glycoprotein gene leads to a complete absence of phospholipid from bile and to liver disease. Cell 75: 451–462.
40. Jung Y, Witek RP, Syn WK, Choi SS, Omenetti A, et al. (2010) Signals from dying hepatocytes trigger growth of liver progenitors. Gut 59: 655–665.
41. Rangwala F, Guy CD, Lu J, Suzuki A, Burchette JL, et al. (2011) Increased production of sonic hedgehog by ballooned hepatocytes. J Pathol 224: 401–410.
42. Yang L, Wang Y, Mao H, Fleig S, Omenetti A, et al. (2008) Sonic hedgehog is an autocrine viability factor for myofibroblastic hepatic stellate cells. J Hepatol 48: 98–106.
43. Das S, Harris LG, Metge BJ, Liu S, Riker AI, et al. (2009) The hedgehog pathway transcription factor GLI1 promotes malignant behavior of cancer cells by up-regulating osteopontin. J Biol Chem 284: 22888–22897.
44. Omenetti A, Choi S, Michelotti G, Diehl AM (2011) Hedgehog signaling in the liver. J Hepatol 54: 366–373.
45. Machado MV, Cortez-Pinto H (2011) Osteopontin: a missing link between hedgehog signaling and fibrosis in nonalcoholic steatohepatitis. Hepatology 53: 382–384.
46. Rangwala F, Omenetti A, Diehl AM (2011) Cancer stem cells: repair gone awry? J Oncol 2011: 465343.

47. Haramaki M, Yano H, Fukuda K, Momosaki S, Ogasawara S, et al. (1995) Expression of CD44 in human hepatocellular carcinoma cell lines. Hepatology 21: 1276–1284.
48. Dennler S, Andre J, Verrecchia F, Mauviel A (2009) Cloning of the human GLI2 Promoter: transcriptional activation by transforming growth factor-beta via SMAD3/beta-catenin cooperation. J Biol Chem 284: 31523–31531.
49. Dennler S, Andre J, Alexaki I, Li A, Magnaldo T, et al. (2007) Induction of sonic hedgehog mediators by transforming growth factor-beta: Smad3-dependent activation of Gli2 and Gli1 expression in vitro and in vivo. Cancer Res 67: 6981–6986.
50. Friedman SL (2008) Hepatic stellate cells: protean, multifunctional, and enigmatic cells of the liver. Physiol Rev 88: 125–172.
51. Olive KP, Jacobetz MA, Davidson CJ, Gopinathan A, McIntyre D, et al. (2009) Inhibition of Hedgehog signaling enhances delivery of chemotherapy in a mouse model of pancreatic cancer. Science 324: 1457–1461.
52. Ankoma-Sey V, Wang Y, Dai Z (2000) Hypoxic stimulation of vascular endothelial growth factor expression in activated rat hepatic stellate cells. Hepatology 31: 141–148.
53. Lee JS, Semela D, Iredale J, Shah VH (2007) Sinusoidal remodeling and angiogenesis: a new function for the liver-specific pericyte? Hepatology 45: 817–825.
54. Witek RP, Yang L, Liu R, Jung Y, Omenetti A, et al. (2009) Liver cell-derived microparticles activate hedgehog signaling and alter gene expression in hepatic endothelial cells. Gastroenterology 136: 320–330 e322.
55. Song Z, Yue W, Wei B, Wang N, Li T, et al. (2011) Sonic hedgehog pathway is essential for maintenance of cancer stem-like cells in human gastric cancer. PLoS One 6: e17687.
56. Katoh Y, Katoh M (2009) Hedgehog target genes: mechanisms of carcinogenesis induced by aberrant hedgehog signaling activation. Curr Mol Med 9: 873–886.
57. Tanaka H, Nakamura M, Kameda C, Kubo M, Sato N, et al. (2009) The Hedgehog signaling pathway plays an essential role in maintaining the CD44+CD24−/low subpopulation and the side population of breast cancer cells. Anticancer Res 29: 2147–2157.
58. Jung Y, Brown KD, Witek RP, Omenetti A, Yang L, et al. (2008) Accumulation of hedgehog-responsive progenitors parallels alcoholic liver disease severity in mice and humans. Gastroenterology 134: 1532–1543.
59. Sicklick JK, Li YX, Melhem A, Schmelzer E, Zdanowicz M, et al. (2006) Hedgehog signaling maintains resident hepatic progenitors throughout life. Am J Physiol Gastrointest Liver Physiol 290: G859–870.
60. Jung Y, McCall SJ, Li YX, Diehl AM (2007) Bile ductules and stromal cells express hedgehog ligands and/or hedgehog target genes in primary biliary cirrhosis. Hepatology 45: 1091–1096.
61. Omenetti A, Syn WK, Jung Y, Francis H, Porrello A, et al. (2009) Repair-related activation of hedgehog signaling promotes cholangiocyte chemokine production. Hepatology 50: 518–527.
62. Fleig SV, Choi SS, Yang L, Jung Y, Omenetti A, et al. (2007) Hepatic accumulation of Hedgehog-reactive progenitors increases with severity of fatty liver damage in mice. Lab Invest 87: 1227–1239.

14

Oral Methylthioadenosine Administration Attenuates Fibrosis and Chronic Liver Disease Progression in *Mdr2−/−* Mice

M. Ujue Latasa[1], Carmen Gil-Puig[1,2], Maite G. Fernández-Barrena[1,3], Carlos M. Rodríguez-Ortigosa[1,3], Jesús M. Banales[1,3], Raquel Urtasun[1], Saioa Goñi[1], Miriam Méndez[1], Sara Arcelus[3], Nerea Juanarena[1], Juan A. Recio[4], Sophie Lotersztajn[5,6], Jesús Prieto[1,3], Carmen Berasain[1], Fernando J. Corrales[1], Jon Lecanda[1,2¶], Matías A. Ávila[1*¶]

1 Division of Hepatology and Gene Therapy, CIMA, University of Navarra, Pamplona, Spain, **2** Digna Biotech, Madrid, Spain, **3** CIBERehd, University Clinic, University of Navarra, Pamplona, Spain, **4** Vall d'Hebron Research Institute, Institute of Oncology and Hospital, Barcelona, Spain, **5** Inserm, U955, Créteil, France, **6** Université Paris-Est, Faculté de Médecine, UMR-S955, Créteil, France

Abstract

Background: Inflammation and fibrogenesis are directly related to chronic liver disease progression, including hepatocellular carcinoma (HCC) development. Currently there are few therapeutic options available to inhibit liver fibrosis. We have evaluated the hepatoprotective and anti-fibrotic potential of orally-administered 5′-methylthioadenosine (MTA) in *Mdr2*$^{-/-}$ mice, a clinically relevant model of sclerosing cholangitis and spontaneous biliary fibrosis, followed at later stages by HCC development.

Methodology: MTA was administered daily by gavage to wild type and *Mdr2*$^{-/-}$ mice for three weeks. MTA anti-inflammatory and anti-fibrotic effects and potential mechanisms of action were examined in the liver of *Mdr2*$^{-/-}$ mice with ongoing fibrogenesis and in cultured liver fibrogenic cells (myofibroblasts).

Principal Findings: MTA treatment reduced hepatomegaly and liver injury. α-Smooth muscle actin immunoreactivity and collagen deposition were also significantly decreased. Inflammatory infiltrate, the expression of the cytokines IL6 and Mcp-1, pro-fibrogenic factors like TGFβ2 and tenascin-C, as well as pro-fibrogenic intracellular signalling pathways were reduced by MTA *in vivo*. MTA inhibited the activation and proliferation of isolated myofibroblasts and down-regulated cyclin D1 gene expression at the transcriptional level. The expression of JunD, a key transcription factor in liver fibrogenesis, was also reduced by MTA in activated myofibroblasts.

Conclusions/Significance: Oral MTA administration was well tolerated and proved its efficacy in reducing liver inflammation and fibrosis. MTA may have multiple molecular and cellular targets. These include the inhibition of inflammatory and pro-fibrogenic cytokines, as well as the attenuation of myofibroblast activation and proliferation. Downregulation of JunD and cyclin D1 expression in myofibroblasts may be important regarding the mechanism of action of MTA. This compound could be a good candidate to be tested for the treatment of (biliary) liver fibrosis.

Editor: Massimo Federici, University of Tor Vergata, Italy

Funding: This work was supported by the agreement between FIMA and the "UTE project CIMA"; RTICC-RD06 00200061 (CB, FJC, MAA), CiberEhd (MGF-B, JB, CRO, JP), FIS-PI070392 and PI070402 (CB, MAA); SAF2008-01540 (FJC); Instituto de Salud Carlos III Fellowship (SG); Ramón y Cajal Program (MUL) and Torres Quevedo Program (CG-P, RU); INSERM, Université Paris-Est, the Agence Nationale de la Recherche and the Fondation pour la Recherche Medicale (SL). The funders had no role in study design, data collection and analysis, decision to publish, or preparation of the manuscript.

Competing Interests: The authors have declared that no competing interests exist.

* E-mail: maavila@unav.es

These authors contributed equally to this work.

¶ These authors also contributed equally to this work.

Introduction

Liver diseases are currently the fifth cause of mortality in the Western world, and as opposed to other major causes of mortality their incidence is increasing [1,2]. The principal causes of the most common liver ailments are well known, and include chronic alcohol consumption, infection by hepatitis viruses, genetic conditions such as hemochromatosis or α1-antitrypsin deficiency, autoimmune hepatitis and metabolic disorders [1,2]. Regardless of the etiology, chronic tissue injury and inflammation are increasingly recognized as driver mechanisms in liver disease progression from fibrosis, characterized by the excessive accumulation of extracellular matrix (ECM), to hepatocellular carcinoma (HCC) [1–3]. The molecular links in the so-called inflammation-fibrosis-cancer axis in the liver are currently being elucidated in experimental models of acute and chronic injury. These links include a variety of intracellular pathways triggered by extracellular mediators like the cytokines interleukin 1 (IL1), IL6 and tumour necrosis factor alpha (TNFα), platelet-derived growth factors and transforming growth factor beta (TGFβ), among others [3–5]. These growth factors and cytokines stimulate ECM synthesis by the activation of hepatic stellate cells and myofibroblasts in the hepatic parenchyma [3–5]. Targeted interference with these and other mediators has clearly shown a beneficial effect on the course of the experimental disease, lending support to their pathological role [6,7]. However, in spite of these remarkable advances the availability of safe and efficacious therapies to halt the progression of fibrosis and liver disease in humans is still limited [8,9]. The use of experimental models of chronic liver injury resembling the human pathology is important to evaluate candidate drugs with chances of succeeding in the clinical setting. One such experimental model are the *Mdr2/Abcb4*-deficient mice (*Mdr2*$^{-/-}$), which lack the canalicular phosphatidylcholine flippase [10]. The absence of phosphatidylcholine from bile occurring in these mice leads to bile regurgitation into the portal tracts, causing periportal inflammation and injury early in life (2–3 weeks), periportal fibrosis (4 weeks), and the appearance of preneoplastic lesions (at 4–6 months) [10–12]. These pathogenic characteristics resemble what occurs in human primary sclerosing cholangitis and biliary fibrosis, making these mice an excellent model to study disease mechanisms, and a test ground for hepatoprotective and antifibrotic therapies [10–13]. In analogy to the situation found in humans, protracted injury and inflammation lead to HCC development in virtually 100% of *Mdr2*$^{-/-}$ mice by 16 months [14].

We and others have previously demonstrated the *in vivo* anti-inflammatory effects of 5′-methylthioadenosine (MTA), a sulphur-containing adenine nucleoside produced from S-adenosylmethionine (SAMe) during polyamine biosynthesis [15]. Parenteral MTA administration reduces the production of inflammatory mediators triggered by bacterial lipopolysaccharide or pro-inflammatory peptides in mice [16–18], and protects from liver injury in rats treated with CCl_4 or with the carcinogen diethylnitrosamine [19,20]. MTA is therefore a compound with an attractive pharmacological profile for the treatment of chronic liver disease. Using the *Mdr2*$^{-/-}$ mice as a model, here we show for the first time that orally administered MTA attenuates liver injury and inflammation, and inhibits the progression of hepatic fibrosis. The mechanism of action of MTA is likely to be multifaceted. MTA reduced the production of inflammatory and pro-fibrogenic mediators and inhibited the proliferation and activation of fibrogenic cells. These observations gathered in the *Mdr2*$^{-/-}$ mouse model indicate that MTA could be useful for the treatment of biliary fibrosis and conditions such as primary sclerosing cholangitis, a severe disease frequently associated with hepatobiliary cancer and with limited therapeutic options.

Methods

Ethics statement

Animals received humane care and study protocols complied with our institution's guidelines and the recommendations of the European Accreditation of Laboratory Animal Care. The protocol was approved by the Committee on the Ethics of Animal Experiments of the University of Navarra (protocol number: 025-10).

Animal studies

Male *Mdr2*$^{-/-}$ and *Mdr2*$^{+/+}$ mice (The Jackson Laboratory, Bar Harbor, ME) were fed standard laboratory diet. Two groups of mice per genotype were established (2 months old, n = 8 per group). One group received a daily oral dose of 30 mg/Kg body weight of MTA dissolved in 0.2% dimethylsulfoxide by gavage for three weeks, the control group received the same volume of vehicle (0.2% dimethylsulfoxide). MTA was from Enantia S.L. (Barcelona, Spain). This dose of MTA has been used previously, but was administered intraperitoneally [16,17]. Liver enzymes and bilirrubin levels were analyzed in serum (Cobas® analyzer, Roche). Livers were excised, weighted, and were either snap frozen or fixed in formalin and paraffin-embedded.

Metabolite measurement in liver tissues

Glutathione (GSH) was measured using the Gluthatione Assay Kit (Sigma, St. Louis, USA). Tissue samples were processed as recommended by the manufacturer. SAMe was measured as previously described [21].

Tissue staining and immunohistochemistry

Tissue sections were stained with Picro-Sirius Red to visualize collagen deposition as reported [22]. For morphometric analysis images were captured at 100X magnification (Nikon Eclipse 1000), and percentage of collagen cover per field was estimated with an Arkon software (Arkon Resources Inc. Arcadia, CA) as described [22]. Values are the means of five fields taken from different tissue sections per mouse. Immunodetection of α-smooth muscle actin (αSMA) on liver sections was carried out as described using a monoclonal anti-αSMA antibody (#A2547) from Sigma (St. Louis, MO) [22]. Tenascin-C and Ki-67 immunostainings were performed using rabbit polyclonal antibodies from Millipore (#AB1951) (Millipore Iberica, Madrid, Spain) and Abcam (#ab833) (Cambridge, UK) respectively. Immunostaining for CD45 was performed with a rat-anti-mouse CD45 antibody (clone 30-F11, #103101) from BioLegend (San Diego, CA).

Cell culture and treatments

Liver myofibroblasts were isolated from wild type and *Mdr2*−/− mice by collagenase perfusion and density-gradient purification in Nycodenz, and cultured in Dulbecco's Modified Eagle's medium (DMEM) containing 10% fetal calf serum (FCS) as described [23]. For [^{3}H]thymidine incorporation myofibroblasts were incubated under the specified conditions for 24 h with 2 μCi/ml [^{3}H]thymidine. Cells were lysed and radioactivity measured as described [22]. Human recombinant platelet derived growth factor BB (PDGF) was from Calbiochem (#521225) (Merck KGaA, Darmstadt, Germany). MTA showed no cytotoxic effects, as determined by measuring lactate-dehydrogenase in culture media using the Cytotox assay (Promega, Madison, WI). Apoptosis was measured in cultured myofibroblasts using the Cell Death Detection Assay from Roche (Barcelona, Spain) as previously described [22].

The murine monocyte/macrophage RAW 264.7 cells (American Type Culture Collection, ATCC) were cultured in DMEM supplemented with 10% FCS. Where indicated cells were treated with *Salmonella typhymurium* lipopolysaccharide (LPS) (50 mg/mL) from Sigma (#L6511, Lot#3944110). The adenosine receptor agonist 5′-(N-Ethylcarboxamido) adenosine (NECA) and the adenosine A2B receptor antagonist MRS 1754 were from Sigma, the adenosine A2A receptor antagonist ZM 241385 was purchased from Tocris Bioscience (Bristol, UK). TNFα concentration in conditioned media was measured using an enzyme-linked immunosorbent assay (ELISA) kit from BD Biosciences (San Diego, CA).

RNA isolation and quantitative real-time RT-PCR

Total RNA was extracted using the TRI Reagent (Sigma). Real time PCR was performed using an iCycler (BioRad, Hercules, CA)

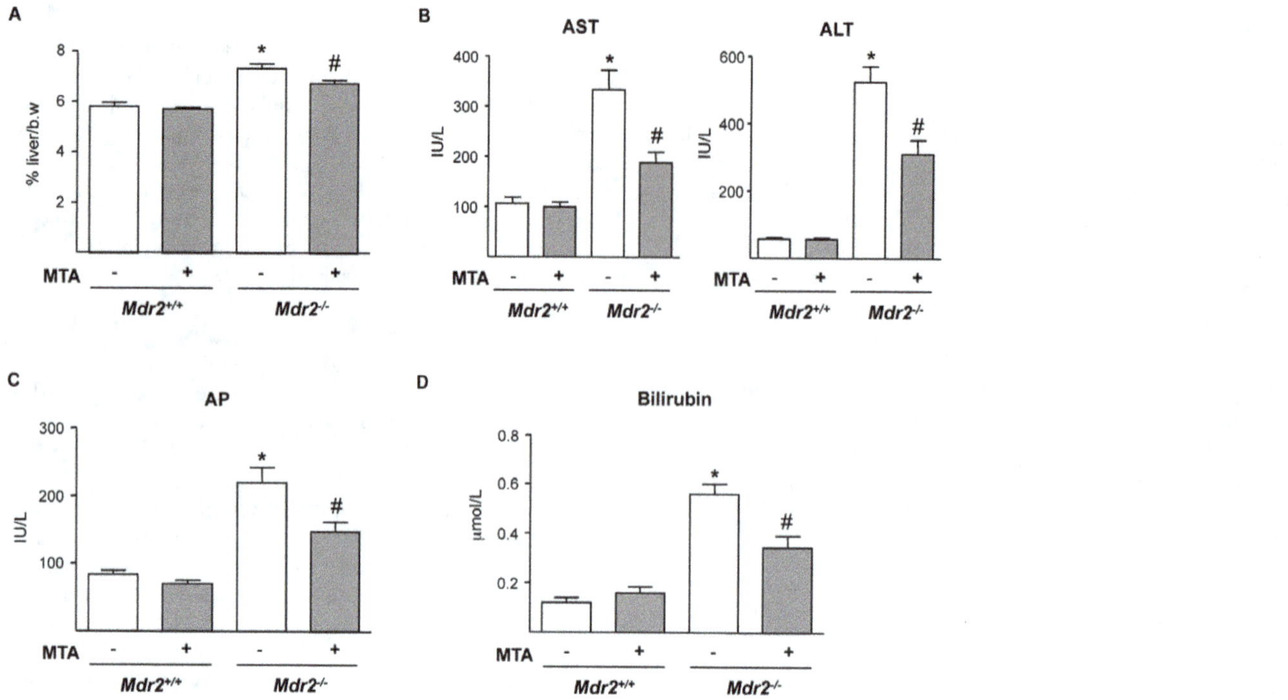

Figure 1. Oral administration of MTA to *Mdr2*$^{-/-}$ mice reduces hepatomegaly and serum parameters of liver injury. *Mdr2*$^{+/+}$ and *Mdr2*$^{-/-}$ mice were treated with MTA during three weeks. Increased liver-to-body weight ratio (%) in *Mdr2*$^{-/-}$ mice was reduced by MTA (A). Serum transaminases (B), alkaline phosphatase (C) and bilirubin (D), levels that are increased in *Mdr2*$^{-/-}$ mice were attenuated by MTA. **P*<0.05 *vs* untreated *Mdr2*$^{+/+}$ mice, #*P*<0.05 *vs* untreated *Mdr2*$^{-/-}$ mice.

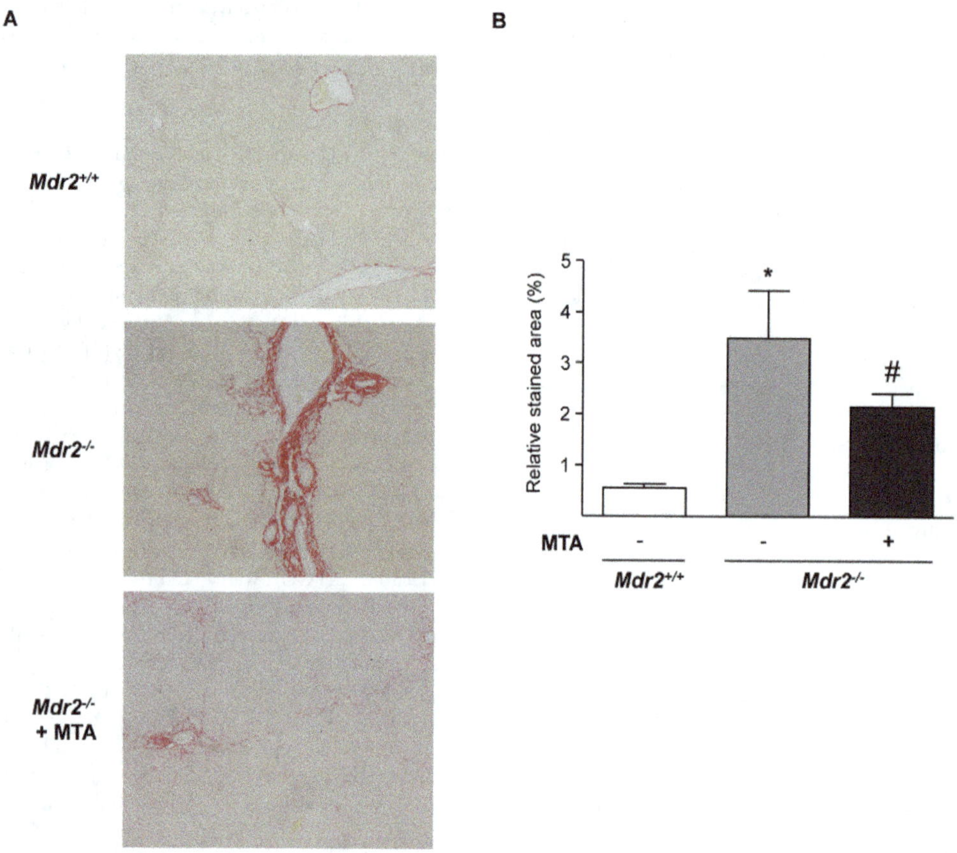

Figure 2. MTA administration reduces the spontaneous fibrosis that develops in *Mdr2*$^{-/-}$ mice. Representative Sirius Red-stained liver sections from *Mdr2*$^{+/+}$, control *Mdr2*$^{-/-}$ and MTA-treated *Mdr2*$^{-/-}$ mice (*Mdr2*$^{-/-}$ + MTA) (A). Fibrosis was quantified as function of mean percentage of stained area (B). **P*<0.05 *vs* *Mdr2*$^{+/+}$ mice, #*P*<0.05 *vs* untreated *Mdr2*$^{-/-}$ mice.

and the iQ SYBR Green Supermix (BioRad) as reported [22]. Gene expression was determined using the ΔΔCT calculation as described [21,22]. We designed all primers to distinguish between genomic and cDNA amplification and sequenced all PCR products to confirm the specificity. Primers for α1(I)-procollagen, matrix metalloprotease-13 (MMP13) and TIMP1 determination were described previously [22]. αSMA, TGFβ1 and TGFβ2 primers were as reported [11], TNFα, IL6 and inducible NO synthase (iNOS) primers were as described [17], tenascin-C primers were as reported [24]. Monocyte chemotactic protein-1 (Mcp-1) primers were: sense 5′-CCACTCACCTGCTGCTACTC-3′, antisense 5′-TTCACATTCAAAGGTGCTGAAG-3′. JunD primers were: sense 5′-CGCCCATCGACATGGACAC-3′, antisense 5′-GT-TGACGTGGCTGAGGACTT-3′. Adenosine A2B receptor primers were: sense 5′-TGGCGCTGGAGCTGGTTA-3′, antisense 5′-GCAAAGGGGATGGCGAAG-3′.

Western blot analysis

Tissues and cells were homogenized and analyzed by Western blotting as described [22]. The antibodies used were: anti-cyclin-D1 (#sc-450), anti-c-Jun N-terminal kinase (JNK) (#sc-571), anti-phospho-extracellular signal-regulated kinase (Tyr^{204}) (pErk1/2) (#sc7383), anti-Smad1/5/8 (#sc-6031-R), anti-JunD (#sc-74) from Santa Cruz Biotechnology (Santa Cruz, CA); anti-phospho-JNK(Thr^{183}/Tyr^{185}) (#9251), anti-c-Jun (#9165), anti-phospho-c-Jun (Ser^{63}) (#9261), and anti-phospho-S6 ribosomal protein (Ser^{235}/Ser^{236})(#4857) were from Cell Signaling Technology (Danvers, MA); anti-phospho-Smad2 ($Ser^{465/467}$) (#AB3849), anti-Smad2/3 (#05-914), anti-phospho-Smad1/5/8($Ser^{463/465}$) (#AB3848), anti-Erk1/2 (#06-182) were from Millipore (Billerica, MA). GAPDH antibodies (#MCA4739) were from AbD-Serotec (Dusseldorf, Germany).

Chromatin immunoprecipitation (ChIP)

ChIP assay was performed in mouse myofibroblasts essentially as described [18], using anti-JunD (#sc-74x) (Santa Cruz Biotechnology) or anti-tri-methyl-H3K4 (#ab8580) (Abcam) antibodies, or a control rabbit IgG (Santa Cruz Biotechnology). The promoter region −905 to −725 of the murine cyclin D1 gene, which includes a growth factor-responsive binding site for activator protein 1 (AP1) factors [25], was analyzed by RT-PCR with the following primers: 5′-AACGAAGCCAATCAAGAAGC-3′, 5′-CAGTATCCCCCTCCTCCACT-3′. Values were normalized to average values of inputs.

Statistical analysis

Data are means ±SEM. Analyses were performed using GraphPad Prism version 5.00 (GraphPad Software, San Diego, USA). Data were compared among groups using the Student *t* test. A P value of <0.05 was considered significant.

Results

MTA treatment reduces liver injury in *Mdr2*$^{-/-}$ mice

By three months of age *Mdr2*$^{-/-}$ mice typically display hepatomegaly and elevated serum levels of hepatic enzymes

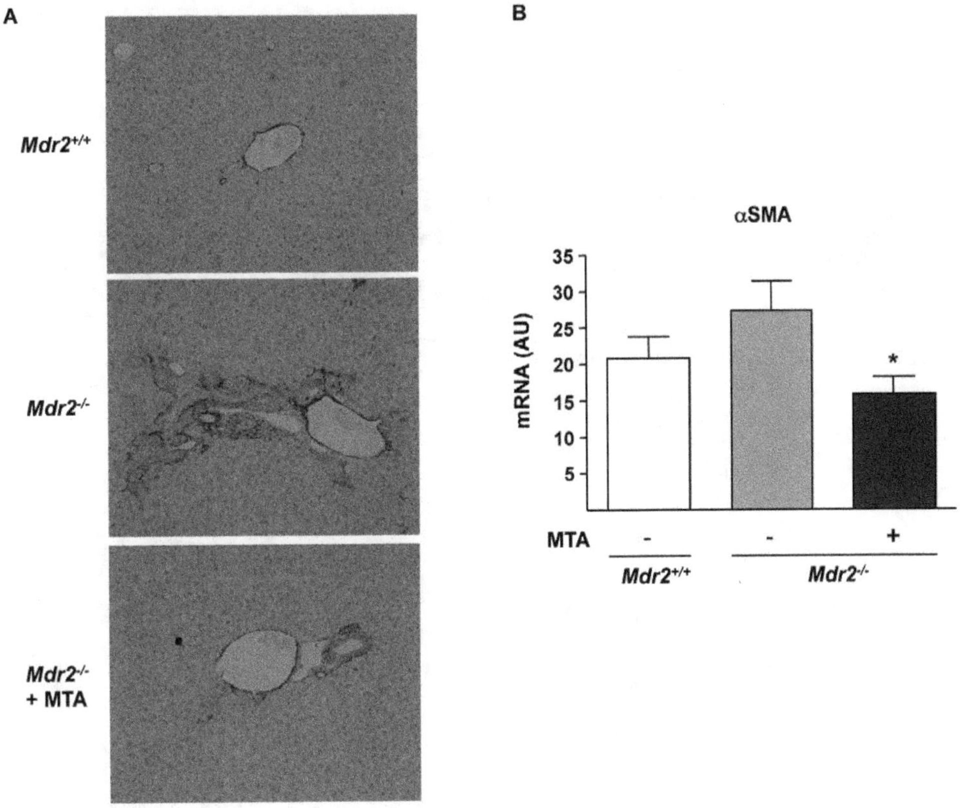

Figure 3. MTA administration reduces αSMA expression in *Mdr2*$^{-/-}$ mice. Immunohistochemical staining of αSMA in representative liver sections from wild type, control *Mdr2*$^{-/-}$ mice, and MTA-treated *Mdr2*$^{-/-}$ mice (*Mdr2*$^{-/-}$ + MTA). The increased number of positive periductal myofibroblasts was reduced upon MTA administration (A). αSMA mRNA levels in *Mdr2*$^{+/+}$, control *Mdr2*$^{-/-}$, and MTA-treated *Mdr2*$^{-/-}$ mice (B). AU: arbitrary units. *$P<0.05$ *vs* untreated *Mdr2*$^{-/-}$ mice.

[10,11,14]. MTA administration was well tolerated, and treated animals gained similar weight as controls. MTA reduced the liver to body weight ratio (Fig. 1A), and improved aspartate aminotransferase (AST) and alanino aminotransferase (ALT) serum levels (Fig. 1B). Circulating levels of alkaline phosphatase (AP) and bilirubin were also lowered by MTA (Fig. 1C and 1D).

MTA treatment attenuates liver fibrosis in *Mdr2*$^{-/-}$ mice

MTA significantly reduced the periductal fibrosis that spontaneously develops in these mice [11], as determined by Sirius Red staining of crosslinked collagen in liver sections and morphometric quantitation of stained areas (Fig. 2A and B). MTA administration to *Mdr2*$^{+/+}$ mice had no effect on collagen levels (not shown). As previously described [11], we found an increase in periductal αSMA-positive cells and αSMA mRNA levels, which were also reduced by MTA treatment (Fig. 3A and B). In accordance with the histology, the expression of α1(I)procollagen mRNA was reduced in MTA treated mice (Fig. 4A). As reported [11], the expression of the interstitial collagenase MMP13, and that of its inhibitor TIMP1, was significantly increased in *Mdr2*$^{-/-}$ mice (Fig. 4B and C). MTA reduced MMP13 expression, and although not statistically significant there was a tendency towards decreased TIMP1 mRNA levels (Fig. 4B and C).

MTA reduces hepatic levels of inflammatory and pro-fibrogenic mediators in *Mdr2*$^{-/-}$ mice

Although the expression of inflammatory cytokines in the liver of *Mdr2*$^{-/-}$ mice is maximal between 2–8 weeks [10,11], we still detected elevated TNFα and IL6 mRNA levels (Fig. 5A and B). MTA tended to reduce TNFα mRNA, and significantly lowered IL6 expression (Fig. 5A and B). Consistently, the expression of iNOS gene, a transcriptional target of pro-inflammatory cytokines, was decreased by MTA (Fig. 5C). Importantly, upon MTA administration we observed reduced Mcp-1 expression (Fig. 5D), a pro-fibrogenic chemokine up-regulated in *Mdr2*$^{-/-}$ mice [12]. TGFβ1 and TGFβ2 expression is elevated in the liver of these animals, particularly during the first 8 weeks of life [10–12]. Accordingly we found that by 11 weeks TGFβ1 expression in *Mdr2*$^{-/-}$ mice was similar to wild types, while TGFβ2 levels were still high, and were attenuated by MTA (Fig. 5E and F). These findings were accompanied by a significant decrease in inflammatory infiltrate, as assessed by staining for the leukocyte marker CD45 (Fig. 6).

Tenascin-C is a TGFβ-inducible extracellular protein expressed in liver fibrogenic cells that participates in inflammation and fibrogenesis [24,26]. As described in other models of chronic liver injury [24], we found increased tenascin-C staining around portal areas in *Mdr2*$^{-/-}$ mice (Fig. 7A). MTA treatment reduced

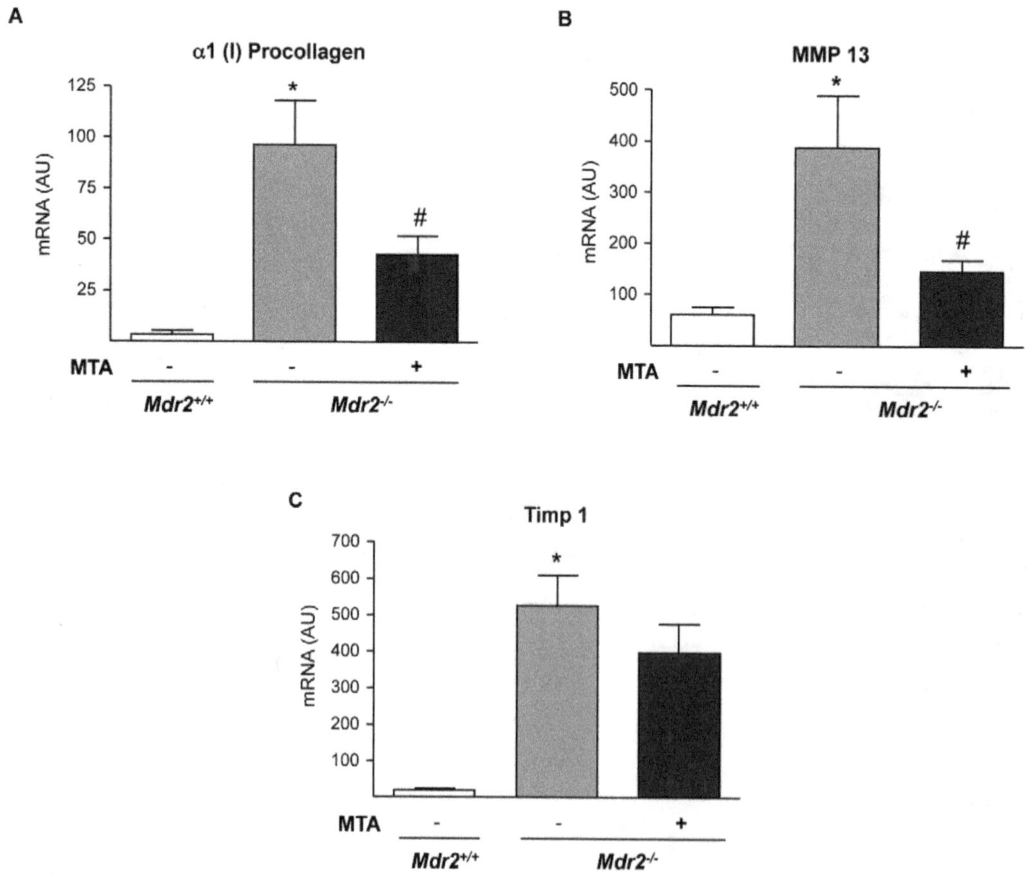

Figure 4. Fibrosis-related gene expression in *Mdr2*$^{-/-}$ mouse liver is attenuated by MTA treatment. mRNA levels of α1(I) procollagen (A), MMP13 (B) and TIMP1 (C), were measured in the liver of *Mdr2*$^{+/+}$, control *Mdr2*$^{-/-}$, and MTA-treated *Mdr2*$^{-/-}$ mice. AU: arbitrary units. *$P<0.05$ *vs* *Mdr2*$^{+/+}$ mice, #$P<0.05$ *vs* untreated *Mdr2*$^{-/-}$ mice.

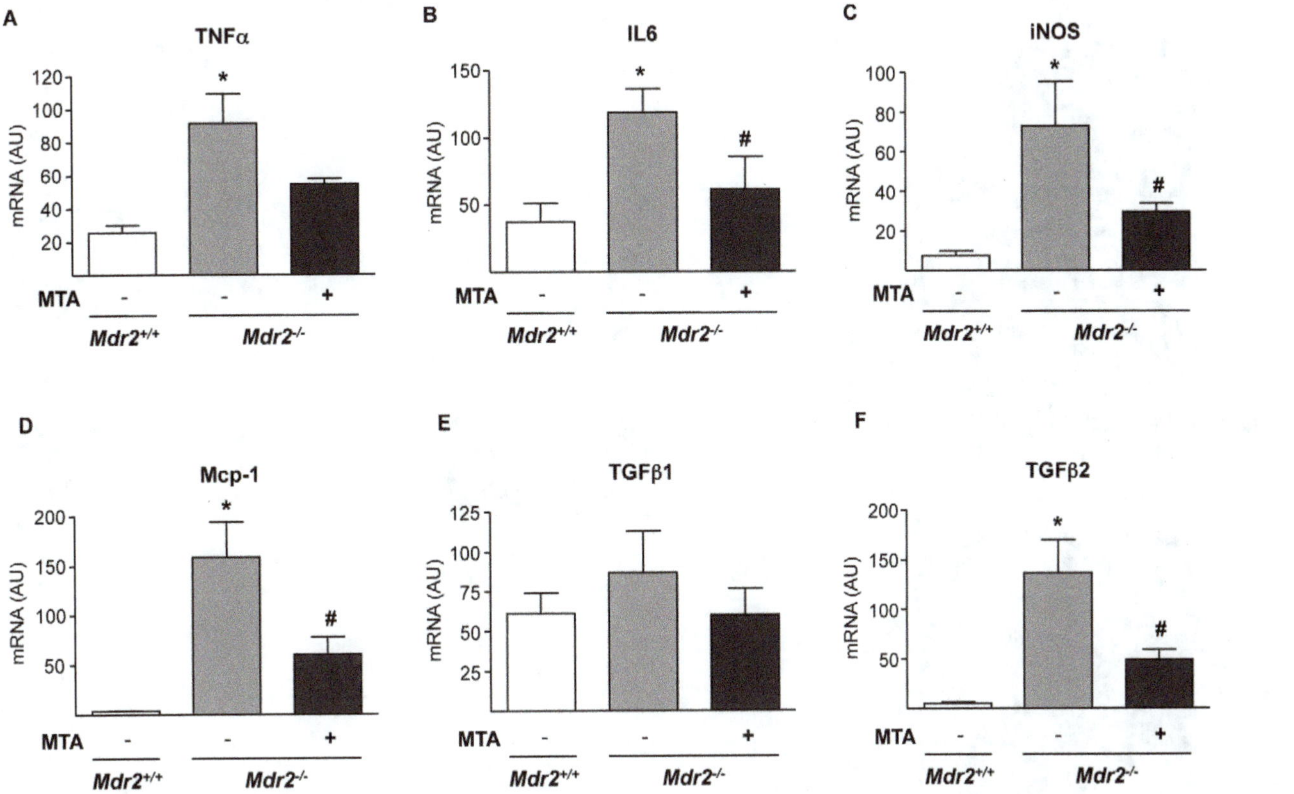

Figure 5. Effect of MTA on the expression of inflammatory cytokines and iNOS in *Mdr2*$^{-/-}$ mouse liver. mRNA levels of TNFα (A), IL6 (B), iNOS (C), Mcp-1 (D), TGFβ1 (E) and TGFβ2 (F) were measured in the liver of *Mdr2*$^{+/+}$, control *Mdr2*$^{-/-}$, and MTA-treated *Mdr2*$^{-/-}$ mice. **P*<0.05 *vs* *Mdr2*$^{+/+}$ mice, #*P*<0.05 *vs* untreated *Mdr2*$^{-/-}$ mice.

tenascin-C immunostaining and mRNA levels (Fig. 7A and B). However, the expression of αvβ6 integrin, which is induced in *Mdr2*$^{-/-}$ mice biliary epithelia and binds tenascin-C [13], was unaffected by MTA (not shown).

Effect of MTA on signalling pathways involved in fibrosis and hepatocellular proliferation in the *Mdr2*$^{-/-}$ mouse liver

To further explore the mechanism of action of MTA we examined the activation of signalling pathways associated with fibrogenesis and disease progression, including the Smad and mitogen-activated protein kinase (MAPK) pathways [3,6,9,27–30]. We found that total and phosphorylated Smad1/5/8 and Smad2 levels were increased in *Mdr2*$^{-/-}$ mouse liver extracts, and that MTA treatment reduced Smad2 and p-Smad2 contents (Fig. 8A and B). We also observed increased MAPK pathway activity in *Mdr2*$^{-/-}$ mice, as evidenced by elevated levels of p-Erk1/2, p-JNK and p-c-Jun. These pathways were also inhibited by MTA (Fig. 8C and D). No changes were observed in MTA-treated *Mdr2*$^{+/+}$ mice (not shown).

In agreement with the hyperactivation of pro-mitogenic signalling pathways, and confirming previous reports [6,30], we

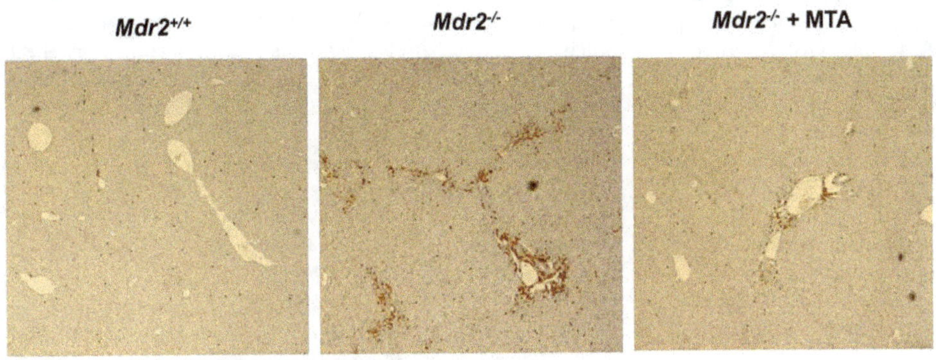

Figure 6. MTA reduces the recruitment of leukocytes to the portal fields of *Mdr2*$^{-/-}$ mice. Representative staining for the pan-leukocyte marker CD45 showing increased accumulation of CD45 positive cells in the portal field of *Mdr2*$^{-/-}$ mice compared to WT animals. Treatment with MTA reduced CD45 positive leukocyte accumulation. Representative images are shown.

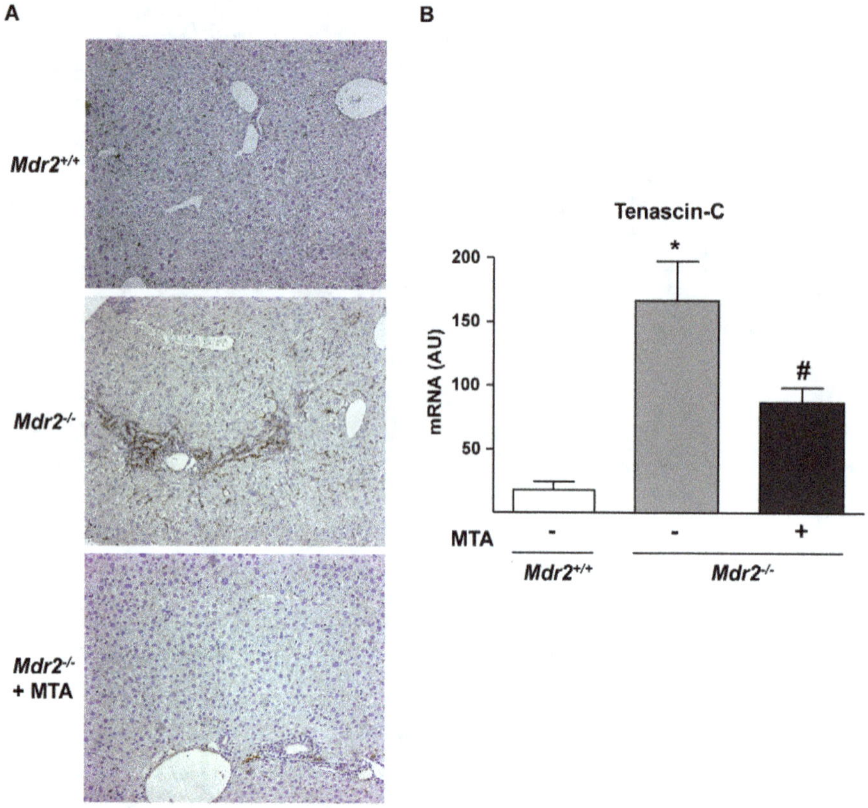

Figure 7. Expression of the fibrosis-associated protein tenascin-C, up-regulated in *Mdr2$^{-/-}$* mice, is attenuated by MTA administration. Immunohistochemistry of tenascin-C in representative liver sections shows increased staining around portal areas in *Mdr2$^{-/-}$* mice and its downregulation by MTA (A). Tenascin-C mRNA levels in the liver of *Mdr2$^{+/+}$*, control *Mdr2$^{-/-}$*, and MTA-treated *Mdr2$^{-/-}$* mice (B). *$P<0.05$ *vs* *Mdr2$^{+/+}$* mice, #$P<0.05$ *vs* untreated *Mdr2$^{-/-}$* mice.

found enhanced hepatocellular proliferation in *Mdr2$^{-/-}$* mice, as evidenced by increased hepatocyte staining with the proliferation marker Ki-67 (Fig. 9A and B). MTA reduced hepatocellular proliferation (Fig. 9A and B) and cyclin D1 protein levels (Fig. 9C), markedly elevated in the liver parenchymal cells of these animals [14].

MTA effects on liver SAMe and GSH levels in *Mdr2$^{-/-}$* mice

In vivo MTA is produced from SAMe during polyamine metabolism, and subsequently MTA can be metabolically recycled back to methionine [15,31]. Methionine metabolism in turn is necessary for the production of SAMe and GSH, and it is impaired in liver injury [31]. The expression of key genes in methionine metabolism is down-regulated in *Mdr2$^{-/-}$* mice [32]. In view of this we measured MTA effects on liver SAMe levels. We observed that SAMe was not reduced in *Mdr2$^{-/-}$* mice, and was unaffected by MTA treatment (82.9±10.6 in *Mdr2$^{+/+}$*; 110.6±9.7 in *Mdr2$^{-/-}$* and 103.2±12.3 in MTA-treated *Mdr2$^{-/-}$*, values are nmol/g tissue). GSH levels were not altered either in *Mdr2$^{-/-}$* mice compared to *Mdr2$^{+/+}$*, and were not affected by MTA (6.49±0.57 in *Mdr2$^{+/+}$*; 5.92±0.68 in *Mdr2$^{-/-}$* and 5.61±0.51 in MTA-treated *Mdr2$^{-/-}$*, values are µmol/g tissue).

Effects of MTA on inflammatory cells

Our current *in vivo* observations indicate that MTA administration significantly attenuated the inflammatory response found in the liver of *Mdr2−/−* mice. MTA is structurally very close to adenosine, a potent endogenous immune regulatory molecule produced mainly by cells of the immune system during tissue injury and inflammation [33]. Adenosine mediates its cellular effects through the interaction with cell surface receptors such as A2A and A2B, which are expressed in monocytes/macrophages and play a major role in the anti-inflammatory and immunomodulatory actions of this nucleoside [33,34]. In view of this and considering the ability of MTA to interact with adenosine receptors [35], we decided to explore the potential implication of A2A and A2B receptors in MTA anti-inflammatory effects. To directly address this issue we took advantage of the murine monocyte/macrophage cell line RAW 264.7, which has been widely used in mechanistic studies on the anti-inflammatory effects of adenosine upon bacterial lipopolysaccharide (LPS) challenge [36,37]. First we evaluated the expression and release of TNFα in LPS-stimulated RAW 264.7 cells in the presence of MTA. As shown in Fig. 10A, and in agreement with our previous findings [16], we found a potent inhibitory effect of MTA on TNFα expression. We also observed that the inhibitory effect of MTA was preserved when RAW 264.7 cells were incubated in the presence of the A2A or A2B specific antagonists ZM 241385 and MRS 1754 respectively (Fig. 10A and B). On the other hand, and in accordance with the literature [38,39], the inhibition of LPS-elicited TNFα production by the stable adenosine analogue NECA was attenuated by the A2A antagonist ZM 241385 (Fig. 10A). These observations suggested that the effect of MTA on the activation of inflammatory cells was not dependent on its potential direct interaction with adenosine receptors. However, although

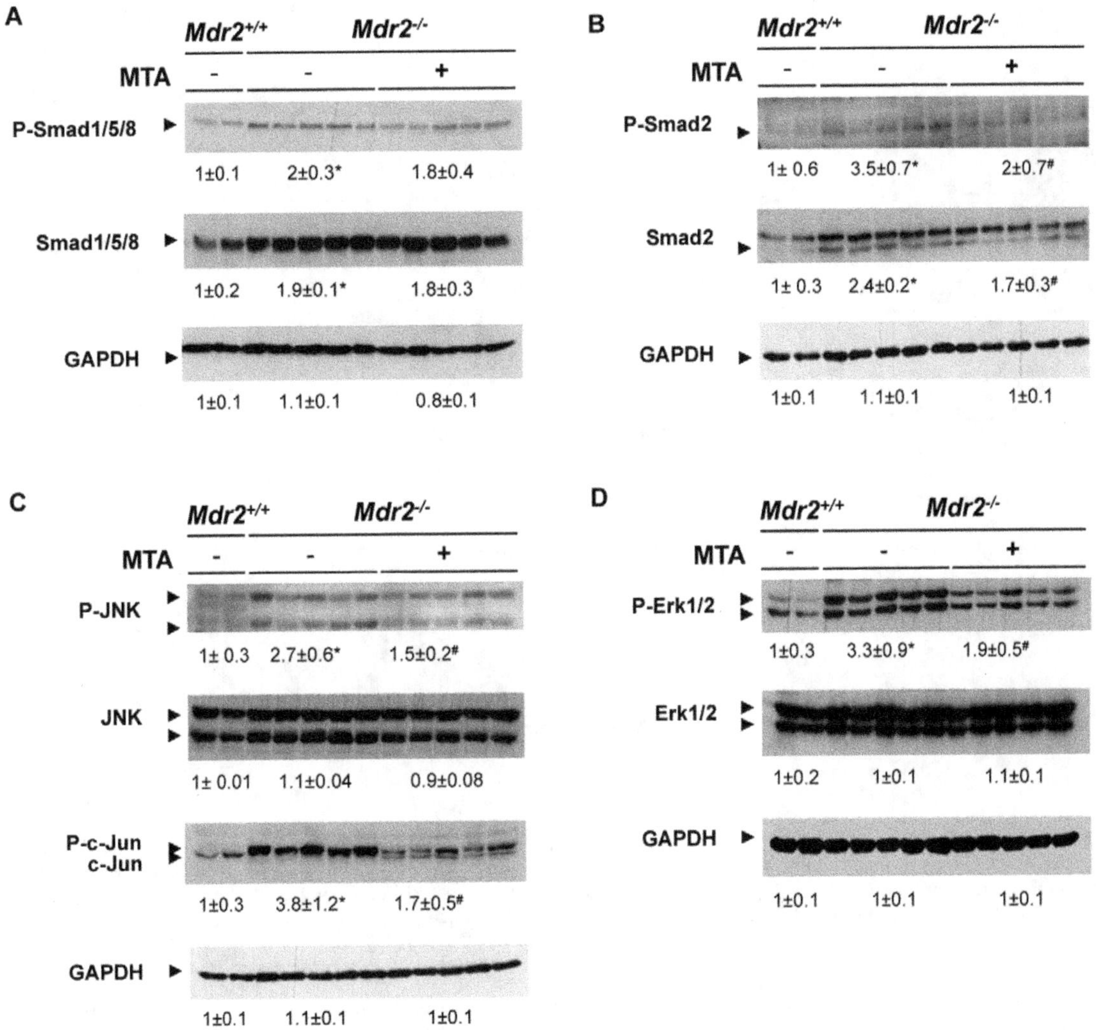

Figure 8. MTA modulates intracellular signalling pathways activated in *Mdr2*$^{-/-}$ mouse liver. Phosphorylation levels of Smad1/5/8 (A), Smad2 (B), JNK and c-Jun (C) and Erk1/2 (D) were analyzed by western blotting in liver extracts from *Mdr2*$^{+/+}$, control *Mdr2*$^{-/-}$, and MTA-treated *Mdr2*$^{-/-}$ mice. *$P<0.05$ *vs* *Mdr2*$^{+/+}$ mice, #$P<0.05$ *vs* untreated *Mdr2*$^{-/-}$ mice.

apparently MTA was not acting as an A2B receptor agonist we found that this molecule dramatically synergized with LPS in the up-regulation of A2B mRNA levels (Fig. 10C). Increased A2B expression has been linked to the activation of anti-inflammatory responses [37,39,40]. Interestingly this effect of MTA was not reproduced by the adenosine analogue NECA (Fig. 10C).

Effect of MTA on cultured liver myofibroblasts

Next we tested whether MTA had a direct effect on liver myofibroblasts, which participate in biliary fibrosis and represent a relevant source of extracellular matrix in *Mdr2*$^{-/-}$ mice [9,30,41]. Given that isolated myofibroblasts display high proliferation and activity upon *in vitro* culture, we pre-incubated the cells in serum free medium for 12 h to attenuate activation and proliferation, and subsequently cultures were stimulated with 10% FCS to promote myofibroblast activation in the presence or absence of MTA. We observed that the expression of the fibrogenic markers α1(I)procollagen and αSMA elicited by FCS treatment was inhibited by MTA (Fig. 11A and B). Similar observations were made when myofibroblasts were challenged with TGFβ (not shown). Additionally, TGFβ1 and TGFβ2 expression triggered by FCS was also attenuated by MTA (Fig. 11C and D). In agreement with previous reports [30] we found that FCS treatment increased Mcp-1 expression, and this response was also reduced by MTA (Fig. 11E), while IL6 expression was unaltered (Fig. 11F).

We also examined whether MTA could affect myofibroblast proliferation. Figure 12A shows that MTA reduced FCS-triggered DNA synthesis, without causing any toxicity (determined by lactate dehydrogenase release, not shown). Additionally we observed that MTA did not induce apoptosis in cultured myofibroblasts (data not shown). Our [^{3}H]thymidine incorporation experiments suggested that MTA inhibited cell cycle progression through the S phase (DNA synthesis), therefore we examined the expression of cyclin D1, a key cyclin in the transition from G_0/G_1 to S phase. We found that cyclin D1 expression was reduced by MTA treatment both at the mRNA and protein levels (Figure 12B). The expression of cyclin D1 can be regulated by AP-1 transcription factors, and among the components of the AP-1 complex JunD has been identified as a critical transcription factor in liver fibrogenesis [27,42]. Therefore we examined the binding of JunD to a region of the cyclin D1 promoter that contains a key AP-1 binding site [25] by ChIP

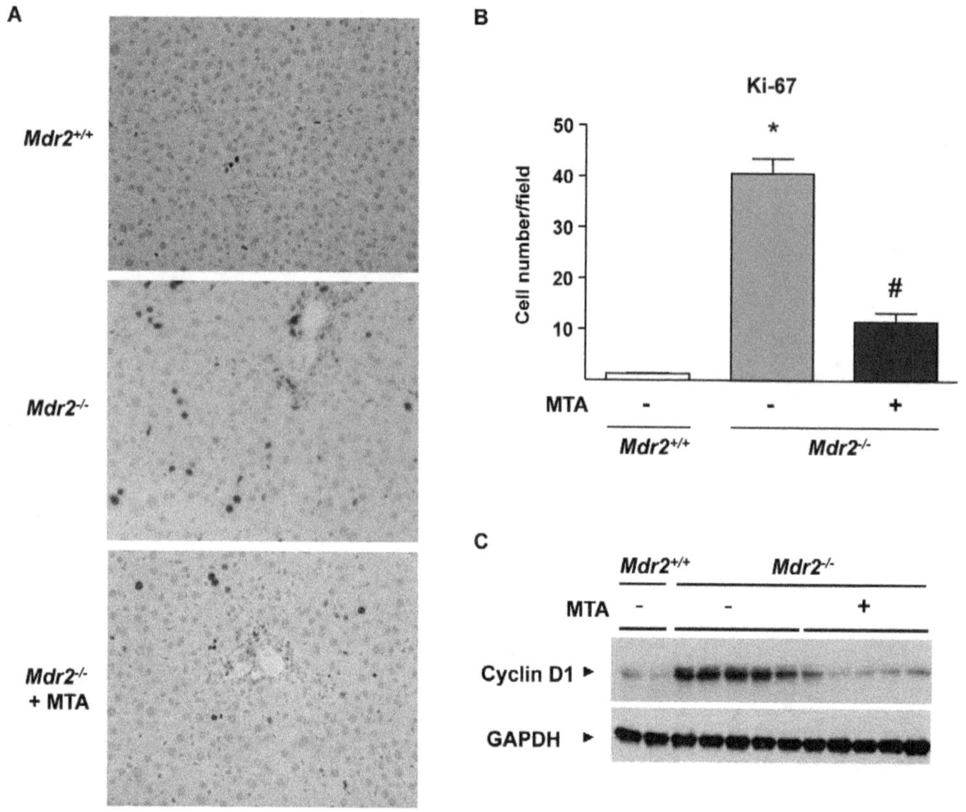

Figure 9. Increased hepatocellular proliferation in *Mdr2*$^{-/-}$ mice is attenuated by MTA administration. Immunohistochemical staining of Ki-67 in liver sections from *Mdr2*$^{+/+}$, control *Mdr2*$^{-/-}$, and MTA-treated *Mdr2*$^{-/-}$ mice (*Mdr2*$^{-/-}$+MTA)(A). Ki-67 positive hepatocytes were counted in 30 high-power fields per mouse, n = 5 per group (B). *$P<0.01$ *vs* *Mdr2*$^{+/+}$ mice, #$P<0.05$ *vs* untreated *Mdr2*$^{-/-}$ mice. Western blot analysis of cyclin-D1 protein in liver extracts from *Mdr2*$^{+/+}$ mice, untreated *Mdr2*$^{-/-}$ and MTA-treated *Mdr2*$^{-/-}$ mice (C).

analysis. As depicted in Figure 12C, MTA treatment almost completely blunted JunD association with cyclin D1 promoter in this regulatory region. In view of this response we examined the expression of JunD in cultured myofibroblasts treated with MTA, and observed that MTA significantly reduced JunD protein levels (Fig. 12D). These data suggested that the reduction of cyclin D1 expression by MTA could be mediated in part through the downregulation of JunD levels. Nevertheless, in spite of this effect of MTA on JunD cellular contents this compound almost totally inhibited cyclin D1 expression, and our ChIP experiment showed a near complete inhibition of JunD binding to the cyclin D1 promoter. This suggested that MTA could also affect the interaction of the remaining JunD protein with this cyclin D1 regulatory region. MTA is a well known inhibitor of methylation reactions [15], and it has been shown to inhibit H3K4 trimethylation, a hallmark of open chromatin conformation and transcriptional activation [43], in different cell types [18,44]. In view of this we examined the levels of tri-methylated-H3K4 in chromatin associated with this region of the cyclin D1 promoter. We detected increased levels of tri-methylated-H3K4 upon FCS stimulation, and observed that this modification was lowered by MTA treatment (Fig. 12E).

The relevance of these *in vitro* effects of MTA on the expression of fibrogenic and cell proliferation-related genes was supported by the observation of reduced α1(I)procollagen, αSMA, tenascin-C, TGFβ1, TGFβ2, JunD and cyclin D1 expression in myofibroblasts isolated from *Mdr2−/−* mice treated for 3 weeks with MTA when compared to cells isolated from untreated mice (Fig.13).

Finally, to gain additional insight into the mechanisms of the antifibrogenic effects of MTA we explored the direct effects of this molecule on the activity of intracellular signalling pathways related to the proliferation and fibrogenic activation of myofibroblasts [27–30]. As depicted in Fig. 14A, while MTA treatment was not able to directly modify the phosphorylation of Erk1/2 elicited by FCS, it reduced the levels of phospho-c-Jun, a target of the pro-fibrogenic JNK signalling pathway in liver extracellular matrix producing cells [29]. Interestingly, MTA significantly attenuated the phosphorylation of the mTOR and $p70^{S6}$ kinase downstream target S6 ribosomal protein triggered by the pro-fibrogenic growth factor PDGF (Fig. 14B). $p70^{S6}$ kinase activity is required for G_1 cell cycle progression, and it has been also identified as a signal transducer for liver fibrogenic cell growth [45].

Discussion

We have shown that oral administration of the nucleoside MTA significantly ameliorates liver injury in *Mdr2*$^{-/-}$ mice. These mice represent a clinically relevant model of spontaneous chronic liver disease, spanning from peribiliary inflammation and fibrosis to HCC development [9–14]. MTA was well tolerated and a significant improvement in serum markers of hepatic injury and function was observed. This was accompanied by reduced hepatic fibrosis and fibrogenic cell abundance. Accordingly, α1(I)procollagen mRNA levels were lowered, and TIMP1 expression tended to decrease. The fact that MTA also reduced the expression of MMP13, the interstitial collagenase in rodents, suggests that MTA

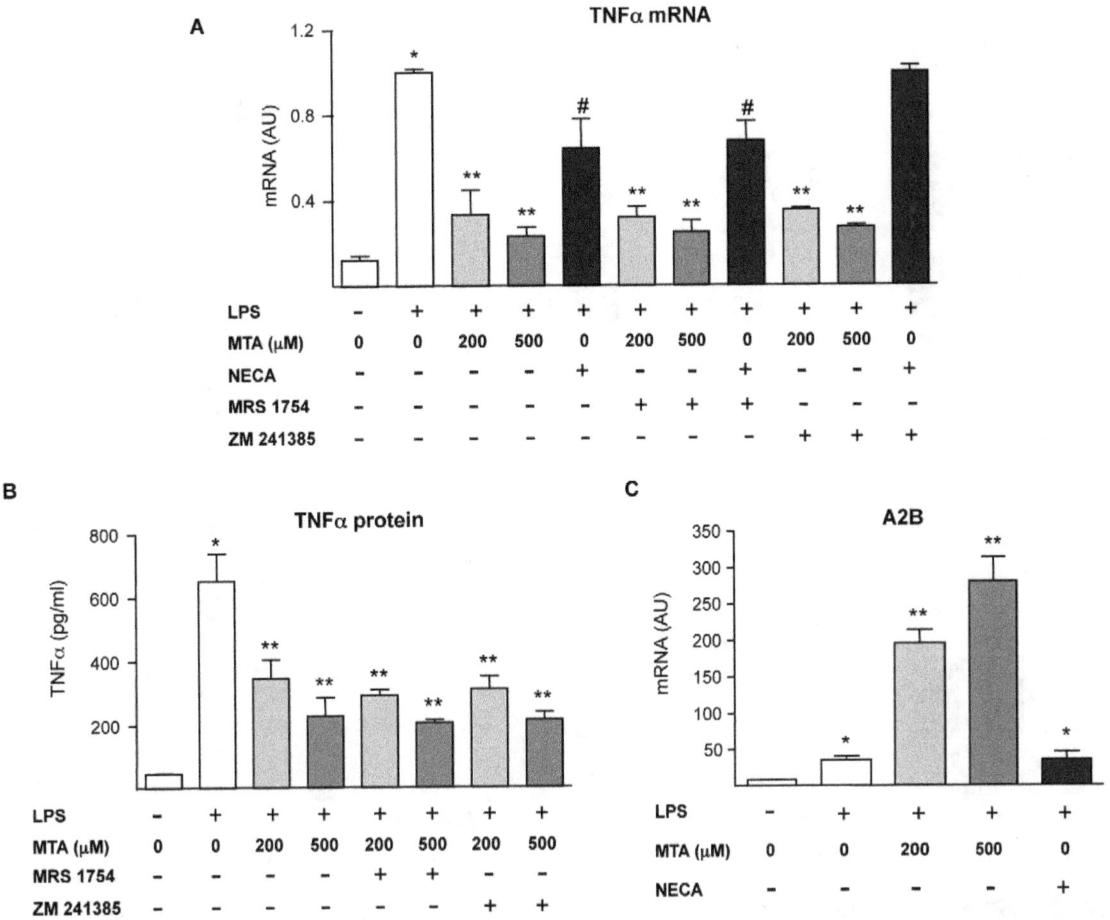

Figure 10. Effect of MTA on the activation of inflammatory cells: interaction with adenosine receptors. As indicated in the figure serum-starved murine monocyte/macrophages RAW 264.7 cells were pre-treated for 30 min with the A2A receptor antagonist ZM 241385 (10 μM) or the A2B receptor antagonist MRS 1754 (1 μM), then MTA or the adenosine receptor agonist NECA (20 μM) where added to the cultures for another 30 min. Subsequently and where indicated cells were treated with LPS (50 ng/ml) for up to 5 h. TNFα mRNA levels in cell lysates (A) and TNFα protein contents in conditioned media (B) were measured. *$P<0.01$ *vs* control, **$P<0.01$ *vs* LPS, #$P<0.05$ *vs* LPS. The expression of the adenosine A2B receptor was measured in RAW 264.7 cells pre-treated with MTA or the adenosine agonist NECA (20 μM) for 30 min and then where indicated with LPS (50 ng/ml) for up to 5 h (C). *$P<0.01$ *vs* control, **$P<0.01$ *vs* LPS.

down-regulates overall tissue remodelling activity, inhibiting fibrosis progression rather than stimulating fibrosis resolution [3].

Previous studies have shown that MTA exerts remarkable biological effects, its pharmacologic administration modulates different pathways and cellular responses, including gene expression, cell cycle progression and inflammation [15–20]. Therefore, the mechanisms behind MTA therapeutic action on a complex model such as *Mdr2*$^{-/-}$ mice are likely multifaceted. Our current findings agree with those reported by Simile et al., who showed that parenteral MTA administration to rats undergoing chronic CCl_4-induced liver injury reduced fibrosis [19]. This effect was mechanistically related to MTA antioxidant properties, that counteracted the oxidative stress and subsequent injury generated by CCl_4 metabolism [19]. However, oxidative stress is not a prominent feature in *Mdr2*$^{-/-}$ mice [14]. Accordingly, we found that GSH levels were unaltered in *Mdr2*$^{-/-}$ mouse liver, and were not affected by MTA, suggesting that MTA effects were not attributable to its antioxidant potential. *In vivo* MTA is metabolized to methionine in the so called methionine salvage pathway, and in the liver methionine is efficiently metabolized into SAMe [15]. SAMe is a key methyl donor with significant hepatoprotective properties, including antifibrotic activity in experimental cholestasis [31,46]. In view of the metabolic links between MTA and SAMe, we measured SAMe levels in control and MTA-treated *Mdr2*$^{-/-}$ mouse liver but did not observe major differences, indicating that MTA effects were not likely mediated through its potential contribution to the SAMe pool. Moreover, this may suggest that the antifibrotic effects of SAMe in experimental cholestasis [46] could be mediated in part by the metabolic or non-enzymatic conversion of SAMe into MTA [15].

Interestingly, MTA reduced the expression of the extracellular matrix protein tenascin-C in the liver of *Mdr2*$^{-/-}$ animals. This may be directly related to MTA antifibrotic effects, since tenascin-C is required for the development of experimental liver fibrosis [24]. Furthermore, tenascin-C is up-regulated in chronic hepatitis C, and its expression in peritumoral activated stellate cells in HCC associates with poor clinical prognosis [26,38,47]. In view of this, tenascin-C may be a previously unrecognized player in fibrosis and HCC development in *Mdr2*$^{-/-}$ mice, and its attenuation by MTA a key event in the anti-fibrotic and anti-neoplastic properties of this molecule [20]. Moreover, tenascin-C binds and activates αvβ6 integrin, a recently identified pharmacological target in biliary fibrosis [13].

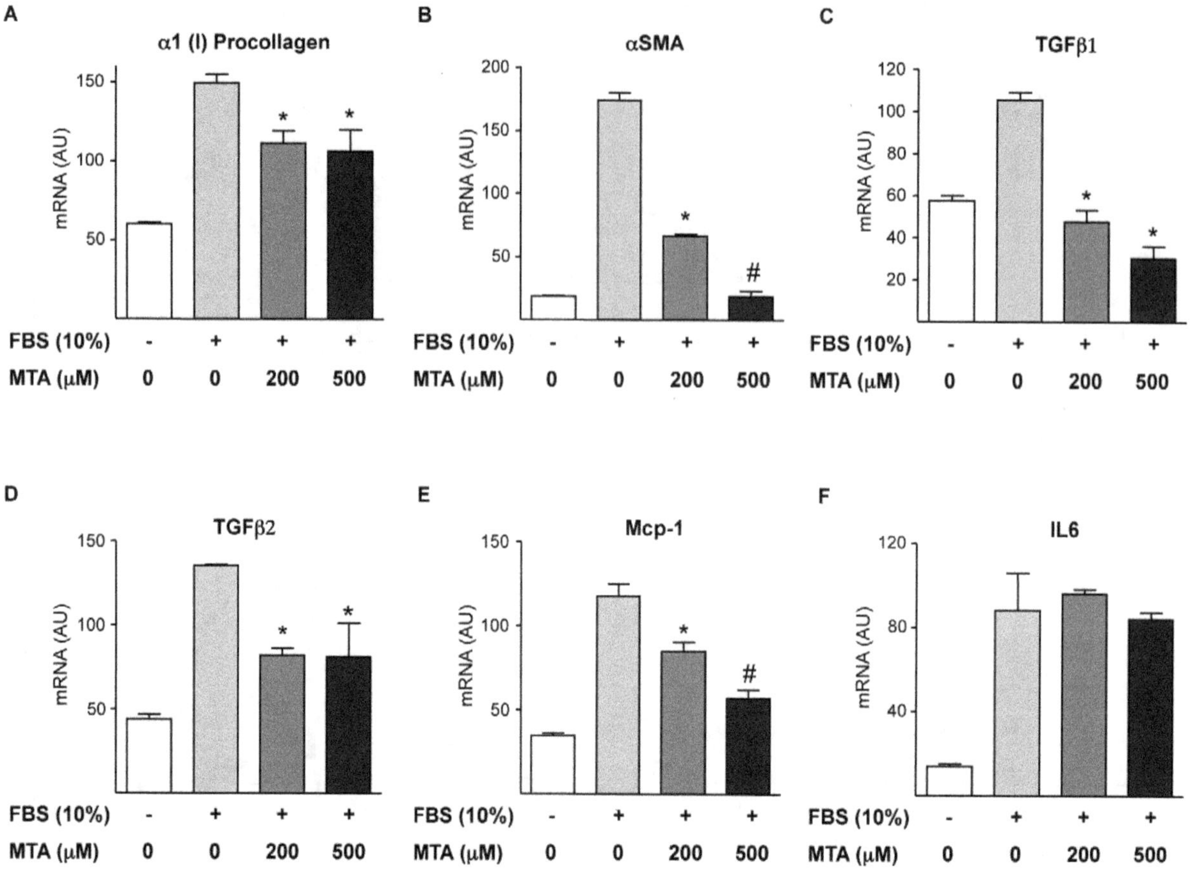

Figure 11. Effects of MTA on liver myofibroblast activation and cytokine expression. Primary myofibroblasts were serum starved (12 h) and then treated (12 h) with 10% FCS and MTA as indicated. mRNA levels of α1(I)procollagen (A), αSMA (B), TGFβ1 (C), TGFβ2 (D), Mcp-1 (E) and IL6 (F) were measured at the end of treatments. *$P<0.05$ *vs* FCS, #$P<0.05$ *vs* FCS+MTA 200 μM.

As occurs in human chronic liver disease, progression of liver injury in $Mdr2^{-/-}$ mice is associated with persistent inflammation. The observation that anti-inflammatory compounds like ibuprofen or curcumin ameliorate injury and fibrosis in $Mdr2^{-/-}$ mice [6,30], and that TNFα blockade prevents hepatocarcinogenesis in these animals [6], underscore the role played by inflammation in this model. We and others have previously shown that MTA has a significant immunomodulatory potential. MTA inhibits NF-κB mediated signalling, reduces inflammatory cytokine production by macrophages and lymphocytes, and attenuates the cellular effects of these cytokines [16–18]. We now observed that in $Mdr2^{-/-}$ mice MTA reduced the expression of IL6, Mcp-1, the NO-generating enzyme iNOS, and the profibrogenic factor TGFβ2. Accordingly MTA attenuated the activation of Erk1/2, JNK and Smad2, intracellular pathways triggered by these cytokines and which are directly implicated in fibrogenesis [3,5,27–30]. Therefore, interference with inflammatory cytokine and NO generation likely contributes to MTA hepatoprotective and anti-fibrogenic effects in this model [10,48].

From a mechanistic perspective, and in view of the remarkable anti-inflammatory effects of MTA, we cannot overlook the fact that this molecule is structurally very close to adenosine, a purine nucleoside released form cells with notorious anti-inflammatory properties [15,33]. Adenosine interacts with different G-protein-coupled cell surface receptors including the A1, A2A, A2B and A3 receptors. Until recently adenosine anti-inflammatory effects were mainly attributed to its interaction with the high affinity A2A receptor subtype [49], however an important role for the low affinity A2B receptor in the anti-inflammatory response to adenosine is currently emerging [34,38,40]. Using specific pharmacological antagonists of the A2A and A2B receptors we evaluated their potential implication in the immunomodulatory effects of MTA on mouse RAW 264.7 monocytes/macrophages challenged with bacterial LPS, a prototypic model of the inflammatory response. We found that the inhibition of LPS-elicited TNFα production by MTA was not impaired in the presence of these drugs, suggesting that MTA effects were not mediated through these receptors. Nevertheless, the involvement of the adenosine signalling system in the biological effects of MTA cannot be completely disregarded. Interestingly we observed that MTA treatment resulted in a remarkable potentiation of the expression of A2B receptors triggered by LPS, and this effect was not shared by the adenosine receptor agonist NECA. As previously mentioned A2B receptors display low affinity for adenosine, but their expression is up-regulated during tissue injury and inflammation, conditions in which interstitial adenosine concentrations raise. The expression of A2B receptors seems to be very important for the attenuation of the systemic inflammatory response, as illustrated by the fact that A2B knockout mice show enhanced cytokine production and overall mortality during sepsis [39,50]. Therefore the stimulatory effect of MTA on A2B receptor expression could also contribute to dampen inflammation in the chronically injured *Mdr2−/−* mouse liver.

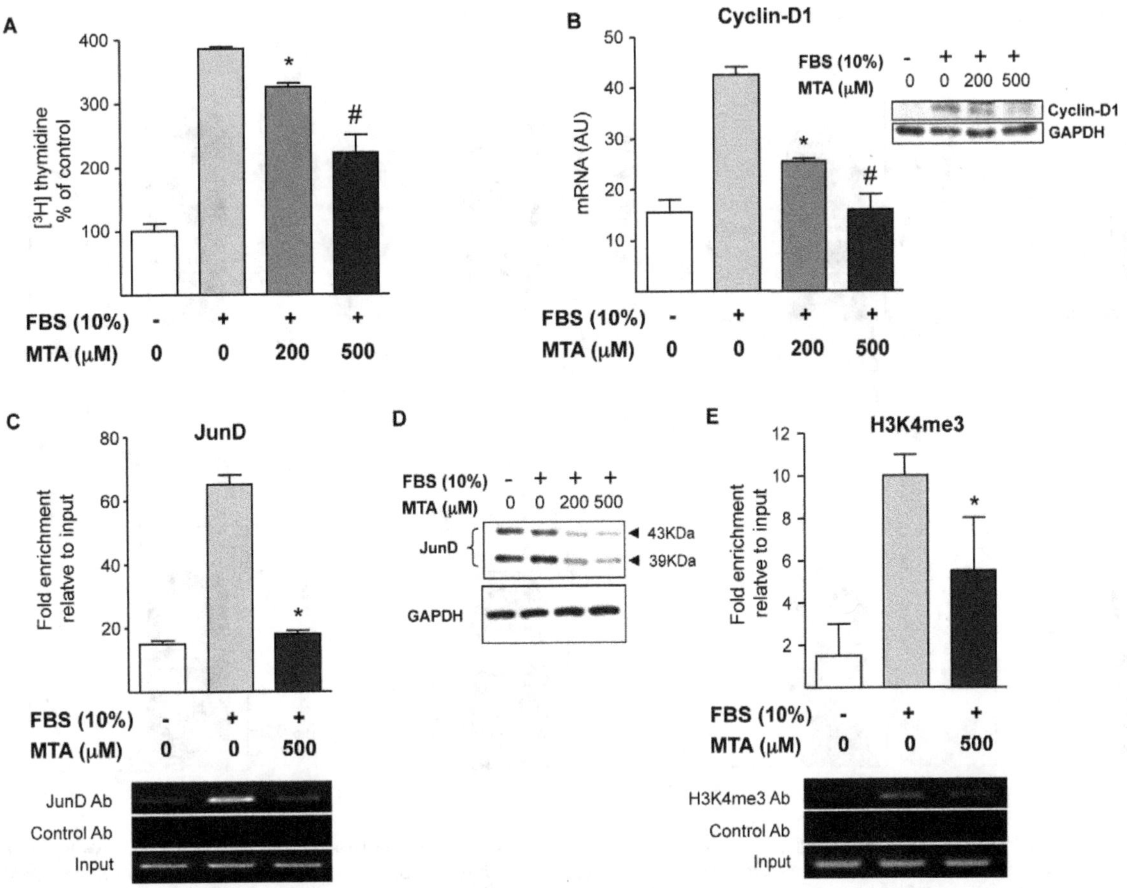

Figure 12. MTA inhibits DNA synthesis in myofibroblasts. MTA Effects on cyclin D1 and JunD expression. Effect of MTA on FCS-induced [^{3}H]thymidine incorporation in myofibroblasts treated as indicated (24 h) (A). Cyclin D1 mRNA expression in myofibroblasts treated (12 h) with 10% FCS and MTA as indicated. Inset shows a Western blot analysis of cyclin D1 protein (B). ChIP assay measuring the binding of JunD to the −905 to −725 cyclin D1 promoter region encompassing a key AP-1 binding site in myofibroblasts treated as indicated (12 h). Immunoprecipitated genomic DNA corresponding to the −905 to −725 cyclin D1 promoter region was quantified by real time PCR as indicated in Methods section. A representative gel picture of amplified DNA fragments is shown (C). Western blot analysis of JunD protein levels in myofibroblasts treated as indicated for 6 h (D). ChIP assay measuring the binding of tri-methylated-H3K4 (H3K4me3) to the same cyclin-D1 promoter region in myofibroblasts treated as indicated (12 h). A representative gel picture of amplified DNA fragments is shown (E). *$P<0.05$ *vs* FCS, #$P<0.05$ *vs* FCS+MTA 200 μM.

In addition to these responses, a direct cytoprotective effect of MTA on hepatocytes may also be involved, as we previously observed that MTA can prevent hepatocyte death *in vitro* [51,52]. Mechanistically, the attenuation of JNK activity found in MTA-treated *Mdr2*$^{-/-}$ mice could be related to the hepatoprotective effects of this molecule, given that inhibition of JNK has been demonstrated to prevent liver damage in different *in vitro* and *in vivo* experimental models of hepatocellular injury [53–55]. In this context the reduced hepatocyte proliferation found in MTA-treated mice may be related in part to the attenuation of liver damage, since liver regeneration occurs in response to injury.

We also observed that MTA has direct effects on liver fibrogenic cells. A previous study had reported that MTA could reduce collagen gene expression in primary hepatic stellate cells [56]. Here we confirmed this observation in liver myofibroblasts, and we also found that MTA down-regulated also the expression of αSMA, TGFβ1 and TGFβ2, and Mcp-1, all markers of activated fibrogenic cells [3,6,57]. However, MTA did not modify IL6 mRNA levels in myofibroblasts. This supports the specificity of MTA effects on gene expression, and indicates that the downregulation of IL6 observed *in vivo* could be attributed to the interaction of MTA with other cell types, likely inflammatory cells. The reduction of TGFβ isoforms and Mcp-1 expression by MTA found *in vivo* as well as in cultured myofibroblasts may be important effects regarding the mechanisms of action of this molecule. TGFβ1 and TGFβ2 are key cytokines in the development of liver fibrosis that can be expressed in a variety of cells including activated stellate cells, myofibroblats, macrophages and activated cholangiocytes [58,59]. The inhibition of TGFβ1 and TGFβ2 expression and activation has been demonstrated to attenuate liver fibrosis, including biliary fibrosis [59]. On the other hand, Mcp-1 participates in the recruitment of inflammatory cells during liver injury, and has been cogently demonstrated to contribute to hepatic parenchymal damage [60]. Moreover, besides expressing Mcp-1 liver fibrogenic cells can be activated and induced to proliferate by this chemokine [61,62]. Together these findings suggest that attenuation of TGFβ1/2 and Mcp-1 expression could have important mechanistic roles in the therapeutic action of MTA.

Increased proliferation and survival of ECM-producing cells are central events in the development of liver fibrosis [5,58]. MTA has been shown to induce apoptosis of different cell types, including HCC cells [51]. However, we did not observe any pro-apoptotic or cytotoxic effect of MTA in liver myofibroblasts. What we found

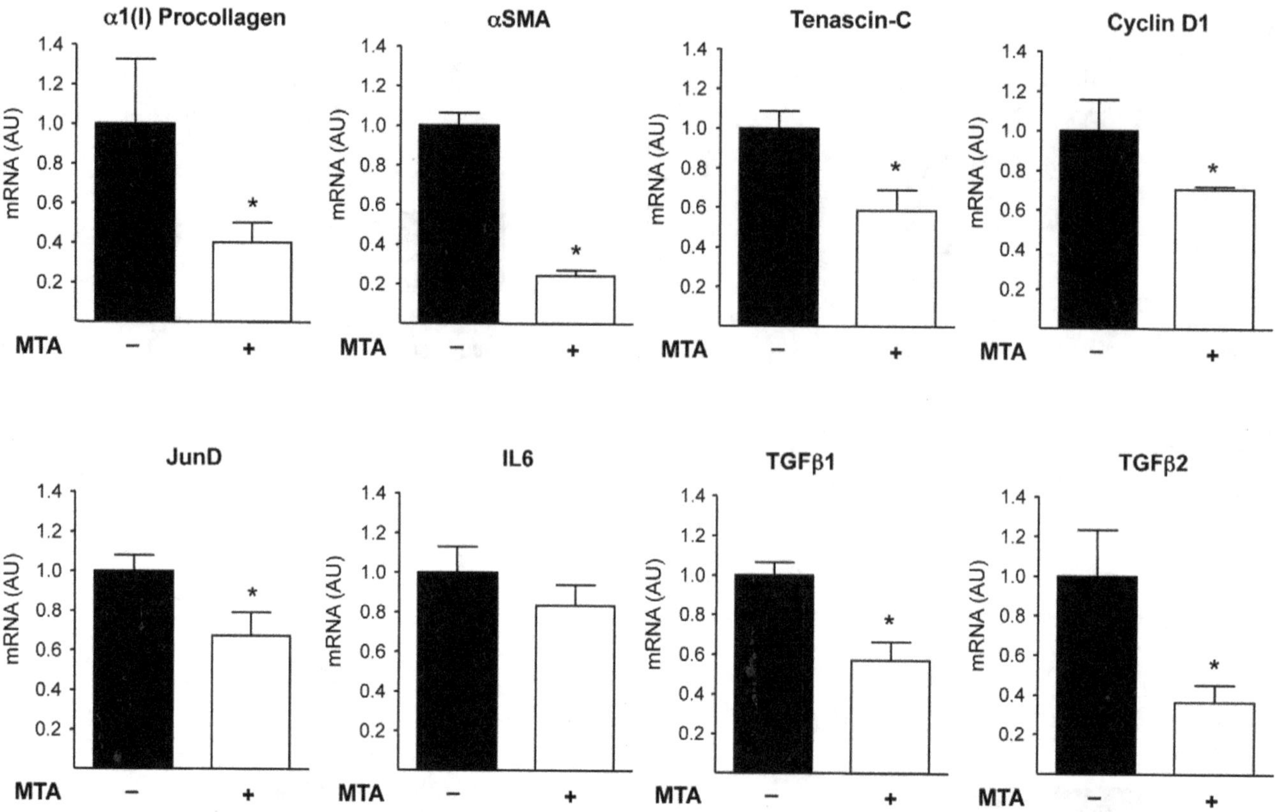

Figure 13. Expression of fibrogenic activation and cellular proliferation-related genes in myofibroblasts isolated from the liver of control and MTA-treated *Mdr2−/−* mice. *Mdr2−/−* mice were treated for three weeks with MTA or vehicle as described in the Methods section. At the end of the treatments hepatic myofibroblasts were isolated and the mRNA levels of the indicated genes were measured. Data are means ±SEM of three independent cell preparations per condition. $^*P<0.05$ *vs* vehicle-treated *Mdr2−/−* mice.

was a significant inhibition by MTA of FCS-stimulated DNA synthesis. In line with this response we observed that MTA reduced the expression of cyclin D1, a key G_1 cyclin associated with liver fibrogenic cell proliferation [63]. AP-1 transcription factors can stimulate the expression of genes involved in the activation and proliferation of liver fibrogenic cells, and among

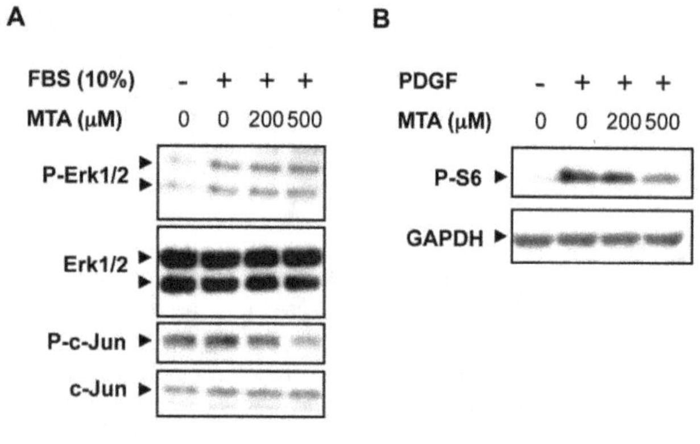

Figure 14. Effect of MTA on liver myofibroblast intracellular signalling pathways. Liver myofibroblasts were pre-treated with MTA for 30 min in the absence of serum and then stimulated with 10% FCS for 30 min or PDGF (20 ng/ml) for 60 min. Phosphorylation levels of Erk1/2 and c-Jun upon FCS stimulation (A), and S6 ribosomal protein after PDGF treatment (B) were analyzed by western blotting. Representative blots are shown.

them JunD is known to play an important role in liver fibrogenesis [27,42]. To gain further insight into the mechanism of action of MTA, we examined the binding of JunD to cyclin D1 promoter and found that it was markedly reduced in myofibroblasts treated with this compound. This can be due in part to the observed downregulation of JunD levels in MTA-treated cells, and therefore reduction of JunD expression may be a relevant mechanism in the antifibrogenic action of MTA.

In order to better understand the mechanisms behind the antiproliferative effects of MTA, we examined the activity of three signalling pathways that are involved in fibrogenic cell proliferation. We found that while MTA did not affect FCS-triggered Erk1/2 phosphorylation, it reduced phopho-c-Jun levels and significantly attenuated PDGF elicited ribosomal S6 protein phosphorylation. Both, the JNK and the mTOR and $p70^{S6}$ kinase pathways have been demonstrated as key regulators of hepatic fibrogenic cell proliferation [29,45], and therefore their inhibition by MTA could be relevant in the mechanism of action of this compound. The selective interaction of MTA with protein kinase-mediated intracellular signalling pathways as described here is likely to have profound effects on cellular behaviour and thus deserves further examination.

We also noticed that MTA could attenuate the increase in H3K4 trimethylation elicited by FCS stimulation in the cyclin D1 promoter. H3K4 trimethylation is a marker of transcriptional active chromatin, and this modification contributes to gene activation [64]. MTA is an inhibitor of methylation reactions [15], including histone methylation [18], our observations suggest

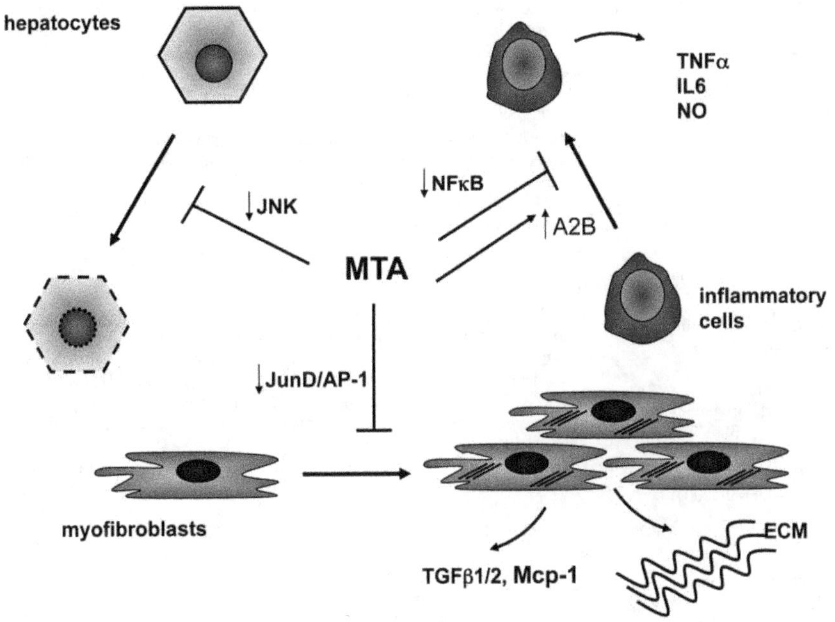

Figure 15. Potential mechanisms of action of MTA in *Mdr2*$^{-/-}$ mice. Our *in vivo* and *in vitro* observations indicate that MTA displays different actions that may underlie its beneficial effects on the course of liver injury and fibrosis in *Mdr2*$^{-/-}$ mice. MTA may exert a direct cytoprotective effect on hepatocytes by reducing JNK activity, preventing hepatocellular death and further inflammation. MTA also inhibits the production of cytokines by inflammatory cells, likely through interference with NFκB activity as described before [16–18]. In addition, enhanced expression of adenosine A2B receptors may contribute to the anti-inflammatory pharmacological profile of MTA. This compound can also exert direct effects on extracellular matrix (ECM) producing cells (myofibroblasts), reducing their activation, proliferation and the production of pro-fibrogenic factors. Inhibition of JunD expression may be an important event in the antifibrogenic action of MTA.

that interference with this epigenetic mechanism could account in part for the effects of MTA on cyclin D1 gene expression. Moreover, this finding makes it tempting to speculate that MTA could exert its antifibrogenic effects also through an overall action on the epigenetic programming. In this regard 3 deazaneplanocin, another methyltransferase inhibitor, has been recently reported to prevent the activation of liver fibrogenic cells, however its efficacy and tolerability in chronic *in vivo* models of liver fibrosis have not been tested yet [65]. Together these findings suggest that the antifibrogenic effects of MTA observed *in vivo* may be mediated in part through the direct inhibition of myofibroblast activation and proliferation. Nevertheless, a direct effect of MTA on bile duct epithelial cell damage and cholangiocyte activation, important events in the pathogenesis of liver injury in *Mdr2*$^{-/-}$ mice [30], cannot be discarded and merit future evaluation. Figure 15 summarizes the proposed mechanisms of action of MTA in *Mdr2*$^{-/-}$ mice mainly based on the observations reported in this study.

In summary, here we have demonstrated that oral MTA administration is an effective therapeutic strategy to attenuate disease progression in a relevant model of liver injury and fibrosis. In addition to our current study, MTA has been previously tested in *in vivo* experimental models never showing untoward effects [16,17,66,67], and an ID_{50} of 2.9±0.4 g/kg was estimated when administered intramuscularly to rats [19]. In humans MTA administration is also well tolerated [68,69]. These considerations, together with the efficacy described herein, suggest that MTA could be a good candidate to be clinically tested in the context of liver injury and fibrosis.

Author Contributions

Conceived and designed the experiments: MAA. Performed the experiments: MUL CG-P MGF-B CMR-O MM JMB SG SA NJ RU JL FJC. Analyzed the data: FJC MUL RU JP JL CB MAA. Contributed reagents/materials/analysis tools: JMB SL JAR. Wrote the paper: JL MAA.

References

1. Williams R (2006) Global challenges in liver disease. Hepatology 44: 521–6.
2. Siegel AB, Zhu AX (2009) Metabolic syndrome and hepatocellular carcinoma. Cancer 115: 5651–5661.
3. Bataller R, Brenner DA (2005) Liver fibrosis. J Clin Invest 115: 209–218.
4. Elsharkawy AM, Mann DA (2007) Nuclear factor-κB and the hepatic inflammation-fibrosis-cancer axis. Hepatology 46: 590–597.
5. Lotersztajn S, Julien B, Teixeira-Clerc F, Grenard P, Mallat A (2005) Hepatic fibrosis: molecular mechanisms and drug targets. Annu Rev Pharmacol Toxicol 45: 605–628.
6. Pikarski E, Porat RM, Stein I, Abramovitch R, Amit S, et al. (2004) NF-κB functions as a tumour promoter in inflammation-associated cancer. Nature 431: 461–466.
7. Berasain C, Castillo J, Perugorria MJ, Latasa MU, Prieto J, et al. (2009) Inflammation and liver cancer: new molecular links. Ann NY Acad Sci; 1155: 206–221.
8. Pinzani M, Rombouts K, Colagrande S (2005) Fibrosis in chronic liver diseases: diagnosis and management. J Hepatol 42(Suppl): S22–S36.
9. Popov Y, Schuppan D (2009) Targeting liver fibrosis: strategies for development and validation of antifibrotic therapies. Hepatology 50: 1294–1306.
10. Fickert P, Fuchsbichler A, Wagner M, Zollner G, Kaser A, et al. (2004) Regurgitation of bile acids from leaky bile ducts causes sclerosing cholangitis in *Mdr2* (*Abcb4*) knockout mice. Gastroenterology 127: 261–274.
11. Popov Y, Patsenker E, Fickert P, Trauner M, Schuppan D (2005) Mdr2 (*Abcb4*)-/- mice spontaneously develop severe biliary fibrosis via massive dysregulation of pro- and antifibrogenic genes. J Hepatol 43: 1045–1054.
12. Nakken KE, Nygård S, Haaland T, Berge KE, Arnkværn K, et al. (2007) Multiple inflammatory-, tissue remodelling- and fibrosis genes are differentially transcribed in the livers of Abcb4 (-/-) mice harbouring chronic cholangitis. Scand J Gastroenterol 42: 1245–1255.

13. Patsenker E, Popov Y, Stickel F, Jonczyk A, Goodman SL, et al. (2008) Inhibition of integrin αvβ6 on cholangiocytes blocks transforming growth factor-β activation and retards biliary fibrosis progression. Gastroenterology 135: 660–670.
14. Katzenellenbogen M, Pappo O, Barash H, Klopstock N, Mizrahi L, et al. (2006) Multiple adaptive mechanisms to chronic liver disease revealed at early stages of liver carcinogenesis in the Mdr2-knockout mice. Cancer Res 66: 4001–4010.
15. Avila MA, Garcia-Trevijano ER, Lu SC, Corrales FJ, Mato JM (2004) Methylthioadenosine. Int J Biochem Cell Biol 36: 2125–2130.
16. Hevia H, Varela-Rey M, Corrales FJ, Berasain C, Martínez-Chantar ML, et al. (2004) 5′-Methythioadenosine modulates the inflammatory response to endotoxin in mice and in rat hepatocytes. Hepatology 39: 1088–1098.
17. Moreno B, Hevia H, Santamaria M, Sepulcre J, Muñoz J, et al. (2006) Methylthioadenosine reverses brain autoimmune disease. Ann Neurol 60: 323–334.
18. Iglesias-Ara A, Xia M, Ramani K, Mato JM, Lu SC (2008) S-Adenosylmethionine inhibits lipopolysaccharide-induced gene expression via modulation of histone methylation. Hepatology 47: 1655–1666.
19. Simile MM, Banni S, Angioni E, Carta G, De Miglio MR, et al. (2001) 5′-Methylthioadenosine administration prevents lipid peroxidation and fibrogenesis induced in rat liver by carbon-tetrachloride intoxication. J Hepatol 34: 386–394.
20. Pascale RM, Simile MM, De Miglio MR, Feo F (2002) Chemoprevention of hepatocarcinogenesis: S-adenosyl-L-methionine. Alcohol 27: 193–198.
21. Berasain C, Hevia H, Fernández-Irigoyen J, Larrea E, Caballería J, et al. (2004) Methylthioadenosine phosphorylase gene expression is impaired in human liver cirrhosis and hepatocarcinoma. Biochim Biophys Acta 1690: 276–284.
22. Perugorria MJ, Latasa MU, Nicou A, Cartagena-Lirola H, Castillo J, et al. (2008) The epidermal growth factor receptor ligand amphiregulin participates in the development of mouse liver fibrosis. Hepatology 48: 1251–1261.
23. Li LY, Grenard P, Van Nhieu JT, Julien B, Mallat A, et al. (2003) Heme oxygenase-1 is an antifibrogenic protein in human hepatic myofibroblasts. Gastroenterology 125: 460–469.
24. El-Karef A, Yoshida T, Gabazza EC, Nishioka T, Inada H, et al. (2007) Deficiency of tenascin-C attenuates liver fibrosis in immune-mediated chronic hepatitis in mice. J Pathol 211: 86–94.
25. Eto I. Molecular cloning and sequence analysis of the promoter region of mouse cyclin D1 gene. Cell Prolif 2000; 33: 167–187.
26. El-Karef A, Kaito M, Tanaka H, Ikeda K, Nishioka T, et al. (2007) Expression of large tenascin-C splice variants by hepatic stellate cells/myofibroblasts in chronic hepatitis C. J Hepatol 46: 664–673.
27. Mann J, Mann DA (2009) Transcriptional regulation of hepatic stellate cells. Adv Drug Delivery Rev 61: 497–512.
28. Tao J, Mallat A, Gallois C, Belmadani S, Méry PF, et al. (1999) Biological effects of C-type natriuretic peptide in human myofibroblastic hepatic stellate cells. J Biol Chem 274: 23761–23769.
29. Kluwe J, Pradere JP, Gwak GY, Mencin A, De Minicis S, et al. (2010) Modulation of hepatic fibrosis by c-Jun-N-terminal kinase inhibition. Gastroenterology 138: 347–359.
30. Baghdasaryan A, Claudel T, Kosters A, Gumhold J, Silbert D, et al. (2010) Curcumin improves sclerosing cholangitis in Mdr2-/- mice by inhibition of cholangiocyte inflammatory response and portal myofibroblast proliferation. Gut 59: 521–530.
31. Mato JM, Martínez-Chantar ML, Lu SC (2008) Methionine metabolism and liver disease. Annu Rev Nutr 28: 273–293.
32. Katzenellenbogen M, Mizrahi L, Pappo O, Klopstock N, Olam D, et al. (2007) Molecular mechanisms of liver carcinogenesis in the Mdr2-knockout mice. Mol Cancer Res 5: 1159–1170.
33. Jacobson KA, Gao Z (2006) Adenosine receptors as therapeutic targets. Nat Rev Drug Discovery 5: 247–264.
34. Haskó G, Csóka B, Németh ZH, Vizi ES, pacher P (2009) A_{2B} adenosine receptors in immunity and inflammation. Trends Immunol. 30: 263–270.
35. Munshi R, Clanachan AS, Baer HP (1988) 5′-deoxy-5′-methylthioadenosine: a nucleoside which differentiates between adenosine receptor types. Biochem Pharmacol 37: 2085–2089.
36. Németh ZH, Leibovich SJ, Deitch EA, Vizi S, Szabó C, et al. (2003) cDNA Microarray analysis reveals a nuclear factor-κB-independent regulation of macrophage function by adenosine. J Pharmacol Exp Ther 306: 1042–1049.
37. Németh ZH, Lutz CS, Csóka B, Deitch EA, Leibovich SJ, et al. (2005) Adenosine augments IL-10 production by macrophages through an A_{2B} recptor-mediated posttranscriptional mechanism. J Immunol 175: 8260–8270.
38. Kreckler LM, Wan TC, Ge Z, Auchampach JA (2006) Adenosine inhibits tumor necrosis factor-α release from mouse peritoneal macrophages via A_{2A} and A_{2B} but not the A_3 adenosine receptor. J Pharmacol Exp Ther 317: 172–180.
39. Ryzhov S, Zaynagetdinov R, Goldstein AE, Novitskiy SV, Blackburn MR, et al. (2008) Effetc of A_{2B} adenosine receptor gene ablation on adenosine-dependent regulation of proinflammatory cytokines. J Pharm Exp Ther 324: 694–700.
40. Aherne CM, Kewley EM, Eltzschig HK (2010) The resurgence of A2B adenosine receptor signalling. Biochim Biophys Acta May 27. [Epub ahead of print].
41. Dranoff JA, Wells RG (2010) Portal fibroblasts: underappreciated mediators of biliary fibrosis. Hepatology 51: 1438–1444.
42. Smart DE, Green K, Oakley F, Weitzman JB, Yaniv M, et al. (2006) JunD is a profibrogenic transcription factor regulated by Jun N-terminal kinase-independent phosphorylation. Hepatology 44: 1432–1440.
43. Guenther MG, Levine SS, Boyer LA, Jaenisch R, Young RA (2007) A chromatin landmark and transcription initiation at most promoters in human cells. Cell 130: 77–88.
44. Song M-R, Ghosh A (2004) FGF2-induced chromatin remodelling regulates CNTF-mediated gene expression and astrocyte differentiation. Nat Neurosci 7: 229–235.
45. Gäbele E, Reif S, Tsukada S, Bataller R, Yata Y, et al. (2005) The role of $p70^{S6K}$ in hepatic stellate cell collagen gene expression and cell proliferation. J Biol Chem 280: 13374–13382.
46. Yang H, Ramani K, Xia M, Ko KS, Li TWH, et al. (2009) Dysregulation of glutathione synthesis during cholestasis in mice: molecular mechanisms and therapeutic implications. Hepatology 49: 1982–1991.
47. Ju M, Qiu S, Fan J, Xiao Y, Gao Q, et al. (2009) Peritumoral activated hepatic stellate cells predict poor clinical outcome in hepatocellular carcinoma. Am J Clin Pathol 131: 498–510.
48. Spirli C, Fabris L, Duner E, Fiorotto R, Roskams T, et al. (2003) Cytokine-stimulated nitric oxide production inhibits adenylyl cyclase and cAMP-dependent secretion in cholangiocytes. Gastroenterology 124: 737–753.
49. Sitkovsky MV (2003) Use of the A_{2A} adenosine receptor as a physiological immunosuppressor and to engineer inflammation in vivo. Biochem Pharmacol 65: 493–501.
50. Csóka B, Németh ZH, Rosenberger P, Eltzschig HK, Spolarics Z, et al. (2010) A_{2B} adenosine receptors protect against sepsis-induced mortality by dampening excessive inflammation. J Immunol 185: 542–550.
51. Ansorena E, Garcia-Trevijano ER, Martinez-Chantar ML, Huang Z, Chen L, et al. (2002) S-Adenosylmethionine and methylthioadenosine are antiapoptotic in cultured rat hepatocytes but proapoptotic in human hepatoma cells. Hepatology 35: 274–280.
52. Ansorena E, Berasain C, López Zabalza MJ, Avila MA, García-Trevijano ER, et al. (2006) Differential regulation of the JNK/AP-1 pathway by S-adenosylmethionine and methylthioadenosine in primary rat hepatocytes versus HuH7 hepatoma cells. Am J Physiol Gastrointest Liver Physiol 290: G1186–G1193.
53. Marderstein EL, Bucher B, Guo Z, Feng X, Reid K, et al. (2003) Protection of rat hepatocytes from apoptosis by inhibition of c-Jun N-terminal kinase. Surgery 134: 280–284.
54. Uehara T, Bennett B, Sakata ST, Satoh Y, Bilter G, et al. (2005) JNK mediates hepatic ischemia reperfusion injury. J Hepatol 42: 850–859.
55. Gunawan BK, Liu ZX, Hanawa N, Gaarde WA, Kaplowitz N (2006) c-Jun N-terminal kinase plays a major role in murine acetaminophen hepatotocicity. Gastroenterology 131: 165–178.
56. Nieto N, Cederbaum AI, S-Adenosylmethionine blocks collagen I production by preventing transforming growth factor-β induction of the COL1A2 promoter (2005) J Biol Chem 280: 30963–30974.
57. Marra F, DeFranco R, Grappone C, Milani S, Pastacaldi S, et al. (1998) Increased expression of monocyte chemotactic protein-1 during active hepatic fibrogenesis: correlation with monocyte infiltration. Am J Pathol 152: 423–430.
58. Friedman SL (2008) Mechanisms of hepatic fibrogenesis. Gastroenterology 134: 1655–1669.
59. Schuppan D, Popov Y (2009) Rationale and targets for antifibrotic therapies. Gastroenterol Clin Biol 33: 949–957.
60. Zamara E, Galastri S, Aleffi S, Petrai I, Aragno M, et al. (2007) Prevention of severe toxic liver injury and oxidative stress in MCP-1-deficient mice. J Hepatol 46: 230–238.
61. Marra F, Valente AJ, Pinzani M, Abboud HE (1993) Cultured human liver fat-storing cells produce monocyte chemotactic protein-1. Regulation by proinflammatory cytokines. J Clin Invest 92: 1674–1680.
62. Kruglov EA, Nathanson RA, Nguyen T, Dranoff JA (2006) Secretion of MCP-1/CCL2 by bile duct epithelia induces myofibroblastic trasndifferentiation of portal fibroblasts. Am J Physiol Gastrointest Liver Physiol 290: G765–G771.
63. Kawada N, Ikeda K, Seki S, Kuroki T (1999) Expression of cyclins D1, D2 and E correlates with proliferation of rat stellate cells in culture. J Hepatol 30: 1057–1064.
64. Wysoka J, Swigut T, Xiao H, Milne TA, Kwon SY, et al. (2006) A PHD finger of NURF couples histone H3 lysine 4 trimethylation with chromatin remodelling. Nature 442: 86–90.
65. Mann J, Chu DCK, Maxwell A, Oakley F, Zhu N, Tsukamoto H, Mann DA. MeCP2 controls an epigenetic pathway that promotes myofibroblast transdifferentiation and fibrosis. Gastroenterology 2010; 138: 705–714.
66. Chen H, Xia M, Lin M, Yang H, Kuhlenkamp J, et al. (2007) Role of methionine adenosyltransferase 2A and S-adenosylmethionine in mitogen-induced growth of human colon cancer cells. Gastroenterology 133: 207–219.
67. Andreu-Perez P, Hernandez-Losa J, Moline T, Gil R, Grueso J, et al. (2010) Methylthioadenosine (MTA) inhibits melanoma cell proliferation and *in vivo* tumor growth. BMC Cancer 10: 265.
68. Stramentinoli G, Gennari F. Adenosine derivatives of anti- inflammatory and analgesic activity, and therapeutic compositions which contain them as their active principle. Stramentinoli patent 4,454,122. Filed: Aug 6, 1982; Issued: Jun 12, 1984.
69. Moratti E. Pharmaceutical compositions containing 5-deoxy-5-methylthioadenosine s-adenosylmethionine and their salts for reducing seborrhoea. Moratti patent 5,753,213. Filed: Mar 13, 1990; Issued: May 19, 1998.

15

Non-Coding Keratin Variants Associate with Liver Fibrosis Progression in Patients with Hemochromatosis

Pavel Strnad[1*], Ozlem Kucukoglu[1], Mariia Lunova[1], Nurdan Guldiken[1], Tim C. Lienau[2], Felix Stickel[3], M. Bishr Omary[4]

1 Department of Internal Medicine I, University Medical Center Ulm, Ulm, Germany, **2** Medizinische Klinik mit Schwerpunkt Hepatologie und Gastroenterologie, Charite, Universitätsmedizin Berlin, Berlin, Germany, **3** Department of Medicine I, University of Erlangen-Nuremberg, Erlangen, Germany, **4** Department of Molecular and Integrative Physiology, University of Michigan Medical School, Ann Arbor, Michigan, United States of America

Abstract

Background: Keratins 8 and 18 (K8/K18) are intermediate filament proteins that protect the liver from various forms of injury. Exonic K8/K18 variants associate with adverse outcome in acute liver failure and with liver fibrosis progression in patients with chronic hepatitis C infection or primary biliary cirrhosis. Given the association of K8/K18 variants with end-stage liver disease and progression in several chronic liver disorders, we studied the importance of keratin variants in patients with hemochromatosis.

Methods: The entire K8/K18 exonic regions were analyzed in 162 hemochromatosis patients carrying homozygous C282Y HFE (hemochromatosis gene) mutations. 234 liver-healthy subjects were used as controls. Exonic regions were PCR-amplified and analyzed using denaturing high-performance liquid chromatography and DNA sequencing. Previously-generated transgenic mice overexpressing K8 G62C were studied for their susceptibility to iron overload. Susceptibility to iron toxicity of primary hepatocytes that express K8 wild-type and G62C was also assessed.

Results: We identified amino-acid-altering keratin heterozygous variants in 10 of 162 hemochromatosis patients (6.2%) and non-coding heterozygous variants in 6 additional patients (3.7%). Two novel K8 variants (Q169E/R275W) were found. K8 R341H was the most common amino-acid altering variant (4 patients), and exclusively associated with an intronic KRT8 IVS7+10delC deletion. Intronic, but not amino-acid-altering variants associated with the development of liver fibrosis. In mice, or ex vivo, the K8 G62C variant did not affect iron-accumulation in response to iron-rich diet or the extent of iron-induced hepatocellular injury.

Conclusion: In patients with hemochromatosis, intronic but not exonic K8/K18 variants associate with liver fibrosis development.

Editor: Rafael Aldabe, Centro de Investigación en Medicina Aplicada (CIMA), Spain

Funding: This work was supported by National Institutes of Health (NIH) grant DK52951 and the Department of Veterans Affairs (to MBO) and the Emmy-Noether-Programme funding STR 1095/2-1 (to PS). The funders had no role in study design, data collection and analysis, decision to publish, or preparation of the manuscript.

Competing Interests: The authors have declared that no competing interests exist.

* E-mail: pavel.strnad@uniklinik-ulm.de

These authors contributed equally to this work.

Introduction

Intermediate filaments (IFs), together with microtubules and the actin-containing microfilaments constitute the three major components of eukaryotic cytoskeleton [1]. Keratins (*KRT* genes, K proteins) represent the IFs of epithelial cells and are further subdivided into subtypes II (including K1–K8 and K71–K80) and I (K9–K28), which are both required to form obligate heteropolymers [2,3]. Consequently, each epithelial cell expresses at least one type I and one type II keratin [2,3]. Adult hepatocytes are unique, in that they contain K8/K18 as their only cytoplasmic IFs, while most other cell types display a more complex keratin composition [3]. The simple hepatocellular keratin expression pattern accounts for the observation that animals either lacking K8/K18 or expressing mutant K8/K18 display a predominant hepatic phenotype [4]. These animal findings spurred human association studies, which identified K8/K18 variants to be overrepresented in patients with cryptogenic and non-cryptogenic liver cirrhosis [4]. Subsequent reports showed that the presence of K8/K18 variants predisposes to liver fibrosis development in patients with chronic hepatitis C and primary biliary fibrosis as well as to adverse outcome of acute liver failure [5,6,7]. Keratin variants display ethnicity-specific distribution with K8 G62C/R341H and K8 Y54H/G434S being the most common amino-acid altering variants in Caucasians and African-American patients, respectively [7].

The pathogenesis of keratin variants was supported by the transgenic mice overexpressing K8 G62C variant, which are susceptible to Fas-induced apoptosis and microcystin-induced liver injury [8]. Presence of keratin variants predisposes to selective types of liver insults such as Fas but not TNF-α induced apoptotic injury; and thioacetamide- but not carbon tetrachloride-induced liver fibrosis development [9,10]. This suggests that the presence of keratin variants may predispose to specific liver diseases, while other liver disorders might be resistant to keratin mutation. To test this hypothesis, we studied the role of keratin variants in patients with hereditary hemochromatosis (HHC).

Hereditary hemochromatosis (HHC) comprises genetic disorders leading to iron overload [11]. The most frequent cause of HHC is the homozygous C282Y mutation in the *HFE* gene, which is as frequent as 1:200 in Caucasians of northern European descent [11,12]. Homozygous carriers of this mutation present with elevated transferrin saturation, ferritin and serum iron levels [11,12]. Epidemiological studies demonstrated that the clinical penetrance of *HFE* mutations is highly variable and does not necessarily lead to a clinically-manifest iron overload or even development of end-stage liver disease [11,12]. Additional modifying factors including gender, alcohol consumption or co-infection with hepatitis C virus are involved [11,12]. In addition, polymorphic variants of genes coding for modulators of iron metabolism, oxidative stress and certain cytokines were also shown to affect disease development [13,14,15].

In a study that examined candidate gene variants that may associate with the presence of HHC, the K8 R341H heterozygous variant was identified in 3 of 13 iron overload subjects but not in 5 controls [16]. This K8 variant was then examined in 119 subjects with the C282Y/C282Y *HFE* mutation and 116 age-, sex- and ethnic background matched controls. In that group, 9 patients in the HHC cohort carried the K8 R341H variant but none in the controls [16]. However, the frequency of the K8 R341H in more than 800 controls was 3.1% [5]. Notably, iron overload in HHC patients is known to generate reactive oxygen species [17,18], and earlier findings demonstrate that mice that overexpress the K18 R90C variant manifest upregulation of hepatic oxidative injury gene products under basal conditions [17,18]. These collective findings led us to analyze a cohort of 162 HHC patients from central Europe for the presence of keratin variants, and to evaluate the impact of iron overload in previously established transgenic mice overexpressing the human K8 G62C variant.

Methods

Ethics statement

The study protocol was reviewed and approved by the local ethics committees of the participating centers Austria (Vienna, Salzburg, and Innsbruck) and Germany (Regensburg, Erlangen) between 1991–2005, and all recruited patients gave informed and written consent.

All animal experiments were conducted with the approval of UCUCA under animal protocol number 10081 (Michigan, USA) for animal welfare.

Hemochromatosis Patient Cohort and Control Subjects

To determine the impact of keratin variants on liver disease development in HHC, we analyzed a previously described cohort of 162 homozygous carriers of the *HFE* C282Y mutation [19,20]. The analyzed subjects were recruited in five medical centers in Austria (Vienna, Salzburg, and Innsbruck) and Germany (Regensburg, Erlangen) between 1991–2005. The presence of the *HFE* mutation of the analyzed subjects was confirmed by standard genetic testing [21]. All patients underwent liver biopsy and the liver sections were evaluated by two independent pathologists [19,20] as described by Ishak et al. [22], with fibrosis stages 5 and 6 being considered as cirrhosis. Serum iron, ferritin, and transferrin levels were measured by routine commercial testing. Hepatic iron concentration (HIC) was measured by atomic absorption spectrometry [23], and is expressed as μg/g of dry liver tissue weight. The hepatic iron index (HII) was calculated by dividing the HIC by the age of the patients (in years) and by the molecular weight of iron. Transferrin saturation was calculated as follows: (serum iron×70.9)/(serum transferrin). Reference ranges are: serum iron, 40–150 μg/dL; serum ferritin in men, 18–440 ng/mL; serum ferritin in premenopausal women, 8–120 ng/mL; serum ferritin in postmenopausal women, 30–300 ng/mL; HIC, 300–1400 μg iron/g of dry liver tissue weight; transferrin saturation, 16–45%. The cut-off criteria for significant alcohol consumption were: <20 g/day (females) and <60 g/day (males) [19,20]. The presence of major liver disorders (e.g., viral hepatitis, heavy alcohol consumption, Wilson disease, primary biliary cirrhosis) was excluded by the appropriate clinical workup [20]. Informed consent was obtained from all subjects and the study was approved by the Ethics Committees of the participating centers. The liver-healthy control subjects were recruited in the medical centers of Bern (Switzerland) and Erlangen (Germany).

Mutation Detection

Genomic DNA was isolated from peripheral whole blood using an established DNA isolation kit (Qiagen GmbH, Hilden, Germany). For hemochromatosis patients, all 15 K8 and K18 exons and their adjacent exon-intron boundaries were amplified using previously described primers and a mixture of T Taq and Optimase Polymerases (Transgenomic, Omaha, NE) [24], while only K8 exons 1 and 6 were analyzed in control subjects. All amplicons were pre-screened with denaturing high pressure liquid chromatography (DHPLC) [24]. Probes with abnormal elution peak were purified with a QIAquick PCR purification kit (Qiagen) and sequenced in both directions using an ABI PRISM 377 DNA Sequencer (Applied Biosystems, Foster City, CA). The location of the coding *KRT8/KRT18* variants was assigned based on the mRNA sequences NM 002273.2 and NM 000224.2, respectively, while genomic sequences M34482.1 and AF179904.1 were employed for assignment of non-coding variants (www.ncbi.nlm.nih.gov). New genetic variants were reported in GenBank (accession numbers for K8 Q169E, R275W and E339A are rs199422323, rs199422324 and rs144044115, respectively).

Mouse Experiments

To study whether the presence of keratin variants affects hepatic iron accumulation, previously described transgenic mice (3–4 months old, four male/group) overexpressing human wild-type K8 (K8 WT) or the K8 G62C variant [8] were fed *ad libitum* with 3% carbonyl iron (Sigma-Aldrich, Germany)-containing diet (5001 Labdiet, Brentwood, MO) for one month. Age-matched male mice kept on a standard diet were used as controls. Mice were euthanized by CO_2 inhalation and blood was collected by intracardiac aspiration to measure serum alanine aminotransferase (ALT) levels. Livers were removed and cut into pieces for: (i) fixation in 10% formaldehyde for histological staining, (ii) snap freezing to measure hepatic iron concentration (HIC), or submerging into RNAlater stabilization reagent (Qiagen) for RNA analysis. Histological images were taken by Olympus BX40 with spot insight QE camera. The mRNA was transcribed into cDNA using oligo-dT primers and Superscript II reverse transcriptase (Invitrogen, Germany). Quantitative real-time polymerase chain reaction (RT-PCR) was carried out with SYBR green Master Mix (Applied Biosystems; Foster City, CA) and performed in duplicate using specific mouse hepcidin (encoded by *Hamp* gene), collagen1 (*Col1a1*), smooth muscle α-actin (*SMA*) and transforming growth factor-β (*TGF-β*) primers and *L7* ribosomal protein as an internal control (Table S2). All animals received humane care and their use was approved by the Institutional Animal Care Committee.

Determination of Hepatocellular Iron Toxicity

To test whether the presence of keratin variants influences hepatocellular iron toxicity, we isolated primary hepatocytes from K8 WT and G62C males as described before [8]. Briefly, the portal vein was cannulated and perfused with preheated liver Perfusion medium (Gibco 17701, Invitrogen, Darmstadt, Germany) then with pre-warmed 67 µ/mg Worthington type I collagenase-containing DMEM medium (CellSystems Biotechnologie Vertrieb GmbH, Troisdorf, Germany). The cell suspension was collected from extirpated livers, filtered through 100 µm-cell strainers (BD Falcon 9322799, Heidelberg, Germany) and centrifuged at 50 g for 1 min. The pellet was washed three times, and the isolated cells were cultured in hepatocyte culture medium (Gibco Hepatozym-SFM 17705, Darmstadt, Germany) supplemented with 10% FCS, 1% penicillin-streptomycin and L-Glutamine. To mimic the acute iron toxicity, hepatocytes were subjected to 100 µM iron-nitrilotriacetic acid complex (FeNTA) for 48 hours with the molar ratio of NTA/Fe^{3+} of 2:1 [25,26]. Untreated cells or cells treated with 100 µM nitrilotriacetic acid (NTA) without Fe were used as controls. Cell viability was determined using a commercially available MTT (3-(4,5-Dimethylthiazol-2-yl)-2,5-diphenyltetrazolium bromide) assay (Roche Cell Proliferation Kit I). Lactate dehydrogenase (LDH) and ALT were measured from cell supernatants.

Statistical Analysis

The unpaired two-tailed t or chi-square tests were used, and P values less than 0.05 were considered statistically significant.

Results

Patient Demographics

The clinical characteristics of the previously described cohort of 162 subjects carrying homozygous *HFE* C282Y mutation are displayed in Table 1; [19,20]. Most patients were males and harbored a significantly higher risk to develop liver cirrhosis than females ($p<0.0001$). Similarly, all assessed parameters of iron metabolism were markedly higher in males compared to females (Table 1) (ferritin $p<0.0001$, HIC $p = 0.001$, HII $p = 0.003$). Only a minority of patients had significant alcohol consumption.

Analysis for Presence of Coding K8/K18 Variants

Genetic analysis of the entire coding regions of K8/K18 identified 10 heterozygous K8 variants that result in amino acid substitution (overall variant frequency 6.2%, Table 2). K8 G62C and K8 R341H were the most frequent amino-acid-altering variants and were found in three and four independent patients, respectively. One patient harbored two heterozygous amino-acid altering K8 variants (K8 A319S+R341H). Two novel variants were detected that had not been described before. One of the novel variants, *KRT8* 505 C→G resulting in a K8 Q169E substitution within the rod domain (subdomain 1B), was found in two patients. The other novel variant, *KRT8* 823 C→T that codes for a K8 R275W substitution in the L2 linker sequence of *KRT8*, was found in one patient. The novel variants were detected in non-cirrhotic patients, and the involved amino acid residues are remarkably conserved among species and among some type II keratins (Figure S1). In addition to amino-acid-altering variants, a previously described common K8 L227L polymorphism was observed (not shown) [27].

An analysis of K8 variant hotspots in 234 liver healthy Central European subjects revealed a comparable variant frequency of 8.1% with K8 R341H and G62C variants being found in nine and six subjects respectively. One novel variant (E339A) was detected that had not been described before. The frequency of amino-acid-altering variants was similar in cirrhotic and non-cirrhotic patients (6.6% vs. 6.1%). Among the described keratin variants, only K8 G62C and R341H were previously clearly implicated in liver disease development [4] and the frequency of these two variants was somewhat higher in cirrhotic versus non-cirrhotic patients (6.6% vs 3.0%; "significant variants" in Table 2). This was mainly due to the K8 G62C variant, which was found exclusively in patients with liver cirrhosis (Table 2) but the numbers were too small to reach statistical significance.

Characterization of the Non-Coding K8/K18 Variants

Our genetic analysis identified 9 non-coding heterozygous K8 variants (Table 3). Among these, an intronic KRT8 IVS7+10delC deletion was the most common variant and exclusively associated with K8 R341H substitution as described before [28]. IVS6+46A>T intronic variant was the only intronic variant found in the control group and was seen in one subject (out of 234). The presence of additional intronic variants (IVS7+20G>A and IVS8+31C>T) was not analyzed in the control group. When compound exonic-intronic variants were excluded, "pure" intronic variants (labeled as "total intronic variants in Table 3) were

Table 1. Patient Demographics and Biochemical Values.

Demographics	Male	Female	Total	# Patients without data (%)
# of patients (%)	120 (74.5)	41 (25.5)	162 (100)	1(0.6)
Age at LBx, mean ± SD (years)	50±13	52±12	50±13	-
Cirrhosis yes/no (%)	58/60 (49/51)	3/38 (7/93)	61/99(38/62)	-
Alcohol consumption (yes/no)	6/104	4/31	10/135	19 (11.7)
Serum iron (µg/dL), mean± SD	213±43	195±35	208±41	38 (23.5)
Transferrin Saturation (%), mean± SD	87±17	74±19	84±18	29 (17.9)
Serum ferritin (ng/mL), mean± SD**	2501±1953	711±592	2081±1891	17 (10.5)
HIC (µg/g dry weight), mean± SD	13339±8537	7416±6945	11671±8518	59 (36.4)
HII, mean± SD	5.2±3.6	2.9±3.2	4.6±3.7	55 (34.0)

Abbreviations: LBx:liver biopsy; SD: standard deviation; HIC: hepatic iron concentration; HII:hepatic iron index.

Table 2. Distribution of Exonic Keratin Variants.

KRT8			Cirrhosis (# and % of patient)		Total # of variant (%)	Total # of control (%)
Variant	**Nucleotide**	**Location**	**Yes (61/38)**	**No (99/62)**	**162**	**234**
G62C	GGC→TGC	Exon 1	3	0	3 (1.85)	6 (2.6)
I63V*	ATC→GTC	Exon 1	0	0	0	2 (0.8)
Q169E†	CAG→GAG	Exon 2	0	2	2 (1.23)	N.T.
R275W†	CGG→TGG	Exon 5	0	1	1 (0.62)	N.T.
A319S*	GCT→TCT	Exon 5	0	1$	1 (0.62)	N.T.
E339A†,*	GAG→GCG	Exon 6	0	0	0	1 (0.4)
R341H	CGT→CAT	Exon 6	1	3$	4 (2.50)	9 (3.8)
# Patients with any variant (%)			**4 (6.56)**	**6& (6.06)**	**10 (6.17)**	**19 (8.1)**
# Patients with significant variant (%)			**4 (6.56)**	**3 (3.03)**	**7 (4.32)**	**15 (6.4)**

The table displays the number of patients with and without liver cirrhosis for the listed keratin variants.
*The highlighted variant is considered to be a "polymorphism" rather than a "mutation" that is likely to have biologic significance.
†Novel variants which were not previously described.
$One female patient harbored 2 independent amino acid altering KRT8 variants (R341H+A319S). N.T.not tested.

seen in 6 hemochromatosis patients (variant frequency 3.7%). Five patients carrying "pure" intronic variants displayed liver cirrhosis (8.2%), while only one subject did not have cirrhosis. Consequently, the non-coding *KRT8* variants were significantly over-represented in cirrhotic patients ($p = 0.02$). However, neither intronic nor exonic keratin variants associated with iron accumulation in hemochromatosis patients as suggested by similar levels for serum iron, transferrin, transferrin saturation, ferritin and HIC and HII indices (Table 4). On the other hand, cirrhotic subjects were older and had higher transferrin saturation than non-cirrhotic patients (Table S1).

The K8 G62C Variant Does Not Alter Experimental Iron Accumulation

Given that all patients harboring the K8 G62C variant displayed liver fibrosis, we used previously-characterized transgenic mice that overexpress K8 G62C and control mice that overexpress WT K8 [8] to test whether K8 G62C affects iron accumulation. As expected, both untreated and iron-fed K8 WT and K8 G62C mice had normal ALT levels (Figure 1A), and did not display any histological signs of liver damage (not shown). Iron-feeding led to a dramatic increase in hepatic iron, which were slightly more pronounced in K8 WT animals; however, the difference between genotypes is not statistically significant (p = 0.08; Figure 1B). Furthermore, both genotypes expressed nearly identical levels of the iron uptake-regulating hormone hepcidin (*Hamp*) and comparable levels of fibrosis-associated genes collagen 1 (*Col1a1*), smooth muscle α-actin (*SMA*) and transforming growth factor-β (*TGF-β*) (Figure S2). In addition, Perl's Prussian blue staining revealed a similar pattern of iron accumulation in both genotypes (Figure 1C).

The K8 G62C Variant Does Not Increase Mouse Hepatocyte Iron Toxicity Ex-Vivo

To test whether the presence of K8 G62C variant affects hepatocellular iron toxicity, primary hepatocytes from K8 WT and G62C mice were treated with FeNTA. FeNTA exposure led to significant increase in the release of ALT and LDH into the cell culture supernatant; which, however, did not differ significantly between the genotypes (Figure 2A, B). Similarly, addition of FeNTA reduced cell viability in both K8 WT and G62C hepatocytes to a similar extent (Figure 2C), thereby suggesting that the presence of K8 G62C does not enhance hepatocyte iron toxicity.

Discussion

In the study herein, we first analyzed HHC samples for the presence of K8/K18 variants. Amino-acid-altering keratin vari-

Table 3. Distribution of Non-Coding Keratin Variants.

KRT8		Cirrhosis (# and % of patient)		Total # of variant (%)
Variant	**Location**	**Yes (61/38)**	**No (99/62)**	**162**
IVS7+10delC*	Intronic	1	3	4
IVS6+46A>T†	Intronic	1	1	2 (1.23)
IVS7+20G>A	Intronic	3	0	3 (1.85)
IVS8+31C>T	3′-UTR	1	0	1 (0.62)
Total intronic variant (%)		**5 (8.20)****	**1 (1.01)****	**6 (3.70)**

The table displays the number of patients with and without liver cirrhosis for the listed keratin variants.
*IVS7+10delC variant completely associates with KRT8 R341H variant and is not included in the count of total intronic variants.
†The highlighted variant was found only in one control subject (out of 234).
**$p = 0.02$.

Table 4. The Clinical Features of Hemochromatosis Patients Harboring Exonic and Intronic Keratin 8 Variants.

	Presence of Exonic Variants		Presence of Intronic Variants	
Demographics	**YES (n = 10)**	**NO (n = 152)**	**YES (n = 6)**	**NO (n = 156)**
Sex (M/F)	7/3	113/38	5/1	115/40
Age at LBx, mean ± SD (years)	55±11	50±13	59±8	50±13
Cirrhosis (yes/no)	4/6	57/93	5/1	56/98
Alcohol consumption (yes/no)	0/6	10/127	0/6	10/127
Serum iron (μg/dl), mean± SD	216±31	208±42-	202±29	209±42
Transferrin Saturation (%), mean± SD	84±20	84±18	95±6	84±18
Serum ferritin (μg/l), mean± SD	2377±2147	2409±4703	2166±1786	2077±1901
HIC (μg/g), mean± SD	14012±8560	11552±8543	12765±9145	11627±8539
HII, mean± SD	5.4±3.6	4.5±3.7	3.7±2.3	4.6±3.7

Abbreviations: LBx:liver biopsy; SD: standard deviation; HIC: hepatic iron concentration; HII: hepatic iron index.
Note that intronic keratin variants were preferentially found in male subjects ($p = 0.09$ for distribution among the sexes).

ants were detected in 10 of 162 HHC patients (variant frequency 6.2%) and a similar frequency of keratin variants was seen in the control group (8.1%). In contrast, substantially higher keratin variant frequencies (>10%) were previously described in patients with end-stage liver disease or acute liver failure, which is likely due to the enrichment of keratin variants in patients with severe liver disease [5,7]. On the other hand, comparable keratin variant frequencies were seen in two European studies, which analyzed patients with chronic hepatitis C infection and primary biliary cirrhosis that included patients with all ranges of liver disease severity [6,28].

Among single point mutations, we identified four patients with K8 R341H variant (variant frequency 2.5%), which is comparable with the frequency seen in liver-healthy Caucasians [7] and hitherto analyzed control subjects (variant frequency 3.8%), but lower than a previously analyzed US HHC patient cohort (variant frequency 7.6%, p = 0.08, [16]). Furthermore, we observed a novel K8 Q169E variant in two unrelated HHC patients, which we had

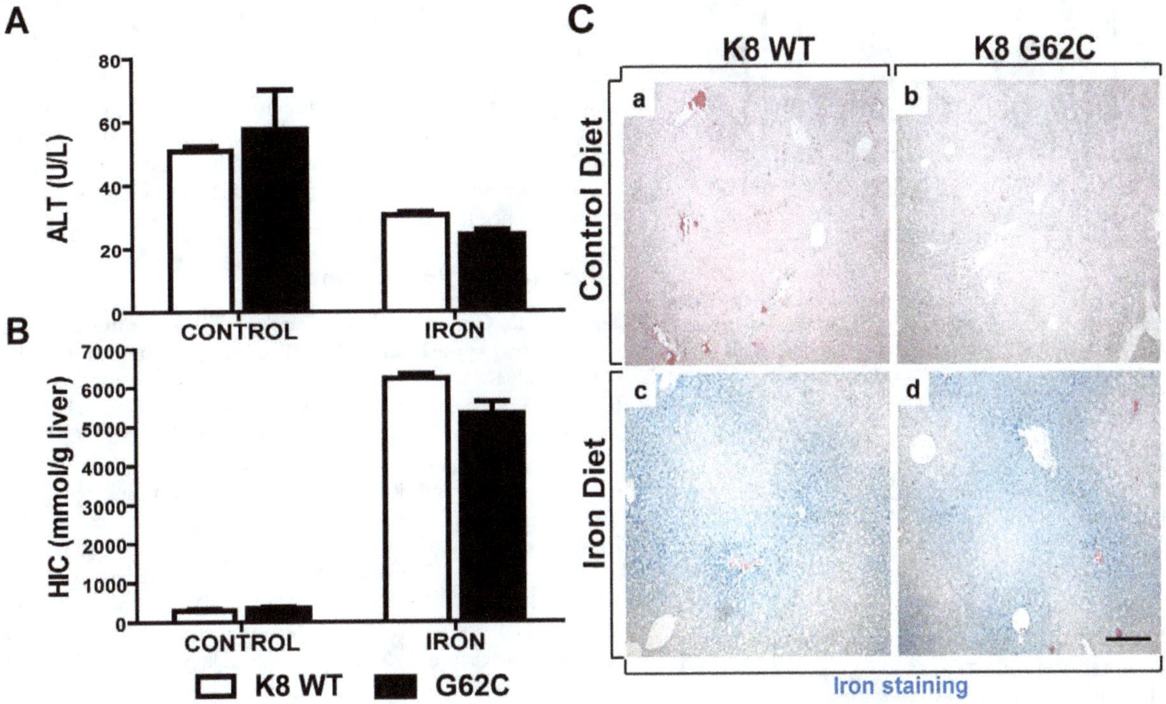

Figure 1. The K8 G62C variant does not influence the extent of hepatocellular iron accumulation. To test, whether hepatocellular iron accumulation is affected by the presence of keratin variants, transgenic mice overexpressing wild-type human keratin 8 (K8 WT) or K8 G62C variant were fed with 3% carbonyl iron-containing diet for one month (Iron) and compared to age-matched animals kept on standard diet (Control) (n = 4 mice/group). Iron-feeding did not lead to an increase in serum ALT (**A**), but caused a significant elevation in hepatic iron concentration (HIC) (**B**). There was no significant difference in ALT or HIC levels between K8 WT and G62C mice after iron feeding. (**C**) Perl's Prussian blue staining revealed a similar pattern of iron deposition in both mouse lines. Scale bar = 200 μm.

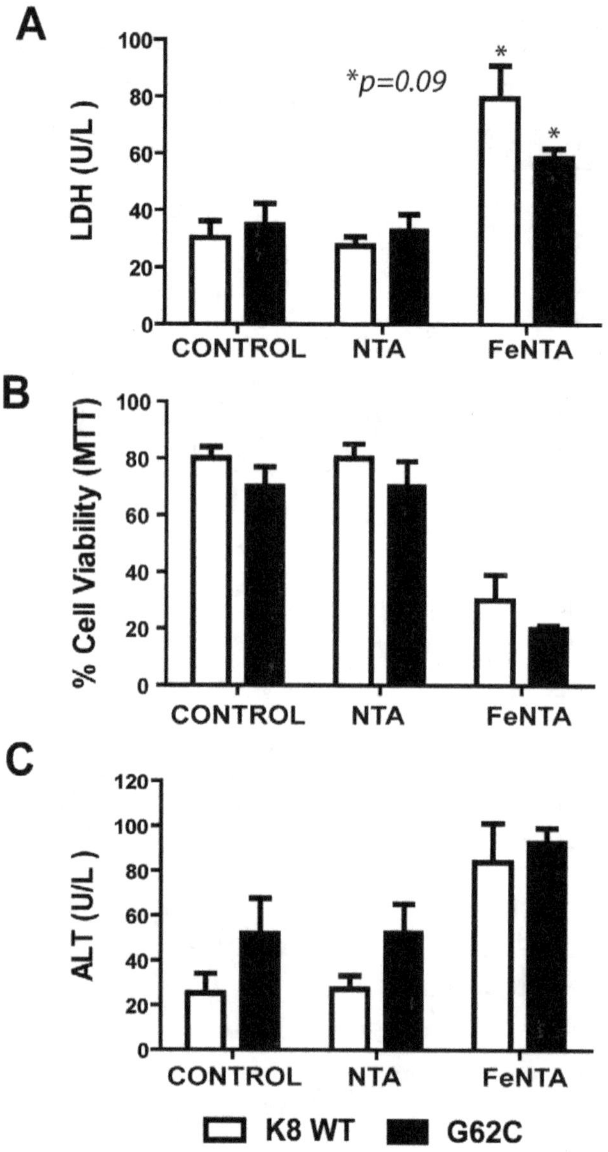

Figure 2. The K8 G62C variant does not affect iron toxicity in ex vivo cultured hepatocytes. To study the hepatocellular iron toxicity, primary hepatocytes from transgenic animals overexpressing K8 WT or K8 G62C were cultured in normal media (Control) or media supplemented with 100 μM nitrilotriacetic acid (NTA) or 100 μM iron-NTA (FeNTA) for 24 hours. FeNTA, but not NTA treatment led to a significant increase in LDH (**A**) and ALT levels (**C**) in cell culture supernatants together with significant decrease in cell viability as assessed by MTT assay (**B**). The enzyme levels and cell viability did not differ significantly between K8 WT and K8 G62C hepatocytes.

not detected in >1000 subjects analyzed to date with various liver diseases [5,7]. The K8 Q169E variant introduces a charged amino acid, and leads to replacement of the highly conserved K8 Q169. Given that no mutations have been reported in homologous keratin residues among other type II keratins (http://www.interfil.org/), further studies are needed to address the potential pathogenic role of this variant.

While the amino-acid altering K8/K18 variants exhibited similar frequencies in HHC patients with and without liver cirrhosis, all patients harboring the K8 G62C variant had liver cirrhosis. This mutation might therefore be of particular relevance in HHC. This hypothesis is further supported by the fact that this variant introduces a cysteine into the K8 backbone, which normally lacks cysteines, and leads to keratin crosslinking and impairment of keratin filament reorganization upon oxidative stress [29]. Given the established role of oxidative stress in HHC development as well as the finding that an introduction of cysteine into otherwise cysteine-less K18 predisposes mice to oxidative injury [17,18], we used previously described transgenic mice overexpressing K8 G62C to study the importance of K8 G62C in iron-overload [24]. However, K8 G62C presence did not accelerate iron accumulation or augment iron-induced hepatocellular damage and apoptosis (Figure 1, 2). We posit that if K8 G62C does indeed predispose to liver disease progression, then it does so in a manner that is independent of iron accumulation.

In summary, the combination of genetic and experimental data suggests that in contrast to hepatitis C, primary biliary cirrhosis and acute liver failure [5,7], amino-acid altering variants may not contribute to liver disease development in HHC. This finding is not surprising since different liver disorders were shown to posses their unique genetic disease-modifiers [30]. For example, factors modifying iron accumulation might be particularly important in hereditary hemochromatosis, while genes affecting inflammatory response and lipid metabolism may contribute to disease progression in patients with hepatitis C infection and alcoholic/non-alcoholic liver disease, respectively [13–15] [30].

Unlike the exonic variants, the intronic variants were shown to be overrepresented in HHC patients with liver cirrhosis. This finding represents the first such liver disease association since intronic K8/K18 variants did not associate with liver fibrosis development in patients with chronic hepatitis C infection [28]. However, intronic variants may very well be functional, given that introns harbour multiple functional elements that regulate alternative splicing or transcription [31]. Furthermore, there was a trend for intronic variants to be more abundant in primary biliary cirrhosis patients as compared with the control group; however their association with liver disease progression was not analyzed [6]. Given the limited number of patients analyzed in the present study and the fact that there are no available data about the biological significance of the observed intronic variants, further studies are needed to determine their role in liver disease.

Supporting Information

Figure S1 Conservation of novel K8 variants among species and type II keratins. The sequences surrounding the amino acids K8 Q169 (A, B) and K8 R275W (C, D) are displayed for selected species (A, C) and type II keratins (B, D). The sequences illustrate the single nucleotide variations leading to the highlighted amino acid change (E, F). Note that K8 Q169 is highly conserved among species and among type II keratins, while K8 R275 amino acid is highly conserved among species, and is also conserved from a charge perspective among type II keratins. The figures were assembled using the following reference sequences: K8: NM 002273.3 (Homo sapiens), NM 19937.1 (Rattus norvegicus), NM 031170.2 (Mus musculus), BC 044116.1 (Xenopus laevis) and NM 200080.2 (Danio rerio); Type II Keratins: NM 006121.3 (*KRT1*), NM 000423.2 (*KRT2a*), NM 015848.4 (*KRT2p*), NM 057088.2 (*KRT3*), NM 002272.3 (*KRT4*), NM 000424.3 (*KRT5*), NM 005554.3 (*KRT6A*), NM 005555.3 (*KRT6B*), NM 005556.3 (*KRT7*).

Figure S2 mRNA expression of fibrosis-related genes and hepcidin does not differ among K8 WT and G62C fed iron-rich diet. WT mRNA levels are set at 1.0 and G62C mRNA levels of the indicated transcripts are displayed relative to WT. mRNA was isolated from 4 independent livers per genotype.

Table S1 The clinical characteristics of the previously described cohort of 162 subjects carrying homozygous HFE C282Y mutation (cirrhotic patients vs non-cirrhotic patients).

Table S2 Sequence of primers used for quantitative real time-PCR and length of the amplified products.

Acknowledgments

The authors are indebted to the patients whose participation in the study made this work possible.

Author Contributions

Conceived and designed the experiments: PS OK MBO. Performed the experiments: PS OK ML NG. Analyzed the data: PS OK FS. Contributed reagents/materials/analysis tools: PS TCL MBO. Wrote the paper: PS OK.

References

1. Ku NO, Zhou X, Toivola DM, Omary MB (1999) The cytoskeleton of digestive epithelia in health and disease. Am J Physiol 277: G1108–1137.
2. Coulombe PA, Kerns ML, Fuchs E (2009) Epidermolysis bullosa simplex: a paradigm for disorders of tissue fragility. J Clin Invest 119: 1784–1793.
3. Omary MB (2009) "IF-pathies": a broad spectrum of intermediate filament-associated diseases. J Clin Invest 119: 1756–1762.
4. Omary MB, Ku NO, Strnad P, Hanada S (2009) Toward unraveling the complexity of simple epithelial keratins in human disease. J Clin Invest 119: 1794–1805.
5. Ku NO, Strnad P, Zhong BH, Tao GZ, Omary MB (2007) Keratins let liver live: Mutations predispose to liver disease and crosslinking generates Mallory-Denk bodies. Hepatology 46: 1639–1649.
6. Zhong B, Strnad P, Selmi C, Invernizzi P, Tao GZ, et al. (2009) Keratin variants are overrepresented in primary biliary cirrhosis and associate with disease severity. Hepatology 50: 546–554.
7. Strnad P, Zhou Q, Hanada S, Lazzeroni LC, Zhong BH, et al. (2010) Keratin variants predispose to acute liver failure and adverse outcome: race and ethnic associations. Gastroenterology 139: 828–835, 835 e821–823.
8. Ku NO, Omary MB (2006) A disease- and phosphorylation-related nonmechanical function for keratin 8. J Cell Biol 174: 115–125.
9. Strnad P, Tao GZ, Zhou Q, Harada M, Toivola DM, et al. (2008) Keratin mutation predisposes to mouse liver fibrosis and unmasks differential effects of the carbon tetrachloride and thioacetamide models. Gastroenterology 134: 1169–1179.
10. Ku NO, Soetikno RM, Omary MB (2003) Keratin mutation in transgenic mice predisposes to Fas but not TNF-induced apoptosis and massive liver injury. Hepatology 37: 1006–1014.
11. Pietrangelo A (2011) Hepcidin in human iron disorders: therapeutic implications. J Hepatol 54: 173–181.
12. Alexander J, Kowdley KV (2009) HFE-associated hereditary hemochromatosis. Genet Med 11: 307–313.
13. Wood MJ, Powell LW, Ramm GA (2008) Environmental and genetic modifiers of the progression to fibrosis and cirrhosis in hemochromatosis. Blood 111: 4456–4462.
14. Weiss G (2010) Genetic mechanisms and modifying factors in hereditary hemochromatosis. Nat Rev Gastroenterol Hepatol 7: 50–58.
15. Rochette J, Le Gac G, Lassoued K, Ferec C, Robson KJ (2010) Factors influencing disease phenotype and penetrance in HFE haemochromatosis. Hum Genet 128: 233–248.
16. Lee P, Gelbart T, West C, Halloran C, Beutler E (2002) Seeking candidate mutations that affect iron homeostasis. Blood Cells Mol Dis 29: 471–487.
17. Ramm GA, Ruddell RG (2005) Hepatotoxicity of iron overload: mechanisms of iron-induced hepatic fibrogenesis. Semin Liver Dis 25: 433–449.
18. Zhou Q, Ji X, Chen L, Greenberg HB, Lu SC, et al. (2005) Keratin mutation primes mouse liver to oxidative injury. Hepatology 41: 517–525.
19. Osterreicher CH, Datz C, Stickel F, Hellerbrand C, Penz M, et al. (2005) Association of myeloperoxidase promotor polymorphism with cirrhosis in patients with hereditary hemochromatosis. J Hepatol 42: 914–919.
20. Stickel F, Osterreicher CH, Datz C, Ferenci P, Wolfel M, et al. (2005) Prediction of progression to cirrhosis by a glutathione S-transferase P1 polymorphism in subjects with hereditary hemochromatosis. Arch Intern Med 165: 1835–1840.
21. Kazemi-Shirazi L, Datz C, Maier-Dobersberger T, Kaserer K, Hackl F, et al. (1999) The relation of iron status and hemochromatosis gene mutations in patients with chronic hepatitis C. Gastroenterology 116: 127–134.
22. Ishak K, Baptista A, Bianchi L, Callea F, De Groote J, et al. (1995) Histological grading and staging of chronic hepatitis. J Hepatol 22: 696–699.
23. Di Bisceglie AM, Axiotis CA, Hoofnagle JH, Bacon BR (1992) Measurements of iron status in patients with chronic hepatitis. Gastroenterology 102: 6.
24. Strnad P, Lienau TC, Tao GZ, Ku NO, Magin TM, et al. (2006) Denaturing temperature selection may underestimate keratin mutation detection by DHPLC. Hum Mutat 27: 444–452.
25. White GP, Jacobs A (1978) Iron uptake by Chang cells from transferrin, nitriloacetate and citrate complexes: the effects of iron-loading and chelation with desferrioxamine. Biochimica Et Biophysica Acta 543: 217–225.
26. Morel I, Lescoat G, Cillard J, Pasdeloup N, Brissot P, et al. (1990) Kinetic evaluation of free malondialdehyde and enzyme leakage as indices of iron damage in rat hepatocyte cultures. Involvement of free radicals. Biochemical Pharmacology 39: 1647–1655.
27. Hesse M, Berg T, Wiedenmann B, Spengler U, Woitas RP, et al. (2004) A frequent keratin 8 p.L227L polymorphism, but no point mutations in keratin 8 and 18 genes, in patients with various liver disorders. J Med Genet 41: e42.
28. Strnad P, Lienau TC, Tao GZ, Lazzeroni LC, Stickel F, et al. (2006) Keratin variants associate with progression of fibrosis during chronic hepatitis C infection. Hepatology 43: 1354–1363.
29. Ku NO, Gish R, Wright TL, Omary MB (2001) Keratin 8 mutations in patients with cryptogenic liver disease. N Engl J Med 344: 1580–1587.
30. Zimmer V, Lammert F (2011) Genetics in liver disease: new concepts. Curr Opin Gastroenterol 27: 231–239.
31. Cooper DN, Chen JM, Ball EV, Howells K, Mort M, et al. (2010) Genes, mutations, and human inherited disease at the dawn of the age of personalized genomics. Hum Mutat 31: 631–655.

Hepatic Deletion of Smad7 in Mouse Leads to Spontaneous Liver Dysfunction and Aggravates Alcoholic Liver Injury

Lu Zhu, Lingdi Wang, Xiao Wang, Xiaolin Luo, Ling Yang, Rui Zhang, Hongkun Yin, Dong Xie, Yi Pan, Yan Chen*

Key Laboratory of Nutrition and Metabolism, Institute for Nutritional Sciences, Shanghai Institutes for Biological Sciences, Graduate School of the Chinese Academy of Sciences, Chinese Academy of Sciences, Shanghai, China

Abstract

Background: TGF-β has been known to play an important role in various liver diseases including fibrosis and alcohol-induced fatty liver. Smad7 is an intracellular negative regulator of TGF-β signaling. It is currently unclear whether endogenous Smad7 has an effect on liver function and alcoholic liver damage.

Methodology/Principal Findings: We used Cre/loxP system by crossing Alb-Cre mice with Smad7$^{loxP/loxP}$ mice to generate liver-specific deletion of Smad7 with loss of the indispensable MH2 domain. Alcoholic liver injury was achieved by feeding mice with a liquid diet containing 5% ethanol for 6 weeks, followed by a single dose of ethanol gavage. Deletion of Smad7 in the liver was associated with increased Smad2/3 phosphorylation in the liver or upon TGF-β treatment in primary hepatocytes. The majority of mice with liver specific deletion of Smad7 (Smad7$^{liver\text{-}KO}$) were viable and phenotypically normal, accompanied by only slight or no reduction of Smad7 expression in the liver. However, about 30% of Smad7$^{liver\text{-}KO}$ mice with high efficiency of Smad7 deletion had spontaneous liver dysfunction, demonstrated as low body weight, overall deterioration, and increased serum levels of AST and ALT. Degeneration and elevated apoptosis of liver cells were observed with these mice. TGF-β-induced epithelial to mesenchymal transition (EMT) was accelerated in Smad7-deleted primary hepatocytes. In addition, alcohol-induced liver injury and steatosis were profoundly aggravated in Smad7 deficient mice, associated with upregulation of critical genes involved in lipogenesis and inflammation. Furthermore, alcohol-induced ADH1 expression was significantly abrogated by Smad7 deletion in hepatocytes.

Conclusion/Significance: In this study, we provided *in vivo* evidence revealing that endogenous Smad7 plays an important role in liver function and alcohol-induced liver injury.

Editor: Bing Sun, Institut Pasteur of Shanghai, China

Funding: This work was supported by research grants from National Natural Science Foundation of China (30830037 and 81021002) and the Ministry of Science and Technology of China (2007CB947100 and 2006CB943900) to Y.C. The work was also supported by Ministry of Science and Technology of China (2010CB529506), National Natural Science Foundation of China (30971660) and a grant from Shanghai Institutes for Biological Sciences (2009KIP207) to YP. The funders had no role in study design, data collection and analysis, decision to publish, or preparation of the manuscript.

Competing Interests: The authors have declared that no competing interests exist.

* E-mail: ychen3@sibs.ac.cn

Introduction

Liver dysfunction is a life-threatening medical scenario that demands clinical care. Severe liver dysfunction leads to liver failure that occurs when the majority of liver tissue is damaged beyond repair and the liver is no longer able to perform normal functions [1]. In most cases, liver dysfunction occurs gradually over many years. However, a rare condition known as acute liver failure such as fulminant hepatitis can occur rapidly. Transforming growth factor-β ((TGF-β) plays an important role in liver diseases [2]. TGF-βs belong to a large family of growth and differentiation factors that utilize complex signaling networks to regulate numerous cellular activities including differentiation, proliferation, motility, adhesion, and apoptosis [3]. The TGF-β family members regulate gene expression via serine/threonine kinase receptors at the cell surface and a group of intracellular transducers called Smad proteins including R-Smads (receptor-specific Smad, including Smad1, 2, 3, 5 and 8), Co-Smad or Smad4 (a common-Smad), and I-Smads (inhibitory Smads, including Smad6 and Smad7) [3,4,5,6]. The signaling starts by binding of the ligand to the cognate transmembrane receptor kinase, followed by phosphorylation of R-Smad and complex formation between R-Smad with Co-Smad. The Smad complex transduces the signal from the plasma membrane into the nucleus in which Smad proteins and their transcriptional partners directly regulate gene expression [3,6]. Smad7 is a member of the I-Smad subfamily that is able to directly interact with the TGF-β type I receptor [7], whereas blocking the phosphorylation of R-Smads Smad2 and Smad3 and inhibiting TGF-β signaling.

Alterations in the production of TGF-β or mutations within the genes involved in TGF-β signaling pathway are associated with the pathogenesis of many diseases including fibrotic disease of the kidney, liver and lung. The *in vivo* functions of the Smad proteins as well as their association with diseases are revealed by targeted deletion of the corresponding genes in mice [8]. Deletions of Smad1, Smad2 and Smad4 lead to embryonic lethality of the mouse, indicating the importance of these genes in early development [9,10,11]. Deletion of Smad3 gives rise to abnormalities in mucosal immune system, related to development of colorectal cancers [12,13]. Mouse deletion studies also indicate that Smad5 is involved in angiogenesis during embryogenesis [14]. A recent *in vivo* study indicates that Smad8 is involved in pulmonary vascular remodeling [15]. Interestingly, deletion studies of inhibitory Smads suggest that both Smad6 and Smad7 are involved in cardiovascular development in the mouse. Deletion of the indispensable MH2 domain of Smad6 results in multiple cardiovascular defects during early development [16]. On the other hand, deletion of the MH2 domain of Smad7 leads to defects in the development of atrioventricular cushion [17], while hypomorphic Smad7 deficiency with deletion of the MH1 domain of Smad7 is associated with altered B-cell response [18].

A few studies have emerged to reveal the role of Smad7 in liver diseases. Overexpression of Smad7 in mouse liver could attenuate TGF-β signaling and improve carbon tetrachloride (CCl_4)-provoked liver fibrosis [19]. On the other hand, hypomorphic Smad7 deficiency enhances CCl_4-induced liver damage and fibrosis [20]. In this study, we established a mouse model with liver-specific deletion of the MH2 domain of Smad7. Interestingly, we found that deletion of Smad7 is associated with development of spontaneous liver dysfunction in the mouse.

The most common causes of chronic liver injury include virus infection, long term alcohol consumption, cirrhosis, inherited disorders, and malnutrition. Among these major factors that cause chronic liver injury, alcohol drinking is a major etiologic one in chronic liver disease worldwide, causing fatty liver, alcoholic hepatitis, cirrhosis, and eventually hepatocellular carcinoma. In the past few decades, major progress has been made in our understanding about the molecular mechanisms underlying alcoholic liver injury, such as the functional roles of STAT3 [21]. We also found that Smad7 deficiency is able to enhance formation of alcohol-induced fatty liver. These results, combining with the studies from other laboratories, pinpoint an important role of Smad7 in liver functionalities and liver diseases.

Results

Generation and characterization of liver-specific Smad7 deletion mouse

To investigate the potential function of Smad7 in the liver, we crossed Albumin-Cre transgenic mice with Smad7$^{loxP/loxP}$ mice that contain two loxP fragments flanking the 5′ half of exon 4 of Smad7 gene [17]. The Albumin-Cre transgenic mice specifically express *Cre* recombinase in hepatocytes under control of a rat albumin promoter/enhancer. Specific deletion of the MH2 domain (encoded by the 5′ half of exon 4) of Smad7 in the mouse liver was confirmed by RT-PCR (Figure 1A). As expected, we found that the mRNA region corresponding to exon 1–3 was not deleted in the liver-specific Smad7-deleted mouse (Smad7$^{liver-KO}$ mouse). However, only the mRNA region corresponding to exon 3–4 was lost in the liver of Smad7$^{liver-KO}$ mouse, but not changed in the other tissues such as brain, lung, heart, and kidney, indicating liver-specific deletion of Smad7 MH2 domain. To verify Smad7 deletion, the protein level of Smad7 was also examined by immunohistochemistry staining in the liver sections. The result revealed that the protein level of Smad7 was markedly decreased in the liver of Smad7$^{liver-KO}$ mouse in comparison with wide type animals (Figure 1B).

As the major cellular function of Smad7 is to inhibit TGF-β signaling, we analyzed whether deletion of Smad7 is associated with an enhancement of Smad2/3 phosphorylation in the mouse liver. By immunohistochemistry using liver sections from either wild type or Smad7$^{liver-KO}$ mice, we found that Smad2 phosphorylation was significantly increased in the liver from the Smad7$^{liver-KO}$ mice in comparison with the wild type animals (Figure 1C). Furthermore, we analyzed the phosphorylation levels of Smad2 and Smad3 using cultured primary hepatocytes isolated from the mice. TGF-β1-induced Smad2 and Smad3 phosphorylation appeared to be enhanced by Smad7 deletion by an immunoblotting assay (Figure 1D). Collectively, these results indicate that Smad7 deficiency is associated with enhancement of TGF-β signaling in the liver, consistent with the notion that Smad7 is an intracellular inhibitory protein to negatively modulate TGF-β signaling pathway [7].

Deletion of Smad7 causes spontaneous liver dysfunction in the mouse

Interestingly, the phenotype of Smad7$^{liver-KO}$ mice varied from mouse to mouse. While the majority of Smad7$^{liver-KO}$ mice had no apparent phenotypical change, a small portion of the mice had obvious growth retardation and the overall condition started to deteriorate at 2–3 months of age (Figure 2A). We monitored the changes of liver enzymes together with the mRNA level of Smad7 corresponding to the region encoded by exon 4 in the liver (Figure 2B). In comparison with the wild type controls, ~30% of Smad7$^{liver-KO}$ mice had over 50% of reduction of the mRNA level of Smad7 exon 4, while ~70% Smad7$^{liver-KO}$ mice had only slight or no reduction of Smad7 exon 4 mRNA. The variation of Smad7 deficiency observed in the study is likely caused by incomplete expression of Cre recombinase driven by the albumin promoter (Figure S1). Interestingly, only those Smad7$^{liver-KO}$ mice with significant deletion of Smad7 had severely decreased body weight (Figure 2C, left panel), accompanied by robustly elevated blood levels of aspartate aminotransferase (AST) and alanine aminotransferase (ALT) (Figure 2B and 2C). The blood levels of both AST and ALT were inversely correlated with the mRNA level of Smad7 exon 4 (Figure 2C, middle and right panels). Together, these data indicate that marked deletion of Smad7 expression is associated with spontaneous liver dysfunction in the mouse.

Deletion of Smad7 increases apoptosis in hepatocytes

The observed spontaneous liver damage in Smad7$^{liver-KO}$ mice was further investigated by histological and immunohistochemical analyses. In comparison with the wild type littermate, the liver sections from the Smad7$^{liver-KO}$ mouse with significant reduction of Smad7 expression had features of cell degeneration (Figure 3A), accompanied by elevation of apoptosis (Figure 3B and 3C, marked by arrows). Furthermore, we analyzed TGF-β-induced apoptosis in primary hepatocytes isolated from the wild type and Smad7$^{liver-KO}$ mice. TGF-β1 treatment itself could increase the number of apoptotic hepatocytes (Figure 3D, left panel). However, the TGF-β1-induced hepatocyte apoptosis was significantly enhanced by Smad7 deletion (Figure 3D, right panel). Collectively, these results indicate that deletion of Smad7 in the liver is able to induce apoptosis of hepatocytes, leading to spontaneous liver failure in the mouse.

Smad7 deficiency enhances TGF-β-induced EMT in hepatocytes

We next analyzed the cellular function of Smad7 on epithelial to mesenchymal transition (EMT) in hepatocytes as TGF-β plays a pivotal role in EMT [22]. We isolated primary hepatocytes from

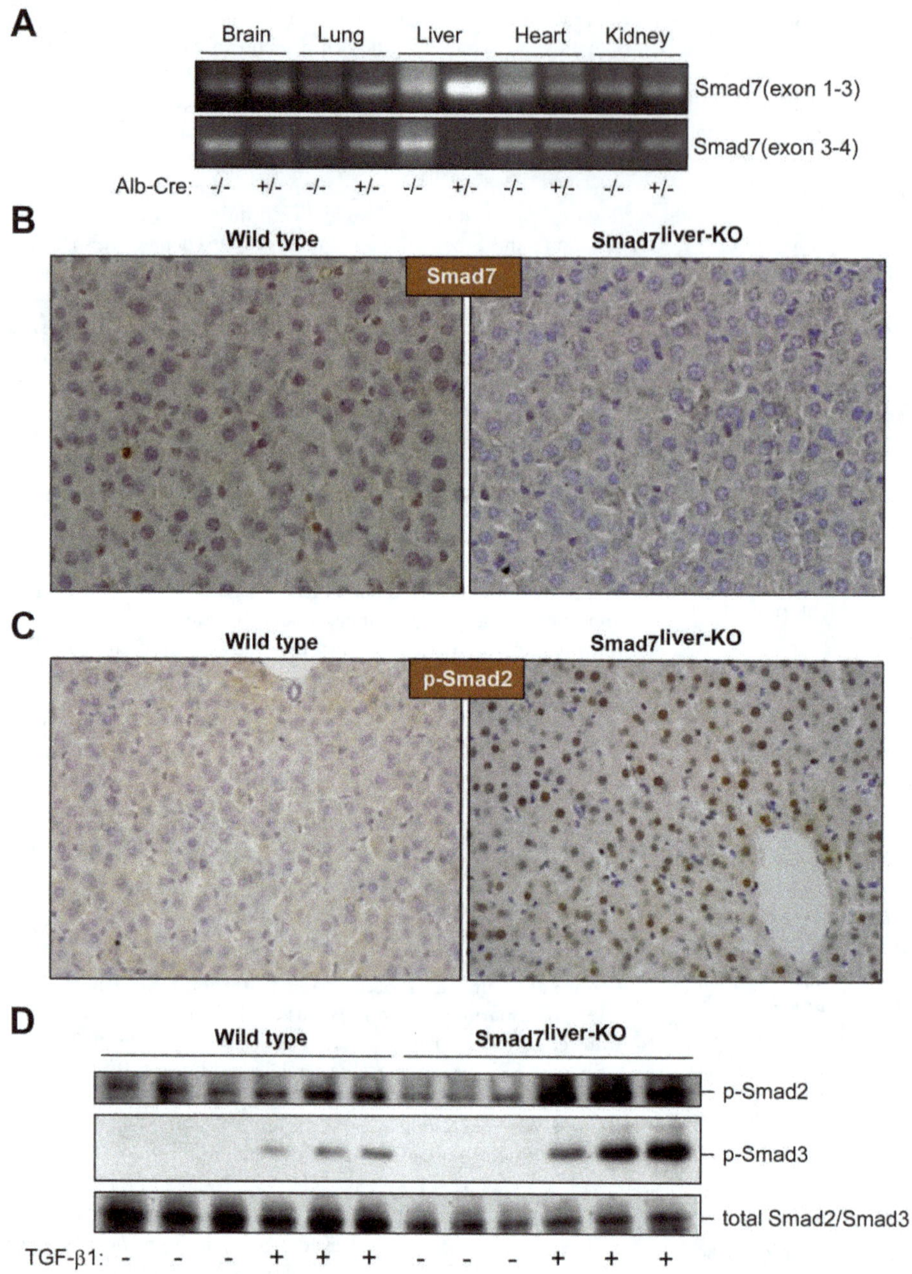

Figure 1. Characterization of Smad7$^{liver-KO}$ mice. (A) Liver-specific deletion of Smad7. RT-PCR analysis was performed with total RNA isolated from multiple tissues in Alb-Cre heterozygous or wild type mice (all mice having Smad7$^{loxP/loxP}$) with specific primers that amplify mRNA regions corresponding to exons 1–3 or exons 3–4 of Smad7 respectively. (B) Analysis of the Smad7 by immunohistochemistry staining. Representative liver sections (400 X) from wild type and Smad7$^{liver-KO}$ mice were used in immunohistochemistry staining with an anti-Smad7 antibody. The nuclei were stained with haematoxylin. (C) Smad2 phosphorylation is elevated in the liver of Smad7$^{liver-KO}$ mice. Smad2 phosphorylation was analyzed by immunohistochemistry using liver sections from either wild type or Smad7$^{liver-KO}$ mice. The nuclei were stained with hematoxylin. Note that nuclear phospho-Smad2 staining is increased in the liver of Smad7$^{liver-KO}$ mice. (D) TGF-β-induced Smad2 and Smad3 phosphorylation is enhanced by Smad7 deletion in primary hepatocytes. Immunoblotting was performed using total protein lysate extracted from primary hepatocytes using antibodies as indicated. The cells were treated with or without 5 ng/ml of TGF-β1 for 24 hours as indicated after overnight serum starvation.

wild type and Smad7$^{liver-KO}$ mice. The cultured hepatocytes isolated from Smad7$^{liver-KO}$ mice did have significant reduction of the mRNA encoded by Smad7 exon 4 (Figure 4A), confirming that Smad7 was successfully deleted in these cells. When the cultured primary hepatocytes were treated with TGF-β1, the cells underwent morphological changes characteristic of EMT (Figure 4B). Untreated hepatocytes exhibited a cuboidal phenotype, while TGF-β1 treatment induced a fibroblastic transition resulting in elongated and spindle-like cell morphology. Interestingly, the TGF-β1-induced EMT morphology was robustly enhanced by Smad7 deletion (Figure 4B, right panel). We also analyzed the cell motility using standard scratch-wound assays as previously described [23]. At 48 h after wounding, the untreated cells from both wild type and Smad7-deleted mice were unable to migrate into the wound area (Figure 4C). TGF-β1 treatment was able to induce migration of the cells and such effect was

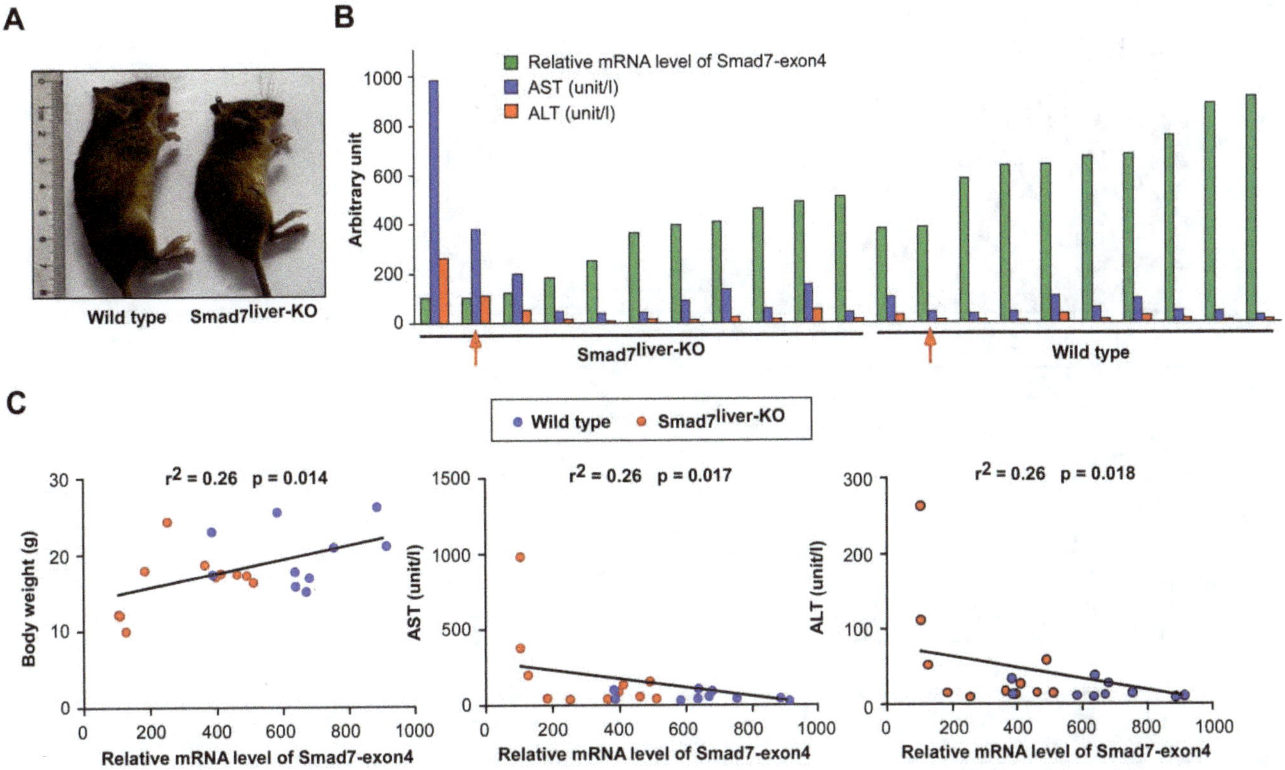

Figure 2. Deletion of Smad7 causes spontaneous liver failure. (A) Representative images of 12-week-old wild type and Smad7$^{liver-KO}$ mice. (B) Relative mRNA level of Smad7 exon4 (green) as comparison with the serum AST (blue) and ALT (red) values. The arrows indicate the mice that were used in histological and immunohistochemical analyses performed in Figure 3. (C) Correlation analyses of body weight, AST and ALT levels with the mRNA level of Smad7 exon4. The values of body weight, AST and ALT values were plotted against the relative mRNA level of Smad7 exon4 for each mouse (red for Smad7$^{liver-KO}$ mice and blue for wild type mice) and subjected to linear regression analysis. n = 11 for Smad7$^{liver-KO}$ and n = 10 for wild type mice.

significantly accelerated when Smad7 was deleted (Figure 4C). TGF-β-induced EMT was further analyzed by immunoblotting to detect expression of E-cadherin and vimentin, two well-recognized markers for EMT [22]. We found that TGF-β1-induced reduction of E-cadherin and increase of vimentin was profoundly enhanced by Smad7 deletion (Figure 4D). These data, therefore, reveal that Smad7 deficiency is able to enhance TGF-β-induced EMT in hepatocytes.

Smad7$^{liver-KO}$ mice are more susceptible to alcohol-induced liver injury and steatosis than wild type mice

We further investigated the potential function of Smad7 deletion on alcohol-induced liver damage. Both the wild type and Smad7$^{liver-KO}$ mice at 10 to 12 weeks old were fed with a liquid diet containing 5% ethanol or a control diet for up to 6 weeks. On the day of animal sacrifice, a single dose of gavage with 10% ethanol or isocaloric maltose dextrin was administered. We first analyzed the expression level of mRNA encoded by exon 4 of Smad7 gene to confirm that Smad7 expression was indeed significantly reduced in the Smad7$^{liver-KO}$ mice (Figure 5A). We tracked the alteration of food intake and body weight for the entire 6-week period and found that there were no significant differences among the four groups in food intake (data not shown), except for a slightly reduced body weight gain in Smad7$^{liver-KO}$ mice (Table 1). Alcohol exposure significantly increased the liver/body weight ratio in both wild type and Smad7$^{liver-KO}$ mice (Table 1). Alcohol exposure decreased the levels of serum triglyceride and cholesterol in wild type mice, while Smad7-deleted mice only had a significant reduction of serum triglyceride but not cholesterol after alcohol administration (Table 1). As expected, alcohol exposure could increase serum ALT and AST activities in the mice (Figure 5B and 5C). However, the alcohol-induced raise of these enzymes was more significant in Smad7$^{liver-KO}$ mice than the wild type animals (Figure 5B and 5C).

We also analyzed the histological changes of the liver. As shown in Figure 5D and 5E, H&E staining and Oil-Red-O staining revealed that hepatic steatosis was induced by chronic alcohol exposure. Furthermore, the alcohol-induced liver steatosis was profoundly enhanced by Smad7 deletion. Consistently, Smad7 deletion led to a significant increase in the content of triglyceride level in the liver upon alcohol exposure (Figure 5F). Together, these data suggest that the liver injury and steatosis induced by chronic alcohol administration were enhanced by Smad7 deletion, further indicating that Smad7 deletion has a deteriorating effect on liver functions.

Smad7 deficiency reduces alcohol-induced ADH1 expression in hepatocytes

Recently, it was reported that over-activation of TGF-β signaling may enhance alcohol-mediated liver damage by reducing expression of alcohol dehydrogenase 1 (ADH1) [24]. In wild type mice, alcohol administration significantly increased the mRNA level of ADH1 in the liver (Figure 6A). Interestingly, alcohol-induced ADH1 upregulation in the liver was slightly reduced in Smad7-deleted mice (Figure 6A). To further confirm the effect of Smad7 deletion on ADH1 expression, we isolated primary

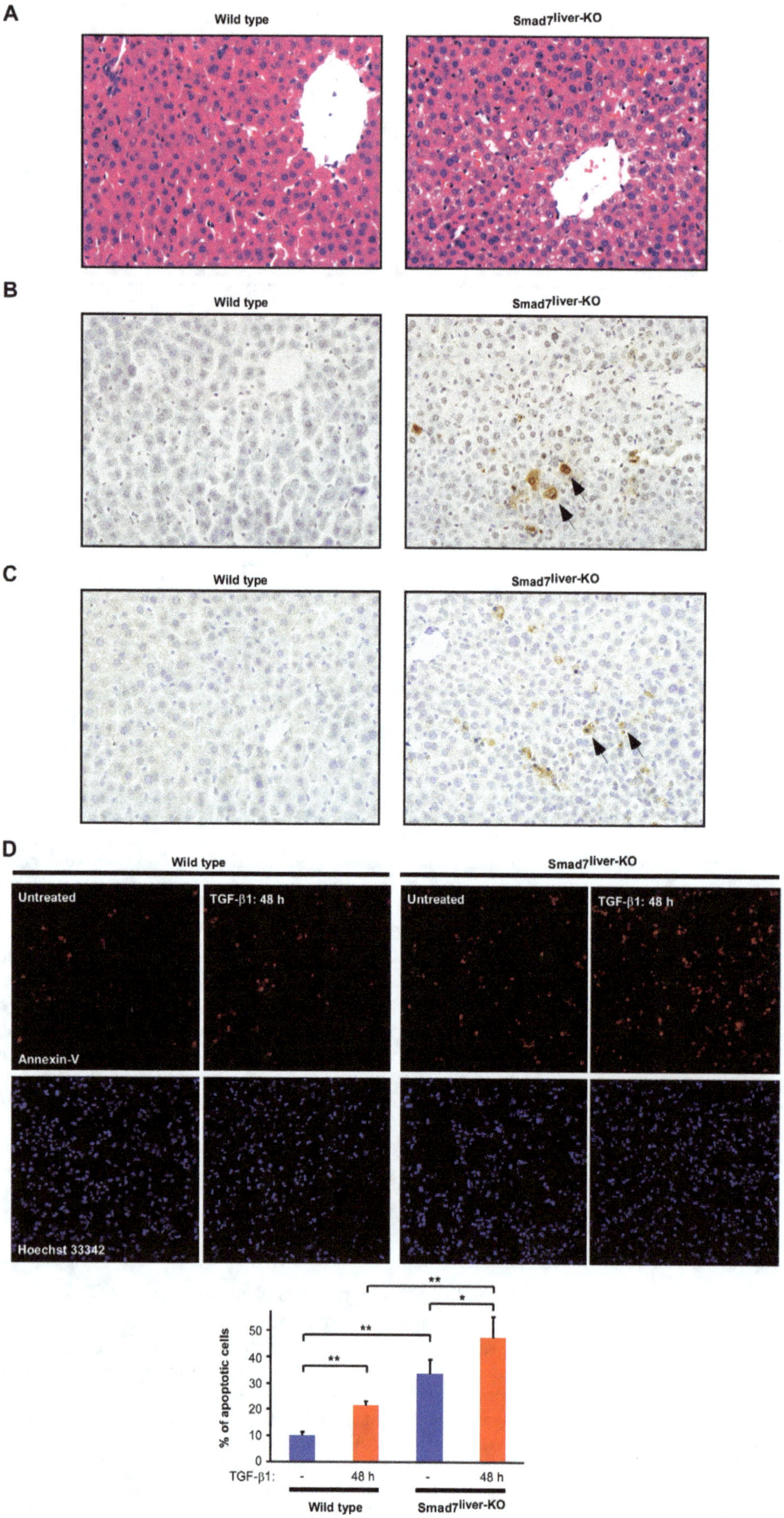
A
Wild type
Smad7liver-KO
B
Wild type
Smad7liver-KO
C
Wild type
Smad7liver-KO
D
Wild type
Smad7liver-KO
Untreated
TGF-β1: 48 h
Untreated
TGF-β1: 48 h
Annexin-V
Hoechst 33342
% of apoptotic cells
50
40
30
20
10
0
**
**
**
*
TGF-β1:
-
48 h
-
48 h
Wild type
Smad7liver-KO

Figure 3. Deletion of Smad7 leads to liver degeneration and apoptosis. (A) Representative images of H&E staining of liver sections are shown with the magnification at X 400. (B) TUNEL assay of liver sections with methyl green as a counter-stain. Representative apoptotic cells are marked by arrows. Note that the Smad7$^{liver\text{-}KO}$ mouse (with liver failure) displayed an increase of apoptosis-positive cells. (C) Immunohistochemistry with an antibody against cleaved caspase-3 to identify apoptotic cells in the liver sections. The arrows indicate apoptotic cells in the liver of Smad7$^{liver\text{-}KO}$ mouse. (D) TGF-β-induced apoptosis is enhanced by Smad7 deletion in hepatocytes. Primary hepatocytes were treated without or with TGF-β1 (5 ng/ml) for 48 h as indicated, followed by immunofluorescence staining with Annexin V for apoptosis (Red) and Hoechst 33342 for nuclei (blue). Quantitation of the percentage of apoptotic cells in each group is shown in the bottom panel as mean ± SD. * indicate $p<0.05$ and ** for $p<0.01$ as comparison between the groups as indicated by Student's t-test.

hepatocytes from the wild type and Smad7$^{liver\text{-}KO}$ mice. The level of mRNA region corresponding to exon 4 of Smad7 gene was significantly reduced in Smad7-deleted hepatocytes, confirming that Smad7 was deleted in these cells (Figure 6C). Alcohol treatment could significantly elevate Smad7 expression (Figure 6B). Furthermore, alcohol administration could stimulate the expression of ADH1 in hepatocytes (Figure 6C). However, the expression level of ADH1 was significantly reduced in Smad7-deleted hepatocytes under both basal and alcohol-treated conditions (Figure 6C), further indicating that Smad7 deletion can reduce AHD1 expression in the liver. As Smad7 deletion is associated with activation of TGF-β signaling (Figure 1), our observation is also constant with the hypothesis that hyperactivity of TGF-β signaling aggravates alcohol-mediated liver injury through down-regulation of ADH1 [24].

Upregulation of lipogenesis- and inflammation-related genes in Smad7$^{liver\text{-}KO}$ mice

It was previously reported that SREBP1c, a key regulator of fatty acid synthesis, is implicated in the development of fatty liver [25,26]. Intriguingly, we found that the expression levels of SREBP1c as well as the critical lipogenic genes controlled by SREBP1c (including fatty acid synthase, stearoyl-CoA desaturase 1, and acetyl-CoA carboxylase-1) were all upregulated by ethanol treatment and by Smad7 deletion (Figure 7A). These results not only indicate that SREBP1c pathway is involved in ethanol-induced hepatic steatosis, but also suggest that Smad7 deletion may aggravate fatty liver formation through upregulation of SREBP1c.

We also analyzed hepatic expression of a series of pro-inflammatory cytokines and chemokines (Figure 7B). We found that chemokines (including CCR2 and F4/80) and a number of proinflammatory cytokines (including TNF-α, IFN-γ, IL-1β, IL-6, MCP-1, MIP1α, and MIP1β) were significantly increased by ethanol feeding in wild type mice, confirming that ethanol is able to successfully induced inflammatory response in the liver. We also found that Smad7 deletion led to significant increase of chemokines (including CCR2 and F4/80) and proinflammatory cytokines (including TNF-α, IFN-γ, IL-1β, IL-6, MCP-1, MIP1α, and MIP1β. These data indicate that deletion of Smad7 is associated with an elevation of inflammatory response in the liver, likely contributing to the observed hepatic dysfunction in Smad7-deleted mice in this study. Furthermore, the ethanol-induced expression of F4/80, IFN-γ and IL-6 was further elevated by Smad7 deletion, indicating that changes of these factors may underlie the aggravated liver dysfunction in Smad7-deleted mice upon ethanol administration.

Discussion

In this study, we established a mouse model with liver-specific deletion of Smad7. We found that functional loss of Smad7 in the liver is associated with hyperactivity of TGF-β signaling, as TGF-β1-induced Smad2/3 phosphorylation and EMT was significantly enhanced by Smad7 deletion (Figure 1 and Figure 4). The Smad7$^{liver\text{-}KO}$ mice with high efficiency of Smad7 deletion had spontaneous liver dysfunction, demonstrated as general deterioration of the body condition and increased serum levels of AST and ALT (Figure 2), accompanied by liver degeneration and an increase in hepatocyte apoptosis (Figure 3). Furthermore, hepatic injury and steatosis induced by chronic alcohol exposure were accelerated by Smad7 deletion (Figure 5). These data, therefore, reveal for the first time that loss of endogenous Smad7 in the liver can result in spontaneous liver dysfunction and enhance ethanol-induced liver injury.

Our results are consistent with a few recent studies pinpointing the functional role of Smad7 in liver diseases. Overexpression of Smad7 in mouse liver could attenuate TGF-β signaling and TGF-β-induced EMT, while improve CCl_4-provoked liver fibrosis [19]. On the other hand, hypomorphic Smad7 deficiency could enhance CCl_4-induced liver damage and fibrosis [20]. The liver damage imposed by Smad7 deletion as observed in this study and by Hamzavi, *et al* is likely mediated by hyperactivity of TGF-β signaling, as overexpression of TGF-β1 specifically in mouse liver leads to increases in hepatic fibrosis and hepatocyte apoptosis [27]. However, unlike this study, spontaneous liver dysfunction was not observed with hypomorphic Smad7 deficiency [20]. We speculate that the difference is dependent on the magnitude of Smad7 deletion. Deletion of the MH1 domain of Smad7 gene only leads to partial loss of Smad7 function [18]. In our study, we found that spontaneous liver dysfunction only occur in Smad7$^{liver\text{-}KO}$ mice with high degree of Smad7 deletion (Figure 2). It is speculated that the function of Smad7 needs to be lost to certain degree to initiate spontaneous liver damage in the mouse.

TGF-β is considered one of the most important growth factors that induce EMT process [22,28,29]. Activated Smad proteins upon binding of TGF-β to its receptors act as transcription factors to induce expression of EMT-inducing transcription factors within the Snail, ZEB and bHLH families [29]. It has been reported that EMT plays a critical role in the repair of liver tissues after damage and the pathogenesis of liver fibrosis [30]. In this study, we found that loss of Smad7 is associated with enhancement of TGF-β-induced EMT in hepatocytes, consistent with the idea that Smad7 deletion is associated with hyperactivity of TGF-β signaling. Our results are also consistent with the report demonstrating that partial loss of Smad7 function can increase EMT in the liver and accelerates CCl_4-induced liver fibrosis [20]. It is also in agreement with the finding that overexpression of Smad7 in the liver can inhibit EMT and attenuate TGF-β-mediated fibrogenesis [19]. However, it is noteworthy that whether hepatocytes can directly convert into mesenchymal cells is still controversial. Recently, it was reported that neither hepatocytes nor cholangiocytes could undergo EMT and contribute to liver fibrosis *in vivo* [31,32].

It is well known that liver is the major organ for detoxification of many chemicals including alcohol. It was recently found that there exist a functional interplay between alcohol-induced liver damage and TGF-β signaling [24]. TGF-β is induced in the mouse liver upon chronic alcohol administration. Interestingly, TGF-β is able to downregulate a key alcohol metabolizing enzyme ADH1 and it is proposed that TGF-β imposes its pro-steatotic action by decreasing the expression of ADH1 in the liver [24]. In our study, we also found that loss of Smad7 function is accompanied by enhancement of

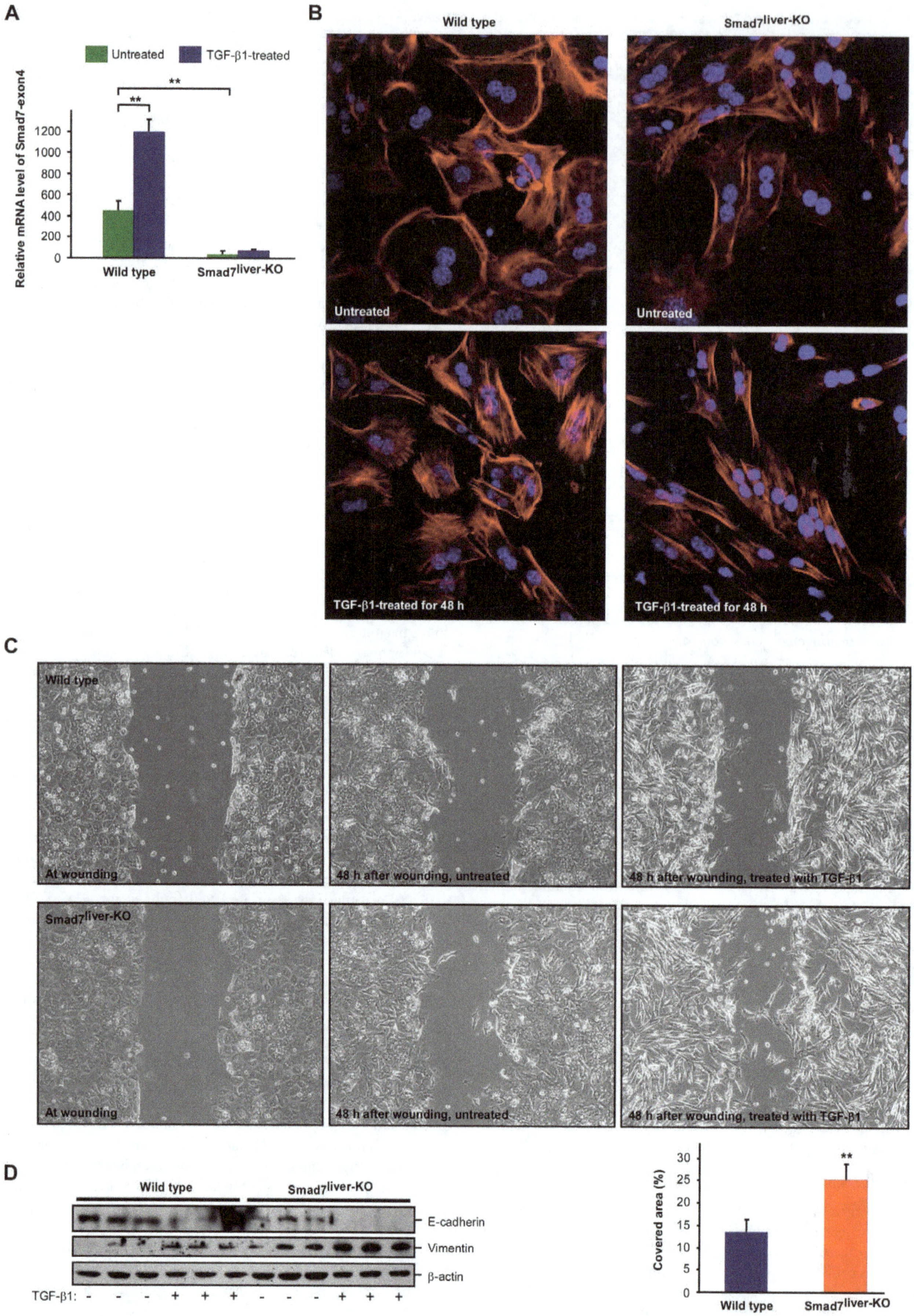
A
Untreated
TGF-β1-treated
Relative mRNA level of Smad7-exon4
**
**
1200
1000
800
600
400
200
0
Wild type
Smad7liver-KO
B
Wild type
Smad7liver-KO
Untreated
Untreated
TGF-β1-treated for 48 h
TGF-β1-treated for 48 h
C
Wild type
At wounding
48 h after wounding, untreated
48 h after wounding, treated with TGF-β1
Smad7liver-KO
At wounding
48 h after wounding, untreated
48 h after wounding, treated with TGF-β1
Covered area (%)
30
25
20
15
10
5
0
**
Wild type
Smad7liver-KO
D
Wild type
Smad7liver-KO
E-cadherin
Vimentin
β-actin
TGF-β1: - - - + + + - - - + + +

Figure 4. Deletion of Smad7 enhances TGF-β-induced EMT. (A) Confirmation of Smad7 deletion in primary hepatocytes isolated from $Smad7^{liver\text{-}KO}$ mouse. Real time RT-PCR was performed with total RNA isolated from wild type or $Smad7^{liver\text{-}KO}$ mice with primers to detect the mRNA region corresponding to exon4 of Smad7 gene. The data are shown as mean ± SD and ** indicates $p<0.01$ as comparison between the groups as indicated by Student's t-test. (B) TGF-β-induced EMT-like morphology changes. Immunofluorescence labeling were performed with wild type or $Smad7^{liver\text{-}KO}$ hepatocytes treated with or without TGF-β1 (5 ng/ml) for 48 h. F-actin was stained with fluorescein isothiocyanate-labeled phalloidin (Red) and the nuclei were labeled by Hoechst 33342 (Blue). (C) Analysis of cell motility by a wound-healing assay. Cultured primary hepatocytes were analyzed by phase contrast microscopy. The cells were treated with or without TGF-β1 (5 ng/ml) for 48 h. Quantitation of the cell motility is shown in lower right panel as mean ± SD and ** indicates $p<0.01$ by Student's t-test. (D) Analysis of EMT markers E-cadherin and vimentin. Primary hepatocytes were treated with or without TGF-β1 (5 ng/ml) for 48 h and the cell lysate was used in immunoblotting with the antibodies as indicated.

alcoholic hepatic steatosis (Figure 5), further indicating the importance of TGF-β signaling in the development of alcohol-induced liver damage. Furthermore, we found that Smad7 deletion is associated with significant reduction of alcohol-induced ADH1 expression in the liver (Figure 6), underscoring the importance of ADH1 in mediating liver injury imposed by hyperactivity of TGF-β signaling.

In addition to the regulation of ADH1 by Smad7 in the liver, we also found that ethanol treatment and Smad7 deletion had evident effects on the expression of a series of genes involved in lipogenesis and inflammatory response (Figure 7). On the one hand, ethanol administration was able to significantly elevate the expression of SREBP1c and its target genes involved in fatty acid synthesis (Figure 7A). This finding is consistent with the notion that SREBP1c is a key regulator of fatty acid synthesis and implicated in the development of fatty liver [25,26]. Interestingly, the expression of SREBP1c and its target genes involved in fatty acid synthesis was also elevated by Smad7 deletion, indicating that Smad7 deletion may aggravate fatty liver development through upregulation of SREBP1c. On the other hand, we observed that the expression of a series of inflammation-related genes was altered by ethanol treatment and Smad7 deletion (Figure 7B). Chemokines (including CCR2 and F4/80) and a number of proinflammatory cytokines (including TNF-α, IFN-γ, IL-1β, IL-6, MCP-1, MIP1α, and MIP1β) were all elevated by either ethanol treatment or Smad7 deletion. Furthermore, ethanol treatment and Smad7 deletion had a synergistic effect to induce expression of F4/80, IFN-γ and IL-6, indicating that these factors may underlie the aggravated liver dysfunction in Smad7-deleted mice upon ethanol

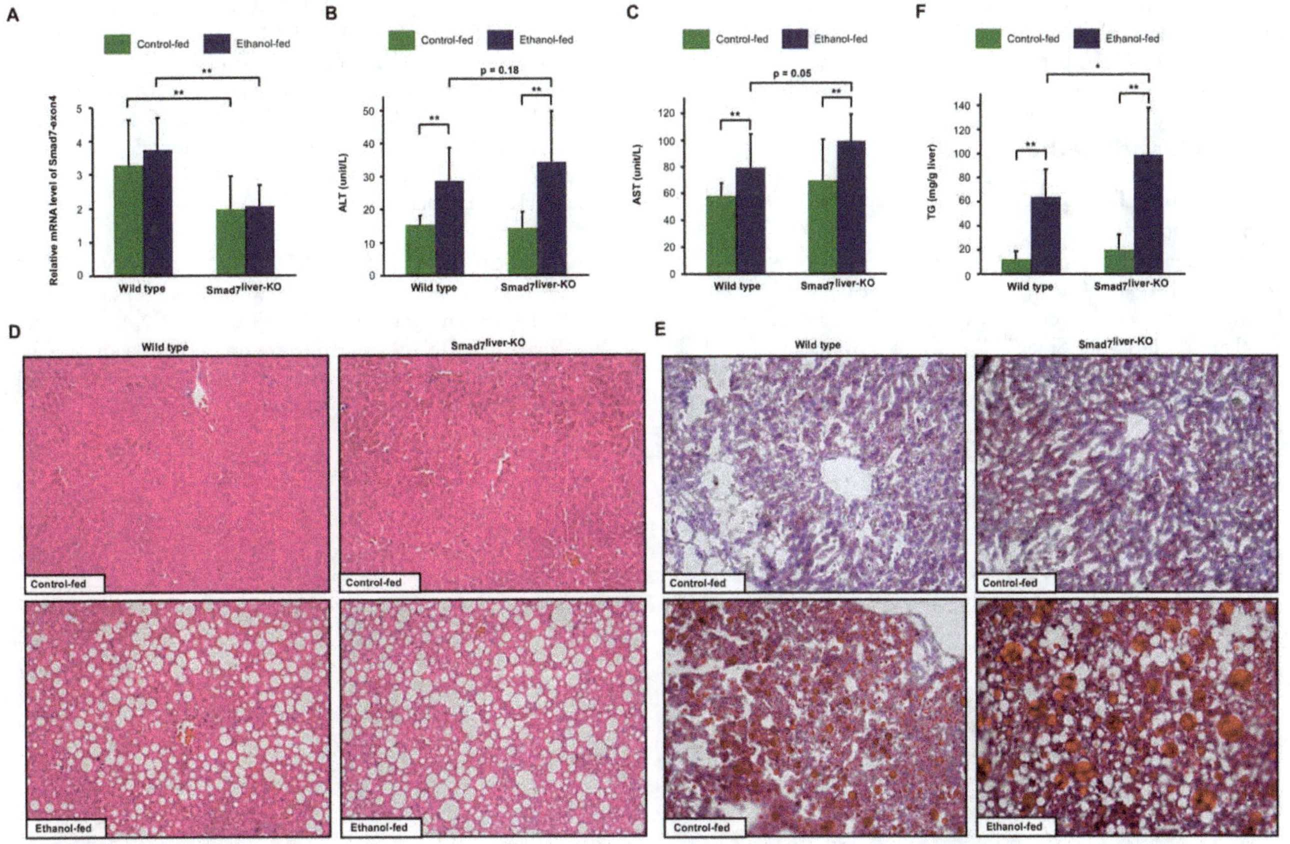

Figure 5. Alcohol-induced liver injury and steatosis were aggravated in $Smad7^{liver\text{-}KO}$ mice. (A) Confirmation of Smad7 deletion. Wild type and $Smad7^{liver\text{-}KO}$ mice were fed with control or ethanol-containing diet for 6 weeks, followed by a single gavage of 10% ethanol or maltose respectively (8 mice per group). Real time RT-PCR was performed with total RNA isolated from the mice with primers to detect the mRNA region corresponding to exon4 of Smad7 gene. (B) and (C) Measurement of serum ALT and AST. The data are shown as mean ± SD and ** indicates $p<0.01$ by Student's t-test. (D) Histological analysis of the liver. Representative images of H&E staining are shown for each group of mice. Please note that fatty liver degeneration induced by alcohol administration is enhanced in $Smad7^{liver\text{-}KO}$ mice. (E) Oil-Red-O staining of the liver. (F) Triglyceride level of the liver. The data are shown as mean ± SD. * and ** indicates $p<0.05$ and $p<0.01$ respectively.

Table 1. Physiological and serum parameters of mice upon chronic-binge alcohol exposure.

Parameters	Wild type		Smad7$^{liver-KO}$	
	Control-fed	Ethanol-fed	Control-fed	Ethanol-fed
Body weight-initial (g)	23.68±2.65	23.74±3.04	23.46±2.35	22.58±2.03
Body weight-end (g)	24.85±2.78	24.28±4.20	26.61±4.24	23.13±2.65
Body weight-gain (g)	1.18±2.59	0.54±2.24	3.15±2.21	0.55±1.71$^{\$\$}$
Liver weight (g)	0.93±0.10	1.11±0.24	0.98±0.18	1.09±0.11
Liver weight/body weight (%)	3.70±0.34	4.64±0.63$^{\#\#}$	3.61±0.54	4.80±0.56$^{\$\$}$
EWAT (g)	0.65±0.28	0.49±0.24	0.71±0.32	0.56±0.20
EWAT/body weight (%)	2.52±0.88	1.95±0.72	2.52±0.77	2.40±0.67
Blood triglyceride (mg/ml)	0.73±0.27	0.45±0.22$^{\#}$	0.80±0.35	0.47±0.10$^{\$}$
Blood cholesterol (mmol/L)	2.41±0.50	1.72±0.22$^{\#\#}$	2.17±0.52	1.89±0.47

EWAT: Epididymal white adipose tissue.
The data are shown as means ± SD (n = 8 for each group).
$^{\#}$and $^{\#\#}$: comparison between control-fed and ethanol-fed wild type mice. $^{\#}$ for $p<0.05$ and $^{\#\#}$ for $p<0.01$.
$^{\$}$and $^{\$\$}$: comparison between control-fed and ethanol-fed Smad7$^{Liver-KO}$ mice. $^{\$}$ for $p<0.05$ and $^{\$\$}$ for $p<0.01$.

administration. Combining these results, we propose that the alteration of ethanol metabolism, lipogenesis and inflammatory response caused by Smad7 deletion may act together to contribute to severe alcoholic liver injury and steatosis in Smad7-deleted mice. In this regard, our model of liver-specific deletion of Smad7 can serve as a useful tool to comprehend the biological function of endogenous Smad7 in the liver as well as in liver diseases.

Materials and Methods

Generation of liver-specific Smad7 deletion mice and genotyping

All animal procedures and protocols were approved by the Institutional Animal Care and Use Committee of the Institute for Nutritional Sciences, Chinese Academy of Sciences with approval number 2010-AN-8. Smad7$^{loxP/loxP}$ mice were developed as previously described [17]. Liver specific deletion of Smad7 mice (Smad7$^{liver-KO}$) were generated by crossing Smad7$^{loxP/loxP}$ mice with Alb-Cre mice that contain a *Cre* recombinase driven by albumin promoter (the Jackson Laboratory, Bar Harbor, ME, USA). Tail biopsies of the mice were analyzed by genomic PCR. The presence of Smad7-loxP allele was detected by primer A (5′-TGTCCCGCTTGTCTTGTTCTTTGAG-3′) and primer G (5′-CAGAGCAGCCGATTGTCTGTTGTGC-3′), resulting in a ~500-bp PCR product. The wild-type allele was detected by primers A and B (5′-TGCTGACTCTCGTTTCCTGTCTTCG-3′), giving rise to a 154-bp product. The genotyping of Alb-Cre transgenic mouse was performed following the protocol provided by the Jackson Laboratory.

RNA isolation, RT-PCR and real-time quantitative PCR

Total RNA from mouse tissues was isolated using TRIzol reagent (Invitrogen, Carlsbad, CA, USA). The RNA was treated with RNase-free DNase I and reverse-transcribed with oligo(dT) primer using the SuperScript First-Strand Synthesis System for RT-PCR (Invitrogen). Oligonucleotide primers used for RT-PCR to

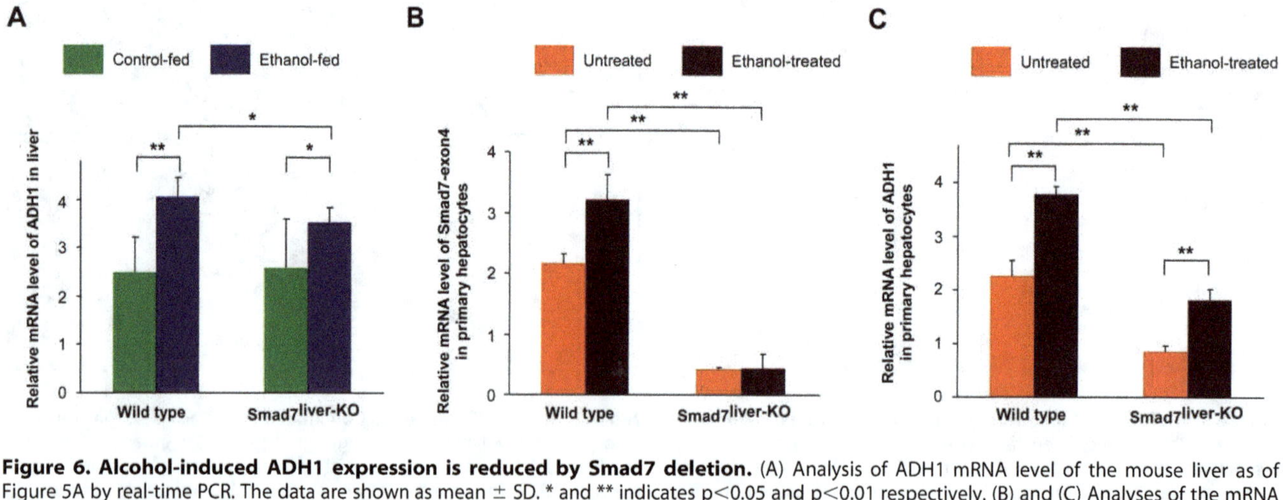

Figure 6. Alcohol-induced ADH1 expression is reduced by Smad7 deletion. (A) Analysis of ADH1 mRNA level of the mouse liver as of Figure 5A by real-time PCR. The data are shown as mean ± SD. * and ** indicates $p<0.05$ and $p<0.01$ respectively. (B) and (C) Analyses of the mRNA levels of Smad7 and ADH1 in primary hepatocytes. Primary hepatocytes isolated from wild type and Smad7$^{liver-KO}$ mice were incubated with or without ethanol (100 mmol/L) for 24 h. The mRNA were isolated and used in real-time PCR. The data are shown as mean ± SD with * for $p<0.05$ and ** for $p<0.01$ between the groups as indicated.

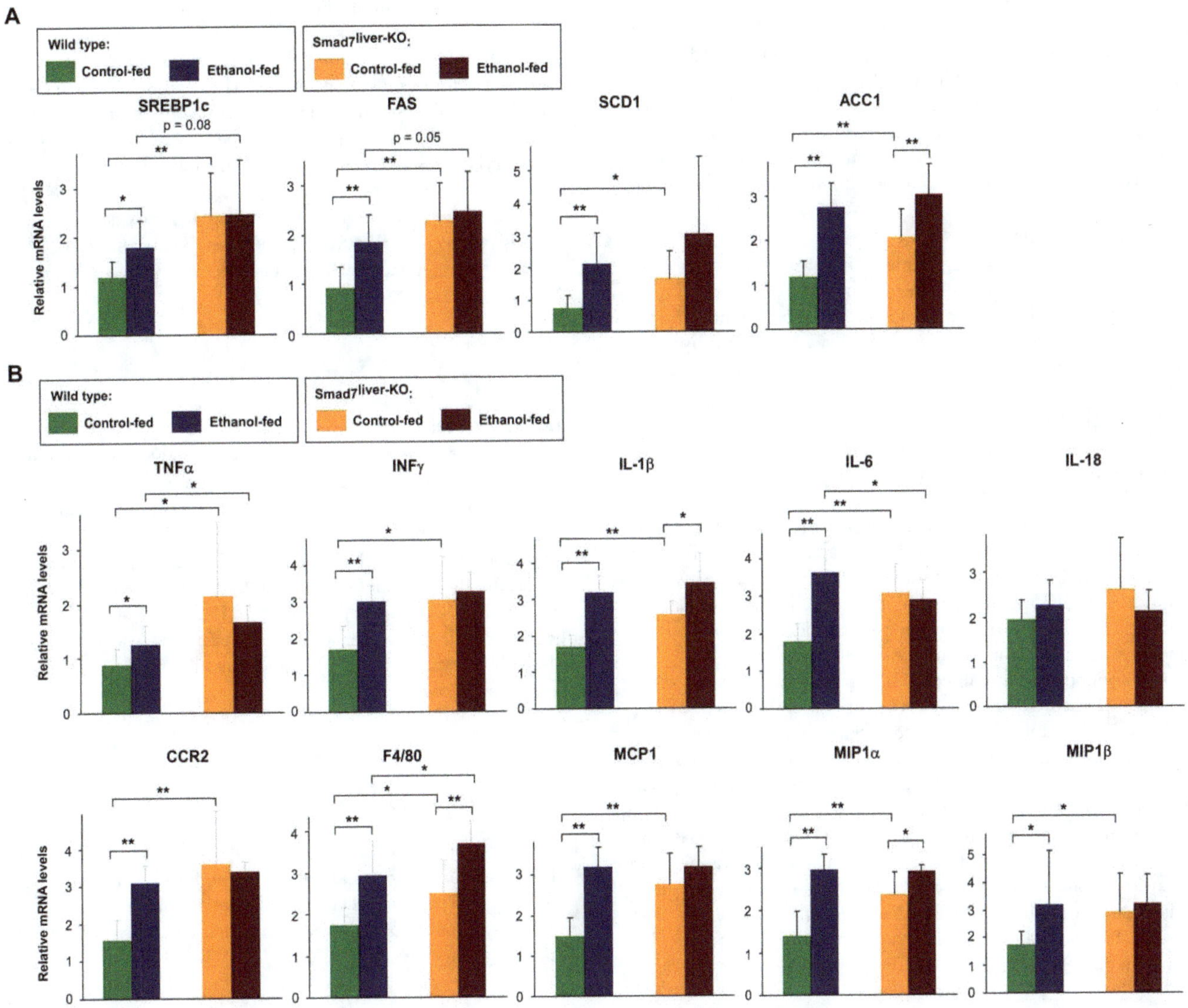

Figure 7. Upregulation of lipogenesis- and inflammation-related genes by ethanol treatment and Smad7 deletion. (A) Analysis of the mRNA levels of critical lipogenic genes of the mouse liver by real-time RT-PCR. Alcohol-feeding of the mice was as described in Figure 5A. The data are shown as mean ± SD. * and ** indicates $p<0.05$ and $p<0.01$ respectively. (B) Analysis of the mRNA levels of a series of inflammation-related factors by real-time RT-PCR with the samples as in Figure 5A. The data are shown as mean ± SD with * for $p<0.05$ and ** for $p<0.01$ between the groups as indicated.

detect Smad7 mRNA were: 5′-AAGTGTTCAGGTGGCCG-GATCTCAG-3′ and 5′-ACAGCATCTGGACAGCCTGCAGT-TG-3′ for exon 1-3 of Smad7, 5′-CAACTGCAGGCTGTCCA-GATGCTGTAC-3′ and 5′-GTAAACCCACACGCCATCCAC-TTCC-3′ for exon 3–4 of Smad7. Quantitative real-time PCR was done with the SYBR Green PCR system (Applied Biosystems, Foster City, CA, USA), using actin as an internal control for normalization. Primers used for each gene are listed as follows: 5′-CTCCTCCTTTCTCGTCATCC-3′ and 5′- CACACACACAA-CCCAACAAA-3′ for the mRNA region corresponding to exon 4 of Smad7, 5′-GGCCGCCTTGACACCAT-3′ and 5′-GCACTCC-TACGACGACGCTTA-3′ for ADH-1, 5′-GATCATTGCTCC-TCCTGAGC-3′ and 5′-ACTCCTGCTTGCTGATCCAC-3′ for β-actin. Other primers used in this study are listed in Table S1.

Mouse model of chronic-binge ethanol consumption

The chronic alcohol-fed mouse model was established as previously described with minor modification [21,33]. In brief, 10 to 12 weeks old male mice were fed with a nutritionally adequate liquid diet containing 5% ethanol or a control diet for up to 6 weeks (Dyets, Inc., Bethlehem, PA, USA). Both diets were dispensed in glass liquid-diet feeding tubes. Ethanol was introduced gradually by increasing the content by 1% (vol/vol) every day until the mice were consuming diet containing 5% (vol/vol) ethanol for up to 6 weeks. After that, the mice of ethanol-treated group were gavaged with a single doses of ethanol (5 g/kg body weight, 10% ethanol), whereas mice in control groups were gavaged with isocaloric dextrin maltose. After gavage, mice were kept on control or ethanol diet and euthanized 6 hours later.

Isolation of primary mouse hepatocytes

Mouse hepatocytes were isolated from livers of 8-week-old mice by a modified two-step collagenase perfusion protocol [34]. In brief, the hepatocytes were plated on collagen I coated 6-well plates (3×10^5 cells/well) in Dulbecco modified Eagle medium-F-12 (DMEM, from GIBCO-BRL, Gaithersburg, MD, USA) with supplements as described previously [35]. The medium was changed after 4 h with DMEM supplemented with 1% penicillin/streptomycin. For TGF-β1 treatment, the cell culture medium was changed to serum-free DMEM with 1% penicillin/streptomycin and 5 ng/ml TGF-β1 (Sigma–Aldrich, St. Louis, MO, USA) was added as indicated. For ethanol treatment, 100 mmol/L ethanol was added in fresh medium for 24 hours. The plates were sealed with parafilm to prevent evaporation after the addition of ethanol.

Cell motility assay

Primary hepatocytes were plated on collagen I-coated 6-well plates (3×10^5 cells/well) and then "wounded" by scratching the cells with a 200 µl pipette tip in the presence or absence of TGF-β1 after attachment and then monitored in 24 and 48 h by phase-contrast microscope photography as described previously [23].

Immunoblotting analysis

For Western blotting analysis, the cells and tissues were lysed in a radioimmunoprecipitation assay (RIPA) buffer (150 mmol/L NaCl, 1% Triton X-100, 0.5% sodium deoxycholate, 0.1% SDS, 50 mmol/L Tris-HCl at pH 7.4) containing phosphatase inhibitors and a protease inhibitor cocktail (Sigma-Aldrich). The lysate was subjected to SDS-PAGE, transferred to polyvinylidene fluoride (PVDF) membranes, and incubated with the primary antibodies, followed by horseradish peroxidase-conjugated secondary antibody (Amersham, Little Chalfont, Bucks, UK). The bound antibody was visualised using enhanced chemiluminescence reagents (Pierce, Rockford, USA). The antibodies used were as follows: rabbit anti-actin antibody (Santa Cruz Biotechnology, Santa Cruz, CA, USA), goat anti-Smad7 antibody (Santa Cruz Biotechnology), rabbit anti-phosphorylated-Smad2 antibody (Cell Signaling Technology, Beverly, MA, USA), rabbit anti-phosphorylated-Smad3 antibody (Cell Signaling Technology), goat anti-Smad2/3 antibody (Santa Cruz Biotechnology), rabbit anti-cleaved-caspase-3 antibody (Cell Signaling Technology), mouse anti-E-cadherin antibody (BD Transduction Laboratories, New Jersey, USA), and mouse anti-vimentin antibody (Santa Cruz Biotechnology).

Analysis of blood and tissue samples

The serum levels of alanine transaminase (ALT), aspartate transaminase (AST) and total cholesterol (TC) were determined by a kit from ShenSuoYouFu (Shanghai, China). Triglycerides were determined by the Serum Triglyceride Determination Kit (Sigma-Aldrich). The measurement of hepatic triglyceride was following a protocol as previously reported [36]. About 40–60 mg of liver tissue was homogenized in a total of 4 ml of a mixture of $CHCl_3$-CH_3OH (2:1, v/v). After addition of 1 ml 0.88% NaCl, the homogenate was centrifuged at 3700 rpm for 10 min at room temperature. The portion at the lower organic phase was transferred to a new tube and dried under nitrogen. The dried residue was resuspended in 1 ml of 1% Triton X-100 in absolute ethanol.

Histology and immunohistochemistry

Following fixation of the livers with 10% formalin/phosphate-buffered saline, paraffin-embedded sections were subjected to standard Hematoxylin & Eosin (H&E) staining. Hepatic lipid content was determined by 10 µm thick frozen sections stained with Oil Red O (Sigma–Aldrich). The immunohistochemistry was performed with 5 µm sections using SABC (mouse/rabbit IgG) kit according to the manufacturer's instruction (Boster, Wuhan, Hubei, China). The primary antibodies used were as follows: phosphorylated Smad2 (1:200, Cell Signaling Technology) and cleaved caspase-3 (1:1000, Cell Signaling Technology). TUNEL assay was carried out using ApopTagH Peroxidase In Situ Apoptosis Detection Kit (from Chemicon, Temecula, CA, USA) following the manufacturer's instructions.

Annexin V staining

Hepatocytes were plated on coverslips (~80,000 cells per well in 6 well plates). After overnight serum starvation, cells were treated with 5 ng/mL TGF-β1 as indicated. Residual culture medium was washed off the cells with phosphate-buffered saline. Cells were stained for 5 minutes with Annexin V-PE Apoptosis Detection Kit (BioVision Inc., Mountain View, CA, USA) and 5 µg/mL Hoechst 33342 (Molecular Probes, Eugene, OR, USA) in phosphate-buffered saline. Unbound stain was washed off the cells with phosphate-buffered saline, and fluorescent signal was detected immediately.

Immunofluorescence

Immunofluorescence staining was performed as described previously [37]. Fluorescein isothiocyanate-phalloidin (Sigma-Aldrich) was used to detect F-actin. Cell nuclei were counter-stained with Hoechst 33342.

Statistical analysis

Statistically significance was assessed by one-way ANOVA or Student's t test.

Author Contributions

Conceived and designed the experiments: LZ YC. Performed the experiments: LZ LW XW XL LY RZ YP. Analyzed the data: LZ YC. Contributed reagents/materials/analysis tools: HY DX. Wrote the paper: LZ YC.

References

1. Murray KF, Hadzic N, Wirth S, Bassett M, Kelly D (2008) Drug-related hepatotoxicity and acute liver failure. J Pediatr Gastroenterol Nutr 47: 395–405.
2. Castilla A, Prieto J, Fausto N (1991) Transforming growth factors beta 1 and alpha in chronic liver disease. Effects of interferon alfa therapy. N Engl J Med 324: 933–940.
3. Massague J (1998) TGF-beta signal transduction. Annu Rev Biochem 67: 753–791.
4. Heldin CH, Miyazono K, ten Dijke P (1997) TGF-beta signalling from cell membrane to nucleus through SMAD proteins. Nature 390: 465–471.

5. Miyazono K, Kusanagi K, Inoue H (2001) Divergence and convergence of TGF-beta/BMP signaling. J Cell Physiol 187: 265–276.
6. Wrana JL, Attisano L, Carcamo J, Zentella A, Doody J, et al. (1992) TGF beta signals through a heteromeric protein kinase receptor complex. Cell 71: 1003–1014.
7. Hayashi H, Abdollah S, Qiu Y, Cai J, Xu YY, et al. (1997) The MAD-related protein Smad7 associates with the TGFbeta receptor and functions as an antagonist of TGFbeta signaling. Cell 89: 1165–1173.
8. Weinstein M, Yang X, Deng C (2000) Functions of mammalian Smad genes as revealed by targeted gene disruption in mice. Cytokine Growth Factor Rev 11: 49–58.
9. Tremblay KD, Dunn NR, Robertson EJ (2001) Mouse embryos lacking Smad1 signals display defects in extra-embryonic tissues and germ cell formation. Development 128: 3609–3621.
10. Waldrip WR, Bikoff EK, Hoodless PA, Wrana JL, Robertson EJ (1998) Smad2 signaling in extraembryonic tissues determines anterior-posterior polarity of the early mouse embryo. Cell 92: 797–808.
11. Takaku K, Oshima M, Miyoshi H, Matsui M, Seldin MF, et al. (1998) Intestinal tumorigenesis in compound mutant mice of both Dpc4 (Smad4) and Apc genes. Cell 92: 645–656.
12. Zhu Y, Richardson JA, Parada LF, Graff JM (1998) Smad3 mutant mice develop metastatic colorectal cancer. Cell 94: 703–714.
13. Yang X, Letterio JJ, Lechleider RJ, Chen L, Hayman R, et al. (1999) Targeted disruption of SMAD3 results in impaired mucosal immunity and diminished T cell responsiveness to TGF-beta. EMBO J 18: 1280–1291.
14. Chang H, Huylebroeck D, Verschueren K, Guo Q, Matzuk MM, et al. (1999) Smad5 knockout mice die at mid-gestation due to multiple embryonic and extraembryonic defects. Development 126: 1631–1642.
15. Huang Z, Wang D, Ihida-Stansbury K, Jones PL, Martin JF (2009) Defective pulmonary vascular remodeling in Smad8 mutant mice. Hum Mol Genet 18: 2791–2801.
16. Galvin KM, Donovan MJ, Lynch CA, Meyer RI, Paul RJ, et al. (2000) A role for smad6 in development and homeostasis of the cardiovascular system. Nat Genet 24: 171–174.
17. Chen Q, Chen H, Zheng D, Kuang C, Fang H, et al. (2009) Smad7 is required for the development and function of the heart. J Biol Chem 284: 292–300.
18. Li R, Rosendahl A, Brodin G, Cheng AM, Ahgren A, et al. (2006) Deletion of exon I of SMAD7 in mice results in altered B cell responses. J Immunol 176: 6777–6784.
19. Dooley S, Hamzavi J, Ciuclan L, Godoy P, Ilkavets I, et al. (2008) Hepatocyte-specific Smad7 expression attenuates TGF-beta-mediated fibrogenesis and protects against liver damage. Gastroenterology 135: 642–659.
20. Hamzavi J, Ehnert S, Godoy P, Ciuclan L, Weng H, et al. (2008) Disruption of the Smad7 gene enhances CCI4-dependent liver damage and fibrogenesis in mice. J Cell Mol Med 12: 2130–2144.
21. Horiguchi N, Wang L, Mukhopadhyay P, Park O, Jeong WI, et al. (2008) Cell type-dependent pro- and anti-inflammatory role of signal transducer and activator of transcription 3 in alcoholic liver injury. Gastroenterology 134: 1148–1158.
22. Kalluri R, Weinberg RA (2009) The basics of epithelial-mesenchymal transition. J Clin Invest 119: 1420–1428.
23. Cano A, Perez-Moreno MA, Rodrigo I, Locascio A, Blanco MJ, et al. (2000) The transcription factor snail controls epithelial-mesenchymal transitions by repressing E-cadherin expression. Nat Cell Biol 2: 76–83.
24. Ciuclan L, Ehnert S, Ilkavets I, Weng HL, Gaitantzi H, et al. (2010) TGF-beta enhances alcohol dependent hepatocyte damage via down-regulation of alcohol dehydrogenase I. J Hepatol 52: 407–416.
25. Horton JD, Goldstein JL, Brown MS (2002) SREBPs: activators of the complete program of cholesterol and fatty acid synthesis in the liver. J Clin Invest 109: 1125–1131.
26. Ji C, Chan C, Kaplowitz N (2006) Predominant role of sterol response element binding proteins (SREBP) lipogenic pathways in hepatic steatosis in the murine intragastric ethanol feeding model. J Hepatol 45: 717–724.
27. Sanderson N, Factor V, Nagy P, Kopp J, Kondaiah P, et al. (1995) Hepatic expression of mature transforming growth factor beta 1 in transgenic mice results in multiple tissue lesions. Proc Natl Acad Sci U S A 92: 2572–2576.
28. Miettinen PJ, Ebner R, Lopez AR, Derynck R (1994) TGF-beta induced transdifferentiation of mammary epithelial cells to mesenchymal cells: involvement of type I receptors. J Cell Biol 127: 2021–2036.
29. Xu J, Lamouille S, Derynck R (2009) TGF-beta-induced epithelial to mesenchymal transition. Cell Res 19: 156–172.
30. Choi SS, Diehl AM (2009) Epithelial-to-mesenchymal transitions in the liver. Hepatology 50: 2007–2013.
31. Taura K, Miura K, Iwaisako K, Osterreicher CH, Kodama Y, et al. (2010) Hepatocytes do not undergo epithelial-mesenchymal transition in liver fibrosis in mice. Hepatology 51: 1027–1036.
32. Scholten D, Osterreicher CH, Scholten A, Iwaisako K, Gu G, et al. (2010) Genetic labeling does not detect epithelial-to-mesenchymal transition of cholangiocytes in liver fibrosis in mice. Gastroenterology 139: 987–998.
33. Ki SH, Park O, Zheng M, Morales-Ibanez O, Kolls JK, et al. (2010) Interleukin-22 treatment ameliorates alcoholic liver injury in a murine model of chronic-binge ethanol feeding: role of signal transducer and activator of transcription 3. Hepatology 52: 1291–1300.
34. Neufeld DS (1997) Isolation of rat liver hepatocytes. Methods Mol Biol 75: 145–151.
35. Bottinger EP, Factor VM, Tsang ML, Weatherbee JA, Kopp JB, et al. (1996) The recombinant proregion of transforming growth factor beta1 (latency-associated peptide) inhibits active transforming growth factor beta1 in transgenic mice. Proc Natl Acad Sci U S A 93: 5877–5882.
36. Yang L, Zhang Y, Wang L, Fan F, Zhu L, et al. (2010) Amelioration of high fat diet induced liver lipogenesis and hepatic steatosis by interleukin-22. J Hepatol 53: 339–347.
37. Zavadil J, Cermak L, Soto-Nieves N, Bottinger EP (2004) Integration of TGF-beta/Smad and Jagged1/Notch signalling in epithelial-to-mesenchymal transition. EMBO J 23: 1155–1165.

17

Comprehensive miRNA Expression Analysis in Peripheral Blood can Diagnose Liver Disease

Yoshiki Murakami[1]*, Hidenori Toyoda[2], Toshihito Tanahashi[3], Junko Tanaka[4], Takashi Kumada[2], Yusuke Yoshioka[5], Nobuyoshi Kosaka[5], Takahiro Ochiya[5], Y-h Taguchi[6]

1 Department of Hepatology, Graduate School of Medicine, Osaka City University, Osaka, Japan, **2** Department of Gastroenterology, Ogaki Municipal Hospital, Ogaki, Japan, **3** Department of Medical Pharmaceutics, Kobe Pharmaceutical University, Kobe, Japan, **4** Department of Epidemiology, Infectious Disease Control and Prevention, Hiroshima University Graduate School of Biomedical Sciences, Hiroshima, Japan, **5** Division of Molecular and Cellular Medicine, National Cancer Center Research Institute, Tokyo, Japan, **6** Department of Physics, Chuo University, Tokyo, Japan

Abstract

Background: miRNAs circulating in the blood in a cell-free form have been acknowledged for their potential as readily accessible disease markers. Presently, histological examination is the golden standard for diagnosing and grading liver disease, therefore non-invasive options are desirable. Here, we investigated if miRNA expression profile in exosome rich fractionated serum could be useful for determining the disease parameters in patients with chronic hepatitis C (CHC).

Methodology: Exosome rich fractionated RNA was extracted from the serum of 64 CHC and 24 controls with normal liver (NL). Extracted RNA was subjected to miRNA profiling by microarray and real-time qPCR analysis. The miRNA expression profiles from 4 chronic hepatitis B (CHB) and 12 non alcoholic steatohepatitis (NASH) patients were also established. The resulting miRNA expression was compared to the stage or grade of CHC determined by blood examination and histological inspection.

Principal Findings: miRNAs implicated in chronic liver disease and inflammation showed expression profiles that differed from those in NL and varied among the types and grades of liver diseases. Using the expression patterns of nine miRNAs, we classified CHC and NL with 96.59% accuracy. Additionally, we could link miRNA expression pattern with liver fibrosis stage and grade of liver inflammation in CHC. In particular, the miRNA expression pattern for early fibrotic stage differed greatly from that observed in high inflammation grades.

Conclusions: We demonstrated that miRNA expression pattern in exosome rich fractionated serum shows a high potential as a biomarker for diagnosing the grade and stage of liver diseases.

Editor: Xiao-Ping Miao, MOE Key Laboratory of Environment and Health, School of Public Health, Tongji Medical College, Huazhong University of Science and Technology, China

Funding: Y.M, J.T, and T.K. were financially supported by the Ministry of Health, Labour and Welfare of Japan (H22-general-008)and Y.M, J.T, T.K, and Y.T received Grants-in-Aid for scientific research from the Ministry of Education, Culture, Sports, Science and Technology (22590727). The funders had no role in study design, data collection and analysis, decision to publish, or preparation of the manuscript.

Competing Interests: The authors have declared that no competing interests exist.

* E-mail: m2079633@med.osaka-cu.ac.jp

Introduction

MicroRNAs (miRNAs) are a gene family that is evolutionarily conserved and have important roles in the control of many biological processes, such as cellular development, differentiation, proliferation, apoptosis, and metabolism [1]. Aberrant expression of miRNAs in liver tissue has been implicated in the progression of liver fibrosis, and hepatocarcinogenesis [2,3,4]. Recently, two independent groups showed that miR-122 plays a critical role in the maintenance of liver homeostasis and anti-tumor formation [5,6].

Exosome in one of the endoplasmic reticulum carries mRNAs and miRNAs [7]. Recently, it has become clear that exosome perform intercellular signaling through miRNA. miRNAs are released through a ceramide-dependent secretory machinery and are then transferred and become functional in the recipient cells [8]. In a prior study using human blood and cultured cells, several miRNAs were selectively packaged into microvesicle (MV) and actively secreted [9]. In another study, miRNAs originating from EBV was transported by exosome and then participated in the immune response of host cells [10]. In HCC cells as well, this type of exosome-mediated miRNA transfer is an important mechanism of intercellular communication [11].

It has also become clear that exosome can adjust to immune function, control infection or carry the virus itself. Exosomes of T, B and dendritic immune cells contain a repertoire of miRNAs that differ from that of their parent cells [12,13]. Exosomes released from nasopharyngeal carcinoma cells harboring latent EBV were shown to contain LMP1, signal transduction molecules, and virus-encoded miRNAs [14]. Retroviruses evade adaptive immune responses by using nonviral or host exosome biogenesis pathways to form infectious particles and as a mode of infection [15].

Recent evidence has shown that the expression patterns of serum or plasma miRNAs are altered in several diseases, in particular heart disease, sepsis, malignancies, and autoimmune diseases (reviewed in [16]). Discoveries such as this is encouraging and has propelled further research leading to the hypothesis that circulating miRNAs are detectable in serum and plasma in a form sufficiently stable to serve as biomarkers [17,18]. One such example is that tumour-associated miRNAs were found in the serum of diffuse large B-cell lymphoma patients [19]. In other examples, serum levels of miR-34a and miR-122 were associated with histological disease severity in patients with CHC or non-alcoholic fatty-liver disease (NAFLD) [20]. In fact, the serum level of miR-122 strongly correlates with serum ALT activity and with necro-inflammatory activity in patients with CHC and elevated ALT levels. However, there seems to be no significant correlation between fibrosis stage and functional capacity of the liver [21]. The expression levels of miR-122 and miR-194 correlated negatively with age in patients with CHB and HBV associated acute-on-chronic liver failure [22]. The expression level of miR-122 in serum was found to be closely related to non drug-induced acute liver injury [23]. Based on the above, it comes as no surprise that recently, the expression profile from extracellular miRNA is being used clinically to diagnose various diseases.

Here, in order to obtain data with high resolution that is reproducible, we extracted MVs from serum using exoquick and then performed a comprehensive microarray analysis. We attempted to diagnose HCV infection, and ascertain the degree of liver inflammation and fibrosis stage using exosome-rich fractioned miRNA. In short, we investigate if serum-derived miRNAs had the potential to serve as non-invasive bio-markers for various liver diseases.

Results

Reproducible Gene-analysis Using Microarray

In microarray experiments, serum analysis is comparatively easy; however, the downside is that the accuracy and reproducibility of the results are usually not satisfactory. To circumvent this drawback, we devised a procedure that would give us higher accuracy and reproducibility. Serum samples from NL subjects were prepared and divided into two groups; for the first, RNA was extracted using exoquick treated serum, and in the second, RNA was extracted from total serum. Next, miRNA expression was analyzed using Agilent miRNA microarray. The above procedure was performed independently twice (**Fig. 1A**). We compared the miRNA expression pattern among the four microarray results (**Fig. 1B**) and found that miRNA expression analysis using exoquick was the more reliable and reproducible (**Fig. 1C**).

Exosome from normal human prostatic cell lines PNT-2, was yielded by the conventional ultra-centrifugation method [8]. We prepared serums with and without exoquick treatment and performed immunoblot analysis with anti-CD63 (**Fig. 1D**). Bands of the expected relative sizes were detected in serum treated with exoquick. We designated RNA extracted using exoquick treated serum as exosome-rich fractionated RNA.

Unique Expression Pattern of miRNA in CHC

We attempted to diagnose CHC using the miRNA expression pattern found in the peripheral blood samples from 64 CHC and 24 NL. The expression of nine miRNAs (miR-1225-5p, miR-1275, miR-638, miR-762, miR-320c, miR-451, miR-1974, miR-1207-5p, and miR-1246) allowed us to categorize patients as CHC or NL with 96.59% accuracy (**Fig. 2, 3** Table 1 and Table S1). As shown in **Fig. 2C**, CHC and NL were well differentiated due to their distinct miRNA expression patterns. The expression pattern of 12 miRNAs led to the distinction of CHC, CHB, NASH, and NL with 87.50% accuracy (**Fig. 4, S1A,** and Table S1). The accuracy of determining whether samples were CHC or CHB, CHC or NASH, CHB or NASH was 98.35%, 97.37%, and 87.50%, respectively. The accuracy of judging whether samples were NL or CHB, NL or NASH, was 89.29% and 88.89%, respectively (**Fig. 3, S1B** and Table S1). Unlike CHC and NL, there were relatively fewer analyses done of CHB and NASH (due to a small sample size), therefore, we used *"in silico"* resampling to overcome any possible bias. With *"in silico"* we found that it was highly reproducible to determine with high accuracy whether samples were CHC, CHB, NASH, or NL, CHC or CHB, CHC or NASH, CHC or NL, CHB or NASH, CHB or NL, or finally NASH or NL (**Fig. S2 to S8** and Supporting Information).

In order to validate our above-mentioned classifications, we prepared a separate independent sample consisting of 31 CHC, 16 CHB, and 8 NASH. We established miRNA expression patterns using microarray for each of these chronic liver disease groups. We tried to discriminate among the classifications in the independent cohort using the semi-supervised learning method [24] based only on the labels in the original sample group and the selected miRNAs shown in Table S1. The accuracy of judging whether samples were CHB or CHC, CHC or NASH, CHB or NASH, was 74.47%, 87.18%, and 79.19%, respectively (**Fig. S9**, Table 1, and Supporting Information). During the process of obtaining these results, we noticed that different versions of the Feature Extraction (FE) Software provided slightly different results, however it was not possible to fully unify these versions of FE. This may explain the relatively lower performance of the independent group compared with the original samples that mostly used the same FE Software versions.

miRNA Expression Correlates with the Grade of Liver Inflammation

The grade of inflammation for CHC patients was ascertained by liver histological examination, and then samples were divided into four groups A0, A1, A2, and A3 based on their fibrosis stage. miRNA expression profiles were then established for CHC according to each of their inflammation grade. From the four groups (A0 to A3), a combination of six arbitrary pairs is possible. miRNAs which had significant differential expression in five or more of the six pairs were extracted ($p<0.05$). Five miRNAs (miR-1914*, miR-193a-5p, miR-22, miR-659, and miR-711) had expression levels that increased as the severity of liver inflammation progressed. On the other hand, the expression levels of nine miRNAs (miR-1274b, miR-197, miR-1974, miR-21, miR-34a, miR-451, miR-548d-5p, miR-760, and miR-767-3p) significantly decreased with the progression of liver inflammation (**Fig. 5, S10** and Table S2).

The Grade of Liver Fibrosis Corresponded with the Expression Level of miRNAs

As previously noted, CHC samples were divided into F0, F1, F2, and F3 based on patients' fibrotic stage. From these four fibrotic groups, a combination of six arbitrary pairs were possible. miRNAs that had significant differential expression in all six pairs were extracted ($p<0.05$). The expression levels of two miRNAs (miR-483-5p and miR-671-5p) significantly increased the higher the fibrotic stage and the expression level of 14 miRNAs (let-7a, miR-106b, miR-1274a, miR-130b, miR-140-3p, miR-151-3p, miR-181a, miR-19b, miR-21, miR-24, miR-375, miR-548l, miR-93, and miR-941) became progres-

A

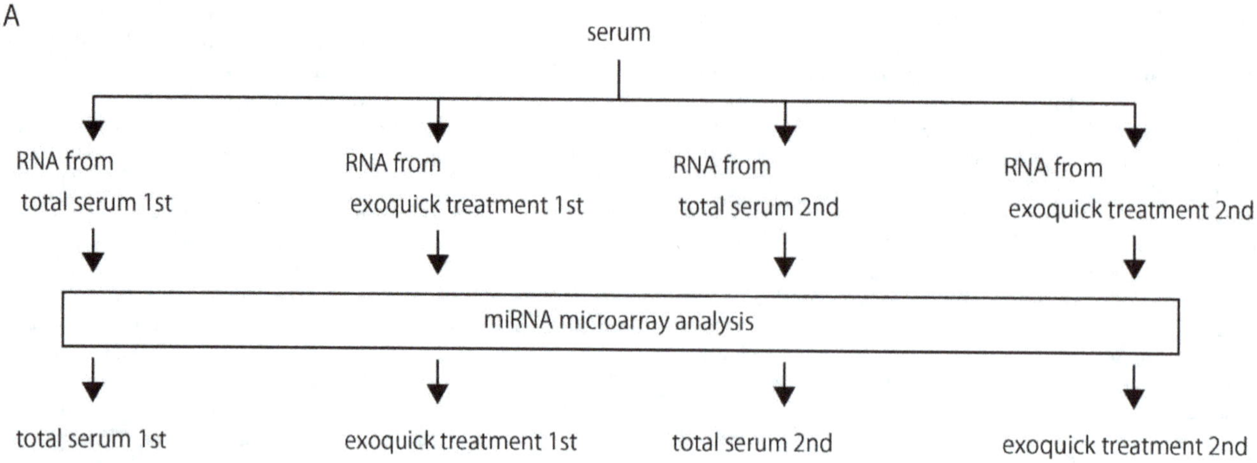

B

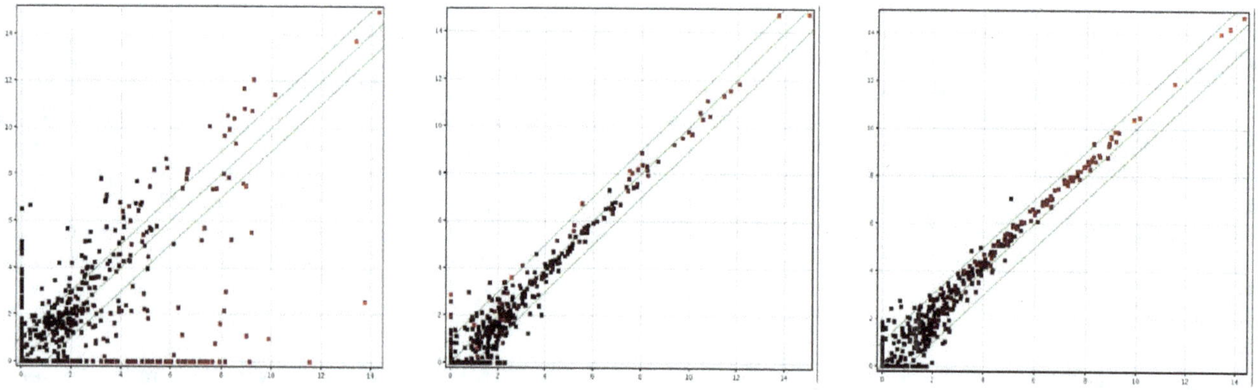

C

	exoquick 1st	total serum 1st	exoquick 2nd	total serum 2nd
exoquick 1st	1	0.836	0.998	0.809
total serum 1st	–	1	0.831	0.930
exoquick 2nd	–	–	1	0.821
total serum 2nd	–	–	–	1

D

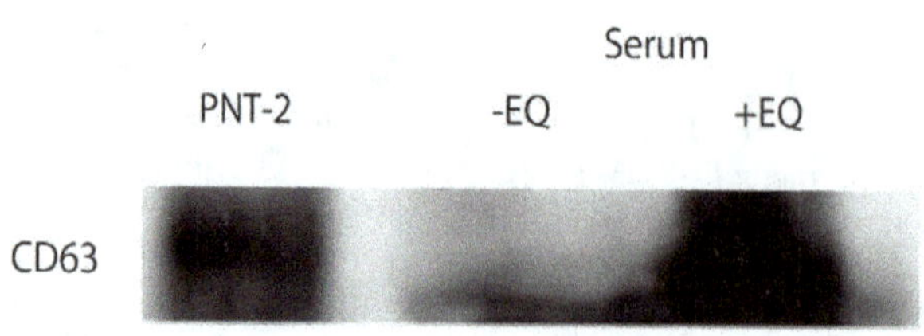

Figure 1. The method used to obtain reproducible data for microarray analysis conducted on serum-extracted samples. A. NL patients' serum were sampled twice. In the first, RNA was extracted first from untreated serum, and then extracted again from serum treated with exoquick. In the second serum sample, RNA was also extracted from both untreated serum and serum treated with exoquick. Microarray analysis was conducted for RNA in a total of four samples. B. Reproducibility test of microarray data. Scatter plots comparing non- normalized signal intensities of miRNAs in two independent experiments from human total serum and exosome rich fraction. Red and black denotes high and low miRNA expressions respectively. Total serum extracted first, versus exosome rich fraction first (left), total serum extracted first versus second (middle), and exosome rich fraction extracted first versus second (right). C. Pearson's pairwise correlations of signal intensities of miRNAs from human total serum and exosome rich fraction. D. Western blot was performed for untreated serum, serum extracted by exoquick and exosome fraction from PNT-2, using anti-CD63.

A

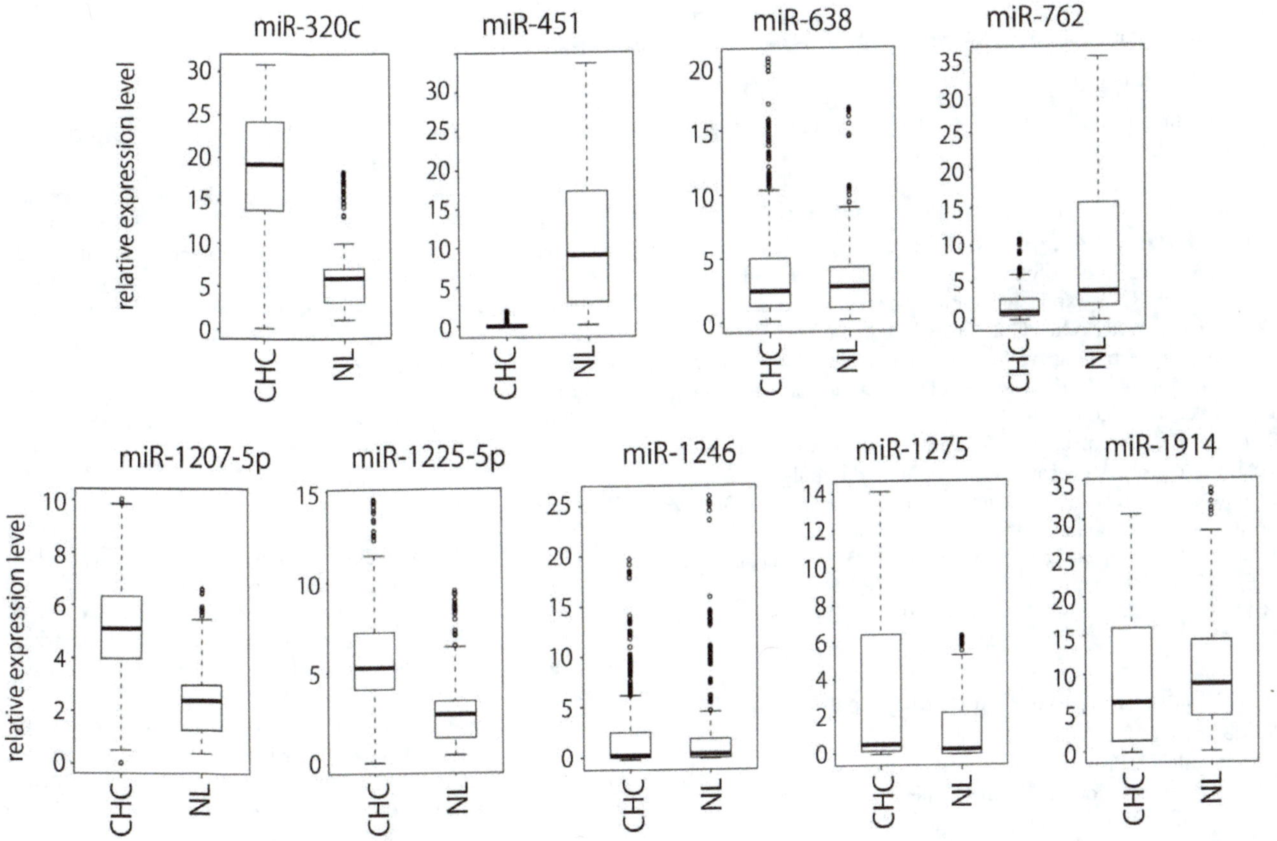

B

		result	
		CHC	NL
prediction	CHC	64	3
	NL	0	21

accuracy 96.6%

C

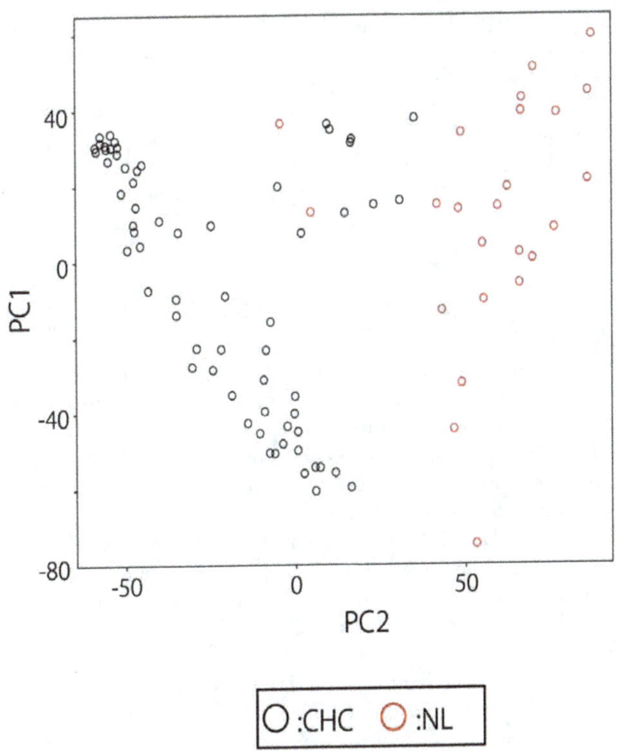

Figure 2. Expression patterns of miRNA used for discriminating between CHC and NL. A. Box plots of expression patterns of the nine miRNAs used for discriminating between CHC and NL. B. Classification of CHC and NL using LOOCV from miRNA expression profile. C. PCA in CHC and NL. The two dimensional embedding of CHC and NL by PCA. The first and second principal component scores computed (not selected for discrimination) of normalized miRNA expression were employed for this plot. Computation was done with ALL.

sively downregulated as liver fibrotic stage increased (**Fig. 6, S11** and Table S2).

Classification of Liver Inflammation Grade and Fibrotic Stage Using miRNA Expression Pattern

We attempted to classify liver inflammation grade and fibrosis stage using miRNA expression pattern. Liver inflammation was diagnosed by Leave One Out Cross-Validation (LOOCV); the accuracy of determining A1 from other inflammation grade was 71.88% and its odds ratio was 7.08. The accuracy of determining A2 and A3 was 75.00% and 82.81%, and their odds ratios were 9.50 and 11.08, respectively. In our study, we were unable to accurately classify A0 because we were limited to only one sample for that grade (**Fig. 7A**). Diagnosis of liver fibrosis by LOOCV showed that determining F0 from the other fibrotic stages had an accuracy of 87.50% and an odds ratio of 14.25. The classification of F1, F2, and F3 had accuracy rates of 65.63%, 70.31%, and 73.44% and odds ratio of 3.16, 6.39 and 5.80, respectively (**Fig. 7B**).

miRNA Expression Level Detected by Real-time qPCR Validated the Microarray Result

Four miRNAs (miR-1207-5p, miR-134, miR-1249, and miR-1183) with expression levels that differed among liver inflammation grades and liver fibrotic stages were chosen in order to confirm the microarray results using stem-loop based real-time qPCR. miRNAs that correlated with other clinical characteristics besides liver fibrosis and inflammation were listed using the Wilcoxon test. We performed two Wilcoxon tests and ranked miRNAs based on their p-value from smallest to largest and selected the miRNAs with the four smallest p-values that were common among the two Wilcoxon tests.

The real-time qPCR result was consistent with the microarray analysis (**Fig. 8**). Here also, we applied *"in silico"* resampling to compensate for the small number of patients used in the real-time qPCR analysis. The results of the *"in silico"* resampling conferred with the results of the real-time qPCR (**Fig. S12**).

miRNA Expression Pattern was Closely Related to Several Clinical Parameters in CHC

Although we observed that miRNA expression correlated with ALT value, we were unable to identify miRNAs that displayed a strong correlation. 12 miRNAs were chosen sequentially from miRNAs with a high absolute correlation coefficient. One to 12 of these selected miRNAs were used to compare the canonical correlation coefficient of the above. When the expression patterns of six of the 12 miRNAs were compared with serum ALT value, the correlation coefficient and p-value were 0.44 and 4.91E−02, respectively. Similarly, when serum Albumin value was compared with the expression pattern of all 12 miRNAs, the correlation coefficient and p-value were 0.59 and 2.04E−02, respectively. Finally when the amount of serum HCVRNA was compared with the expression pattern of 12 miRNAs, the resulting correlation coefficient and p-value were 0.59 and 1.89E−02, respectively (**Fig. 9, S13** and Table S3).

Expression Pattern of a Several miRNAs Correlated to Serum and Hepatic Tissue

In a previous report, we described the miRNA expression pattern found in liver tissues obtained from 105 CHC [2]. From this group, we analyzed the miRNA expression of hepatic tissue and serum in 60 samples. We observed that the expression pattern of three miRNAs (miR-134, miR-200b, miR-324-5p) in hepatic tissue negatively correlated with that in serum, and the expression pattern of miR-370 in hepatic tissue positively correlated with that in serum ($p<0.05$) (Table S4). However, there was no significant correlation between the expression pattern of miR-122 in the hepatic tissue and serum (**Fig. S14** and Table S4).

Discussion

In this comprehensive miRNA analysis in various chronic liver diseases, we observed that aberrant expression of miRNAs was closely related to disease progression. Based on this, we believe that these miRNAs are potential readily accessible biomarkers, useful for diagnosing hepatic viral infection and for grading or staging liver diseases.

Many investigators have elected to use miRNA from serum instead of miRNA from exosome as the candidate for diagnosing diseases [18,20,22,25,26]. In our study, when exoquick was used, exosome could not be isolated therefore other MVs similar in size to exosome were also extracted. In other words, exoquick not only collected miRNAs contained in exosome, but also miRNA that were or were not combined with protein. Despite this, we found that exoquick delivered results that were superior to those obtained without exoquick. Therefore, although the process of analyzing miRNA from serum is simple, we chose to analyze miRNA from exosome rich fraction since it has a higher rate of reproducibility. Moreover, since exosome is closely related to intercellular signaling [14,27], it is expected that data obtained by exosome analysis can clarify the mechanism of chronic infection and inflammation [28].

When we extended our analysis from miR-122 to all miRNAs, it became clear that the expression level of several miRNAs correlated with the progression of liver fibrosis. In fact, recent studies have stated that when the expression levels of adequate numbers of miRNAs is used to identify disease, diagnostic ability is significantly higher than using a single miRNA [29]. In this study, when liver fibrosis was diagnosed using miRNA expression, distinguishing between F0 and F1-3 was done with 87.50% accuracy. Since F0 cannot be distinguished from other stages of chronic liver disease using blood examination, we propose that using miRNA expression pattern may be useful for diagnosing chronic liver disease that is in the early stage.

Previous studies have shown that the level of miR-122 in blood plasma increased earlier than in ALT in the presence of toxic liver injury in rodents [30]. Serum levels of miR-122 in patients with CHC are frequently elevated compared with healthy individuals [21]. Bihrer et al. mentioned that variations in the concentration of miR-122 in serum or plasma tend to be more specific for liver diseases than ALT and AST. This is because miR-122 is almost exclusively expressed in the liver, whereas ALT and AST originate from skeletal muscles and other tissues, therefore their diagnostic value is low [31]. In our study, the expression level of miR-122 had

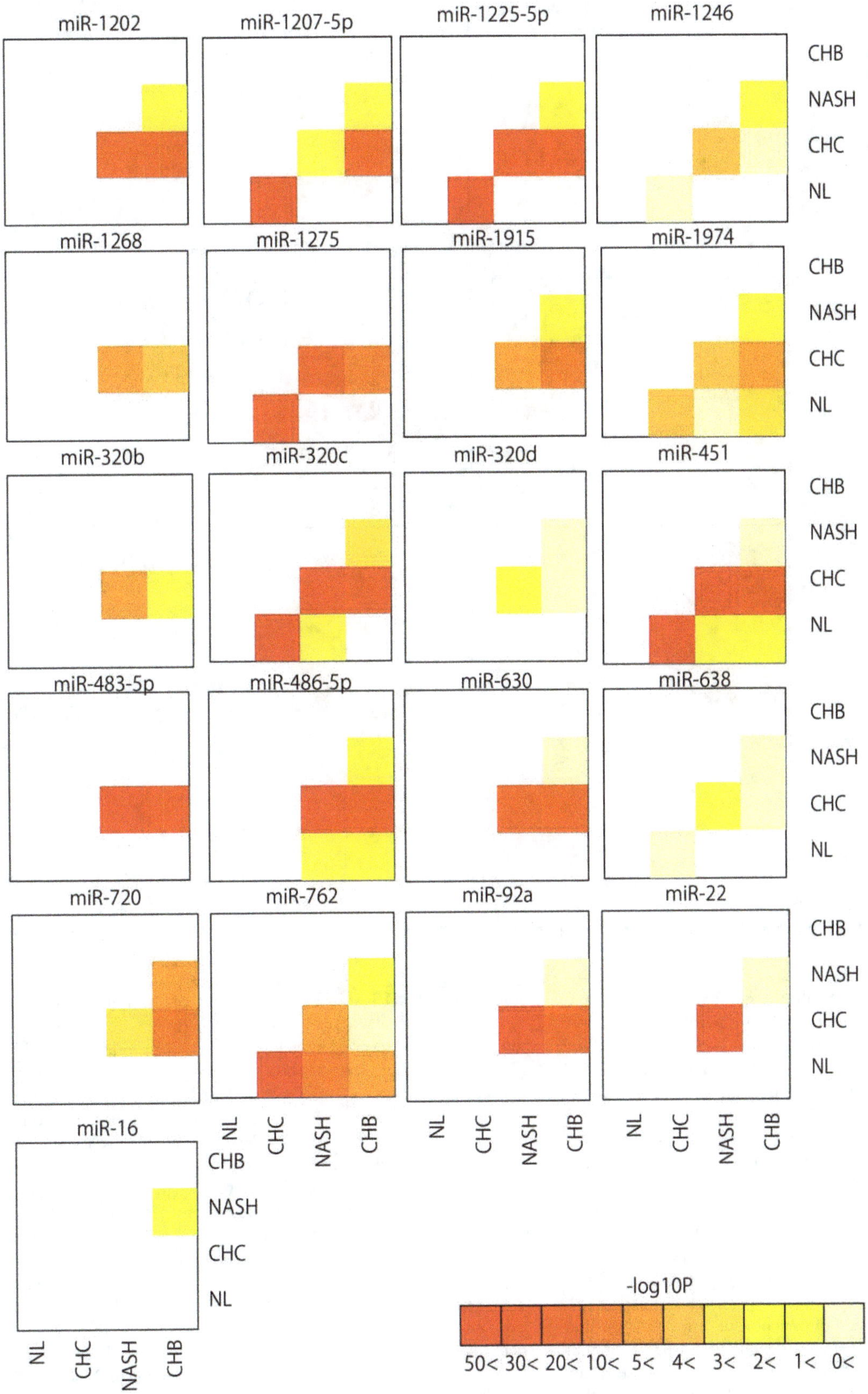

Figure 3. Pairwise heatmap of the miRNAs used for classifying two arbitrary groups. Pairwise heatmap showed the miRNAs and their p-value of two arbitrary groups.

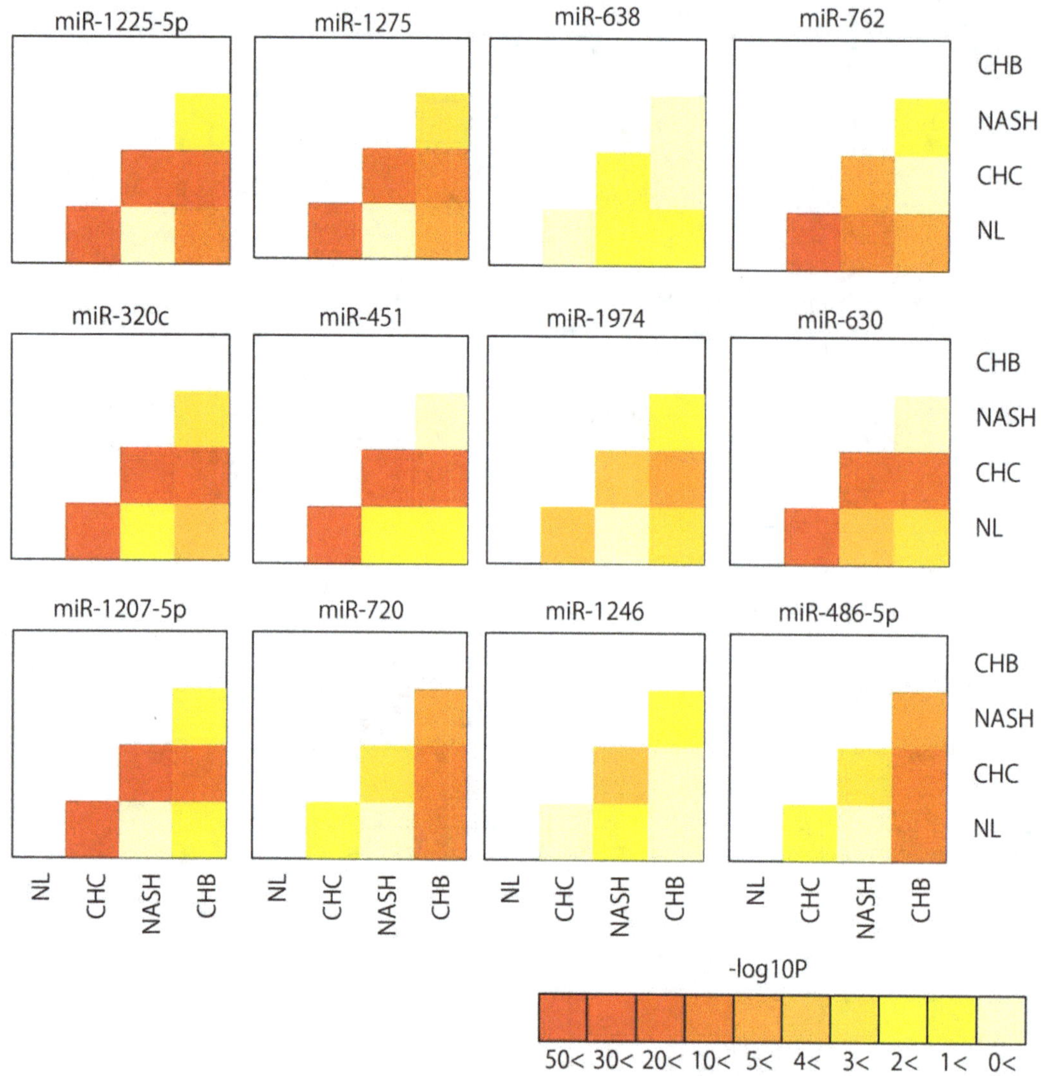

Figure 4. Pairwise heatmap of the miRNAs used for classifying among four groups.

a significant positive correlation with the grade of liver inflammation, serum albumin value, or serum HCVRNA value. However, miR-122 expression did not significantly correlate with liver fibrosis stage. Moreover, there was no correlation between the expression level of miR-122 in liver tissue, and that in serum in the same 60 samples (**Fig. S14**). The expression pattern of only four miRNAs out of total liver tissue miRNAs correlated with the expression patterns of miRNA found in the serum (Table S4). Most serum miRNA had expression patterns that differed from those observed in hepatic tissue samples. Moreover, we observed differences in miRNAs expression between various tissues [32]. These differences were observed even in tissues taken from the same subject; at present we are unclear as to the reason for this phenomenon.

In regards to the progression of liver fibrosis and the expression pattern of miR-21, previous studies concur with our result that miR-21 expression level significantly decreased in response to the progression of liver fibrosis [20]. Taken together, this suggests that any miRNAs that may have been emitted from liver tissue cannot be detected in serum after hepatic cell injury.

The expression pattern of many miRNAs in serum positively correlated with serum ALT, albumin, and HCVRNA levels in this study (**Fig. 9, S13** and Table S3). This result contradicts prior assumptions that no correlation exists between serum miR-122 and HCVRNA serum levels [21]. Three likely reasons for this difference in results are: 1) the detection method used (real-time qPCR versus microarray), 2) the difference in the subjects' ages (the subjects in this study were older), and 3) the difference in the amount of miRNAs (multiple miRNAs vs. a single miRNA) used to identify the clinical parameters of the disease.

CHC and NL were classified with a high level of accuracy using the expression pattern of miRNA. In order to elucidate if the miRNA expression in CHC is common to other chronic liver diseases including CHB, we compared the miRNA expression pattern of CHC with those of NASH and CHB. The result of this analysis was that CHC could be clearly distinguished from both CHB and NASH. These results demonstrate that the varying forms of chronic liver disease have their own unique miRNA expression pattern. NASH is a histological diagnosis that rests on a combination of features and can only be confirmed by liver biopsy. Recently, NASH was diagnosed by first determining the existence of NAFLD from blood samples and then performing an ultrasound tomography. Finally, liver fibrosis stage was determined by Fibroscan

Table 1. Characteristics of subjects in this study of original samples and independent samples.

Original samples

Characteristics	CHC	CHB	NASH	NL
Gender	F: 34/M: 30	F: 2/M: 2	F: 3/M: 9	F:11/M: 13
Age (years)	59.5±8.3	46.8±14.5	52.3±13.1	50.8±12.0
AST (IU/L)	50.1±29.8	83.3±53.7	46.2±16.0	N.D
ALT (IU/L)	57.6±40.6	167.8±170.3	74.5±34.9	N.D
WBC ($x10^3/mm^3$)	5.1±1.5	4.7±1.5	6.2±1.6	N.D
Platelet ($x10^4/mm^3$)	16.6±5.9	14.8±6.3	24.7±8.0	N.D
Total Bilirubin (mg/dl)	0.65±0.22	0.83±0.40	0.76±0.25	N.D
Weight (kg)	57.9±9.18	58.8±4.3	74.9±24.8	59.6±9.6
ALP (IU/L)	267.0±88.4	223.3±25.0	232.7±36.2	N.D
γGTP (IU/L)	46.9±42.3	77.3±82.2	58.4±20.9	N.D
Hemoglobin (g/dl)	13.8±1.2	14.5±0.59	14.7±1.6	N.D
Albumin (g/dl)	4.1±0.4	4.2±0.5	4.4±0.3	N.D

Independent samples

Characteristics	CHC	CHB	NASH
Gender	F: 18/M: 13	F: 10/M: 6	F: 6/M: 2
Age (years)	59.5±8.3	46.8±14.5	54.8±12.7
AST (IU/L)	50.1±29.8	83.3±53.7	80.9±50.0
ALT (IU/L)	57.6±40.6	167.8±170.3	108.9±76.2
WBC ($x10^3/mm^3$)	5.1±1.5	4.7±1.5	5.5±1.8
Platelet ($x10^4/mm^3$)	16.6±5.9	14.8±6.3	19.3±7.6
Total Bilirubin (mg/dl)	0.65±0.22	0.83±0.40	0.73±0.25
Weight (kg)	57.9±9.18	58.8±4.3	66.4±9.9
ALP (IU/L)	267.0±88.4	223.3±25.0	278.6±100.6
γGTP (IU/L)	46.9±42.3	77.3±82.2	130.1±81.23
Hemoglobin (g/dl)	13.8±1.2	14.5±0.59	13.6±1.4
Albumin (g/dl)	4.1±0.4	4.2±0.5	3.8±0.3

Abbreviations; CHC, chronic hepatitis C; CHB, chronic hepatitis B; NASH, non alcoholic steatohepatitis; NL, normal liver (healthy control); N.D, no data.

(reviewed in [33]). However, when the results of these and other measures fail to yield a diagnosis then a pathology evaluation is necessary. Using "*in silico*" resampling to increase the reliability of our data, has led us to believe that NASH diagnosis may be possibly through blood examination.

We tested the reliability of our analysis in two ways and obtained reproducible results in both cases. First we enrolled an independent sample group, and second, we created virtual cohorts using in silico resampling to overcome our small sample size.

In this study we concluded that miRNA profiling is a promising alternative to diagnosing liver disease. This is based on our demonstration that the following evaluations could be performed using suitable miRNA expression profiles (1) determining the stage or grade of chronic liver disease, (2) ascertaining the clinical status of chronic liver diseases, and (3) distinguishing among various forms of chronic liver diseases. While these results suggest there is great potential and benefit of miRNA profiling, future studies in a larger population of CHC patients are warranted to fully elucidate the diagnostic potential of serum miRNA expression.

Materials and Methods

Patient Selection

A cohort of 64 CHC, 4 CHB, and 12 NASH patients who had undergone liver biopsy, as well as 24 healthy control subjects was enrolled. We also prepared independent samples consisting of 31 CHC, 12 CHB, and 8 NASH to validate our results. Patient characteristics are summarized in Table 1 and detailed clinical data is depicted in Table S5. The criteria for exclusion for CHC, CHB, and NASH were: co-infection with human immunodeficiency virus (HIV) types 1 and 2, decompensated liver disease, organ transplantation, immune suppression, autoimmune disorders, consumption of >20 g/day alcohol, and past history of intravenous drug abuse. Healthy controls were selected if they were not infected with HBV, HCV, nor HIV, had normal liver function tests, and had no history of liver disease.

All patients or their guardians provided written informed consent, and Ogaki Municipal Hospital and Kyoto University Graduate School and Faculty of Medicine's Ethics Committee approved all aspects of this study in accordance with the Helsinki Declaration.

Liver Histology and Blood Examination

A liver biopsy specimen was collected from each patient before anti-viral treatment. Histological grading and staging of CHC liver biopsy specimens were performed according to the Metavir classification system [34]. NASH was diagnosed histologically [35].

Serum HCV RNA was quantified before IFN treatment using Amplicor-HCV Monitor Assay (Roche Molecular Diagnostics Co., Tokyo, Japan), while serum HBV DNA was quantified before treatment using Amplicor HBV Monitor Assay (Roche). Pretreatment blood tests were conducted to determine each patient's level of aspartate aminotransferase (AST), alanine aminotransferase (ALT), total bilirubin, alkaline phosphatase, gamma-glutamyl transpeptidase, white blood cell (WBC), platelets, and hemoglobin.

Blood Sampling

Peripheral blood was collected from all subjects directly into serum tubes before anti-viral treatment. The tubes were centrifuged at 1,500 *g* for 10 min at 4°C, sera were aliquoted and additionally centrifuged at 2,000 *g* to completely remove any remaining cells. Sera were stored at −80°C until use.

RNA Preparation

Total RNA from 200 ul of serum was prepared using miRNeasy mini kit (Qiagen, Hilden Germany) according to the manufacturer's instruction. Exosome rich fractionated RNA was prepared using Exoquick (System Biosciences, CA, USA). Briefly, 900 ul of serum was mixed with 250 ul of Exoquick and incubated for 12 hr at 4°C. The tubes were centrifuged at 1500 g for 30 min at room temperature and then supernatant was discarded. The pellet was dissolved with 200 ul of PBS with vigorous vortex. RNA was extracted using miRNeasy mini kit (Qiagen).

Immunoblot Analysis and Exosome Preparation

The procedure for exosome preparation has been previously described [8]. SDS-PAGE gels, SuperSep Ace 5–20% (194–15021) (Wako, Osaka, Japan), were calibrated with Precision Plus Protein Standards (161–0375) (Bio-Rad), and anti-CD63 (1:200)

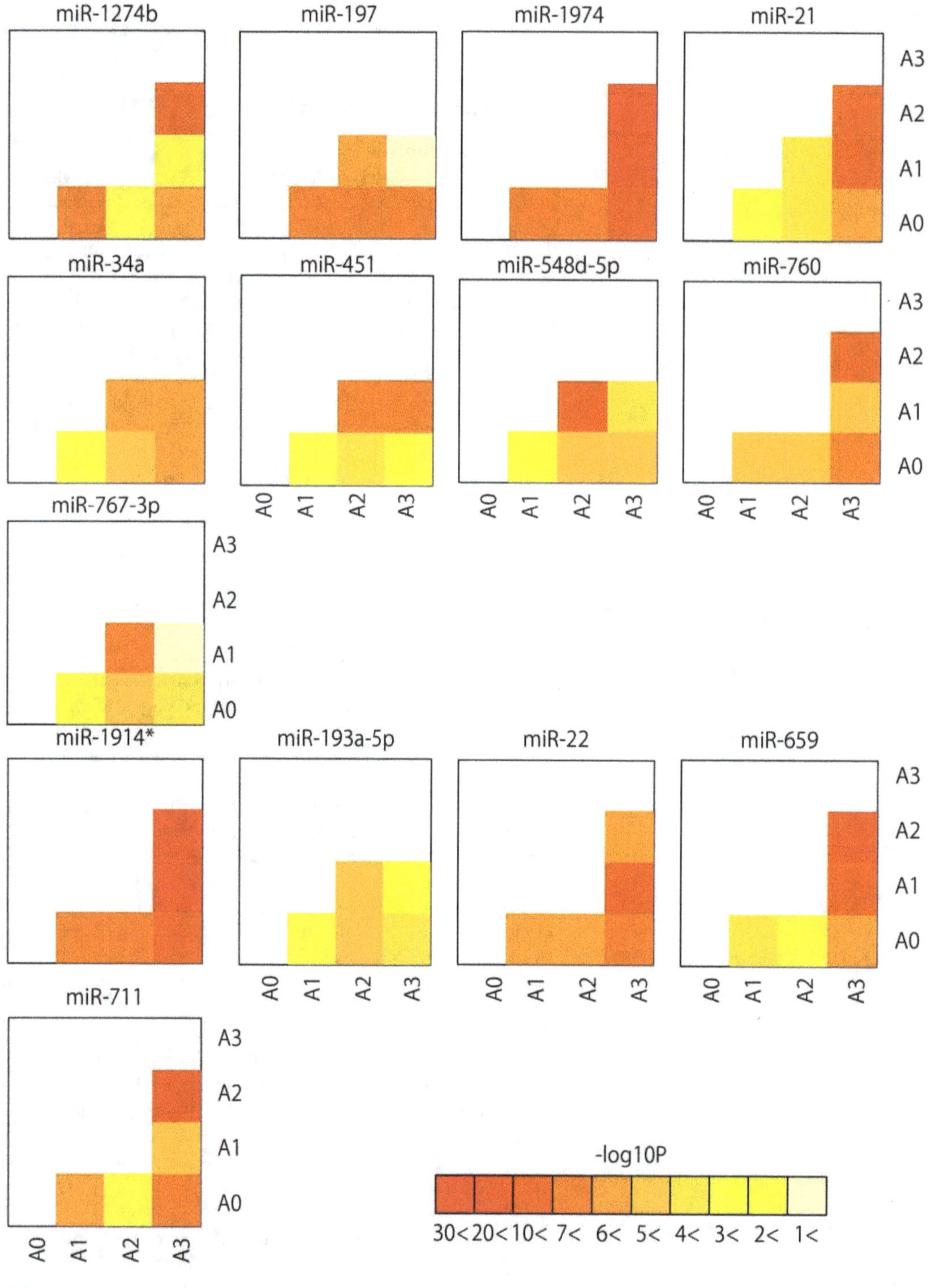

Figure 5. Significantly differentially expressed miRNAs according to liver inflammation grade. Pairwise heatmap showing the miRNAs and p-value of two arbitrary grades.

was used as primary antibodies. The dilution ratio of each antibody is indicated in parentheses. Two secondary antibodies (peroxidase-labeled anti-mouse and anti-rabbit antibodies) were used at a dilution of 1:5000. Bound antibodies were visualized by chemiluminescence using the ImmunoStar LD (Wako) and luminescent images were analyzed by a LuminoImager (LAS-3000; Fuji Film, Inc.). Only gels for CD63 (BD, NJ, USA) detection were run under non-reducing conditions. To exclude the albumin and IgG in serum, Albumin & IgG Depletion SpinTrap kit was used (GE health care, WI, USA). After aliquots isolation, exosome-contained fraction was isolated by Exoquick according to standard instructions.

miRNA Microarray

To detect serum miRNA, 60 ng of RNA was labeled and hybridized using the Human microRNA Microarray Kit (Rel

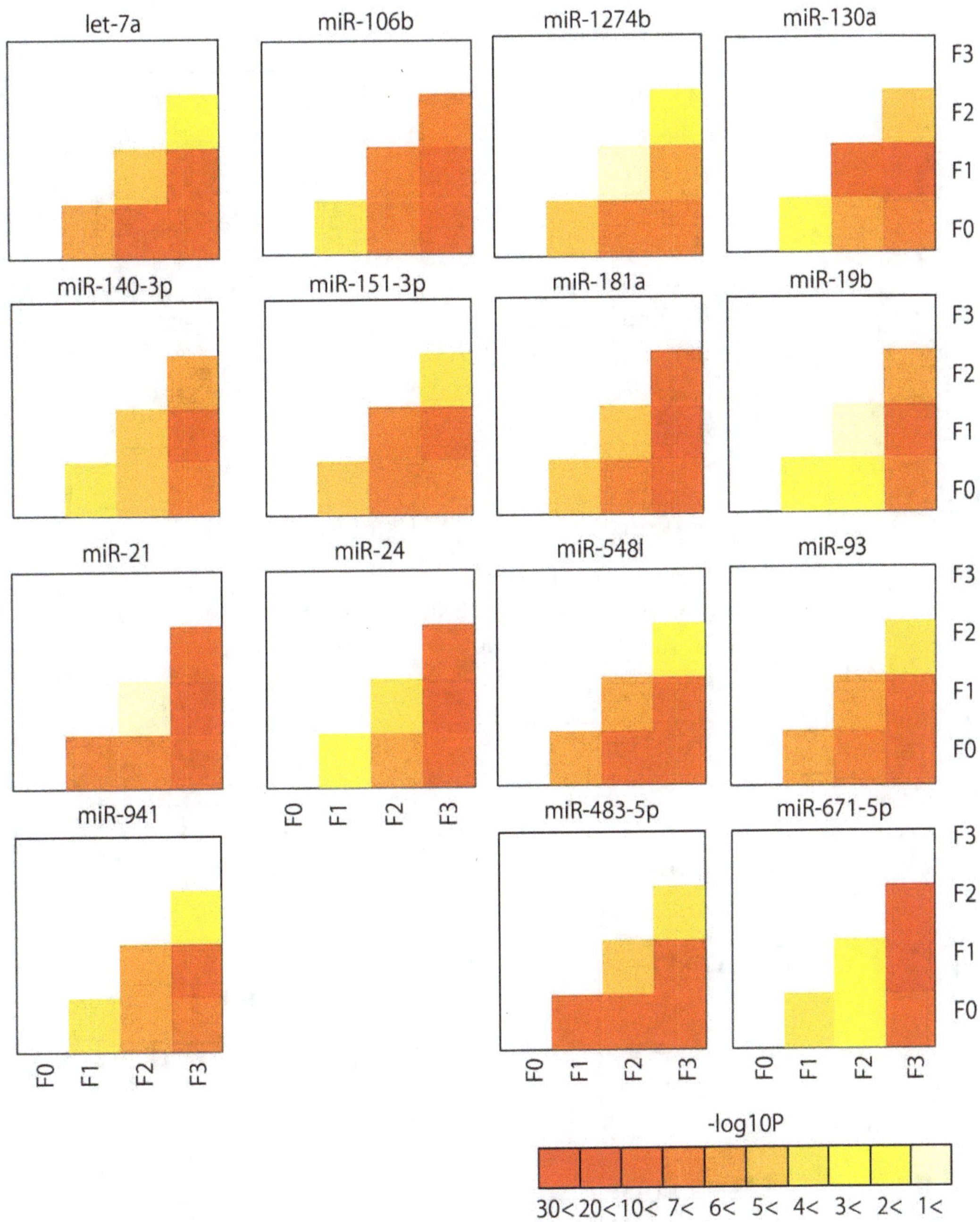

Figure 6. Significantly differentially expressed miRNA according to liver fibrotic stage. Pairwise heatmap showing the miRNAs and p-value of two arbitrary stages.

14.0) (Agilent Technologies, CA, USA) according to the manufacturer's protocol (protocol for use with Agilent microRNA microarrays Version 1.0). Hybridization signals were detected with a DNA microarray scanner G2505B (Agilent Technologies) and the scanned images were analyzed using Agilent feature extraction software (v9.5.3.1). We used raw data (gProcessedSignal) and normalized each expression so as to have zero mean and unit sample variance. The data presented in this manuscript have been deposited in NCBI's Gene Expression Omnibus and are accessible through GEO Series access number GSE33857: http://www.ncbi.nlm.nih.gov/geo/query/acc.cgi?acc = GSE33857.

Real-time qPCR for Human miRNA

To detect miRNA expression level by real-time qPCR, TaqMan® microRNA assay (Applied Biosystems) was used to quantify the relative expression levels of miR-1207-5p (assay ID. 241060), miR-134 (assay ID. 000459), miR-1183 (assay ID. 002841), and miR-1249 (assay ID. 002868). The expression level of miR-16 (assay ID. 000391) was also measured and used as an internal control. cDNA was synthesized using the Taqman miRNA RT Kit (Applied Biosystems). RNA (2 ng/ml) in 5 ml of nuclease free water was added to 3 ml of 5 × RT primer, 10×1.5 μl of reverse transcriptase buffer, 0.15 μl of 100 mM dNTP, 0.19 μl of RNase inhibitor, 4.16 μl of nuclease free water, and 50 U of reverse transcriptase in a total volume of 15 μl. The reaction was performed for 30 min at 16°C, 30 min at 42°C, and 5 min at 85°C.

A

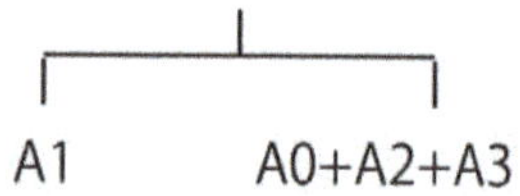

A1 vs A0+A2+A3	
accuracy	71.88%
Fisher's exact test	p-value: 4.07E-04
odds ratio	7.08

		result	
		F	T
prediction	F	22	12
	T	6	24

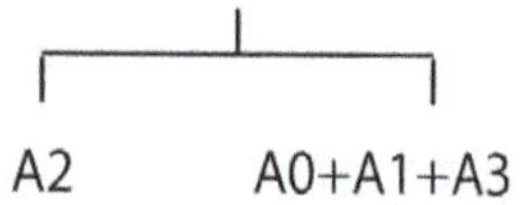

A2 vs A0+A1+A3	
accuracy	75.00%
Fisher's exact test	p-value:2.26E-04
odds ratio	9.50

		result	
		F	T
prediction	F	34	4
	T	12	14

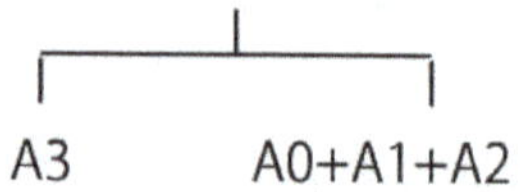

A3 vs A0+A1+A2	
accuracy	82.81%
Fisher's exact test	p-value: 2.30E-03
odds ratio	11.08

		result	
		F	T
prediction	F	47	3
	T	8	6

B

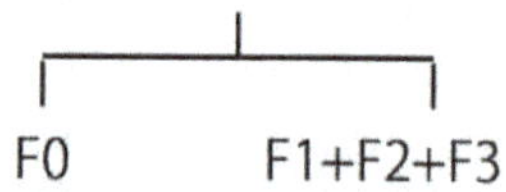

F0 vs F1+F2+F3	
accuracy	87.50%
Fisher's exact test	p-value: 4.95E-02
odds ratio	14.25

		result	
		F	T
prediction	F	54	1
	T	7	2

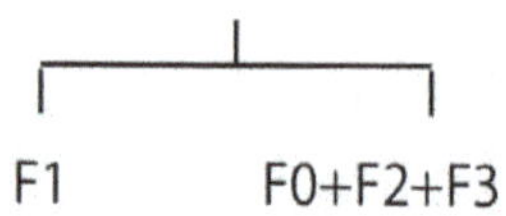

F1 vs F0+F2+F3	
accuracy	64.62%
Fisher's exact test	p-value: 2.73E-02
odds ratio	3.16

		result	
		F	T
prediction	F	21	13
	T	10	20

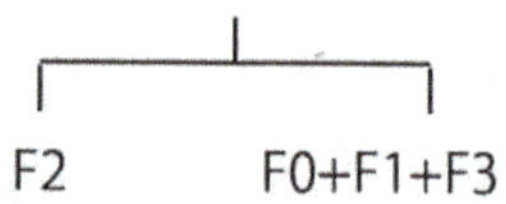

F2 vs F0+F1+F3	
accuracy	70.31%
Fisher's exact test	p-value: 3.24E-03
odds ratio	6.39

		result	
		F	T
prediction	F	33	4
	T	15	12

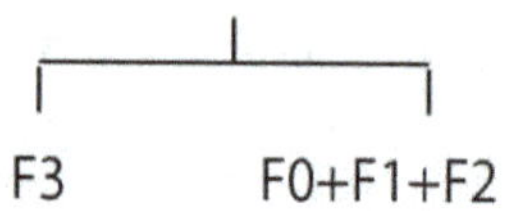

F3 vs F0+F1+F2	
accuracy	73.44%
Fisher's exact test	p-value: 1.35E-02
odds ratio	5.80

		result	
		F	T
prediction	F	39	4
	T	13	8

Figure 7. Determining liver inflammation grade and fibrotic stage using miRNA expression pattern in LOOCV analysis. A. In order to diagnose the grade of liver inflammation, A0 was identified first. Next A1, A2, and A3 were identified in a similar manner as A0. For each, the accuracy rate, P value, and the odds ratio are shown. B. For liver fibrosis stage, F0 was first diagnosed following which the other stages F1, F2, and F3 were diagnosed in a similar manner. For each group the accuracy rate, P value, and the odds ratio are shown.

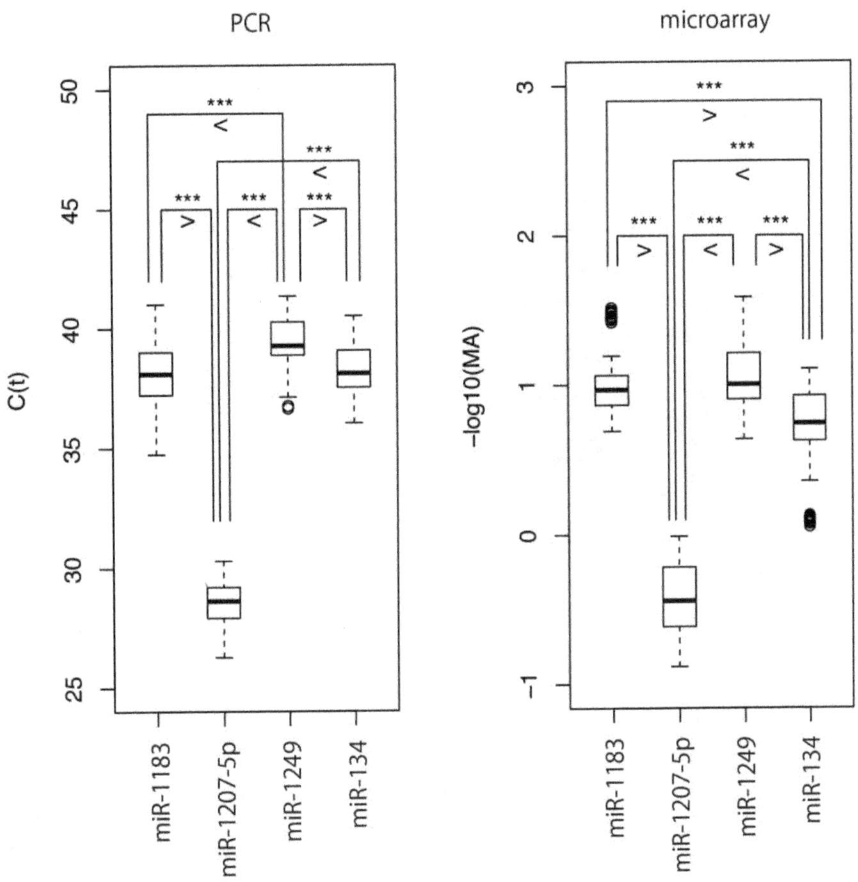

Figure 8. Real-time qPCR validation of microarray analysis. The microarray expression analysis result of four miRNAs was reproduced in real-time PCR analysis. The pairs with $p<0.001$ are marked by "***".

All reactions were run in triplicate. Chromo 4 detector (Bio-rad) was used to detect miRNA expression. To allow for the validation of microarray results with C(t) obtained by qPCR, raw gene expressions were transformed into logarithmic values. P-values were computed via one-sided t test. No averages over probes were taken for the microarray. The above procedures were also done with various packages/functions implemented in R (http://www.r-project.org/).

Statistical Analysis

For symptoms having discrete values, grade pairs were compared with Wilcoxon rank sum test (one-sided); otherwise, P-values were computed from correlation coefficients. In both cases, false discovery rate (FDR) of less then 0.05 computed from the P-value was regarded as significant. Benjamini and Hochberg criterion was used for FDR estimation. All p-values shown are significant even though they are raw numbers. No average over probes was taken before correlation analyses.

The Canonical Correlation Coefficients for miRNA Expression and Clinical Parameters

The canonical correlation coefficients were computed for ALT-miRNA, albumin-miRNA, and HCVRNA-miRNA correlations, using up to 12 miRNA with larger correlation coefficients (see Supporting Information).

Classification Analyses for Liver Fibrosis/inflammation

P-values were computed via one-sided t test using the raw expression values of each miRNA from the samples of CHC and healthy controls. The logarithm of obtained P-values was then transformed into principal components scores via principal components analysis. Following this, grades were discriminated by linear discriminant analysis of CHC ages and the optimal number of principal components.

Selection of miRNAs Required to Diagnose Several Liver Diseases

For specific pairs consisting of one liver disease and a healthy control, their normalized miRNAs expression was transformed into principal components scores via principal components analysis. miRNAs having the larger first and second principal component scores were selected. Following this, the principal component scores of each sample was computed based solely on the selected miRNA expressions. Liver diseases were classified using the optimal number of these principal component scores.

In order to compensate for the relative small number of NASH and CHB patients, we performed "*in silico*" patients resampling analysis of the microarray data (see Supporting Information). All the above procedures were done with various packages/functions implemented in R.

"*In silico*" Resampling

"*In silico*" resampling is a tool often used to overcome the limitation of a small sample size. Using this technique, we combined the clinical traits of existing patients and created various virtual samples. Using these virtual cohorts, we were then able to increase the sample size (see Supporting information).

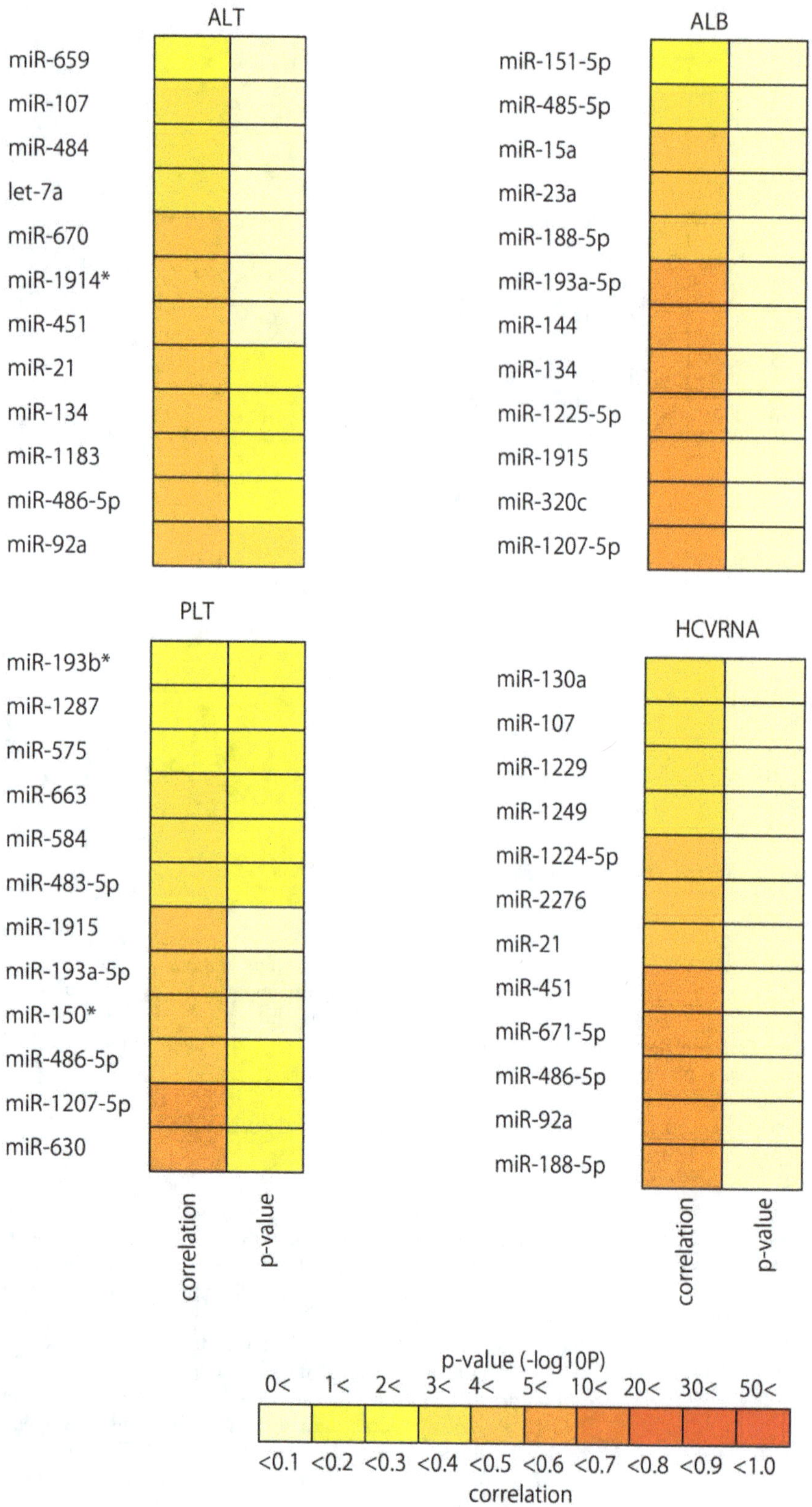

Figure 9. The list of miRNAs used to obtain the maximum correlation coefficient between miRNA expression level, and clinical characteristics. Pairwise heatmap showing miRNAs and their correlation coefficient and p-values.

In order to validate the *"in silico"* resampling results, we prepared another sample set and once again performed *"in silico"* resampling using the microarray data from 99 CHC liver tissue samples [36]. The results proved that *"in silico"* resampling can accurately reproduce an entire population using only a small number of existing samples (see Supporting Information).

Reproducibility Test of Microarray Data

Data were analyzed using the GeneSpring GX10.0.2 (Agilent). Quality control (QC) was applied according to the manufacturer's instructions, and all data were approved by GeneSpring. Following Agilent recommendations, no inter-array normalization was applied because the similarity in miRNA expression among sample arrays was unknown [37]. Scatter plots and Pearson's pairwise correlations were performed with GeneSpring.

Supporting Information

Figure S1 Expression patterns of miRNAs used for discriminating among CHC, NL, CHB, and NASH. Classifying CHC, NL, CHB, and NASH using LOOCV. Distinguishing between two arbitrary groups using LOOCV.

Figure S2 Expression patterns of miRNAs used to discriminate among CHC, CHB, NASH, and NL "in silico" resampling for disease discriminant studies reflected by BMI. A. Box plots of expression pattern of the miRNAs used to discriminate among CHC, CHB, NASH, and NL. B. Discriminating among four groups using LOOCV. Accuracy is 95.25%. C. Two dimensional embedding of CHC, CHB, NASH, and NL by the first and second principle component scores computed with 12 selected miRNAs

Figure S3 The same as Fig.3 for CHC and CHB. A. Box plot of 19 miRNAs used for the discrimination. B. Classification between CHC and CHB. Accuracy is 100%. C. The two dimensional embedding of CHB and CHC by the first and second principal component scores computed with19 selected miRNAs.

Figure S4 The same as Fig.S3 for CHC and NASH. A. Box plots of 20 miRNAs used for the discrimination. B. Classification between CHC and NASH. Accuracy is 100%. C. Two dimensional embedding of CHC and NASH by the first and second principal component scores computed with 19 selected miRNAs

Figure S5 The same as Fig.S3 for CHC and NL. A. Box plots of 9 miRNAs used for the discrimination. B. Classification between CHC and NL. Accuracy is 100%. C. Two dimensional embedding of CHC and NL by the first and second principal component scores computed with 9 selected miRNAs

Figure S6 The same as Fig.S3 for CHB and NL. A. Box plots of 4 miRNAs used for the discrimination. B. Classification between CHB and NL. Accuracy is 93.5%. C. Two dimensional embedding of CHB and NL by the first and second principal component scores computed with 4 selected miRNAs

Figure S7 The same as Fig.S3 for NASH and NL. A. Box plots of 5 miRNAs used for the discrimination. B. Distinguishing between NASH and NL with 84.0% accuracy. C. Two dimensional embedding of NASH and NL by the first and second principal component scores computed with 5 selected miRNAs

Figure S8 The same as Fig.S3 for CHB and NASH pair. A. Box plots of 17 miRNAs used for the discrimination. B. Distinguishing between CHB and NASH with 80.0% accuracy. C. Two dimensional embedding of CHB and NASH by the first and second principal component scores computed with 17 selected miRNAs

Figure S9 Classification of the independent sample using semi-supervised learning based on the labels in the original cohort. A. Classifying CHB and CHC. Accuracy is 74.47%. B. Classifying CHC and NASH. Accuracy is 87.18%. C. Classifying CHB and NASH. Accuracy is 79.19%.

Figure S10 miRNA expression pattern that correlated with the changes in clinical background. miRNAs that were differentially expressed according to the grade of liver inflammation

Figure S11 miRNA expression pattern that correlated with the changes in clinical background. miRNAs that were differentially expressed according to liver fibrosis stage

Figure S12 Real-time qPCR validation of microarray analysis "in silico" resampling for disease discrimination studies reflected by BMI. The result of microarray expression analysis of four miRNAs was reproduced using real-time PCR analysis. Pairs with $p<0.001$ are marked by "***".

Figure S13 The relationship between the expression levels of several miRNAs and serum ALT, albumin, HCVRNA, respectively. Horizontal axis shows the number of miRNAs used in the analysis. Vertical axis shows the correlation index and p-values.

Figure S14 Summary of the relationship between the expression level of miR-122 and several clinical features. A. Expression level of miR-122 positively correlated with an increase in liver inflammatory grade. Asterisk denotes significant differences of $p<0.05$. B. Expression level of miR-122 positively correlated with the serum level of albumin. C. Expression level of miR-122 positively correlated with the amount of serum HCVRNA. D. Expression level of miR-122 in exosome rich fraction did not significantly correlate with that in liver tissues.

Table S1 The list of miRNAs used for classifying arbitrary 2 groups and 4 groups, and their p-values.

Table S2 Significantly differentially expressed miRNAs according liver inflammation grade and liver fibrotic stage.

Table S3 The list of miRNAs used to obtain the maximum correlation coefficient between expression level of miRNAs, and clinical characteristics.

Table S4 List of miRNAs with expression that corresponded in liver tissue and serum.

Table S5 Clinical background of original samples and independent samples in detail.

Table S6 Accuracy of LDA for "in silico" resampling.

Author Contributions

Conceived and designed the experiments: YM NK TO YT. Performed the experiments: YM HT TT YY NK. Analyzed the data: TT YT. Contributed reagents/materials/analysis tools: HT JT TK. Wrote the paper: YM NK TO.

References

1. Ambros V (2004) The functions of animal microRNAs. Nature 431: 350–355.
2. Murakami Y, Toyoda H, Tanaka M, Kuroda M, Harada Y, et al. (2011) The progression of liver fibrosis is related with overexpression of the miR-199 and 200 families. PLoS One 6: e16081.
3. Murakami Y, Yasuda T, Saigo K, Urashima T, Toyoda H, et al. (2006) Comprehensive analysis of microRNA expression patterns in hepatocellular carcinoma and non-tumorous tissues. Oncogene 25: 2537–2545.
4. Braconi C, Henry JC, Kogure T, Schmittgen T, Patel T (2011) The role of microRNAs in human liver cancers. Semin Oncol 38: 752–763.
5. Hsu SH, Wang B, Kota J, Yu J, Costinean S, et al. (2012) Essential metabolic, anti-inflammatory, and anti-tumorigenic functions of miR-122 in liver. J Clin Invest 122: 2871–2883.
6. Tsai WC, Hsu SD, Hsu CS, Lai TC, Chen SJ, et al. (2012) MicroRNA-122 plays a critical role in liver homeostasis and hepatocarcinogenesis. J Clin Invest 122: 2884–2897.
7. Valadi H, Ekstrom K, Bossios A, Sjostrand M, Lee JJ, et al. (2007) Exosome-mediated transfer of mRNAs and microRNAs is a novel mechanism of genetic exchange between cells. Nat Cell Biol 9: 654–659.
8. Kosaka N, Iguchi H, Yoshioka Y, Takeshita F, Matsuki Y, et al. (2010) Secretory mechanisms and intercellular transfer of microRNAs in living cells. J Biol Chem 285: 17442–17452.
9. Zhang Y, Liu D, Chen X, Li J, Li L, et al. (2010) Secreted monocytic miR-150 enhances targeted endothelial cell migration. Mol Cell 39: 133–144.
10. Pegtel DM, Cosmopoulos K, Thorley-Lawson DA, van Eijndhoven MA, Hopmans ES, et al. (2010) Functional delivery of viral miRNAs via exosomes. Proc Natl Acad Sci U S A 107: 6328–6333.
11. Kogure T, Lin WL, Yan IK, Braconi C, Patel T (2011) Intercellular nanovesicle-mediated microRNA transfer: a mechanism of environmental modulation of hepatocellular cancer cell growth. Hepatology 54: 1237–1248.
12. Thery C, Ostrowski M, Segura E (2009) Membrane vesicles as conveyors of immune responses. Nat Rev Immunol 9: 581–593.
13. Mittelbrunn M, Gutierrez-Vazquez C, Villarroya-Beltri C, Gonzalez S, Sanchez-Cabo F, et al. (2011) Unidirectional transfer of microRNA-loaded exosomes from T cells to antigen-presenting cells. Nat Commun 2: 282.
14. Meckes DG Jr, Shair KH, Marquitz AR, Kung CP, Edwards RH, et al. (2010) Human tumor virus utilizes exosomes for intercellular communication. Proc Natl Acad Sci U S A 107: 20370–20375.
15. Gould SJ, Booth AM, Hildreth JE (2003) The Trojan exosome hypothesis. Proc Natl Acad Sci U S A 100: 10592–10597.
16. Kosaka N, Iguchi H, Ochiya T (2010) Circulating microRNA in body fluid: a new potential biomarker for cancer diagnosis and prognosis. Cancer Sci 101: 2087–2092.
17. Mitchell PS, Parkin RK, Kroh EM, Fritz BR, Wyman SK, et al. (2008) Circulating microRNAs as stable blood-based markers for cancer detection. Proc Natl Acad Sci U S A 105: 10513–10518.
18. Chen X, Ba Y, Ma L, Cai X, Yin Y, et al. (2008) Characterization of microRNAs in serum: a novel class of biomarkers for diagnosis of cancer and other diseases. Cell Res 18: 997–1006.
19. Lawrie CH (2007) MicroRNAs and haematology: small molecules, big function. Br J Haematol 137: 503–512.
20. Cermelli S, Ruggieri A, Marrero JA, Ioannou GN, Beretta L (2011) Circulating microRNAs in patients with chronic hepatitis C and non-alcoholic fatty liver disease. PLoS One 6: e23937.
21. Bihrer V, Friedrich-Rust M, Kronenberger B, Forestier N, Haupenthal J, et al. (2011) Serum miR-122 as a biomarker of necroinflammation in patients with chronic hepatitis C virus infection. Am J Gastroenterol 106: 1663–1669.
22. Ji F, Yang B, Peng X, Ding H, You H, et al. (2011) Circulating microRNAs in hepatitis B virus-infected patients. J Viral Hepat 18: e242–251.
23. Starkey Lewis PJ, Dear J, Platt V, Simpson KJ, Craig DG, et al. (2011) Circulating microRNAs as potential markers of human drug-induced liver injury. Hepatology 54: 1767–1776.
24. Chapelle O, Scholkopf B, Zien A (2006) Semi-supervised learning. Cambridge, Mass.: MIT Press. x, 508 p. p.
25. Hunter MP, Ismail N, Zhang X, Aguda BD, Lee EJ, et al. (2008) Detection of microRNA expression in human peripheral blood microvesicles. PLoS One 3: e3694.
26. Marquez RT, Bandyopadhyay S, Wendlandt EB, Keck K, Hoffer BA, et al. (2010) Correlation between microRNA expression levels and clinical parameters associated with chronic hepatitis C viral infection in humans. Lab Invest 90: 1727–1736.
27. Mathivanan S, Ji H, Simpson RJ (2010) Exosomes: extracellular organelles important in intercellular communication. J Proteomics 73: 1907–1920.
28. Simons M, Raposo G (2009) Exosomes–vesicular carriers for intercellular communication. Curr Opin Cell Biol 21: 575–581.
29. Keller A, Leidinger P, Bauer A, Elsharawy A, Haas J, et al. (2011) Toward the blood-borne miRNome of human diseases. Nat Methods 8: 841–843.
30. Laterza OF, Lim L, Garrett-Engele PW, Vlasakova K, Muniappa N, et al. (2009) Plasma MicroRNAs as sensitive and specific biomarkers of tissue injury. Clin Chem 55: 1977–1983.
31. Nathwani RA, Pais S, Reynolds TB, Kaplowitz N (2005) Serum alanine aminotransferase in skeletal muscle diseases. Hepatology 41: 380–382.
32. Landgraf P, Rusu M, Sheridan R, Sewer A, Iovino N, et al. (2007) A mammalian microRNA expression atlas based on small RNA library sequencing. Cell 129: 1401–1414.
33. Dowman JK, Tomlinson JW, Newsome PN (2011) Systematic review: the diagnosis and staging of non-alcoholic fatty liver disease and non-alcoholic steatohepatitis. Aliment Pharmacol Ther 33: 525–540.
34. Bedossa P, Poynard T (1996) An algorithm for the grading of activity in chronic hepatitis C. The METAVIR Cooperative Study Group. Hepatology 24: 289–293.
35. Matteoni CA, Younossi ZM, Gramlich T, Boparai N, Liu YC, et al. (1999) Nonalcoholic fatty liver disease: a spectrum of clinical and pathological severity. Gastroenterology 116: 1413–1419.
36. Murakami Y, Tanaka M, Toyoda H, Hayashi K, Kuroda M, et al. (2010) Hepatic microRNA expression is associated with the response to interferon treatment of chronic hepatitis C. BMC Med Genomics 3: 48.
37. Zhang X, Chen J, Radcliffe T, Lebrun DP, Tron VA, et al. (2008) An array-based analysis of microRNA expression comparing matched frozen and formalin-fixed paraffin-embedded human tissue samples. J Mol Diagn 10: 513–519.

18

Association between Noninvasive Fibrosis Markers and Chronic Kidney Disease among Adults with Nonalcoholic Fatty Liver Disease

Giorgio Sesti*, Teresa Vanessa Fiorentino, Franco Arturi, Maria Perticone, Angela Sciacqua, Francesco Perticone

Department of Medical and Surgical Sciences, University "Magna Graecia" of Catanzaro, Catanzaro, Italy

Abstract

Evidence suggests that nonalcoholic fatty liver disease (NAFLD) and non-alcoholic steatohepatitis (NASH) are associated with an increased risk of chronic kidney disease (CKD). In this study we aimed to evaluate whether the severity of liver fibrosis estimated by NAFLD fibrosis score is associated with higher prevalence of CKD in individuals with NAFLD. To this end NAFLD fibrosis score and estimated glomerular filtration rate (eGFR) were assessed in 570 White individuals with ultrasonography-diagnosed NAFLD. As compared with subjects at low probability of liver fibrosis, individuals at high and intermediate probability showed an unfavorable cardio-metabolic risk profile having significantly higher values of waist circumference, insulin resistance, high sensitivity C-reactive protein, fibrinogen, uric acid and lower insulin-like growth factor-1 levels. Individuals at high and intermediate probability of liver fibrosis have lower eGFR after adjustment for gender, smoking, glucose tolerance status, homeostasis model assessment index of insulin resistance (HOMA-IR index), diagnosis of metabolic syndrome, statin therapy, anti-diabetes and anti-hypertensive treatments ($P=0.001$). Individuals at high probability of liver fibrosis had a 5.1-fold increased risk of having CKD (OR 5.13, 95%CI 1.13–23.28; $P=0.03$) as compared with individuals at low probability after adjustment for age, gender, and BMI. After adjustment for glucose tolerance status, statin therapy, and anti-hypertensive treatment in addition to gender, individuals at high probability of liver fibrosis had a 3.9-fold increased risk of CKD (OR 3.94, 95%CI 1.11–14.05; $P=0.03$) as compared with individuals at low probability. In conclusion, advanced liver fibrosis, determined by noninvasive fibrosis markers, is associated with CKD independently from other known factors.

Editor: Claudia Miele, Consiglio Nazionale delle Ricerche, Italy

Funding: This work was supported by Italian Ministry of University grant FIRB/MERIT RBNE08NKH7_002 to Giorgio Sesti. The funder had no role in study design, data collection and analysis, decision to publish, or preparation of the manuscript.

* E-mail: sesti@unicz.it

Introduction

Renal dysfunction is a worldwide health problem as a consequence of its adverse outcomes including cardiovascular events and all-cause-mortality [1–3]. Increasing evidence suggests that chronic kidney disease (CKD), defined as a sustained reduction in the glomerular filtration rate (GFR), and cardiovascular disease share common risk factors such as the metabolic syndrome and its individual components (elevated blood pressure, high plasma glucose levels, high triglycerides levels, low high density lipoprotein (HDL) levels, and abdominal obesity) [4–6].

Nonalcoholic fatty liver disease (NAFLD) is the most common chronic liver disease in Western countries [7], comprising a large spectrum of disorders ranging from simple steatosis, to non-alcoholic steatohepatitis (NASH) with increasing levels of fibrosis, and, ultimately, cirrhosis [8,9]. While simple liver steatosis is considered as a non-progressive condition, NASH is a potentially harmful disorder associated with increased risk of liver-related morbidity and mortality [10–13]. Like CKD, NAFLD has been linked to the same cluster of cardio-metabolic risk factors including the metabolic syndrome and its individual components [14,15], and is associated with increased risk of incident cardiovascular events [11–13,16,17]. Increasing evidence suggests that NAFLD/NASH and CKD share several traditional and non-traditional cardio-metabolic risk factors including higher plasma inflammatory and hemostatic factors, hyperuricemia, lower circulating insulin-like growth factor-1 (IGF-1) levels, endothelial dysfunction, and oxidative stress biomarkers [17–26]. Additionally, a number of studies has shown that liver biopsy–proven or ultrasonography-diagnosed NAFLD in adult subjects is associated with an increased prevalence [26–29] and incidence [30,31] of CKD. Interestingly, studies that used liver biopsy to diagnose NAFLD have shown that the severity of NASH histology (i.e., fibrosis stage) is associated with a more pronounced kidney dysfunction, independently of potential confounding factors, including the metabolic syndrome and its individual components [28,29]. Liver biopsy is considered the gold standard for the assessment of hepatic fibrosis and inflammation severity in subjects with chronic liver disease but has a number of limitations, including sampling variability, invasiveness, complications, and costs [32] making it unfeasible for large epidemiological studies. In an attempt to overcome these problems, several noninvasive scoring indexes have been developed by combining clinical and biochemical parameters that are useful to categorize subjects with NAFLD in subgroups at low and high risk of advanced fibrosis [33–37]. Recent studies have shown that advanced fibrosis, as determined by the noninvasive NAFLD fibrosis score [34], is a significant predictor of mortality, mainly from cardiovascular causes, in individuals with ultrasonography-diagnosed NAFLD [38,39]. The clinical utility of NAFLD fibrosis score in assessing CKD in individuals with ultrasonography-diagnosed NAFLD is still unsettled. In the present study, we therefore determined whether the severity of liver fibrosis estimated by the NAFLD fibrosis score is associated with higher prevalence of CKD among individuals with ultrasonography-diagnosed NAFLD.

Materials and Methods

The study group comprised 570 White individuals participating to the CATAnzaro MEtabolic RIsk factors (CATAMERI) study, a cross-sectional study assessing cardio-metabolic risk factors in individuals carrying at least one risk factor including dysglycemia, overweight/obesity, hypertension, dyslipidemia, and family history for diabetes [40]. Information regarding medical history, drug use, alcohol, and cigarette consumption were collected. Exclusion criteria included: history of malignant disease, liver cirrhosis, gout, chronic gastrointestinal diseases, chronic pancreatitis, regular use of steatosis-inducing drugs, self-reporting alcohol intake of 3 or more drinks per day, positivity for antibodies to hepatitis C virus (HCV) or hepatitis B surface antigen (HBsAg). Clinical cardiovascular disease was excluded on the basis of medical history and resting electrocardiogram.

All anthropometric and serological measurements were made in the morning after a 12-h fasting using standardized methods. Brachial blood pressure was measured in the left arm of the supine subjects, after 5 min of quiet rest, with a digital electronic tensiometer (regular or large adult cuffs were used according to arm circumference). A minimum of three blood pressure readings were taken on three separate occasions at least 2 weeks apart, and the medians of these three values were used. A 75 g oral glucose tolerance test (OGTT) was performed with sampling for plasma glucose.

Liver ultrasonography was performed in all participants by the same trained operator, who was blinded to participants' details, using a Toshiba Aplio 50 ultrasound apparatus equipped with a 3.5-MHz linear transducer [20,21]. Longitudinal, sub costal, ascending, and oblique scans were performed. The ultrasonographic criteria used to diagnose fatty liver included liver and kidney echo discrepancy, the presence of an increased liver echogenicity or "bright liver", poor echo penetration into the deep portion of the liver, and vascular blurring either singly or in combination.

The protocol was approved by the local ethical committee (Comitato Etico Azienda Ospedaliera "Mater Domini", Catanzaro, Italy), and written informed consent was obtained from all participants in accordance with principles of Helsinki Declaration.

Analytical determinations

Glucose, triglycerides, total and HDL cholesterol concentrations were determined by enzymatic methods (Roche, Basel, Switzerland). Alanine aminotransferase (ALT) and aspartate aminotransferase (AST) levels were measured using the α-ketoglutarate reaction; gamma-glutamyltransferase (GGT) levels with the L-gamma-glutamyl-3-carboxy-4-nitroanilide rate method. Serum creatinine was measured in the routine laboratory by an automated technique based on a Creatinine Jaffè compensated method for serum and plasma (Roche Diagnostics) implemented in an auto-analyzer. Serum uric acid was measured by the URICASE/POD method implemented in an auto-analyzer (Boehringer Mannheim, Mannheim, Germany). Albumin concentration was determined with a Alb2 kit on a Cobas C6000 analyzer (Roche Diagnostics, Milan, Italy). High sensitivity C-reactive protein (hsCRP) levels were measured by automated instrument (CardioPhase® hsCRP, Milan, Italy). An automated nephelometric technology using the BN™ II System analyzer (Siemens Healthcare, Italy) was employed to measure plasma fibrinogen concentrations. Plasma insulin concentration was measured with a chemiluminescence-based assay (Immulite®, Siemens, Italy), and total serum IGF-1 concentrations were determined by chemiluminescent immunoassay (Nichols Institute Diagnostic, San Juan Capistrano, CA).

Definitions

Glucose tolerance status was diagnosed according to the American Diabetes Association (ADA) criteria [41]: normal glucose tolerance (NGT) when fasting plasma glucose (FPG) was <5.6 mmol/l and 2 h post-load <7.8 mmol/l, isolated impaired fasting glucose (IFG) when FPG was 5.6–6.9 mmol/l and 2 h post-load <7.8 mmol/l, impaired glucose tolerance (IGT) when FPG was ≤6.9 mmol/l and 2-h post-load was 7.8–11.0 mmol/l, type 2 diabetes when FPG was ≥7.0 mmol/l and/or 2 h post-load was ≥11.1 mmol/l.

The NAFLD fibrosis score was calculated according to the following formula: −1.675 + 0.0373 x age + 0.0943 x BMI +1.13 x IFG or diabetes (yes = 1, no = 0) + 0.99 x AST/ALT ratio −0.013 x platelet − 0.66 x albumin [20]. Two cutoff points (>0.676 and <−1.455) were used to divide the subjects in three groups: low risk of fibrosis (< −1.455), intermediate risk of fibrosis (−1.455–0.676), and high risk of fibrosis (>0.676) [34].

The homeostasis model assessment index of insulin resistance (HOMA-IR) was calculated as fasting insulin × fasting glucose/22.5 [42].

Estimated glomerular filtration rate (eGFR) was calculated by using the CKD-EPI equation [43]: $eGFR = 141 \times min(Scr/k, 1)^{\alpha} \times max(Scr/k, 1)^{-1.209} \times 0.993^{Age} \times 1.018$ [if female], where Scr is serum creatinine, k is 0.7 for females and 0.9 for males, α is −0.329 for females and −0.411 for males, min indicates the minimum of Scr/k or 1, and max indicates the maximum of Scr/k or 1. CKD was defined as eGFR <60 ml/min/1.73 m^2.

Metabolic syndrome was defined as having three or more of the following criteria [44]: waist circumference >102 cm in men and >88 cm in women, triglycerides >1.69 mmol/l or on treatment for elevated triglycerides, HDL <1.04 mmol/l in men and < 1.3 mmol/l in women or on treatment for reduced HDL, blood pressure >130/85 mmHg or on antihypertensive treatment, fasting glucose ≥5.6 mmol/l.

Statistical analysis

Variables with skewed distribution including triglycerides, hsCRP, GGT, and fasting insulin were natural log transformed for statistical analyses. Continuous data are expressed as means ± SD. Categorical variables were compared by $\chi 2$ test. Anthropometric and metabolic differences between groups were tested after adjusting for gender using a general linear model with *post hoc* Bonferroni correction for multiple comparisons. To avoid overestimation of the model, we excluded those variables used as a part of the NAFLD fibrosis score calculation i.e. age, and BMI. A general linear model was used to determine the independent impact on eGFR values of several variables including smoking habit, glucose tolerance status, HOMA-IR index, diagnosis of metabolic syndrome, statin therapy, medications for diabetes, anti-hypertensive treatments, and gender.

A logistic regression analysis adjusted for gender, age, and BMI was used to determine the association between the study groups and CKD. A second logistic regression model adjusted for glucose tolerance status, statin therapy, and anti-hypertensive treatment in addition to gender was run to determine the association between the study groups and CKD. A P value <0.05 was considered statistically significant. All analyses were performed using SPSS software program Version 16.0 for Windows.

Results

The clinical and biochemical features of the study group are reported in Table 1. The mean age for the entire cohort was 54.1±13.5 yrs. Of the 570 subjects examined, 220 (38.6%) had NGT, 63 (11.1%) had IFG, 112 (19.6%) had IGT, and 175 (30.7%) had type 2 diabetes. Metabolic syndrome was diagnosed in 392 (68.8%) individuals, and 368 (64.6%) subjects had hypertension treated with anti-hypertensive medications. A low probability of advanced liver fibrosis (NAFLD fibrosis score <−1.455) was found in 41.4% of subjects, an intermediate probability of advanced liver fibrosis (NAFLD fibrosis score −1.455–0.676) was found in 48.9% of subjects, and a high probability of advanced liver fibrosis (NAFLD fibrosis score >0.676) was found in 9.6% of subjects. As expected by stratifying subjects according to the NAFLD fibrosis score, individuals classified as at high or intermediate probability of liver fibrosis were older (P<0.0001), had higher BMI (P<0.0001) and AST/ALT ratio (P<0.0001), lower platelet counts (P<0.0001) and albumin levels (P<0.0001), and were more likely to have elevated fasting glucose (P<0.0001) or IFG/IGT/type 2 diabetes (P<0.0001) as compared with those at low probability of liver fibrosis. A lower proportion of individuals classified as at high probability of liver fibrosis were current smokers (P=0.04). Subjects classified as at high or intermediate probability of liver fibrosis were more likely to have metabolic syndrome (P<0.0001) as compared with those at low probability of liver fibrosis. A higher proportion of individuals classified as at high probability of liver fibrosis were treated with insulin (P=0.01) (Table 1). A higher proportion of individuals classified as at high or intermediate probability of liver fibrosis were treated with statins (P<0.0001) (Table 1). In addition, significant differences between the three groups were observed with respect to anti-hypertensive treatments: a higher proportion of individuals classified as at high or intermediate probability of fibrosis were treated with ACE inhibitors, angiotensin receptor blockers and diuretics (P<0.0001) (Table 1).

As compared with individuals at low probability of liver fibrosis, both individuals at high probability of fibrosis and individuals at intermediate probability of fibrosis showed an unfavorable cardio-metabolic risk profile having significantly higher values of waist circumference, insulin resistance, as assessed by the HOMA-IR index, hsCRP, fibrinogen, serum uric acid as well as lower levels of IGF-1 (Table 1). In addition individuals at high probability of fibrosis had higher systolic blood pressure values.

As compared with individuals at low probability of liver fibrosis, both individuals at high and those at intermediate probability of fibrosis exhibited lower value of eGFR (P<0.0001) (Table 1). These differences remained statistically significant after adjustment for smoking habit, glucose tolerance status, HOMA-IR index, diagnosis of metabolic syndrome, statin therapy, medications for diabetes, and anti-hypertensive treatments in addition to gender using a general linear model (P=0.001) (Table 2). Furthermore, the differences remained statistically significant after adjustment for individual components of the metabolic syndrome including waist circumference, blood pressure, HDL, triglycerides, and glucose values in addition to gender (P<0.0001) (Table 3).

When the analysis was restricted to the 175 subjects with IFG or IGT, both individuals at high and those at intermediate probability of fibrosis exhibited lower value of eGFR (95±19 and 100±26 ml/min/1.73 m^2, respectively; P=0.03) as compared with individuals at low probability of liver fibrosis (eGFR = 110±25 ml/min/1.73 m^2). Accordingly, when the analysis was restricted to the 175 subjects with type 2 diabetes, both individuals at high and those at intermediate probability of fibrosis exhibited lower value of eGFR (81±33 and 89±26 ml/min/1.73 m^2, respectively; P=0.001) as compared with individuals at low probability of liver fibrosis (eGFR = 109±42 ml/min/1.73 m^2).

Of the 570 subjects examined, 38 (6.7%) had CKD defined as eGFR <60 ml/min/1.73 m^2. A logistic regression model adjusted for gender, age, and BMI was used to compare the risk of individuals at high and at intermediate probability of fibrosis to have CKD as compared with individuals at low probability of fibrosis (the reference category). Individuals at high probability of fibrosis had a 5.1-fold increased risk of having CKD (OR 5.13, 95%CI 1.13–23.28; P=0.03) and individuals at intermediate probability of fibrosis had a 3.0-fold increased risk of having CKD (OR 3.01, 95%CI 0.87–10.32; P=0.07) as compared with individuals at low probability of fibrosis. After adjustment for glucose tolerance status, statin therapy, and anti-hypertensive treatment in addition to gender, individuals at high probability of fibrosis had a 3.9-fold increased risk of having CKD (OR 3.94, 95%CI 1.11–14.05; P=0.03) as compared with individuals at low probability of fibrosis (Table 4). Increased risk of CKD was also independently associated with glucose tolerance status (P=0.03), and anti-hypertensive treatment (P=0.002) (Table 4).

Discussion

It is increasingly recognized that both NAFLD and CKD are associated with a clustering of traditional and non-traditional cardio-metabolic risk factors, and predict the development of cardiovascular diseases [1–6,10,12–26]. There is also evidence supporting the notion that adverse clinical outcomes are more frequent in patients with NASH rather than in individuals with simple liver steatosis [12–14,17,28,29], thus emphasizing the importance to assess more advanced form of NAFLD in individuals affected by liver steatosis. Several noninvasive scoring indexes combining clinical and laboratory variables have been developed in order to identify advanced fibrosis in individuals with NAFLD [33–37]. Employing one of these liver fibrosis scores, it has been shown that advanced fibrosis is associated with increased risk of cardiovascular mortality in individuals with NAFLD [24,25]. These findings coupled with the accessibility of a carefully characterized cohort of adult subjects have provided the rationale for investigating the relationship between advanced liver fibrosis, as determined by the NAFLD fibrosis score [34], in subjects with ultrasonography-diagnosed NAFLD and CKD. In this cross-sectional study, we report that individuals with high or intermediate probability of advanced liver fibrosis have lower eGFR as compared with individuals at low probability of liver fibrosis. These associations did not change after adjusting for several potential confounders including glucose tolerance status, diagnosis of metabolic syndrome or its individual components, treatments for dyslipidemia or hypertension. Accordingly, individuals with high probability of advanced liver fibrosis showed a 5.1-fold increased risk of having CKD as compared with individuals at low

Table 1. Anthropometric and biochemical characteristics of the study subjects stratified according to fibrosis risk score.

Variables	Whole study subjects	Low probability of fibrosis (< −1.455)	Intermediate probability of fibrosis (−1.455–0.676)	High probability of fibrosis (>0.676)	P
Gender (Male/Female)	319/251	126/110	162/117	31/24	0.56
Age *(yrs)*	54.1±13.5	47.0±12.4	57.7±11.1[d]	66.5±12.9[d]	<0.0001
BMI *(kg/m²)*	32.3±6.5	30.5±5.3	33.0±6.1[b]	36.9±9.3[d]	<0.0001
Waist circumference (cm)	107±14	102±12	109±13[d]	116±17[d]	<0.0001
Current smokers No (%)	102 (17.9%)	50 (21.2%)	48 (17.2%)	4 (7.3%)[a]	0.04
SBP *(mmHg)*	135±18	133±17	136±18	144±23[d]	<0.0001
DBP *(mmHg)*	82±11	82±10	82±11	81±12	0.82
Fasting glucose *(mg/dl)*	113±47	99±35	120±46[d]	143±67[d]	<0.0001
2-h post-load glucose *(mg/dl)*	137±45	123±39	148±48[d]	158±50[d]	<0.0001
Fasting insulin *(μU/ml)*	15±9	14±9	16±9[a]	18±10[a]	0.008
Total cholesterol *(mg/dl)*	197±40	204±37	193±40[b]	181±39[d]	<0.0001
HDL *(mg/dl)*	47±13	48±13	47±13	45±12	0.67
Triglycerides *(mg/dl)*	144±71	137±67	150±73	144±73	0.14
Uric acid *(mg/dl)*	5.5±1.4	5.3±1.3	5.6±1.4	6.3±1.8[d]	<0.0001
IGF-1 *(ng/ml)*	144±57	158±57	137±54[d]	117±46[d]	<0.0001
eGFR (ml/min/1.73m²)	93±25	102 ±27	87±21[d]	82±24[d]	<0.0001
CKD No, (%)	38 (6.7%)	6 (2.5%)	21 (7.5%)	11 (20.0%)	<0.0001
hsCRP *(mg/l)*	4.3±3.9	3.9±3.7	4.3±3.7	5.9±5.1[c]	0.003
Fibrinogen *(mg/dl)*	318±80	307±81	322±78[a]	343±85[b]	0.003
ALT *(UI/l)*	30±18	32±19	29±16[a]	23±16[c]	<0.0001
AST *(UI/l)*	25±14	23±11	25±12	30±25[b]	0.01
AST/ALT ratio	0.94±0.44	0.83±0.27	0.94±0.33[c]	1.41±0.96[d]	<0.0001
GGT *(UI/l)*	36±30	35±26	35±28	46±44	0.25
Platelet count *(x10⁹/l)*	249±71	288±76	230±49[d]	179±43[d]	<0.0001
Albumin *(g/dl)*	4.43±0.35	4.52±0.38	4.41±0.30[d]	4.14±0.29[d]	<0.0001
HOMA-IR index	4.2±3.7	3.5±2.9	4.5±2.9[b]	6.5±7.5[d]	<0.0001
NFG/IFG/IGT/T2DM (No)	220/63/112/175	158/18/29/31	58/39/69/113[d]	4/6/14/31[d]	<0.0001
Metabolic syndrome No (%)	392 (68.8%)	127 (53.8%)	219 (78.5%)[d]	46 (83.6%)[d]	<0.0001
Antidiabetic treatment (No)					
Diet/Oral hypoglycemic agents/Insulin	66/59/50	13/11/7	45/42/26	8/6/17	0.01
Therapy with statins No (%)	144 (25.3%)	38 (16.1%)	82 (29.4%)[c]	24(43.6%)[d]	<0.0001
ACE inhibitor therapy, No (%)	156 (27.4%)	53 (22.5%)	80 (28.7%)[b]	23(41.8%)[d]	<0.0001
Angiotensin receptor blocker therapy, No (%)	132 (23.2%)	38(16.1%)	77 (27.6%)[d]	17 (30.9%)[d]	<0.0001
Calcium channel blockers, No (%)	117 (20.5%)	46 (19.5%)	56 (20.1%)	15(27.3%)	0.42
Diuretics, No (%)	143 (25.1%)	30 (12.7%)	84 (30.1%)[d]	29 (52.7%)[d]	<0.0001

Data are means ± SD. Insulin, triglyceride, hsCRP, and GGT levels were log transformed for statistical analysis, but values in the table represent a back transformation to the original scale. Categorical variables were compared by χ^2 test. *P* values refer to results after analyses with adjustment for gender. M = male; F = female; BMI = body mass index; SBP = systolic blood pressure; DBP = diastolic blood pressure; HDL = high-density lipoprotein; hsCRP = high sensitivity C-reactive protein; ALT = alanine aminotransferase; AST = aspartate aminotransferase; GGT = gamma-glutamyltransferase; HOMA-IR = homeostasis model assessment index of insulin resistance; IGF-1 = insulin-like growth factor-1; eGFR = estimated glomerular filtration rate; CKD = chronic kidney disease; ACE = angiotensin-converting-enzyme; NFG = normal glucose tolerance; IFG = impaired fasting glucose; IGT = impaired glucose tolerance; T2DM = type 2 diabetes.
[a]*P*<0.05 vs. Low risk of fibrosis group.
[b]*P*<0.01 vs. Low risk of fibrosis group.
[c]*P*<0.001 vs. Low risk of fibrosis group
[d]*P*<0.0001 vs. Low risk of fibrosis group.

probability of fibrosis after adjustment for gender, age, and BMI. These data are consistent with those of two previous studies showing that CKD is associated with the severity of liver histopathology in adult individuals with biopsy-proven NAFLD [28,29].

The underlying mechanism(s) by which NAFLD/NASH may contribute to kidney dysfunction are still unsettled. The most

Table 2. General linear model with eGFR as the dependent variable.

Variables	F	*P*
Gender	1.62	0.20
Current smokers No (%)	0.19	0.66
HOMA-IR index	0.03	0.88
Glucose tolerance status	0.13	0.72
Metabolic syndrome diagnosis	0.57	0.45
Antidiabetic treatment	0.42	0.51
Therapy with statins	4.34	0.03
ACE inhibitor therapy	15.2	0.0001
Angiotensin receptor blocker therapy	1.97	0.16
Calcium channel blockers	0.02	0.96
Diuretics	10.6	0.001
Fibrosis risk score	6.99	0.001

eGFR = estimated glomerular filtration rate; HOMA-IR = homeostasis model assessment index of insulin resistance; ACE = angiotensin-converting-enzyme.

obvious explanation is that classical and non-classical cardio-metabolic risk factors, such as abdominal obesity, impaired glucose homeostasis/diabetes, hypertension, dyslipidemia, insulin resistance, metabolic syndrome, elevated serum uric acid, plasma inflammatory and hemostatic factors, all of which are associated with NAFLD/NASH may be also important risk factors for the development of CKD. Accordingly, we found that individuals with high or intermediate probability of advanced liver fibrosis have an unfavorable cardio-vascular risk profile characterized by an increase in visceral adiposity, insulin resistance, inflammatory and pro-coagulant biomarkers such as hsCRP, and fibrinogen. However, the strong relationships between these cardio-metabolic risk factors, NAFLD/NASH, and renal dysfunction make it extremely difficult to determine the precise cause-effect relationship between the two disorders. A potential plausible candidate linking NAFLD/NASH and renal dysfunction merits a comment. A number of evidences suggest that IGF-1 has effects on glomerular hemodynamics by enhancing both renal plasma flow and GFR [19,45–47]. IGF-1 induces NO production in human umbilical vein endothelial cells, an effect that is abolished by a neutralizing IGF-1 receptor antibody [45], and renal vasodilation induced by IGF-1 is completely inhibited by an inhibitor of nitric oxide biosynthesis [46]. Studies in humans have shown that plasma IGF-1 levels are associated with GFR [19], and intravenous infusion of rhIGF-1 increases renal plasma flow and GFR in healthy subjects [47]. We found that individuals with high or intermediate probability of advanced liver fibrosis have lower circulating IGF-1 levels as compared with individuals at low probability of liver fibrosis. These findings are consistent with previous studies showing that plasma IGF-1 concentration is a determinant of eGFR in hypertensive individuals [19], and suggest that lower amounts of circulating IGF-1 associated with NAFLD/NASH [20,21] could contribute to the reduced eGFR observed in individuals with high or intermediate probability of advanced liver fibrosis.

Several strengths and potential limitations of our study deserve comment. The major strengths of the study include the relatively large sample size with detailed anthropometric, clinical, and cardio-metabolic variables, the inclusion of both sexes, the ultrasound diagnosis of NAFLD performed by an experienced

Table 3. General linear model with eGFR as the dependent variable.

Variables	F	*P*
Gender	0.50	0.47
Waist circumference	16.58	0.0001
Fasting glucose	0.57	0.45
HDL	0.70	0.40
Triglycerides	4.20	0.04
Systolic blood pressure	15.57	0.0001
Diastolic blood pressure	7.49	0.006
Fibrosis risk score	17.96	0.0001

eGFR = estimated glomerular filtration rate; HDL = high-density lipoprotein.

examiner who was blinded to the subjects' clinical and biochemical data, the use of the CKD-EPI equation to estimate GFR, which is more accurate than the Modification of Diet in Renal Disease (MDRD) study equation to estimate renal function in obese subjects characterized by a higher GFR, the use of restrictive *post hoc* Bonferroni test to correct for multiple comparisons, and the exclusion of confounding conditions characterized by elevation in liver biomarkers such as heavy drinking, positivity for antibodies to HCV or HBsAg and cirrhosis (thus excluding patients with hepatorenal syndrome).

Nevertheless, the present study has certain limitations that require consideration. First, only serum creatinine levels and estimated GFR were available, introducing inaccuracy into estimates of GFR and, potentially, a misclassification of subjects with impaired kidney function. Although gold standard methods to measure GFR (isotope clearance measurements) may provide a more sensitive estimate of renal function, they are time-consuming and expensive procedures which are not feasible in large-scale studies. However, estimated GFR based on serum creatinine facilitates the detection, evaluation, and management of CKD, and many organizations such as the National Kidney Foundation recommend the use of prediction equations for the evaluation of kidney function in epidemiologic studies and in clinical practice. Thus, our findings may be applicable to public health practice settings. Second, the diagnosis of NAFLD was based on ultrasonography rather than on invasive methods such as percutaneous liver biopsy. Although ultrasonography is the common method of diagnosing for hepatic steatosis in clinical practice, its sensitivity is suboptimal when hepatic fat infiltration of the liver is <30%. However, participants to our study had normal or only mildly elevated serum liver enzymes and, therefore, liver biopsy may be impractical for most of them. Additionally, all laboratory variables, including plasma glucose during OGTT were measured once, and small changes in the variables would therefore be expected if the same measurements were repeated on a different day. Although such an approach is common in clinical practice and in large epidemiologic studies, these assays are subject to intra-individual variability, and, therefore, some inaccuracy in the classification of subjects into glucose tolerance categories might have occurred. Furthermore, the information on alcohol intake was assessed by self-reported questionnaire, thus the real daily alcohol consumption may have been undervalued. Besides, our cohort includes outpatients recruited at a referral university hospital, representing subjects at increased risk for cardio-vascular disease, and, therefore, the present results may not be extendible to the general population. Moreover, all participants to the present

Table 4. Logistic regression analyses adjusted for gender of the association between study group subjects and CKD.

	CKD		
Variables	**OR**	**95%CI**	***P***
Individuals at low probability of fibrosis (reference category)	1	—	—
Individuals at high probability of fibrosis	3.94	1.11–14.05	0.03
Glucose tolerance status	1.33	1.02–1.75	0.03
Statin therapy	1.09	0.51–2.32	0.80
Anti-hypertensive treatment	1.04	1.01–1.06	0.002

CKD = chronic kidney disease.

study were White, and whether these findings also can be extended to other ethnic groups remains to be established. Finally, because of the cross-sectional design of this study, the present findings reflect only an association with prevalent and not incident kidney dysfunction, and therefore no definitive cause and effect relationship can be inferred.

The present cross-sectional findings may have both clinical and public health implications. Impaired renal function and NAFLD/NASH are two worldwide health problems due their devastating adverse outcomes, including end-stage renal disease, cirrhosis, hepatocellular carcinoma, and increased cardiovascular morbidity and mortality. Therefore, it appears necessary to identify those individuals who are at greatest risk for hepatic and renal diseases. The use of noninvasive scoring indexes for the prediction of fibrosis in subjects with NAFLD may be useful to identify those patients who need more stringent clinical surveillance aimed at preventing development or progression of both liver and renal complications.

Author Contributions

Conceived and designed the experiments: GS. Performed the experiments: TVF FA MP AS FP. Analyzed the data: GS. Contributed reagents/materials/analysis tools: GS FP. Wrote the paper: GS.

References

1. Go AS, Chertow GM, Fan D, McCulloch CE, Hsu CY (2004) Chronic kidney disease and the risks of death, cardiovascular events, and hospitalization. N Engl J Med 351:1296–1305.
2. Weiner DE, Tighiouart H, Amin MG, Stark PC, MacLeod B, et al. (2004) Chronic kidney disease as a risk factor for cardiovascular disease and all-cause mortality: a pooled analysis of community-based studies. J Am Soc Nephrol 15:1307–1315.
3. Perticone F, Sciacqua A, Maio R, Perticone M, Laino I, et al. (2009) Renal function predicts cardiovascular outcomes in southern Italian postmenopausal women. Eur J Cardiovasc Prev Rehabil 16:481–486.
4. Fox CS, Larson MG, Leip EP, Culleton B, Wilson PW, et al. (2004) Predictors of new-onset kidney disease in a community-based population. JAMA 291:844–850.
5. Chen J, Muntner P, Hamm LL, Jones DW, Batuman V, et al. (2004) The metabolic syndrome and chronic kidney disease in US adults. Ann Intern Med 140:167–174.
6. Sesti G, Succurro E, Arturi F, Andreozzi F, Laino I, et al. (2011) IGF-1 levels link estimated glomerular filtration rate to insulin resistance in obesity: A study in obese, but metabolically healthy, subjects and obese, insulin-resistant subjects. Nutr Metab Cardiovasc Dis 21:485–491.
7. Browning JD, Szczepaniak LS, Dobbins R, Nuremberg P, Horton JD, et al. (2004) Prevalence of hepatic steatosis in an urban population in the United States: impact of ethnicity. Hepatology 40:1387–95.
8. Angulo P (2002) Nonalcoholic fatty liver disease. N Engl J Med 346:1221–1231.
9. Petta S, Muratore C, Craxi A (2009) Nonalcoholic fatty liver disease pathogenesis: the present and the future. Dig Liver Dis 41:615–25.
10. Bugianesi E, Leone N, Vanni E, Marchesini G, Brunello F, et al. (2002) Expanding the natural history of nonalcoholic steatohepatitis: from cryptogenic cirrhosis to hepatocellular carcinoma. Gastroenterology 123:134–140.
11. Adams LA, Lymp JF, St Sauver J, Sanderson SO, Lindor KD, et al. (2005) The natural history of nonalcoholic fatty liver disease: a population-based cohort study. Gastroenterology 129:113–121.
12. Ekstedt M, Franzen LE, Mathiesen UL, Thorelius L, Holmqvist M, et al. (2006) Long-term follow-up of patients with NAFLD and elevated liver enzymes. Hepatology 44:865–873.
13. Rafiq N, Bai C, Fang Y, Srishord M, McCullough A, et al. (2009) Long-term follow-up of patients with nonalcoholic fatty liver. Clin Gastroenterol Hepatol 7:234–238.
14. Marchesini G, Brizi M, Bianchi G, Tomassetti S, Bugianesi E, et al. (2001) Nonalcoholic fatty liver disease: a feature of the metabolic syndrome. Diabetes 50:1844–1850.
15. Stefan N, Kantartzis K, Haring HU (2008) Causes and metabolic consequences of fatty liver. Endocr Rev 29:939–960.
16. Stepanova M, Younossi ZM (2012) Independent association between nonalcoholic fatty liver disease and cardiovascular disease in the US population. Clin Gastroenterol Hepatol 10:646–50.
17. Targher G, Day CP, Bonora E (2010) Risk of cardiovascular disease in patients with nonalcoholic fatty liver disease. N Engl J Med 363:1341–1350.
18. Perticone F, Maio R, Sciacqua A, Perticone M, Laino I, et al. (2009) Insulin-like growth factor-1 and glomerular filtration rate in hypertensive patients. J Hypertens 27:613–617.
19. Petta S, Cammà C, Cabibi D, Di Marco V, Craxì A (2011) Hyperuricemia is associated with histological liver damage in patients with non-alcoholic fatty liver disease. Aliment Pharmacol Ther 34:757–66.
20. Arturi F, Succurro E, Procopio C, Pedace E, Mannino GC, et al. (2011) Nonalcoholic fatty liver disease is associated with low circulating levels of insulin-like growth factor-I. J Clin Endocrinol Metab 96: E1640–E1644.
21. Hribal ML, Procopio T, Petta S, Sciacqua A, Grimaudo S, et al. (2013) Insulin-Like Growth Factor-1, inflammatory proteins, and fibrosis in subjects with nonalcoholic fatty liver disease. J Clin Endocrinol Metab 98:E304–E308.
22. Sciacqua A, Perticone M, Miceli S, Laino I, Tassone EJ, et al. (2011) Endothelial dysfunction and non-alcoholic liver steatosis in hypertensive patients. Nutr Metab Cardiovasc Dis 21:485–491.
23. Perticone F, Maio R, Perticone M, Sciacqua A, Shehaj E, et al. (2010) Endothelial dysfunction and subsequent decline in glomerular filtration rate in hypertensive patients. Circulation 122:379–384.
24. Targher G, Chonchol M, Miele L, Zoppini G, Pichiri I, et al. (2009) Nonalcoholic fatty liver disease as a contributor to hypercoagulation and thrombophilia in the metabolic syndrome. Semin Thromb Hemost 35:277–287.
25. Weiner DE, Tighiouart H, Elsayed EF, Griffith JL, Salem DN, et al. (2008) The relationship between nontraditional risk factors and outcomes in individuals with stage 3 to 4 CKD. Am J Kidney Dis 51:212–223.
26. Targher G, Chonchol M, Zoppini G, Abaterusso C, Bonora E (2011) Risk of chronic kidney disease in patients with non-alcoholic fatty liver disease: is there a link? J Hepatol 54:1020–9.
27. Targher G, Bertolini L, Rodella S, Zoppini G, Lippi G, et al. (2008) Nonalcoholic fatty liver disease is independently associated with an increased prevalence of chronic kidney disease and proliferative/laser-treated retinopathy in type 2 diabetic patients. Diabetologia 51:444–450.
28. Targher G, Chonchol M, Bertolini L, Rodella S, Lippi G, et al. (2010) Relationship between kidney function and liver histology in subjects with nonalcoholic steatohepatitis. Clin J Am Soc Nephrol 5:2166–2171.
29. Yasui K, Sumida Y, Mori Y, Mitsuyoshi H, Minami M, et al. (2011) Nonalcoholic steatohepatitis and increased risk of chronic kidney disease. Metabolism 60:735–9.

30. Chang Y, Ryu S, Sung E, Woo HY, Oh E, et al. (2008) Nonalcoholic fatty liver disease predicts chronic kidney disease in nonhypertensive and nondiabetic Korean men. Metabolism 57:569–576.
31. Targher G, Chonchol M, Bertolini L, Rodella S, Zenari L, et al. (2008) Increased risk of CKD among type 2 diabetics with nonalcoholic fatty liver disease. J Am Soc Nephrol 19:1564–1570.
32. Myers RP, Fong A, Shaheen AA (2008) Utilization rates, complications and costs of percutaneous liver biopsy: a population-based study including 4275 biopsies. Liver Int 28:705–12.
33. Wai CT, Greenson JK, Fontana RJ, Kalbfleisch JD, Marrero JA, et al. (2003) A simple noninvasive index can predict both significant fibrosis and cirrhosis in patients with chronic hepatitis C. Hepatology 38:518–26.
34. Angulo P, Hui JM, Marchesini G, Bugianesi E, George J, et al. (2007) The NAFLD fibrosis score: a noninvasive system that identifies liver fibrosis in patients with NAFLD. Hepatology 45:846–854.
35. Sterling RK, Lissen E, Clumeck N, Sola R, Correa MC, et al. (2006) Development of a simple noninvasive index to predict significant fibrosis in patients with HIV/HCV coinfection. Hepatology 43:1317–1325.
36. Harrison SA, Oliver D, Arnold HL, Gogia S, Neuschwander-Tetri BA (2008) Development and validation of a simple NAFLD clinical scoring system for identifying patients without advanced disease. Gut 57:1441–1447.
37. Demir M, Lang S, Schlattjan M, Drebber U, Wedemeyer I, et al. (2013) NIKEI: a new inexpensive and non-invasive scoring system to exclude advanced fibrosis in patients with NAFLD. PLoS One 8:e58360.
38. Treeprasertsuk S, Björnsson E, Enders F, Suwanwalaikorn S, Lindor KD (2013) NAFLD fibrosis score: a prognostic predictor for mortality and liver complications among NAFLD patients. World J Gastroenterol 19:1219–29.
39. Kim D, Kim WR, Kim HJ, Therneau TM (2013) Association between noninvasive fibrosis markers and mortality among adults with nonalcoholic fatty liver disease in the United States. Hepatology 57:1357–65.
40. Succurro E, Arturi F, Grembiale A, Iorio F, Fiorentino TV, et al. (2011) One-hour post-load plasma glucose levels are associated with elevated liver enzymes. Nutr Metab Cardiovasc Dis 21:713–718.
41. The Expert Committee on the Diagnosis and Classification of Diabetes Mellitus (2013) Follow-up report on the diagnosis of diabetes mellitus. Diabetes Care 26:3160–3167.
42. Matthews DR, Hosker JP, Rudenski AS, Naylor BA, Treacher DF, et al. (1985) Homeostasis model assessment: insulin resistance and beta-cell function from fasting plasma glucose and insulin concentrations in man. Diabetologia 28:412–419.
43. Levey AS, Stevens LA, Schmid CH, Zhang YL, Castro AF 3rd, et al. (2009) CKD-EPI (Chronic Kidney Disease Epidemiology Collaboration). A new equation to estimate glomerular filtration rate. Ann Intern Med 150:604–612.
44. Alberti KG, Eckel RH, Grundy SM, Zimmet PZ, Cleeman JI, et al. (2009) Harmonizing the metabolic syndrome: a joint interim statement of the International Diabetes Federation Task Force on Epidemiology and Prevention; National Heart, Lung, and Blood Institute; American Heart Association; World Heart Federation; International Atherosclerosis Society; and International Association for the Study of Obesity. Circulation120:1640–1645.
45. Tsukahara H, Gordienko DV, Tonshoff B, Gelato MC, Goligorsky MS (1994) Direct demonstration of insulin-like growth factor-I-induced nitric oxide production by endothelial cells. Kidney Int 45:598–604.
46. Haylor J, Singh I, el Nahas AM (1991) Nitric oxide synthesis inhibitor prevents vasodilation by insulin-like growth factor I. Kidney Int 39:333–335.
47. Giordano M, DeFronzo RA (1995) Acute effect of human recombinant insulin-like growth factor I on renal function in humans. Nephron 71:10–15.

19

Effect of Meal Ingestion on Liver Stiffness in Patients with Cirrhosis and Portal Hypertension

Annalisa Berzigotti[1,2], Andrea De Gottardi[1], Ranka Vukotic[1], Sith Siramolpiwat[1], Juan G. Abraldes[1,2], Juan Carlos García-Pagan[1,2], Jaime Bosch[1,2]*

1 Hepatic Hemodynamic Laboratory, Liver Unit, Hospital Clinic, Institut d'Investigacions Biomediques August Pi i Sunyer (IDIBAPS), Barcelona, Spain, **2** Centro de Investigación Biomédica en Red de Enfermedades Hepáticas y Digestivas (CIBERehd), University of Barcelona, Barcelona, Spain

Abstract

Background and Aims: Liver stiffness is increasingly used in the non-invasive evaluation of chronic liver diseases. Liver stiffness correlates with hepatic venous pressure gradient (HVPG) in patients with cirrhosis and holds prognostic value in this population. Hence, accuracy in its measurement is needed. Several factors independent of fibrosis influence liver stiffness, but there is insufficient information on whether meal ingestion modifies liver stiffness in cirrhosis. We investigated the changes in liver stiffness occurring after the ingestion of a liquid standard test meal in this population.

Methods: In 19 patients with cirrhosis and esophageal varices (9 alcoholic, 9 HCV-related, 1 NASH; Child score 6.9±1.8), liver stiffness (transient elastography), portal blood flow (PBF) and hepatic artery blood flow (HABF) (Doppler-Ultrasound) were measured before and 30 minutes after receiving a standard mixed liquid meal. In 10 the HVPG changes were also measured.

Results: Post-prandial hyperemia was accompanied by a marked increase in liver stiffness (+27±33%; $p<0.0001$). Changes in liver stiffness did not correlate with PBF changes, but directly correlated with HABF changes ($r=0.658$; $p=0.002$). After the meal, those patients showing a decrease in HABF ($n=13$) had a less marked increase of liver stiffness as compared to patients in whom HABF increased ($n=6$; +12±21% vs. +62±29%,$p<0.0001$). As expected, post-prandial hyperemia was associated with an increase in HVPG ($n=10$; +26±13%, $p=0.003$), but changes in liver stiffness did not correlate with HVPG changes.

Conclusions: Liver stiffness increases markedly after a liquid test meal in patients with cirrhosis, suggesting that its measurement should be performed in standardized fasting conditions. The hepatic artery buffer response appears an important factor modulating postprandial changes of liver stiffness. The post-prandial increase in HVPG cannot be predicted by changes in liver stiffness.

Editor: Carlos M. Rodriguez-Ortigosa, CIMA. University of Navarra, Spain

Funding: This work is supported in part by grants from Instituto de Salud Carlos III (FIS 09/1261). CIBERehd is funded by Instituto de Salud Carlos III. The funders had no role in study design, data collection and analysis, decision to publish, or preparation of the manuscript.

Competing Interests: The authors have declared that no competing interests exist.

* E-mail: jbosch@clinic.ub.es

Introduction

Liver stiffness (LS) measurement by transient elastography is a non-invasive ultrasound-based technique increasingly used to estimate the degree of fibrosis in patients with chronic liver diseases [1]. Since liver fibrosis is the major factor contributing to portal hypertension [2], LS is able to predict the presence of portal hypertension in patients with cirrhosis [2]. Interestingly, in this population increasing values of LS are associated [3] and predict [4] clinical end-points such as portal hypertension-related complications and hepatocellular carcinoma [5]. Hence, it is necessary to avoid under- or overestimation of LS in cirrhosis since this would lead to erroneous conclusions about the patients' clinical risk.

On the other hand LS increases transiently and independently of fibrosis in a number of pathological conditions, including cholestasis [6], hepatic inflammation [7] and liver congestion [8,9], and measurement standardization is a major issue.

Meal ingestion causes a physiological increase of splanchnic blood flow, which in patients with cirrhosis is associated with an acute increase in HVPG[10–13]. It has been proposed that meals may influence LS in patients with mild chronic hepatitis [14], but there is no information on the post-prandial variation of LS in patients with cirrhosis, who represent the population at risk of clinical events.

In the present study we aimed at investigating whether a test meal induces changes in LS in patients with cirrhosis and whether these changes are influenced by the post-prandial increase occurring in portal blood flow and HVPG.

Patients and Methods

Patients

This study included 19 patients (14 men and 5 women) with cirrhosis and portal hypertension. The study was performed according to the principles of the Declaration of Helsinki, (revision of Edinburgh 2000) and was approved by the Human Research Ethics Committee of the Hospital Clinic (Comité Ético de Investigación Clínica, CEIC), Barcelona, Spain. The nature of the study was explained to the patients, and written informed consent was obtained in each case.

All patients had cirrhosis diagnosed by clinical, biochemical, ultrasonographic, and/or histological criteria. Table 1 summarizes the clinical features of the studied patients. Patients with alcoholic cirrhosis were abstinent from at least 6 months at the moment of the study.

As shown, the mean Child-Pugh score was 6.9±1.8 points (range 5–10); all patients had esophageal varices, which were small in 6 cases, medium in 10, and large in 3.

12 patients had had previous decompensation of cirrhosis, and 7 were compensated. 2 patients had ascites at the moment of the study, which was minimal and did not preclude LS measurement. Mean body weight was 72±10 Kg.

Exclusion criteria were the following: obesity (BMI>30 Kg/m^2), technical failure of transient elastography or Doppler-ultrasound and previous derivative treatment of portal hypertension (surgery or transjugular intrahepatic porto-systemic shunt).

Portal Blood Flow, Hepatic Artery Blood Flow and Total Hepatic Blood Flow by Doppler US

The patients were transferred to the Hepatic Hemodynamics Laboratory in the morning after fasting for at least 6 h, and were let supine for at least 10 minutes before the baseline assessment. Doppler-ultrasound studies were performed with a Siemens ACUSON Sequoia^{TM} 512 (Acuson, Mountain View, CA, USA) using a 3.75 multifrequency sector probe provided with pulsed, colour and power device, by a single trained operator.

The examination included a standard B-mode scan for the assessment of the diameter of portal vein (PV) and hepatic artery (HA), and a colour and pulsed Doppler examination for the assessment of PV and HA blood velocity. All these parameters were measured in standardized sites of the vessels, as previously reported[15–17]. Portal blood flow (PBF) was calculated as follows:

$$\text{PBF (ml/}min) = (\text{PV diameter }(cm))^2/4 \\ * \pi * \text{PV mean blood velocity (cm/s)} * 60.$$

Hepatic artery blood flow (HABF) was similarly calculated.

Total hepatic blood flow (THBF) by Doppler was calculated as the sum of PBF and HABF. The hepatic artery buffer response was defined as a decrease of HABF of at least 10% from the baseline value after the test meal.

Liver Stiffness by Transient Elastography

After Doppler-US assessment, LS was evaluated by transient elastography (Fibroscan®; Echosens, Paris, France). As previously described [2], measurements of LS were performed by the same experienced operator on the right lobe of the liver through intercostal spaces on patients lying in the dorsal decubitus position with the right arm in maximal abduction. The tip of the probe transducer was placed on the skin between the ribs at the level of the right hepatic lobe. The operator, assisted by an ultrasonic time-motion image, located a liver portion of at least 6 cm thick free of large vascular structures. 10 successful measurements were performed on each patient. Success rate was calculated as the ratio of the number of successful measurements over the total number

Table 1. Main clinical and biochemical characteristics of patients included in the study (n = 19).

Parameter	Values	Values in patients in whom HVPG was measured (n = 10)
Age (yrs)	56±10	60±8
Gender (M/F)	14/5	5/5
Etiology (HCV/alcohol/NASH)	9/9/1	4/5/1
Body Mass Index (Kg/m^2)	26.4±2.6	27.5±2.4
Child-Pugh score	6.9±1.8	7.0±1.9
Child-Pugh class (A/B/C)	10/7/2	6/2/2
MELD score	11±4	12±5
Esophageal varices size (small/large)	6/13	1/9
Ascites (n)	2	2
Hepatic Encephalopathy (n)	0	0
Previous decompensation (n)	12	7
Receiving non-selective beta-blockers (n)	13	7
Dose of NSBB (mg/day)	66±39	65±34
Receiving Furosemide (n)	2	1
Receiving Aldosterone (n)	3	1
Albumin (g/dl)	3.5±0.5	3.4±0.6
INR	1.38±0.27	1.43±0.34
Bilirubin (mg/dl)	1.4±0.3	2.1±1.3
Creatinine (mg/dl)	0.77±0.17	0.70±0.17
ALT (U/l)	44±27	38±18

NSBB: non-selective beta-blockers.

of acquisitions. Only liver stiffness measurements with a success rate of at least 60% and an interquartile range lower than 30% were considered reliable. The results are expressed in kilopascal (kPa) and median value was kept as representative of liver stiffness. The whole examination duration was less than 5 minutes. To ensure a better reproducibility, the site of baseline measurement was pointed out by a marker-pen on the patient's skin.

Test Meal

After baseline examination all patients ingested the liquid test meal, that consisted in a milkshake in the iso-volumetric quantity of 7 ml/Kg of body weight containing both whole milk and sugar (0.08 g of proteins/ml, 0.32 g of carbohydrates/ml, and 0.26 g of lipids/ml for a total of 4 kcal/Kg) and 1 unit of Ensure Plus (237 ml, Abbott Netherlands, containing 13 g of proteins, 50 g of carbohydrates, and 11 g of lipids for a total of 350 kcal). Thus, for a 75 Kg individual, the test meal provided 650 kcal, equivalent to the caloric intake of a continental breakfast or a regular Mediterranean lunch. The test meal was administered in 5 minutes. After 30 minutes of the end of meal ingestion all the above mentioned non-invasive measurements were repeated.

HVPG Measurement

In 10 patients the HVPG response to the standard meal was also assessed. Immediately after baseline ultrasound examination and LS measurement patients underwent hepatic vein catheterisation. Under local anaesthesia, with ultrasonographic guidance (SonoSite Inc, Bothell, WA) a 8F venous catheter introducer (Axcess; Maxxim Medical, Athens, TX, USA) was placed in the right internal jugular vein using the Seldinger technique. Thereafter, a 7F balloon-tipped catheter (Edwards Lifesciences, Irvine, CA, USA) was advanced into the right hepatic vein to measure wedged and free hepatic venous pressures (WHVP and FHVP, respectively) by the connection to external electro-mechanical transducer and polygraph (Mac-Lab®, GE Healthcare, Freiburg, Germany). Hepatic venous pressure gradient (HVPG) was calculated as the difference between wedged and free hepatic venous pressure, as previously described [18]. HVPG measurement was performed at baseline and after 30 minutes of standard liquid meal ingestion; all measurements were performed in triplicate, and permanent tracings were recorded.

Statistical analysis. The comparison between baseline and post-prandial measurements in the study population was assessed by Wilcoxon's test. Comparisons between different groups were performed by Mann-Whitney's U test. Correlations were assessed by Spearman's r test.

The α value was set at 0.05. All p-values are two-sided. Statistical analysis was performed with SPSS 16.0 package (SPSS, Chicago, IL, USA).

Results

The baseline and post-prandial values of the studied parameters are shown in Table 2.

Liver Stiffness Changes after the Standard Meal

LS increased markedly post-prandially, by 27.5±33.3% (p<0.0001). LS increase was observed in 15 out of 19 patients; in the remaining four patients LS was unchanged in 1 and decreased in 3. Individual changes are shown in Figure 1, Panel A.

No differences in LS change were seen between patients with HCV-related cirrhosis vs. other etiologies, compensated vs. decompensated patients, and between patients with small varices vs. those with medium/large varices. LS increased more in the 13 patients on NSBB as compared to untreated patients, although this was not statistically significant (31.5±38.1% vs. 16.3±8.0%, p = 0.308).

Post-prandial Changes of Portal Blood Flow, Hepatic Artery Blood Flow, Total Hepatic Blood Flow and HVPG

PBF increased markedly after the test meal (+33.0±30.9%, p<0.0001 vs. baseline); this increase was observed in all patients except one, in whom PBF did not change.

HABF showed overall a buffer response, decreasing by 20.2±45.4% (p = 0.04 vs. baseline). Nonetheless, HABF decreased in 13 patients (mean change −41.8±24.8%), while it increased in 6 cases (mean change +38.5±5.7%).

The fraction of liver perfusion contributed by the hepatic artery tended to decrease after the meal (−28.8±43.2%, p = 0.12). This was particularly evident in the subgroup exhibiting the expected hepatic artery buffer response (−52.8±20.2% vs. +23.2±63.1% in patients lacking the buffer response, p = 0.001).

As a consequence of the above mentioned results, THBF increased slightly in the whole population, by 13.9±19.3% (p = 0.03 vs. baseline).

In the 10 patients undergoing HVPG measurement (mean HVPG 16.4±4.7 mmHg) the post-prandial hyperemia was associated with a highly significant increase of HVPG (+26.4±13.4%, p = 0.003). In these patients liver stiffness increased similarly to the remaining part of the population (+31.4±32.2% vs. +23.2±34.8%, p = 0.497).

Correlation among Post-prandial Changes of the Studied Parameters

LS changes did not correlate with changes in PBF (r = −0.27, p = 0.272), THBF (r = 0.16, p = 0.647) or HVPG (r = 0.32, p = 0.364).

Conversely, LS changes showed a direct and significant correlation with changes in HABF both in the whole population (r = 0.658; p = 0.002) and in the subgroup in which the HVPG was measured (r = 0.699; p = 0.013). Patients showing the expected decrease in HABF post-prandially (n = 13) had a significantly lower increase in LS as compared to patients in whom HABF increased post-prandially (n = 6) (+11.6±20.9% vs. +61.9±29.3%, p<0.0001) (Figure 1 Panel B).

Discussion

LS is currently the best non-invasive surrogate predictor of portal hypertension in patients with cirrhosis [19], and its prognostic value was recently confirmed by cross-sectional studies about the presence of gastroesophageal varices [3,20,21] and longitudinal studies with hard clinical end-points such as the appearance of clinical decompensation and hepatocellular carcinoma [4,5]. Since LS measurement is increasingly used in clinical practice in patients with cirrhosis as a help for prognostic stratification, physicians should be aware of factors causing misleading LS values.

In the present study we report that LS increases markedly after a meal in patients with cirrhosis and portal hypertension (by over 25%). This observation carries an important practical message, since it implies that LS should be always measured in fasting conditions to guarantee reliable values and avoid overestimation in this population.

Our results differ from those reported in the study by Mederacke et al. [14] since, contrarily to what we observed, in their study patients with cirrhosis (baseline values >10 kPa) LS did not increase after a standard meal (600 kcal). All our patients

Table 2. Hemodynamic data at baseline and after the standard meal in the entire studied population (n = 19).

	Baseline	After the standard meal	Change (%)	p
Liver stiffness (kPa)	40.7±16.9	51.2±21.0	27.5±33.3	<0.0001
PBF (ml/min)	893±554	1127±536	33.0±30.9	<0.0001
HABF (ml/min)	278±247	171±116	−20.2±45.4	0.04
HABF (% of THBF)	24.5±14.4	13.9±8.5	−28.8±43.3	0.12
THBF (ml/min)	1171±562	1298±571	13.9±19.3	0.03
HVPG (mmHg) (n = 10)	16.4±4.7	20.2±3.9	26.4±13.4	0.003

Data are shown as mean±SD. p values refer to the comparison between baseline and post-prandial values.

belong to this category, but we observed a marked post-prandial increase of LS. This discrepancy might be due to different factors. First, in our study the timing of the measurements was set at 30 minutes after the test meal, while it was immediately after and 1 hour after the standard meal in the study by Mederacke et al. [14]; our time-point was chosen according to previous observations by our group and others indicating that post-prandial hyperaemia and the post-prandial increase of portal pressure are maximum 30 minutes after meal ingestion [10]. The lack of later time-points is a limitation of the present study that makes difficult to specify for how long the patients should fast before TE. In this regard, it is interesting to note that a ultrasound study on the circadian variation of portal blood flow (PBF) in cirrhosis showed that the hyperaemic response is greater after the morning meal, and that PBF returns to pre-meal values only after circa 4 hours [22]. Therefore, we believe that similarly to what recommended for ultrasound, TE should be performed preferably in the morning after overnight fast or in any case after at least 4 hours fast, until new studies specifically address this issue.

Another potential limitation is that we did not assess in this study the intra-observer variability of Doppler-US and TE measurements. In this regard, previous studies suggest that both inter- and intraobserver variability are low for TE [23]. As for Doppler-US, intraobserver variability is low for experienced operators, as it was in the case of this study, and even inter-observer variability is low if measurements are taken according to standardized protocols [15,24].

Our patients had a severe liver disease, showing established portal hypertension and esophageal varices. We chose studying this homogeneous population since in this setting the effects of meals on splanchnic hemodynamics are well characterized [10,25] and since the presence and extent of collaterals influence the hemodynamic response to a meal [10,25].

As for the relationship between the postprandial increase in portal pressure [10] and LS, we acknowledge that the number of patients studied is small and does not allow driving definite conclusions. With these limits, the lack of correlation between the post-prandial increase in HVPG and the postprandial increase in LS suggests that changes in LS do not mirror the increase in portal pressure, and that factors other than increased PBF and HVPG might modulate the post-prandial increase in LS.

In this regard, we observed that in patients with efficient post-prandial buffer response of the hepatic artery blood flow (physiologic response to increased portal blood flow after a meal) the LS increase was significantly less marked. As a consequence those patients lacking this physiologic adaptative mechanism had a much greater increase of LS, probably reflecting a greater

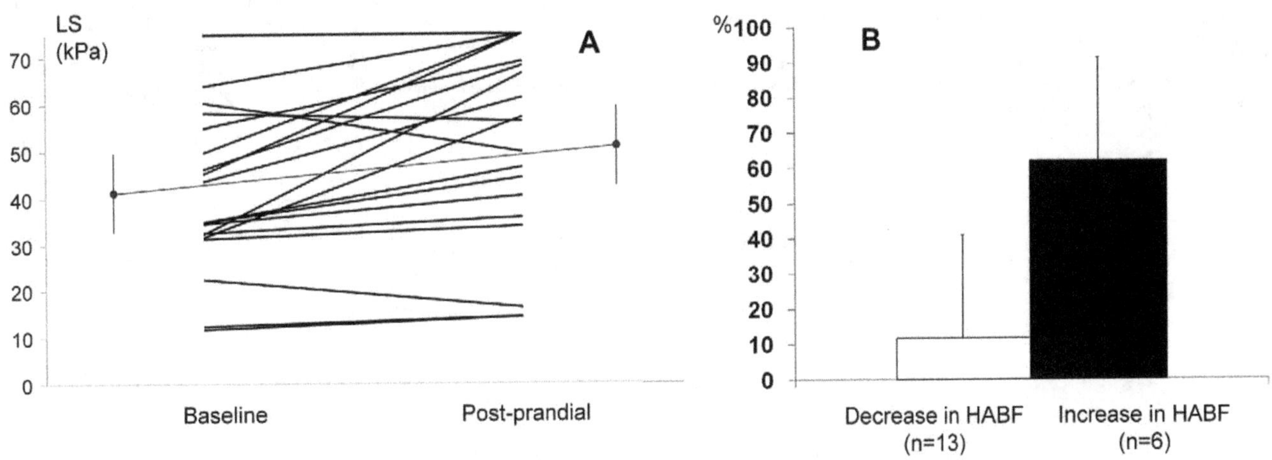

Figure 1. Changes in liver stiffness (LS) after a liquid test meal in the studied population of patients with cirrhosis (n = 19). Panel A. Individual changes of liver stiffness (LS) after the standard meal in the study population (n = 19). Baseline and post-prandial mean value (and standard deviation) are depicted in grey. **Panel B.** Changes in liver stiffness (LS) in patients showing a decrease in hepatic artery blood flow (HABF) post-prandially (column in white, n = 13) vs. HABF increased post-prandially (column in black, n = 6). As shown, patients showing a HABF decrease after the meal had a much lower increase of LS as compared to patients increasing HABF post-prandially (p<0.0001).

contribution of the hepatic arterial blood flow in the total liver perfusion.

Finally, 13/19 patients were receiving propranolol at the moment of the present study. Since propranolol does not blunt postprandial hyperemia [26] and the consequent post-prandial increase in portal pressure [10], it is not surprising that TE increase occurred similarly (and even slightly more pronounced) in patients treated with NSBB.

In conclusion, standard liquid meal ingestion is associated with a marked increase of LS in patients with cirrhosis, suggesting that measurement of LS should be always performed in fasting conditions in this population. LS increase is more pronounced in patients lacking the post-prandial buffer response of hepatic artery blood flow, which appears to be an important factor modulating post-prandial changes in LS.

Acknowledgments

The authors thank Ms. M.A. Baringo, L. Rocabert, and R. Saez for their expert nursing assistance. The authors also express their gratitude to Ms. Clara Esteva for her secretarial support.

Author Contributions

Conceived and designed the experiments: AB JGA JGP JB. Performed the experiments: AB ADG SS RV. Analyzed the data: AB ADG JGP. Contributed reagents/materials/analysis tools: JGP JB. Wrote the paper: AB.

References

1. Friedrich-Rust M, Ong MF, Martens S, Sarrazin C, Bojunga J, et al. (2008) Performance of transient elastography for the staging of liver fibrosis: a meta-analysis. Gastroenterology 134: 960–974.
2. Castera L, Pinzani M, Bosch J (2012) Non invasive evaluation of portal hypertension using transient elastography. J Hepatol 56: 696–703.
3. Foucher J, Chanteloup E, Vergniol J, Castera L, Le Bail B, et al. (2006) Diagnosis of cirrhosis by transient elastography (FibroScan): a prospective study. Gut 55: 403–408.
4. Robic MA, Procopet B, Metivier S, Peron JM, Selves J, et al. (2011) Liver stiffness accurately predicts portal hypertension related complications in patients with chronic liver disease: a prospective study. J Hepatol 55: 1017–1024.
5. Masuzaki R, Tateishi R, Yoshida H, Goto E, Sato T, et al. (2009) Prospective risk assessment for hepatocellular carcinoma development in patients with chronic hepatitis C by transient elastography. Hepatology 49: 1954–1961.
6. Millonig G, Reimann FM, Friedrich S, Fonouni H, Mehrabi A, et al. (2008) Extrahepatic cholestasis increases liver stiffness (FibroScan) irrespective of fibrosis. Hepatology 48: 1718–1723.
7. Arena U, Vizzutti F, Abraldes JG, Corti G, Stasi C, et al. (2008) Reliability of transient elastography for the diagnosis of advanced fibrosis in chronic hepatitis C. Gut 57: 1288–1293.
8. Colli A, Pozzoni P, Berzuini A, Gerosa A, Canovi C, et al. (2010) Decompensated chronic heart failure: increased liver stiffness measured by means of transient elastography. Radiology 257: 872–878.
9. Millonig G, Friedrich S, Adolf S, Fonouni H, Golriz M, et al. (2010) Liver stiffness is directly influenced by central venous pressure. J Hepatol 52: 206–210.
10. Bellis L, Berzigotti A, Abraldes JG, Moitinho E, Garcia-Pagan JC, et al. (2003) Low doses of isosorbide mononitrate attenuate the postprandial increase in portal pressure in patients with cirrhosis. Hepatology 37: 378–384.
11. Brandt JL, Castleman L, Ruskin HD, Greenwald J, Kelly JJ, et al. (1955) The effect of oral protein and glucose feeding on splanchnic blood flow and oxygen utilization in normal and cirrhotic subjects. J Clin Invest 34: 1017.
12. Gaiani S, Bolondi L, Li Bassi S, Santi V, Zironi G, et al. (1989) Effect of meal on portal hemodynamics in healthy humans and in patients with chronic liver disease. Hepatology 9: 815–819.
13. Lee SS, Hadengue A, Moreau R, Sayegh R, Hillon P, et al. (1988) Postprandial hemodynamic responses in patients with cirrhosis. Hepatology 8: 647–651.
14. Mederacke I, Wursthorn K, Kirschner J, Rifai K, Manns MP, et al. (2009) Food intake increases liver stiffness in patients with chronic or resolved hepatitis C virus infection. Liver Int 29: 1500–1506.
15. Sabba C, Merkel C, Zoli M, Ferraioli G, Gaiani S, et al. (1995) Interobserver and interequipment variability of echo-Doppler examination of the portal vein: effect of a cooperative training program. Hepatology 21: 428–433.
16. Sacerdoti D, Gaiani S, Buonamico P, Merkel C, Zoli M, et al. (1997) Interobserver and interequipment variability of hepatic, splenic, and renal arterial Doppler resistance indices in normal subjects and patients with cirrhosis. J Hepatol 27: 986–992.
17. Berzigotti A, Rinaldi MF, Magalotti D, Morelli MC, Zappoli P, et al. (2006) Primary prophylaxis with nadolol in cirrhotic patients: Doppler patterns of splanchnic hemodynamics in good and poor responders. J Hepatol 44: 310–316.
18. Bosch J, Garcia-Pagan JC, Berzigotti A, Abraldes JG (2006) Measurement of portal pressure and its role in the management of chronic liver disease. Semin Liver Dis 26: 348–362.
19. Berzigotti A, Seijo S, Arena U, Abraldes JG, Vizzutti F, et al. (2013) Elastography, spleen size, and platelet count identify portal hypertension in patients with compensated cirrhosis. Gastroenterology 144: 102–111.
20. Castera L, Le Bail B, Roudot-Thoraval F, Bernard PH, Foucher J, et al. (2009) Early detection in routine clinical practice of cirrhosis and oesophageal varices in chronic hepatitis C: comparison of transient elastography (FibroScan) with standard laboratory tests and non-invasive scores. J Hepatol 50: 59–68.
21. Kazemi F, Kettaneh A, N'kontchou G, Pinto E, Ganne-Carrie N, et al. (2006) Liver stiffness measurement selects patients with cirrhosis at risk of bearing large oesophageal varices. J Hepatol 45: 230–235.
22. Schiedermaier P, Koch L, Mojon A, Hermida R, Layer G, et al. (2006) Circadian rhythm of fasting and postprandial portal blood flow in cirrhosis. Scand J Gastroenterol 41: 826–832.
23. Fraquelli M, Rigamonti C, Casazza G, Conte D, Donato MF, et al. (2007) Reproducibility of transient elastography in the evaluation of liver fibrosis in patients with chronic liver disease. Gut 56: 968–973.
24. Berzigotti A, Piscaglia F (2012) Ultrasound in portal hypertension–part 2–and EFSUMB recommendations for the performance and reporting of ultrasound examinations in portal hypertension. Ultraschall Med 33: 8–32.
25. Albillos A, Banares R, Gonzalez M, Catalina MV, Pastor O, et al. (2007) The extent of the collateral circulation influences the postprandial increase in portal pressure in patients with cirrhosis. Gut 56: 259–264.
26. Sabba C, Ferraioli G, Buonamico P, Mahl T, Taylor KJ, et al. (1992) A randomized study of propranolol on postprandial portal hyperemia in cirrhotic patients. Gastroenterology 102: 1009–1016.

20

Complementary Role of HCV and HIV in T-Cell Activation and Exhaustion in HIV/HCV Coinfection

Thijs Feuth[1], Joop E. Arends[1], Justin H. Fransen[1,2], Nening M. Nanlohy[2], Karel J. van Erpecum[3], Peter D. Siersema[3], Andy I. M. Hoepelman[1], Debbie van Baarle[1,2]*

1 Department of Internal Medicine and Infectious Diseases, University Medical Center Utrecht (UMCU), Utrecht, The Netherlands, 2 Department of Immunology, University Medical Center Utrecht (UMCU), Utrecht, The Netherlands, 3 Department of Gastroenterology and Hepatology, University Medical Center Utrecht (UMCU), Utrecht, The Netherlands

Abstract

Objectives: To investigate whether T-cell activation and exhaustion is linked to HCV- and HIV disease parameters in HIV/HCV infected individuals, we studied T-cell characteristics in HIV/HCV coinfected patients and controls.

Methods: 14 HIV/HCV coinfected, 19 HCV monoinfected, 10 HIV monoinfected patients and 15 healthy controls were included in this cross-sectional study. Differences in expression of activation and exhaustion markers (HLA-DR, CD38, PD-1, Tim-3 and Fas) and phenotypic markers on $CD4^+$ and $CD8^+$ T-cells were analysed by flow cytometry and were related to HCV disease parameters (HCV-viremia, ALT and liver fibrosis).

Results: Frequencies of activated $CD4^+$ and $CD8^+$ T-cells were higher in HIV/HCV-coinfected compared to healthy controls and HCV or HIV mono-infected individuals. Coinfected patients also showed high expression of the exhaustion marker PD-1 and death receptor Fas. In contrast, the exhaustion marker Tim-3 was only elevated in HIV-monoinfected patients. T-cell activation and exhaustion were correlated with HCV-RNA, suggesting that viral antigen influences T-cell activation and exhaustion. Interestingly, increased percentages of effector $CD8^+$ T-cells were found in patients with severe (F3–F4) liver fibrosis compared to those with no to minimal fibrosis (F0–F2).

Conclusions: HIV/HCV coinfected patients display a high level of T-cell activation and exhaustion in the peripheral blood. Our data suggest that T-cell activation and exhaustion are influenced by the level of HCV viremia. Furthermore, high percentages of cytotoxic/effector $CD8^+$ T-cells are associated with liver fibrosis in both HCV monoinfected and HIV/HCV coinfected patients.

Editor: Mario A. Ostrowski, University of Toronto, Canada

Funding: The authors have no support or funding to report.

Competing Interests: The authors have declared that no competing interests exist.

* E-mail: dvanbaarle@umcutrecht.nl

Introduction

Co-infection with human immunodeficiency virus (HIV) is relatively common in hepatitis C virus (HCV) infected patients because of shared routes of viral transmission. [1] HIV/HCV-coinfection is associated with an accelerated course of HCV disease progression and increased HCV viral loads compared to HCV-monoinfection, even when HIV is effectively treated.[1–3] Several factors may contribute to this poor prognosis in coinfected patients. Reduced HCV-specific T cell responses have been demonstrated in coinfected patients in the chronic stage of HCV infection, but these studies were limited by either analyzing data of interferon-γ producing cells only [4] or by describing a rather heterogeneous study population including untreated HIV as well as patients on antiretroviral treatment.[4–6] A recent study, investigating the production of interferon-γ (IFN-γ) and tumor necrosis factor-α (TNF-α), found similar HCV-specific T-cell responses in HIV-HCV co-infected patients on antiretroviral treatment compared to HCV monoinfected individuals. [7] Other factors possibly contributing to disease progression in HIV/HCV-coinfection include reduced $CD4^+$ T-cell help in elimination of infected hepatocytes and direct or indirect cytopathic effects of HIV. [8] Increased immune activation has also been proposed as one of the underlying mechanisms of poor clinical outcome of HCV infection in HIV/HCV-coinfected patients. [9].

Next to generalised T cell activation, chronic viral infection is associated with loss of effector and proliferative functions of $CD8^+$ T cells, leading to ineffective viral control. [10] Among other markers of this so-called immune exhaustion, an important function of programmed death receptor 1 (PD-1) has been reported in both HIV and HCV infection and blockage of PD-1 has proved to restore immune function in chronic infection.[10–12] Furthermore, dual expression of exhaustion markers Tim-3 and PD-1 on HCV-specific T cells was shown to be correlated with disease progression in HIV-HCV coinfected patients. [13].

We have previously shown increased expression of the death receptor Fas (CD95) on peripheral CD4+ and CD8+ T-cells in chronic HCV infected patients. [14] This could be a sign of immune activation in these patients similar to the observations of increased immune activation in HIV-patients on effective HAART. [15,16] However, little is known about the additive effect of co-infection with HCV on immune activation in HIV-infected individuals on HAART. A few studies have examined T-cell activation and exhaustion in HIV/HCV co-infection, most of them either lacking a HIV-positive control group or being performed on frozen samples. [5,17,18] To study the contributions of HIV and HCV on T cell activation and exhaustion, we used freshly obtained blood to characterize T-cell phenotypes, activation and exhaustion in HIV/HCV-coinfected patients compared to control groups of healthy individuals, HCV-monoinfected and HIV-monoinfected patients. Additionally, we investigated correlations of T-cell phenotype with HCV disease parameters including stage of liver fibrosis, level of HCV viremia, level of alanine transaminase (ALT) to unravel the contributions of these factors to immune activation.

In the present study we demonstrate that T cell activation and exhaustion are increased in patients with HIV/HCV coinfection compared to control groups. In addition, T-cell activation and exhaustion are correlated with the level of HCV-RNA, suggesting that viral antigen drives T cell activation and exhaustion.

Methods

Ethics Statement

Informed consent was obtained in writing from all patients in accordance with the WMA Declaration of Helsinki and in accordance with the ICH guideline for Good Clinical Practice (6th revision, 2008). The medical ethics committee for research in humans (METC) of the University Medical Center Utrecht, The Netherlands, approved the protocol of this study.

Patients

A total of 58 subjects, including 19 chronic HCV monoinfected patients, 10 HIV-1 monoinfected patients, 14 HIV/HCV coinfected patients and 15 healthy controls were included in this study. All patients were recruited from the Infectious Diseases outpatient clinic or from the Gastroenterology outpatient clinic of the University Medical Center Utrecht (UMCU). All patients were negative for hepatitis B surface antigen (HBsAg). None of the patients received treatment for HCV at the time of inclusion or within 12 months before. All HIV-infected patients were on highly active antiretroviral therapy (HAART), resulting in CD4-counts >200/µL and undetectable HIV viral load (<50 copies/mL). Patients with other diseases possibly interfering with their immune system (e.g. liver disease from non-viral causes, auto-immune disease, malignity or any other severe systemic diseases) were excluded from the study, as well as patients with known prior or present alcohol abuse. In the HCV-monoinfected and the HIV/HCV-coinfected group, liver fibrosis was assessed using transient elastography (Fibroscan® (FS), www.echosens.com, Paris, France). Classification of fibrosis was done using the METAVIR scoring system with F0–F2 being no to mild fibrosis (cut-off <9.5 kPa) and METAVIR F3–F4 being sever fibrosis to cirrhosis (cut-off >9.5 kPa). In patients with recent assessment of fibrosis by liver biopsy (<1 year before inclusion), or known cirrhosis, no fibroscan was required. Levels of HCV-RNA and HIV viral load were measured with COBAS® AmpliPrep/COBAS® TaqMan Polymerase Chain Reaction (PCR; lower limit of detection 15 IU/mL for HCV and 50 copies/ml for HIV). Blood from anonymous healthy controls was requested from the bloodbank Mini Donor Dienst of the UMC Utrecht and was tested negative for hepatitis B, hepatitis C and HIV. All patients and healthy controls were between 18 and 65 years old.

Processing of Blood for Isolation of PBMCs and Analysis with Flow Cytometry

From all patients whole blood was collected by vena puncture in sodium heparin tubes (approximately 27 mL) for PBMCs. Within 8 hours, peripheral blood mononuclear cells (PBMCs) were isolated by standard density centrifugation using Ficoll Hypaque. Per patient, 5 million freshly isolated PBMCs were washed twice with phosphate buffered saline (PBS) and directly stained for markers of T-cell phenotype, activation and exhaustion. The following antibodies were used: anti-CD3 (label: V500; provided by: BD horizon; clone: SP34-2), CD4 (eFluor780; eBioscience; RPA-T4 and PE-Cy7; BioLegend; L3T4), CD8 (PB, BioLegend; RPA-T8 and eFluor780; eBioscience; RPA-T8), CD27 (eFluor780; eBioscience; O323); CD38 (R-PE; Invitrogen; HIT2); CD45RO (APC; BioLegend; UCHL1); CD95 (APC; BP Pharmigen; DX2); PD-1 (PerCP/Cy5.5; BioLegend; EH12.2H7); Tim3 (PE, BioLegend; F38-2E2). Cells were incubated with the antibodies for 20 minutes at 4°C. After washing with PBS/0.5% bovine serum albumin, cells were fixed with Cellfix (BD) and directly analysed by flow cytometry. As an additional marker for effector T-cells, we analysed intracellular perforin expression. To this end, freshly isolated PBMCs were, directly after staining of surface markers, permeabilized and lysed (FACS permeabilizing solution 2 and FACS lysis solution; BD). After permeabilization, cells were incubated with anti-perforin (FITC; δG9; BD). After washing, cells were fixed with Cellfix (BD) and directly analysed on an LSR II FACS machine (BD). Per sample, 100.000 events were acquired. This resulted in exclusion of 2 healthy controls, 4 HCV-monoinfected and 2 HIV/HCV-coinfected patients for the perforin-staining.

Statistical Analysis

Medians were compared with Mann Whitney test or, in case of multiple groups, with one-way ANOVA followed by Dunnett's multiple comparison test. Two-way ANOVA was used for comparing medians with two independent variables. Fisher's exact tests were used to test relation of categorical variables. Dependence of variables was tested using Spearman's one-tailed correlation coefficient. Statistical analysis was performed with IBM SPSS Statistics version 19.0 (SPSS Inc., IBM) and GraphPad Prism 5 for Windows version 5.03 (GraphPad Software, Inc).

Results

Patient Characteristics

Peripheral blood was drawn from a total of 58 subjects, consisting of 14 HIV/HCV-coinfected patients, 19 HCV-monoinfected patients, 10 HIV-monoinfected patients and 15 uninfected healthy controls. Characteristics of the different patient groups are shown in table 1. None of the patients received treatment for HCV at the time of inclusion. However, eight out of nineteen HCV monoinfected patients (42%) and three out of thirteen HIV/HCV coinfected patients (21%) had a history of ineffective HCV treatment more than 1 year before inclusion, while all others were treatment-naïve ($p = 0.07$). All HIV-infected patients (both monoinfected and HCV-coinfected) were on HAART at the time of this study, resulting in $CD4^+$ T-cell counts above 200 cells/mm^3 and HIV-RNA <50 copies/mL. Median duration of HAART was 8 years in the monoinfected and 13 years in the coinfected group ($p = 0.35$). As expected, the ALT value was lower in HIV mono-infected patients (30 IU/L) compared to the

HCV-infected patients (65 IU/L; $p<0.05$), but ALT levels were similar between HIV/HCV coinfected (65 IU/L) and HCV monoinfected patients (69 IU/L; $p=0.92$). There was a trend towards higher level of HCV-viremia in coinfected patients (1.9e6 IU/mL) compared to HCV monoinfected patients (4.5e5 IU/mL; $p=0.07$) (table 1).

HIV/HCV Coinfection is Associated with Increased T-cell Activation and PD-1 Expression

To study T-cell activation and exhaustion in HIV/HCV-coinfected patients, we measured expression of activation markers CD38 and HLA-DR [19], exhaustion markers Programmed Death Receptor-1 (PD-1) and T-cell immunoglobulin domain and mucin domain 3 (Tim-3) and death receptor Fas (CD95) in coinfected patients, HIV- or HCV-monoinfected patients and uninfected healthy controls. Gating strategy and representative plots of a healthy control, HCV-monoinfected, HIV-monoinfected and HIV/HCV-coinfected patient are shown in figure 1A–E. Frequencies of activated $CD4^+$ and $CD8^+$ T-cells, defined by CD38/HLA-DR double positivity, were higher in HIV/HCV-coinfected patients (median 1.9% and 5.6% respectively) compared to healthy controls (medians 0.8%; $p<0.001$ and 1.7%; $p<0.01$). Coinfected patients also displayed higher $CD4^+$ T-cell activation (1.9%) in comparison to HCV- or HIV-monoinfected patients (1.4%, $p<0.01$ and 1.2%, $p<0.01$) (Fig. 2A). Expression of the T-cell exhaustion marker PD-1 was higher on $CD4^+$ T-cells of coinfected patients (13.2%) in comparison with HIV-monoinfected patients (7.8%; $p<0.05$) and healthy controls (5.5%; $p<0.001$). A similar pattern of PD-1 expression was observed in $CD8^+$ T cells (HIV/HCV: 13.3%, healthy controls: 8.1%, HCV: 10.3%, HIV 9.5%; not significant) (Fig. 2B). Interestingly, Tim-3 expression was not significantly increased in HIV/HCV coinfected patients. In contrast, HIV-monoinfected patients depicted significantly higher levels of Tim3 on both $CD4^+$ and $CD8^+$ T cells (1.9% and 2.8%) compared to HIV/HCV coinfected patients (0.8%; $p<0.05$ and 1.1%; $p<0.01$) and healthy controls (0.6%; $p<0.01$ and 0.6%; $p<0.001$) (fig 2C). Numbers of PD-1 and Tim-3 dual positive T cells were too low for reliable analysis.

Furthermore, with high activation and exhaustion in HIV/HCV coinfected patients compared to healthy controls, a higher susceptibility to apoptosis was expected. [20] Indeed, expression of the death receptor Fas on $CD4^+$ T-cells of coinfected patients (median 71%) was significantly increased compared to healthy controls (40%, $p<0.001$) and HIV-infected controls (60%; $p<0.05$). However, in coinfected patients Fas-expression on $CD4^+$ T-cells (71%) did not differ in comparison to HCV monoinfected controls (63%). On $CD8^+$ T-cells, there were no significant differences of Fas expression in coinfected patients (36%) compared to HCV or HIV monoinfected patients (31% and 43%) or healthy controls (16%) (Fig. 2B).

T-cell Activation and Exhaustion are Linked to Level of HCV-RNA in HIV-HCV Co-infection

To elucidate which clinical parameters may contribute to T-cell activation and exhaustion, we investigated correlations of ALT and HCV viremia with expression of HLA-DR/CD38, PD-1, Tim-3, and Fas.

Within all HCV-infected patients, HCV-RNA correlated positively with T cell activation (CD8: $r=0.37$, $p<0.05$; CD4: $r=0.28$, $p=0.08$) as well as with expression of the exhaustion

Table 1. Patient characteristics.

	HCV/HIV	HCV	HIV	
	n = 14	**n = 19**	**n = 10**	**P-value**
General characteristics				
Age, median (IQR), years	48 (14)	55 (7)	46 (6)	0.12
Gender, % male	86%	74%	90%	0.27
ALT, median (IQR), IU/L	65 (80)	69 (85)	30 (22)	<0.001
HCV disease characteristics				
HCV-RNA, median (IQR), IU/mL	1.9e6 (4.8e6)	4.5e5 (1.1e6)		0.07
Genotype, % genotype 1	75%	79%		1.00
History of HCV treatment:				0.07
Naïve, number (%)	3 (21%)	11 (58%)		
Previously failed treatment, n (%)	11 (79%)	8 (42%)		
Liver fibrosis/cirrhosis				0.73
F0–F2, number (%)	8 (57%)	9 (47%)		
F3–F4, number (%)	6 (43%)	10 (53%)		
HIV disease characteristics				
Viral load, copies/mL	All <50		All <50	-
CD4-count, median (IQR),/mm^3	540 (330)		661 (247)	0.11
HAART regimen				0.70
PI-based	7 (50%)		4 (40%)	
Other regimens	7 (50%)		6 (60%)	
Years of HAART, median	13		8	0.35

General and disease-specific characteristics of patient groups. Abbreviations: **ALT**, alanine transaminase; **IQR**, interquartile range; **PI**, protease inhibitor; **HAART**, highly active antiretroviral treatment.

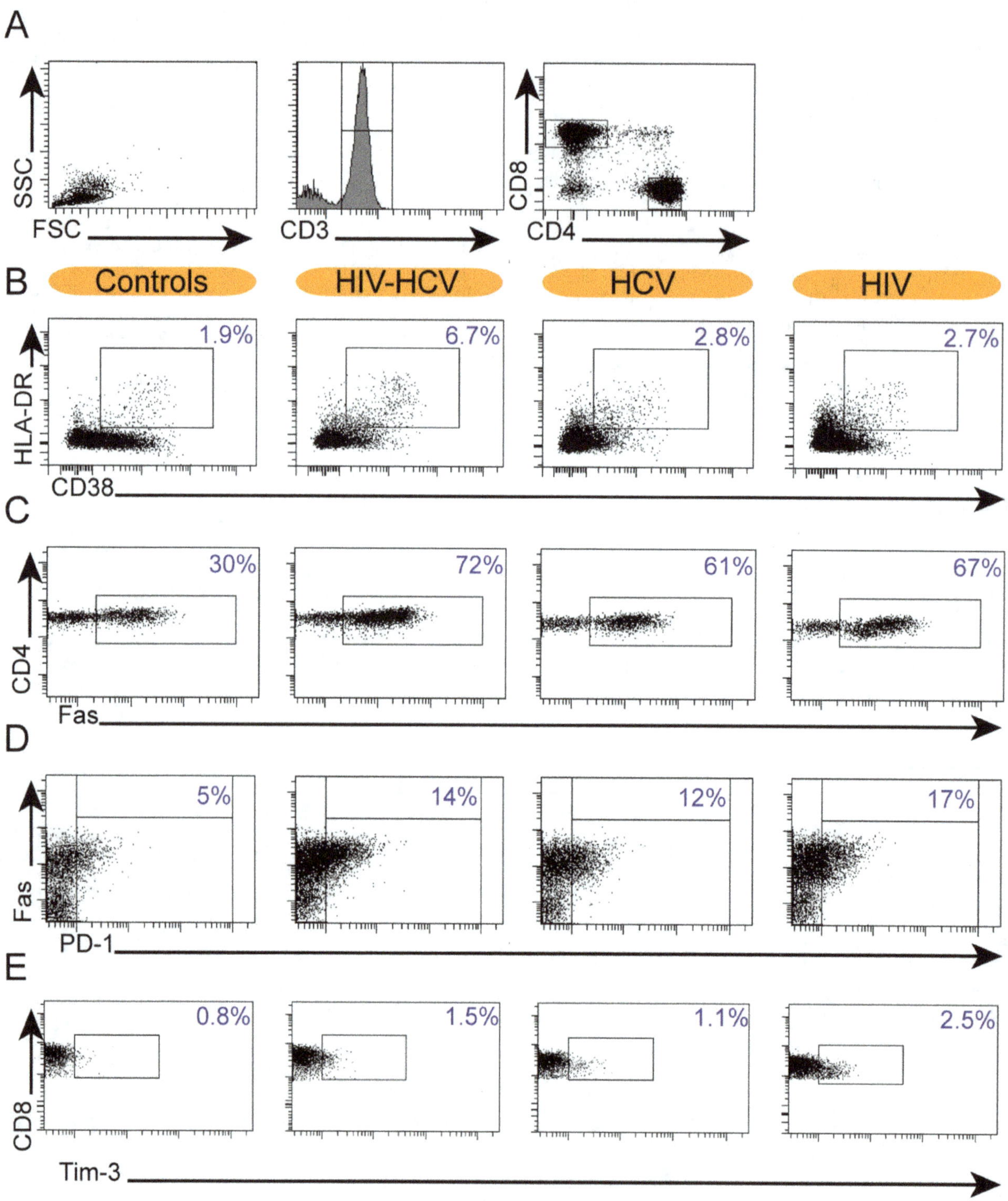

Figure 1. Representative flow cytometry plots. Representative flow cytometry plots of T-cell activation- and exhaustion markers in HIV-HCV coinfected patients, HCV mono- and HIV mono-infected patients and healthy controls. A: gating of $CD4^+$ and $CD8^+$ T-cells by lymphocyte-gate (left panel), CD3-gate (middle panel) and gates for $CD4^+$ or $CD8^+$ T-cells (right panel). B-E: representative flow cytometry plots of a healthy control (left), HIV-HCV coinfected (middle left), HCV monoinfected (middle right) and HIV -monoinfected patient (right) showing (B) activated $CD8^+$ T-cells; (C) Fas-positive $CD4^+$ T-cells; (D) PD-1 positive $CD4^+$ T-cells and (E) Tim-3 positive $CD8^+$ T cells. Percentages are depicted in the right upper corner.

marker PD-1 ($CD4^+$: $r = 0.52$, $p<0.01$ and $CD8^+$: $r = 0.55$, $p<0.001$), whereas there was no correlation with expression of Tim-3. The positive correlation of PD-1 expression was still present when the patients were divided in HCV-monoinfected (CD4: $r = 0.49$, $p = 0.04$; CD8: $r = 0.39$, $p = 0.08$) and HIV/HCV coinfected patients (CD4:0.26, not significant; CD8:0.53, $p = 0.03$). Additionally, a borderline significant correlation of

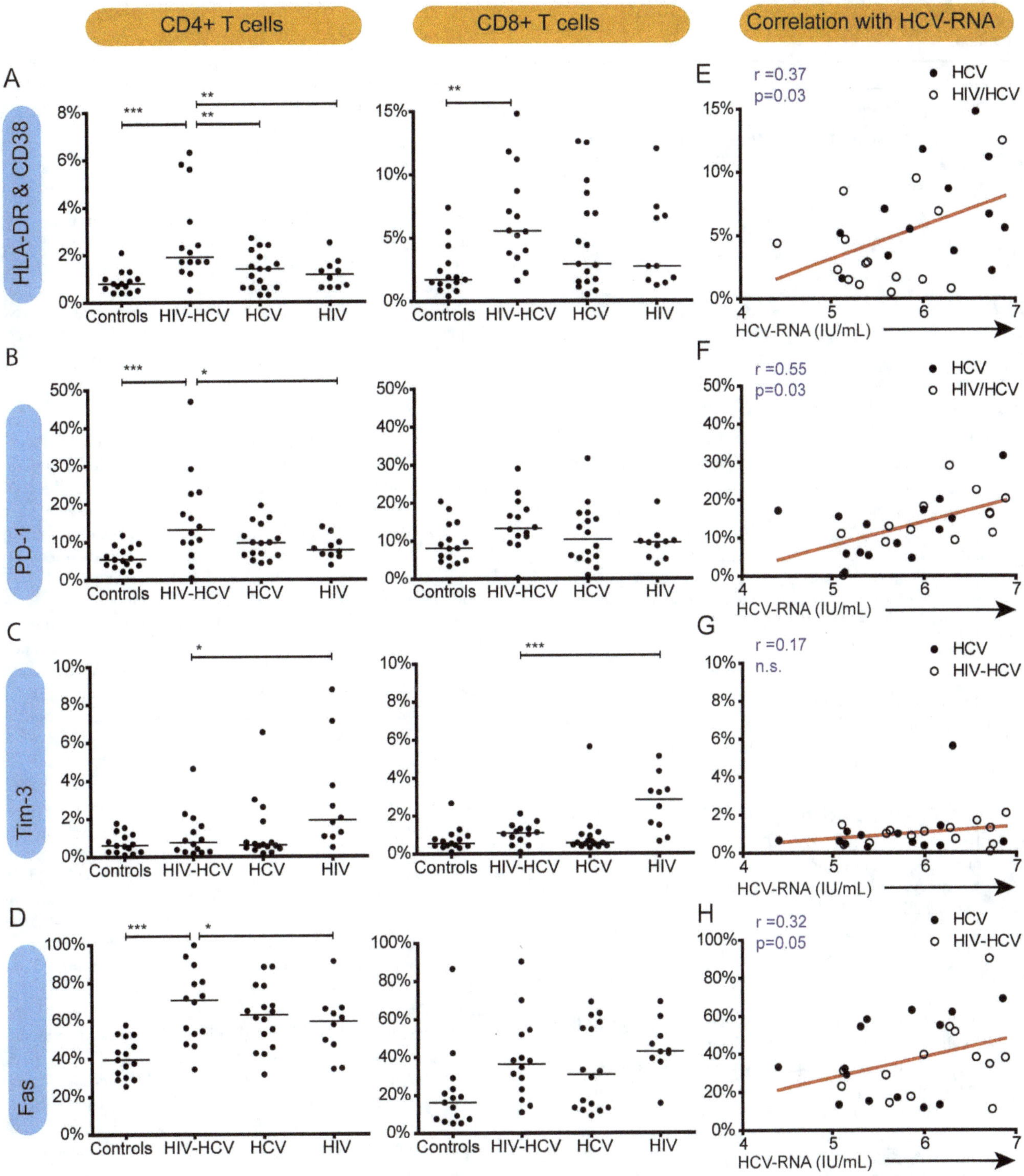

Figure 2. T-cell activation and exhaustion and its correlations with HCV-RNA in HIV/HCV-coinfection and control groups. A: percentages of HLA-DR$^+$CD38$^+$ activated CD4$^+$ (left) and CD8$^+$ T-cells (right). B: percentages of PD-1 positive CD4$^+$ and CD8$^+$ T-cells. C: percentages of Tim3-positive CD4$^+$ and CD8$^+$ T-cells. D: percentage of death receptor Fas positive CD4$^+$ and CD8$^+$ T cells. E-H: correlations of HCV viral load within HIV-HCV coinfected (open dots) and HCV monoinfected patients (closed dots) with percentages of HLA-DR and CD38 positive CD8 T cells (E); PD-1 positive CD8 T cells (F); Tim-3 positive CD8 T cells (G) and Fas positive CD8 T cells (H). HCV viral loads are depicted in IU/mL. P-values are indicated with * ($p<0.05$), ** ($p<0.01$) or *** ($p<0.0001$). Spearman r and p-value of correlations are depicted in the upper left corner of each graph; red lines represent semilog fit lines.

HCV-RNA and death receptor Fas expression on CD8$^+$ T cell was found ($r=0.32$, $p=0.05$) (figure 2; table 2).

In contrast, there was no correlation of T cell activation and exhaustion with ALT (table 2). Furthermore, T-cell activation and

Table 2. Correlations of clinical parameters and T cell markers.

	CD4			CD8		
	Spearman R		p-value	Spearman R		p-value
HCV-RNA						
HLA-DR+CD38+	0.28		0.08	0.37		0.03
PD1+	0.52		<0.01	0.55		0.03
Tim3+	0.01		n.s.	0.17		n.s.
Fas+	0.20		n.s.	0.32		0.05
ALT						
HLA-DR+CD38+	-0.09		n.s.	0.13		n.s.
PD1+	0.16		n.s.	0.26		n.s.
Tim3+	-0.17		n.s.	0.24		n.s.
Fas+	0.24		n.s.	0.12		n.s.
Liver fibrosis	**F0–F2**	**F3–F4**	**P-value**	**F0–F2**	**F3–F4**	**p-value**
HLA-DR+CD38+	1.6%	1.9%	n.s.	4.4%	5.4%	n.s.
PD1+	10.2%	10.4%	n.s.	14.6%	9.8%	n.s.
Tim3+	0.6%	1.1%	n.s.	0.8%	0.7%	n.s.
Fas+	57%	66%	n.s.	34%	32%	n.s.

Spearman correlations of HCV-RNA and ALT with expression of activation and exhaustion markers and median expression of these markers in patients with F0–F2 versus F3–F4 fibrosis in all HCV-monoinfected and HIV/HCV-coinfected patients.

exhaustion as well as level of HCV-viremia were similar in patients with F0–F2 fibrosis or F3–F4 fibrosis (table 2). Lastly, a history of failed HCV-treatment was not associated with differences in T-cell activation or exhaustion.

HCV and HIV are Associated with Differences in Memory and Effector Phenotype of CD8$^+$ T-cells

Chronic viral infections are shown to coincide with changes in T-cell memory and effector phenotype. [21] Therefore, we examined whether HIV/HCV-coinfection drives changes in memory and effector phenotype of CD8$^+$ T-cells, by studying percentages of naïve (CD45RO$^-$CD27$^+$), central memory (CD45RO$^+$CD27$^+$), effector memory (CD45RO$^-$CD27$^+$) and effector (CD45RO$^-$CD27$^-$) CD8$^+$ T-cells. Representative plots of a healthy control, an HCV monoinfected patient and an HIV/HCV coinfected patient are shown in figure 3A.

Mean percentages of T-cell phenotypes in patients compared to healthy controls are depicted as pie graphs in figure 3B. Due to the small percentages of effector T-cells, changes in these subsets are more apparent when depicted as relative increase compared to healthy controls (Fig. 3C). HIV/HCV coinfected patients showed significantly higher frequencies of central memory CD8$^+$ T-cells compared to healthy controls (15.1% versus 11.8% $p<0.05$). The increase of effector CD8$^+$ T-cells was significant in HCV and HIV monoinfection but not in HIV/HCV coinfection (Fig. 3B–C). There was no correlation with levels of HCV-RNA or ALT with memory and effector phenotype.

Liver Fibrosis is Associated with Increased Frequencies of Effector CD8$^+$ T-cells

As T-cell mediated killing of infected hepatocytes is essential in liver fibrogenesis, [22] we investigated whether liver fibrosis was associated with differences in T-cell effector phenotype. Indeed, we found increased effector CD8$^+$ T-cell frequencies in patients with F3–F4 liver fibrosis in both HCV monoinfected patients (median 41.3% versus 21.7% in patients with F0–F2 liver fibrosis) and HIV/HCV-coinfected patients (33.2% versus 25.0%; $p<0.01$) (Fig. 3D). This finding was further confirmed by a positive correlation of percentages effector CD8$^+$ T cells with Fibroscan-score ($r = 0{,}57$; $p = 0.0019$) (data not shown). Additional analysis of intracellular perforin expression within CD8$^+$ T-cells, as an indicator of effector T-cells with a potency to kill, revealed slightly higher frequencies of perforin-positive CD8$^+$ T-cells in mono- and coinfected patients with severe fibrosis, albeit not significant ($p = 0.54$; data not shown). However, frequencies of perforin-positive CD8$^+$ T-cells correlated strongly with effector phenotype ($r = 0.48$; $p<0.001$; Fig. 3E). Altogether, these data suggest a role for perforin-positive/effector phenotype CD8$^+$ T-cells in liver fibrosis.

Discussion

HIV/HCV-coinfection is associated with faster HCV disease progression than HCV-monoinfection. [3] The underlying pathogenic mechanisms for poor clinical outcome in HCV/HIV coinfection remain unclear although various mechanisms have been suggested, including increased immune activation. [9,23] The present study confirms that HIV/HCV coinfected patients on HAART indeed have higher levels of T-cell activation as indicated by CD38/HLA-DR expression. In addition, we show that these T-cells are also high in expression of PD-1 and Fas, both linked to T-cell exhaustion and apoptosis. [24,25] Furthermore, this study shows correlations of concentration between HCV-RNA and markers for T-cell activation and exhaustion, suggesting a role for HCV viremia in influencing T-cell activation and exhaustion in this group of patients.

Recently, it has become clear that HIV-infected patients on antiretroviral treatment still display slightly increased T-cell activation, [26,27] despite its initial decrease upon start of antiretroviral treatment. [28] Interestingly, we observed higher T-cell activation in HIV/HCV coinfected patients compared to HIV-monoinfected patients despite longer history of HAART in coinfected patients. [29] Various underlying mechanisms contributing to T-cell activation in those patients have been proposed in literature, of which the concept of microbial translocation is a currently widely accepted model. [16] As we show that the level of T-cell activation correlates with HCV-RNA, we hypothesize that this concomitant viral infection may well contribute to the observed increase of T-cell activation in HIV-infected individuals. Indeed, in a cohort of HCV monoinfected patients [30] we have previously observed a decrease in CD4 and CD8$^+$ T cell activation after 4 weeks of IFN-α/ribavirin treatment in the subset of patients with rapid viral response (HCV-RNA <50 IU/mL at week 4 of therapy), whereas there was no change in T cell activation in patients without rapid viral response (unpublished data). Since immune activation is thought to play an important role in long-term morbidity and mortality, [31] it can be hypothesized that coinfection with HCV may contribute to long-term extrahepatic morbidity in HIV-infected individuals through increased immune activation. Indeed, a recent study observed a higher prevalence of subclinical carotid plaque formation in HIV-patients coinfected with HCV compared to HIV-monoinfected patients. [32] However, a prospective study is required to examine whether increased peripheral T-cell activation in HCV-monoinfected and HIV/HCV-coinfected patients is indeed associated with mortality and long-term morbidity.

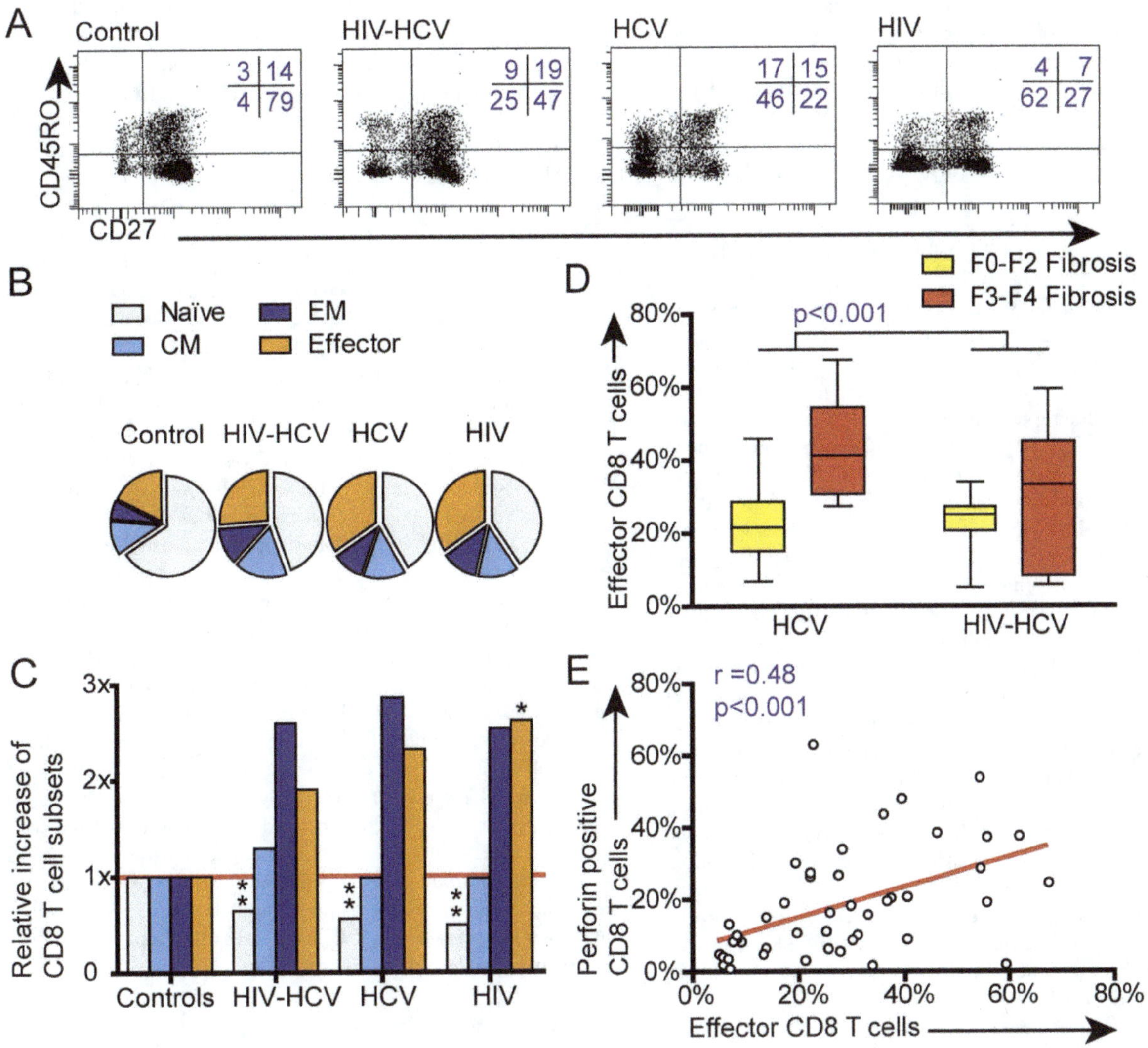

Figure 3. Changes in $CD8^+$ effector and memory phenotype in all patients and healthy controls. A: representative plots of a healthy control, HIV-HCV coinfected, HCV monoinfected and HIV- mono patient showing naïve (right lower quadrant), central memory (right upper quadrant), effector memory (left upper quadrant) and effector (left lower quadrant) $CD8^+$ T-cells by CD27 and CD45RO staining. B: pie charts of mean percentages of naïve (light grey), central memory (CM; light blue), effector memory (EM; dark blue) and effector (orange) $CD8^+$ T-cells in 42 patients and 3 healthy controls. C: relative increase of median percentages of memory subsets compared to healthy controls. D: box plot showing percentages of effector $CD8^+$ T-cells in HCV-monoinfected (left) or HIV/HCV-coinfected patients (right) with fibrosis scores F0–F2 (yellow) versus F3–F4 (red). The depicted p-value was calculated with two way ANOVA and indicates statistical significant difference in percentages of effector $CD8^+$ T cells in F0–F2 fibrosis compared to F3–F4 fibrosis, independent of coinfection with HIV. Liver fibrosis was assessed with Fibroscan in 74% of HCV monoinfected patients and 71% of HIV/HCV coinfected patients. E: correlation of staining for perforin (Y-axis) with effector phenotype (X-axis) in $CD8^+$ T-cells. Box-plots show median, quartiles and range. Line represents linear regression. P-values are depicted as: * (<0.05) and ** (p-value <0.01).

In this study, T cell exhaustion, measured by PD-1 expression, correlated with HCV-RNA in HCV monoinfected and HIV/HCV coinfected patients. This is in line with a rather old study showing a correlation between HCV viral load and decreased T cell function in HCV-monoinfection, but at that time a role for PD-1 was in T cell exhaustion was not yet discovered. [33] Thus, to our knowledge, we are the first to show increased T cell exhaustion indicated by PD-1 expression is linked to HCV viremia. Based on a study evaluating T cell exhaustion upon LCMV-infection in C57BL/6 mice, [34] it can be hypothesised that high level of viremia contributes to increased exhaustion, although it can also be reasoned that T cell exhaustion by itself may lead to higher antigen levels through decreased viral control. [11] In contrast, Tim-3 was lower in HIV-HCV coinfected patients compared to HIV-monoinfected controls. This finding is supported by data from a recent study by Vali *et al.*, in which Tim-3/PD-1 on total $CD4^+$ and $CD8^+$ T cell pools were highest in HIV-monoinfected patients in comparison with HIV-HCV coinfected and HCV monoinfected patients. [13] Although not significant, our data support the observation by *Vali et al.* that Tim-3 expression is increased in HCV-infected patients in comparison to healthy controls. [13] It must be noted that age and gender of healthy volunteers were not characterised do to the anonymous service of the blood bank.

One possible explanation for decreased Tim-3 expression in HIV-HCV coinfected patients compared to HIV-monoinfected patients could be decreased activity of T-bet, a transcription factor classically associated with Th1 phenotype [35] but recently also shown to induce Tim-3 and repress PD-1 expression. [36,37] Persistent antigen exposure was shown to lead to downregulation of T-bet. [37] This suggests that downregulation of T-bet due to persistent HCV antigen may be involved in decreased Tim-3 expression and increased PD-1 expression, as we observed in the present study, next to decreased Th1/Th2 ratio, observed by others, [38] associated with coinfection of HCV in HAART-treated HIV patients.

A second interesting observation in our cross-sectional study is the high level of effector CD8$^+$ T-cells in HCV monoinfected and HIV/HCV-coinfected patients with severe fibrosis. Few other studies investigate changes of memory and effector T-cell memory and effector compartments in HIV/HCV-coinfection. [5,17,18,39] However, these studies did not compare to HCV- or HIV mono-infected controls or were heterogeneous in terms of HIV treatment, including both patients treated with HAART and patients with untreated HIV, [5,17,18,39] which may result in HIV-antigen driven differences in memory and effector phenotype. To our knowledge, no studies relating these T-cell phenotypes to fibrosis progression have been published. Our data suggests that effector T-cells might play a role in liver fibrosis since it has been shown that similar T-cell populations are present in blood as well as in the liver of HCV infected patients. [40] Killing of infected hepatocytes by intrahepatic cytotoxic T-cells may be perforin-dependent [41] and apoptosis of hepatocytes has a strong profibrotic effect through activation of hepatic stellate cells. [42] We therefore postulate that high frequencies of effector CD8$^+$ T-cells may contribute to liver fibrosis by killing infected hepatocytes which in turn activate hepatic stellate cells and promote fibrogenesis. Alternatively, it may be hypothesized that increased percentages in the peripheral blood would reflect an actual decrease at the site of infection due to compartmentalization. However, it has recently been shown that CD27 expression by intrahepatic lymphocytes is reflected by CD27 expression in the peripheral blood. [43] Examination of effector T cell phenotypes in liver biopsies in patients with minimal or severe fibrosis are needed to provide a definite conclusion.

The design of the present study was distinctive for several reasons. First, all stainings for activation and exhaustion markers were performed on freshly isolated PBMCs, thereby eliminating any influence of cryopreservation on expression of activation and exhaustion markers and T-cell phenotype which hampers other studies. [44,45]. Albeit our sample size is somewhat smaller than other studies, we believe that our data closely reflect the actual phenotype of T-cells in the peripheral blood. Furthermore, patients with no or minimal fibrosis as well as patients with severe fibrosis were included enabling us to investigate whether phenotypic differences are correlated to HCV disease progression. The HIV-infected groups were homogenous, including only patients on successful antiretroviral therapy (HIV not detectable, CD4>200). The frequency of HCV treatment experienced patients was higher in the HCV-monoinfected group in comparison to the HIV/HCV-coinfected group, but a minimum of 1 year interferon free period was required before inclusion and no late effects of interferon are known from literature.

The present study is hampered by the fact that we did not investigate antigen-specific T-cells, we cannot be sure whether our findings with respect to T-cell memory subsets, activation and exhaustion are directly influencing HCV-specific T-cell responses. However, various previous studies have convincingly proved that PD-1 and Tim-3 expression suppress HCV-specific immune responses and thereby contribute to viral persistence in HCV. [46] Furthermore, liver infiltrates are largely composed of HCV-nonspecific T cells, suggesting that disease progression may well be affected by non-specific activation. [40,47,48].

From the present study we conclude that T-cells in HIV/HCV-coinfected patients show increased activation and exhaustion surface markers compared to healthy controls as well as to HIV- or HCV (co)infected patients. This suggests that HIV and HCV have a complementary role on T-cell activation in HIV/HCV coinfection. This could at least partly be explained by the level of antigen, since T cell activation and exhaustion correlated with the level of HCV viremia. Furthermore, liver fibrosis is associated with increased frequencies of effector CD8$^+$ T-cells, based on extracellular surface markers and intracellular perforin expression, suggesting that these effector CD8$^+$ T-cells may contribute to liver fibrosis in a perforin dependent manner.

Author Contributions

Conceived and designed the experiments: TF JEA DvB AIMH PDS. Performed the experiments: TF JHF NMN. Analyzed the data: TF DvB JEA. Contributed reagents/materials/analysis tools: KvE JA AIMH. Wrote the paper: MF JA DvB KvE.

References

1. Sherman KE, O'Brien J, Gutierrez AG, Harrison S, Urdea M, et al. (1993) Quantitative evaluation of hepatitis C virus RNA in patients with concurrent human immunodeficiency virus infections. J Clin Microbiol 31: 2679–2682.
2. Bonacini M, Govindarajan S, Blatt LM, Schmid P, Conrad A, et al. (1999) Patients co-infected with human immunodeficiency virus and hepatitis C virus demonstrate higher levels of hepatic HCV RNA. J Viral Hepat 6: 203–208.
3. Koziel MJ, Peters MG (2007) Viral hepatitis in HIV infection. N Engl J Med 356: 1445–1454.
4. Capa L, Soriano V, Garcia-Samaniego J, Nunez M, Romero M, et al. (2007) Influence of HCV genotype and co-infection with human immunodeficiency virus on CD4(+) and CD8(+) T-cell responses to hepatitis C virus. J Med Virol 79: 503–510.
5. Dutoit V, Ciuffreda D, Comte D, Gonvers JJ, Pantaleo G (2005) Differences in HCV-specific T cell responses between chronic HCV infection and HIV/HCV co-infection. Eur J Immunol 35: 3493–3504.
6. Kim AY, Schulze zur WJ, Kuntzen T, Timm J, Kaufmann DE, et al. (2006) Impaired hepatitis C virus-specific T cell responses and recurrent hepatitis C virus in HIV coinfection. PLoS Med 3: e492. 06-PLME-RA-0235R2 [pii];10.1371/journal.pmed.0030492 [doi].
7. Rallon NI, Soriano V, Restrepo C, Garcia-Samaniego J, Labarga P, et al. (2011) HCV-specific T-cell responses in HIV/hepatitis C virus-coinfected patients on highly active antiretroviral therapy are comparable to those observed in hepatitis C virus-monoinfected individuals. J Acquir Immune Defic Syndr 57: 1–8.
8. Rockstroh JK, Spengler U (2004) HIV and hepatitis C virus co-infection. Lancet Infect Dis 4: 437–444. 10.1016/S1473-3099(04)01059-X [doi];S147330990401059X [pii].
9. Page EE, Nelson M, Kelleher P (2011) HIV and hepatitis C coinfection: pathogenesis and microbial translocation. Curr Opin HIV AIDS 6: 472–477.
10. Wherry EJ (2011) T cell exhaustion. Nat Immunol 12: 492–499.
11. Barber DL, Wherry EJ, Masopust D, Zhu B, Allison JP, et al. (2006) Restoring function in exhausted CD8 T cells during chronic viral infection. Nature 439: 682–687.
12. Freeman GJ, Wherry EJ, Ahmed R, Sharpe AH (2006) Reinvigorating exhausted HIV-specific T cells via PD-1-PD-1 ligand blockade. J Exp Med 203: 2223–2227. jem.20061800 [pii];10.1084/jem.20061800 [doi].
13. Vali B, Jones RB, Sakhdari A, Sheth PM, Clayton K, et al. (2010) HCV-specific T cells in HCV/HIV co-infection show elevated frequencies of dual Tim-3/PD-1 expression that correlate with liver disease progression. Eur J Immunol 40: 2493–2505. 10.1002/eji.201040340 [doi].
14. Arends JE, Hoepelman AI, Nanlohy NM, Hoppener FJ, Hirsch KR, et al. (2011) Low doses of the novel caspase-inhibitor GS-9450 leads to lower caspase-3 and -8 expression on peripheral CD4+ and CD8+ T-cells. Apoptosis 16: 959–966.
15. Gonzalez VD, Falconer K, Blom KG, Reichard O, Morn B, et al. (2009) High levels of chronic immune activation in the T-cell compartments of patients coinfected with hepatitis C virus and human immunodeficiency virus type 1 and on highly active antiretroviral therapy are reverted by alpha interferon and ribavirin treatment. J Virol 83: 11407–11411.

16. Brenchley JM, Price DA, Schacker TW, Asher TE, Silvestri G, et al. (2006) Microbial translocation is a cause of systemic immune activation in chronic HIV infection. Nat Med 12: 1365–1371. nm1511 [pii];10.1038/nm1511 [doi].
17. Al-Harthi L, Voris J, Du W, Wright D, Nowicki M, et al. (2006) Evaluating the impact of hepatitis C virus (HCV) on highly active antiretroviral therapy-mediated immune responses in HCV/HIV-coinfected women: role of HCV on expression of primed/memory T cells. J Infect Dis 193: 1202–1210.
18. Nunez M, Soriano V, Lopez M, Ballesteros C, Cascajero A, et al. (2006) Coinfection with hepatitis C virus increases lymphocyte apoptosis in HIV-infected patients. Clin Infect Dis 43: 1209–1212.
19. Hamann D, Baars PA, Rep MH, Hooibrink B, Kerkhof-Garde SR, et al. (1997) Phenotypic and functional separation of memory and effector human CD8+ T cells. J Exp Med 186: 1407–1418.
20. Kondo Y, Machida K, Liu HM, Ueno Y, Kobayashi K, et al. (2009) Hepatitis C virus infection of T cells inhibits proliferation and enhances fas-mediated apoptosis by down-regulating the expression of CD44 splicing variant 6. J Infect Dis 199: 726–736. 10.1086/596739 [doi];10.1086/596739 [pii].
21. Wherry EJ, Ahmed R (2004) Memory CD8 T-cell differentiation during viral infection. J Virol 78: 5535–5545. 10.1128/JVI.78.11.5535-5545.2004 [doi];78/11/5535 [pii].
22. Spengler U, Nattermann J (2007) Immunopathogenesis in hepatitis C virus cirrhosis. Clin Sci (Lond) 112: 141–155.
23. Sandberg JK, Falconer K, Gonzalez VD (2010) Chronic immune activation in the T cell compartment of HCV/HIV-1 co-infected patients. Virulence 1: 177–179.
24. Watanabe T, Bertoletti A, Tanoto TA (2010) PD-1/PD-L1 pathway and T-cell exhaustion in chronic hepatitis virus infection. J Viral Hepat 17: 453–458. JVH1313 [pii];10.1111/j.1365-2893.2010.01313.x [doi].
25. Dianzani U, Bensi T, Savarino A, Sametti S, Indelicato M, et al. (2003) Role of FAS in HIV infection. Curr HIV Res 1: 405–417.
26. Hunt PW, Brenchley J, Sinclair E, McCune JM, Roland M, et al. (2008) Relationship between T cell activation and CD4+ T cell count in HIV-seropositive individuals with undetectable plasma HIV RNA levels in the absence of therapy. J Infect Dis 197: 126–133. 10.1086/524143 [doi].
27. Valdez H, Connick E, Smith KY, Lederman MM, Bosch RJ, et al. (2002) Limited immune restoration after 3 years' suppression of HIV-1 replication in patients with moderately advanced disease. AIDS 16: 1859–1866.
28. Kaufmann GR (2000) Rapid restoration of CD4 T cell subsets in subjects receiving antiretroviral therapy during primary HIV-1 infection.
29. Vrisekoop N, van GR, de Boer AB, Otto SA, Borleffs JC, et al. (2008) Restoration of the CD4 T cell compartment after long-term highly active antiretroviral therapy without phenotypical signs of accelerated immunological aging. J Immunol 181: 1573–1581. 181/2/1573 [pii].
30. Arends JE, Claassen MA, van den Berg CH, Nanlohy NM, van Erpecum KJ, et al. (2010) T-cell responses at baseline and during therapy with peginterferon-alpha and ribavirin are not associated with outcome in chronic hepatitis C infected patients. Antiviral Res 87: 353–360. S0166-3542(10)00635-2 [pii];10.1016/j.antiviral.2010.06.002 [doi].
31. Deeks SG (2009) Immune dysfunction, inflammation, and accelerated aging in patients on antiretroviral therapy. Top HIV Med 17: 118–123.
32. Sosner P, Wangermez M, Chagneau-Derrode C, Le MG, Silvain C (2012) Atherosclerosis risk in HIV-infected patients: The influence of hepatitis C virus co-infection. Atherosclerosis 222: 274–277. S0021-9150(12)00141-4 [pii];10.1016/j.atherosclerosis.2012.02.027 [doi].
33. Hiroishi K, Kita H, Kojima M, Okamoto H, Moriyama T, et al. (1997) Cytotoxic T lymphocyte response and viral load in hepatitis C virus infection. Hepatology 25: 705–712. S0270913997001420 [pii];10.1002/hep.510250336 [doi].
34. Mueller SN, Ahmed R (2009) High antigen levels are the cause of T cell exhaustion during chronic viral infection. Proc Natl Acad Sci U S A 106: 8623–8628. 0809818106 [pii];10.1073/pnas.0809818106 [doi].
35. Szabo SJ, Kim ST, Costa GL, Zhang X, Fathman CG, et al. (2000) A novel transcription factor, T-bet, directs Th1 lineage commitment. Cell 100: 655–669. S0092-8674(00)80702-3 [pii].
36. Anderson AC, Lord GM, Dardalhon V, Lee DH, Sabatos-Peyton CA, et al. (2010) T-bet, a Th1 transcription factor regulates the expression of Tim-3. Eur J Immunol 40: 859–866. 10.1002/eji.200939842 [doi].
37. Kao C, Oestreich KJ, Paley MA, Crawford A, Angelosanto JM, et al. (2011) Transcription factor T-bet represses expression of the inhibitory receptor PD-1 and sustains virus-specific CD8+ T cell responses during chronic infection. Nat Immunol 12: 663–671. ni.2046 [pii];10.1038/ni.2046 [doi].
38. Kang W, Li Y, Zhuang Y, Zhao K, Huang D, et al. (2012) Dynamic analysis of Th1/Th2 cytokine concentration during antiretroviral therapy of HIV-1/HCV co-infected patients. BMC Infect Dis 12: 102. 1471-2334-12-102 [pii];10.1186/1471-2334-12-102 [doi].
39. Roe B, Coughlan S, Dean J, Lambert JS, Keating S, et al. (2009) Phenotypic characterization of lymphocytes in HCV/HIV co-infected patients. Viral Immunol 22: 39–48.
40. Neumann-Haefelin C, Timm J, Spangenberg HC, Wischniowski N, Nazarova N, et al. (2008) Virological and immunological determinants of intrahepatic virus-specific CD8+ T-cell failure in chronic hepatitis C virus infection. Hepatology 47: 1824–1836. 10.1002/hep.22242 [doi].
41. Ando K, Hiroishi K, Kaneko T, Moriyama T, Muto Y, et al. (1997) Perforin, Fas/Fas ligand, and TNF-alpha pathways as specific and bystander killing mechanisms of hepatitis C virus-specific human CTL. J Immunol 158: 5283–5291.
42. Mehal W, Imaeda A (2010) Cell death and fibrogenesis. Semin Liver Dis 30: 226–231. 10.1055/s-0030-1255352 [doi].
43. Heydtmann M, Hardie D, Shields PL, Faint J, Buckley CD, et al. (2006) Detailed analysis of intrahepatic CD8 T cells in the normal and hepatitis C-infected liver reveals differences in specific populations of memory cells with distinct homing phenotypes. J Immunol 177: 729–738.
44. Costantini A, Mancini S, Giuliodoro S, Butini L, Regnery CM, et al. (2003) Effects of cryopreservation on lymphocyte immunophenotype and function. J Immunol Methods 278: 145–155. S0022175903002023 [pii].
45. Fowke KR, Behnke J, Hanson C, Shea K, Cosentino LM (2000) Apoptosis: a method for evaluating the cryopreservation of whole blood and peripheral blood mononuclear cells. J Immunol Methods 244: 139–144. S0022-1759(00)00263-5 [pii].
46. Klenerman P, Thimme R (2011) T cell responses in hepatitis C: the good, the bad and the unconventional. Gut. gutjnl-2011-300620 [pii];10.1136/gutjnl-2011-300620 [doi].
47. He XS, Rehermann B, Lopez-Labrador FX, Boisvert J, Cheung R, et al. (1999) Quantitative analysis of hepatitis C virus-specific CD8(+) T cells in peripheral blood and liver using peptide-MHC tetramers. Proc Natl Acad Sci U S A 96: 5692–5697.
48. Minutello MA, Pileri P, Unutmaz D, Censini S, Kuo G, et al. (1993) Compartmentalization of T lymphocytes to the site of disease: intrahepatic CD4+ T cells specific for the protein NS4 of hepatitis C virus in patients with chronic hepatitis C. J Exp Med 178: 17–25.

21

Glucokinase Regulatory Protein Gene Polymorphism Affects Liver Fibrosis in Non-Alcoholic Fatty Liver Disease

Salvatore Petta[1]*, Luca Miele[2], Elisabetta Bugianesi[3], Calogero Cammà[1], Chiara Rosso[3], Stefania Boccia[2], Daniela Cabibi[4], Vito Di Marco[1], Stefania Grimaudo[1], Antonio Grieco[2], Rosaria Maria Pipitone[1], Giulio Marchesini[5], Antonio Craxì[1]

1 Sezione di Gastroenterologia, Dipartimento Biomedico di Medicina Interna e Specialistica, University of Palermo, Palermo, Italy, **2** Institute of Internal Medicine, School of Medicine, Catholic University of the Sacred Heart, Rome, Italy, **3** Division of Gastroenterology, Dept. of Medical Sciences, University of Turin, Turin, Italy, **4** Cattedra di Anatomia Patologica, University of Palermo, Palermo, Italy, **5** Dipartimento di Medicina e Gastroenterologia, "Alma Mater Studiorum," Università di Bologna, Bologna, Italy

Abstract

Background and Aims: Variant in glucokinase regulatory protein (GCKR), associated with lipid and glucose traits, has been suggested to affect fatty liver infiltration. We aimed to assess whether GCKR rs780094 C→T SNP influences the expression of steatosis, lobular inflammation and fibrosis in NAFLD patients, after correction for PNPLA3 genotype.

Methods: In 366 consecutive NAFLD patients (197 from Sicily, and 169 from center/northern Italy), we assessed anthropometric, biochemical and metabolic features; liver biopsy was scored according to Kleiner. PNPLA3 rs738409 C>G and GCKR rs780094 C>T single nucleotide polymorphisms were also assessed.

Results: At multivariate logistic regression analysis in the entire NAFLD cohort, the presence of significant liver fibrosis (>F1) was independently linked to high HOMA (OR 1.12, 95% CI 1.01–1.23, $p = 0.02$), NAFLD activity score ≥5 (OR 4.09, 95% CI 2.45–6.81, $p < 0.001$), and GCKR C>T SNP (OR 2.06, 95% CI 1.43–2.98, $p < 0.001$). Similar results were observed considering separately the two different NAFLD cohorts. GCKR C>T SNP was also associated with higher serum triglycerides (ANOVA, p = 0.02) in the entire cohort.

Conclusions: In patients with NAFLD, GCKR rs780094 C>T is associated with the severity of liver fibrosis and with higher serum triglyceride levels.

Editor: Erica Villa, University of Modena & Reggio Emilia, Italy

Funding: This study was funded by grants from the FP7/2007–2013 (n°Health-F2-2009-241762), from PRIN 2009 (Prot. N. 2009ARYX4T_004), and from PRIN 2010–2011 (Prot. N. 2010C4JJWB_001). The funders had no role in study design, data collection and analysis, decision to publish, or preparation of the manuscript.

Competing Interests: The authors have declared that no competing interests exist.

* E-mail: petsa@inwind.it

Introduction

Non-alcoholic fatty liver disease (NAFLD) is a frequent and growing cause of chronic liver disease [1,2], affecting about 20%–30% of the general population worldwide [3]. Patients with NAFLD, and especially those with non-alcoholic steatohepatitis (NASH), are at risk of progression to cirrhosis and its complications [1,4], presenting also a high rate of cancer and cardiovascular events [5] compared to subjects without fatty liver. Classical risk factors for liver disease severity and its progression are obesity, insulin resistance (IR) and necroinflammation [6–9].

The above-mentioned conventional risk factors do not entirely explain the occurrence and severity of NAFLD, suggesting that a genetic background might also modulate the spectrum of liver disease and its progression. Accordingly, the severity of disease has been variably associated with different single nucleotide polymorphisms (SNPs) in genes involved in metabolic homeostasis, inflammation, oxidative stress and fibrogenesis [10]. In this context, the patatin-like phospholipase-3 (*PNPLA3)/adiponutrin*, rs738409 C>G SNP remains the most validated risk gene [11–18].

Besides the classical PNPLA3, a recent genome wide study identified other genetic variants associated with computerized tomography (TC)-proven hepatic steatosis in individuals of European ancestry, and validated the results in 592 subjects with biopsy-proven NAFLD from the NASH Clinical Research Network (NASH CRN) database [19]. Among these gene variants, the glucokinase regulatory protein (GCKR) has been further confirmed as linked with steatosis (identified either by ultrasonography, by magnetic resonance, or by computed tomography) in children, in obese patients, and in populations of different ethnicity [20–22]. GCKR seems to interfere with glucose and lipid homeostasis by regulating glucose storage/disposal and by providing substrates for de novo lipogenesis via inhibition of glucokinase, but its potential association with the severity of liver damage has never been tested

Having this in mind, the main outcome of this study was to assess whether GCKR rs780094 was associated with the histological features of liver damage in patients with biopsy-proven NAFLD, after correction for PNPLA3 genotype.

Patients and Methods

Patients

We analyzed data from 366 prospectively recruited Italian patients with a clinical and histological diagnosis of NAFLD, and with blood samples available for genetic analyses. The study cohort included 197 patients from the Gastrointestinal & Liver Unit of the Palermo University Hospital, and 169 central/northern Italy patients from the Department of Internal Medicine Catholic University of the Sacred Heart Rome (n = 114), and from the Gastro-hepatology Division of the University Hospital Torino (n = 55). Other causes of liver disease were ruled out, including alcohol intake (>20 g/day) evaluated by a questionnaire, viral and autoimmune hepatitis, hereditary hemochromatosis and alpha1-antitrypsin deficiency. Patients with advanced cirrhosis, hepatocellular carcinoma and current use of steatosis inducing drugs were excluded.

The study was carried out in accordance with the principles of the Helsinki Declaration, and with local and national laws. Approval was obtained from the hospital Internal Review Boards and their Ethics Committees (UOC Gastroenterologia, AOUP Policlinico of Palermo, Institute of Internal Medicine, Catholic University of the Sacred Heart, Rome, and Division of Gastro-Hepatology, San Giovanni Battista Hospital, University of Torino), and written informed consent for the study was obtained from all patients.

Clinical and Laboratory Assessment

Clinical and anthropometric data were collected at the time of liver biopsy. Body mass index (BMI) was calculated on the basis of weight in kilograms and height in meters. The diagnosis of arterial hypertension was based on the following criteria: systolic blood pressure ≥135 mm Hg and/or diastolic blood pressure ≥85 mm Hg (measured three times within 30 minutes, in the sitting position and using a brachial sphygmomanometer), or use of blood-pressure-lowering agents. The diagnosis of type 2 diabetes was based on the revised criteria of the American Diabetes Association, using a value of fasting cut-off value of blood glucose ≥126 mg/dl on at least two occasions [23]. In patients with a previous diagnosis of type 2 diabetes, current therapy with insulin or oral hypoglycemic agents was documented.

A 12-hour overnight fasting blood sample was drawn at the time of biopsy to determine serum levels of ALT, total cholesterol, HDL-cholesterol, triglycerides, plasma glucose and insulin concentrations. IR was assessed by homeostasis model assessment (HOMA), using the following equation [24]: Insulin resistance (HOMA-IR) = Fasting insulin (μU/mL)×Fasting glucose (mmol/L)/22.5. [25]. HOMAbeta was also assessed as expression of pancreatic beta-cell function [26]

Genetic Analyses

DNA was purified using the QIAmp blood Mini Kit (Qiagen, Mainz, Germany) and DNA samples were quantified using spectrophotometric determination. Genotyping for PNPLA3 *(rs738409), and GCKR (rs780094)* was carried out using the TaqMan SNP genotyping allelic discrimination method (Applied Biosystems, Foster City, CA, USA). Commercial genotyping assays were available for the following SNPs: *rs738409* (cat. C_7241_10), rs780094 (cat. C_2862873_10).

The genotyping call was done with SDS software v.1.3.0 (ABI Prism 7500, Foster City, CA, USA). Genotyping was conducted in a blinded fashion relative to patient characteristics.

Assessment of Histology

Slides were coded and read at each clinical center by one expert pathologist, who was unaware of patients' identity and history. A minimum 15 mm-length of the biopsy specimen or the presence of at least 10 complete portal tracts was required [27]. Steatosis was assessed as the percentage of hepatocytes containing fat droplets (minimum 5%) and evaluated as a continuous variable. Kleiner classification [28] was used to compute steatosis, balloning and lobular inflammation, and to stage fibrosis from 0 to 4. NASH was considered to be present when the NAFLD activity score (NAS) was ≥5 [28].

Statistics

Continuous variables were summarized as mean ± standard deviation, and categorical variables as frequency and percentage. The t-test, ANOVA test, and chi-square test were used when appropriate.

Multiple logistic regression models were used to assess the factors independently associated with severe steatosis, NAS ≥5, and significant fibrosis. In the first model, the dependent variable was steatosis, coded as 0 = mild-moderate (steatosis grade 1–2), 1 = severe (steatosis grade 3). In the second model, the dependent variable was NAS ≥5, coded as 0 = NAS<5 or 1 = NAS ≥5. In the third model, the dependent variable was fibrosis, coded as 0 = no significant fibrosis (F0–F1) or 1 = significant fibrosis (>F1).

As candidate risk factors, we selected age, gender, BMI, the baseline levels of ALT, triglycerides, total and HDL cholesterol, blood glucose, insulin, HOMA score, the presence of diabetes, arterial hypertension, PNPLA3 rs738409, GCKR rs780094, steatosis, lobular inflammation and fibrosis.

In all models, in agreement with literature data, we compared patients homozygous for PNPLA3 G risk allele to all other variants [14], while an additive model was used GCKR C>T SNP [19].

To avoid the effect of colinearity, diabetes, HOMA score, blood glucose and insulin levels, or ALT levels and lobular inflammation were not included in the same multivariate model. Variables associated with the dependent variable at univariate analysis (probability threshold, p≤0.10) were included in the multivariate regression models; PNPLA3 and GCKR SNPs, were forced into the models when not significant associated to the tested dependent variable. Regression analyses were performed using PROC LOGISTIC, PROC REG, and subroutines in SAS [29].

Results

Patient Features and Histology

The baseline characteristics of the 197 Sicilian and the 169 Center/Northern Italian NAFLD patients are shown in Table 1. Patients from Sicily were slightly older and with a moderately lower prevalence of males, were more likely to be obese and to have more severe steatosis and lobular inflammation compared to Center/Northern Italian patients. Nevertheless, histological staging was similar in the two cohorts and significant fibrosis (>F1) was present in approximately half of the patients.

The prevalence of GCKR rs780094 CC, CT and TT genotypes was 16.4%, 48.9% and 34.7% in the entire cohort. When split according to center (Sicily vs. Center/Northern Italy) the prevalence of the single SNPs was similar (16.2%, 50.3% and 33.5% in the Sicilian cohort, vs. 16.6%, 47.3% and 36.1%; p = 0.98). Similarly, the prevalence of PNPLA3 rs738409 CC, CG

Table 1. Baseline Demographic, Laboratory, Metabolic, and Histological Features of 366 Italian Patients with Non-alcoholic Fatty Liver Disease.

Variable	Non-alcoholic Fatty Liver Disease (Sicily n = 197)	Non-alcoholic Fatty Liver Disease (Center/Northern Italy n = 169)	P value
Mean Age - years	45.0±13.3	42.2±11.2	0.03
Male Gender	131 (66.5)	130 (76.9)	0.03
Mean Body Mass Index - kg/m²	29.7±4.6	27.8±4.1	<0.001
Alanine Aminotransferase - IU/L	79.4±55.1	77.8±53.3	0.78
Arterial Hypertension	46 (23.3)	47 (27.8)	0.21
Type 2 Diabetes	28 (14.2)	22 (11.2)	0.39
Cholesterol - mg/dL	205.8±44.8	203.4±45.2	0.74
HDL Cholesterol - mg/dL	49.0±15.4	47.7±11.3	0.38
Triglycerides - mg/dL	147.6±78.7	142.7±86.9	0.57
Blood Glucose - mg/dL	96.1±25.2	94.7±21.5	0.56
Insulin - μU/mL	16.5±9.6	14.5±10.6	0.08
HOMA Score	4.03±2.96	3.57±3.41	0.18
PNPLA3 rs738409 polymorphism			
C/C	62 (31.5)	54 (31.9)	
C/G	94 (47.7)	79 (46.7)	
G/G	41 (20.8)	36 (21.4)	0.98
GCKR rs780094 polymorphism			
C/C	32 (16.2)	28 (16.6)	
C/T	99 (50.3)	80 (47.3)	
T/T	66 (33.5)	61 (36.1)	0.98
Histology			
Lobular inflammation			
2–3			
Balloning	83 (42.1)	20 (11.8)	<0.001
1–2	181 (91.8)	122 (71.7)	<0.001
Steatosis grade			
1 (5%–33%)	72 (36.6)	76 (44.9)	
2 (>33%–66%)	62 (31.5)	62 (36.7)	
3 (>66%)	63 (31.9)	31 (18.4)	0.01
NAS≥5	116 (58.8)	41 (24.2)	<0.001
Stage of Fibrosis			
2–4	86 (43.6)	72 (42.6)	0.84

Abbreviation: IU, international units; HOMA, homeostasis model assessment; HDL, high density lipoprotein. Data are given as mean ± standard deviation, or as number of cases (%).

and GG genotypes was 31.5%, 47.7% and 20.8% in the Sicilian cohort, and 31.9%, 46.7% and 21.4% in the Center/Northern Italy cohort (p = 0.98).

Genetic frequencies of the two polymorphisms fit with Hardy–Weinberg equilibrium.

Influence of GCKR Genotype on Metabolic and Biochemical Parameters

The association of the rs780094 GCKR C→T genotype with anthropometric, metabolic and biochemical parameters in the entire cohort is shown in Table 2. The only significant association was between the TT genotype and higher triglyceride levels, although independent of age, gender distribution, and BMI. When split according to center, broadly similar data were observed in the Center/Northern Italian cohort, where an association between GCKR TT genotype and higher blood glucose levels was also observed (85.5±11.6 for CC, 96.7±24.4 for CT, 96.4±20 for TT; p = 0.03). By contrast, in the Sicilian cohort the rs780094 genotype was not associated with abnormal triglyceride levels.

Factors Associated with Histological Features

In the entire cohort, multivariate logistic regression analysis showed that high BMI (OR 1.10, 95% CI 1.04–1.117, $p = 0.001$), high HOMA considered as continuous variable (OR 1.08, 95% CI 1.00–1.17, $p = 0.04$), and PNPLA3 GG (OR 1.97, 95% CI 1.11–3.51, $p = 0.02$) were independently associated with severe steatosis (table 3 upper panel). Similar results were observed when analyses were split by center (table 3 upper panel).

In the whole NAFLD cohort, NAS score ≥5 was independently associated with female gender (OR 2.55, 95% CI 1.51–4.31,

Table 2. Association of the rs780094 C→T GCKR SNP with anthropometric, biochemical, metabolic and histological features in 366 Patients with Non-alcoholic Fatty Liver Disease.

Variable	GCKR CC N = 60	GCKR CT n = 179	GCKR TT n = 127	Univariate Analysis *p* value °
Mean age - years	42.2±13.0	43.3±12.6	44.9±11.8	0.33
Males	48	127	86	0.22
Mean body mass index - kg/m^2	28.5±4.6	28.7±4.4	29.1±4.5	0.61
Alanine aminotransferase - IU/L	81.6±70.6	81.4±52.1	73.4±48.0	0.40
Cholesterol - mg/dL	198.6±47.9	202.4±40.9	209.5±48.5	0.23
HDL cholesterol - mg/dL	50.2±18.2	48.9±13.2	47.1±12.2	0.32
Triglycerides - mg/dL	139.8±83.3	138.0±69.8	158.3±96.3*	0.09
Blood glucose - mg/dL	91.4±18.6	96.6±27.7	95.8±18.5	0.32
Insulin - μU/mL	15.1±9.8	16.0±9.1	15.4±11.5	0.78
HOMA-score	3.65±3.23	3.96±3.03	3.70±3.05	0.68
HOMAbeta %	144.4±63.7	144.6±71.5	131.8±61.0	0.25
Diabetes	8	21	18	0.81
Arterial hypertension	14	41	38	0.35
Steatosis grade 3	13	44	37	0.49
Lobular Inflammation Grade 2-3	17	53	34	0.86
Ballooning	46	151	105	0.39
NAS ≥5	24	82	51	0.54
Fibrosis >F1	17	71	70	0.001

Data are given as mean ± SD or as number of cases. HDL: high-density lipoprotein; HOMA: homeostasis model assessment.
°by ANOVA;
*p = 0.02 versus GCKR CC/CT.

$p<0.001$), high BMI (OR 1.11 95% CI 1.04–1.17, $p = 0.004$), HOMA (OR 1.13 95% CI 1.03–1.25, $p = 0.01$), and PNPLA3 GG (OR 2.15, 95% CI 1.22–3.77, $p = 0.008$) at multivariate logistic regression analysis (table 3).

Finally, the presence of significant liver fibrosis (>F1) was independently linked to high HOMA (OR 1.12, 95% CI 1.01–1.23, $p = 0.02$), NAS ≥5 (OR 4.09, 95% CI 2.45–6.81, $p<0.001$), and GCKR C>T SNP (OR 2.06, 95% CI 1.43–2.98, $p<0.001$) in the whole study population (table 3 lower panel). When histological variables were removed from the model, >F1 fibrosis was independently linked to female gender (OR 1.77, 95% CI 1.05–2.99, $p = 0.03$), BMI (OR 1.08, 95% CI 1.02–1.14, $p = 0.008$), HOMA (OR 1.16, 95% CI 1.05–1.28, $p = 0.004$), and GCKR C>T SNP (OR 1.88, 95% CI 1.33–2.66, $p<0.001$).

Figure 1 shows the stepwise increased prevalence of significant fibrosis (>F1) according to GCKR genotype. Similar results were observed when the NAFLD cohorts were split by center (table 3 lower panel).

Discussion

The main finding of this study on a large cohort of Italian patients with NAFLD is the association between GCKR rs780094 C>T SNP and high triglyceride levels and the severity of liver fibrosis, independent of other known risk factors for liver damage

The complex interplay between genetic background and environmental factors in the development of NAFLD [26] is progressively unveiled by the recognition of the role of specific SNPs, such as PNPLA3 C>G SNPs. The GCKR C→T SNPs is also emerging as an important genetic determinant of NAFLD. This trait has been initially associated with imaging-based diagnosis of NAFLD in a population of healthy subjects [19], and the association has been further validated in children and in patients of different ethnicity [20–22]. In this study, besides confirming the associations between PNPLA3 C>G SNP and steatosis/lobular inflammation [11–15], for the first time we also highlighted the potential impact of GCKR C→T SNP on liver fibrosis in an European cohort of histologically diagnosed NAFLD patients.

Of importance, this association was independent from other well-known determinants and the severity of liver fibrosis showed a stepwise increase from patients carrying one risk allele to those carrying two risk alleles. It is noteworthy that this trend was observed in both tested cohorts. Our findings are in agreement with the evidence of a link between GCKR C→T SNP and higher ALT levels reported by Hernaez et al [22] in the US Health and Nutrition Examination Survey III, and also agree with preliminary unpublished data from FLIP cohort [30], and published data from a small Asiatic population [31] reporting the association between GCKR gene variant and severity of liver damage in NAFLD.

Although this study was not designed to clarify the pathogenic link between GCKR SNPs and liver fibrosis in NAFLD, some hypotheses can be provided. The GCKR gene product, the glucokinase regulatory protein, acts as an inhibitor of glucokinase (GCK) activity, a key liver enzyme for glucose metabolism, whose hepatic concentrations are increased in fatty liver [32,33]. GCKR rs780094 C>T SNP might facilitate liver fibrogenesis by reducing the inhibitory effect of GCKR, thereby increasing GCK activity. GCKR rs780094 SNP is in linkage disequilibrium with the GCKR rs1260326 SNP, that is associated with an increased GCK liver activity [20,34]. By inducing *de novo* hepatic lipogenesis and by suppressing hepatic fatty acid oxidation, GCK liver activity

Table 3. Association of the GCKR rs780094 genotype and liver damage as evaluated by unadjusted and adjusted models in 366 Patients with Non-alcoholic Fatty Liver Disease.

	Sicilian Cohort n = 197		Center/northern Italy Cohort n = 169		Combined n = 366	
Variable	**OR (95% C.I.)**	**P value**	**OR (95% C.I.)**	**P value**	**OR (95% C.I.)**	**P value**
	Steatosis (1 vs 2 vs 3)					
	Unadjusted Model	**Adjusted Model**	**Unadjusted Model**	**Adjusted Model**	**Unadjusted Model**	**Adjusted Model**
Females	-	-	-	-	1.94 (1.18–3.20) 0.009	1.43 (0.83–2.44) 0.19
Mean BMI - kg/m²	1.09 (1.02–1.17) 0.006	1.08 (1.00–1.16) 0.03	1.15 (1.05–1.27) 0.003	1.12 (1.01–1.25) 0.02	1.13 (1.07–1.19) <0.001	1.10 (1.04–1.17) 0.001
HOMA-score	1.13 (1.01–1.25) 0.02	1.08 (0.97–1.21) 0.14	1.16 (1.03–1.29) 0.01	1.08 (0.96–1.22) 0.17	1.15 (1.06–1.24) <0.001	1.08 (1.00–1.17) 0.04
GCKR CC vs CT vs TT	1.23 (0.79–1.91) 0.35	1.19 (0.75–1.90) 0.44	1.27 (0.72–2.25) 0.40	1.37 (0.74–2.52) 0.31	1.22 (0.87–1.73) 0.24	1.22 (0.85–1.76) 0.27
PNPLA3 CC vs CG vs GG	2.19 (1.08–4.45) 0.02	2.12 (1.02–4.41) 0.04	2.48 (1.05–5.83) 0.03	2.50 (1.03–6.05) 0.04	2.24 (1.31–3.83) 0.003	1.97 (1.11–3.51) 0.02
	NAS≥5					
Mean age - years	-	-	-	-	1.01 (1.00–1.03) 0.05	0.99 (0.97–1.00) 0.79
Females	2.47 (1.30–4.69) 0.006	1.69 (0.83–3.42) 0.14	3.98 (1.83–8.64) <0.001	3.70 (1.62–8.47) 0.002	3.16 (1.97–5.06) <0.001	2.55 (1.51–4.31) <0.001
Mean BMI - kg/m²	1.10 (1.03–1.18) 0.003	1.05 (0.97–1.13) 0.21	1.15 (1.05–1.25) 0.002	1.13 (1.02–1.25) 0.01	1.14 (1.09–1.21) <0.001	1.11 (1.04–1.17) 0.004
HOMA-score	1.38 (1.17–1.64) <0.001	1.28 (1.07–1.53) 0.005	1.14 (1.02–1.27) 0.01	1.03 (0.91–1.17) 0.54	1.24 (1.12–1.36) <0.001	1.13 (1.03–1.25) 0.01
GCKR CC vs CT vs TT	1.14 (0.75–1.73) 0.52	1.10 (0.69–1.75) 0.67	0.76 (0.46–1.27) 0.30	0.75 (0.43–1.30) 0.31	0.96 (0.71–1.29) 0.79	0.91 (0.65–1.26) 0.58
PNPLA3 CC/CG vs GG	3.62 (1.57–8.35) 0.002	3.06 (1.26–7.41) 0.01	2.49 (1.13–5.51) 0.02	2.31 (1.00–5.31) 0.04	2.54 (1.52–4.27) <0.001	2.15 (1.22–3.77) 0.008
	Fibrosis (0–1 versus 2–4)					
Mean age - years	1.03 (1.01–1.06) 0.001	1.03 (1.00–1.05) 0.02	-	-	1.02 (1.01–1.04) 0.001	1.01 (0.99–1.03) 0.28
Females	2.34 (1.28–4.29) 0.006	1.44 (0.68–3.03) 0.33	2.73 (1.30–5.71) 0.007	2.06 (0.86–4.91) 0.10	2.47 (1.55–3.93) <0.001	1.40 (0.80–2.45) 0.23
Mean BMI - kg/m²	1.10 (1.03–1.18) 0.002	1.02 (0.94–1.11) 0.52	1.17(1.07–1.28) <0.001	1.12 (1.01–1.23) 0.02	1.12 (1.07–1.18) <0.001	1.05 (0.98–1.11) 0.10
HOMA-score	1.31 (1.14–1.52) <0.001	1.15 (1.00–1.32) 0.04	1.16 (1.03–1.32) 0.01	1.06 (0.91–1.23) 0.43	1.24 (1.12–1.36) <0.001	1.12 (1.01–1.23) 0.02
Arterial hypertension	-	-	-	-	1.93 (1.20–3.12) 0.007	1.36 (0.76–2.43) 0.29
NAS≥5	7.83 (3.93–15.5) <0.001	7.05 (3.22–15.4) <0.001	5.58 (2.55–12.2) <0.001	4.43 (1.80–10.9) 0.001	5.06 (3.23–7.93) <0.001	4.09 (2.45–6.81) <0.001
GCKR CC vs CT vs TT	1.82 (1.18–2.81) 0.006	2.07 (1.22–3.49) 0.006	1.75 (1.10–2.76) 0.01	2.23 (1.31–3.82) 0.003	1.77 (1.30–2.44) <0.001	2.06 (1.43–2.98) <0.001
PNPLA3 CC/CG vs GG	1.47 (0.73–2.93) 0.27	0.62 (0.26–1.49) 0.29	1.94 (0.92–4.09) 0.07	1.32 (0.54–3.18) 0.53	1.67 (1.01–2.67) 0.04	1.03 (0.56–1.87) 0.92

Unadjusted and adjusted OR were presented for PNPLA3 and GCKR SNPs, and only for clinical, metabolic and histological variables significant at univariate analysis. PNPLA3 and GCKR SNPs, when not significant, were forced into the models.

prompts the hepatic accumulation of triglycerides, causing organ damage. In addition, GCKR rs780094 SNP might favor liver fibrogenesis along two more pathways: a) by affecting the expression of nearby genes, and specifically by increasing the expression of C2orf16 mRNA in the liver [19]; b) by favoring a low grade chronic inflammation as expressed by higher serum levels of C-reactive protein [35].

In our study we also demonstrated that patient homozygous for the T allele of GCKR had higher serum triglycerides levels, in agreement with previous finding by Speliotes et al [19], and with the hypothesis that the GCKR rs780094 SNP could lead to a higher activity of liver glcokinase. In addition we also observed higher triglycerides levels in Sicilian compared with Center/Northern Italy cohort, probably attributable to the more unhealthy lifestyle characterizing the southern population. By contrast we did not identify any association between severity of steatosis and GCKR genotype. Our data are not in contrast with the study of Speliotes et al [19] and more recent studies showing a

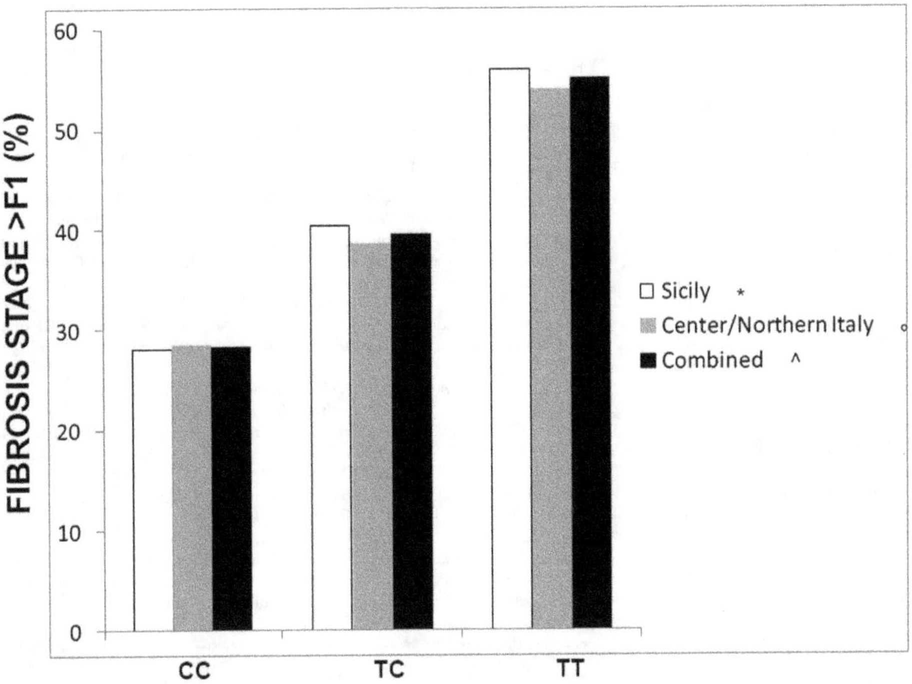

Figure 1. Prevalence of significant fibrosis according to GCKR rs780094 SNP in the Sicilian cohort, in the Center/Northern Italian cohort, and in the combined cohorts of NAFLD patients. *p = 0.02 for prevalence of F2–F4 fibrosis according to GCKR genotype; ° p = 0.04 for prevalence of F2–F4 fibrosis according to GCKR genotype; ^p = 0.001 for prevalence of F2–F4 fibrosis according to GCKR genotype.

link between GCKR SNP and the presence of steatosis [20–22]. We did not test subjects without steatosis of the same geographic area, and therefore we were not able to discriminate between presence/absence of fatty liver infiltration. Obviously, the lack of these data could partially affect the interpretation of our results, and in particular of the significance of the real effect of GCKR SNP on steatosis.

Finally, we did not confirm the reported association between PNPLA3 genotype and severity of liver fibrosis [14]. Differences in the characteristics of the individual study cohorts could explain the lack of association in our cohort.

The main limitation of this study lies in its cross-sectional nature, making it impossible to dissect the temporal relation between genetic background and progression of liver disease over time. This issue should be tested in longitudinal analyses. A further methodological question is the potentially limited external validity of the results for different populations and settings. Our study included cohorts of Italian patients enrolled at tertiary care centers, who may be different, in terms of both metabolic features and severity of liver disease, from the majority of prevalent cases of NAFLD in the general population. However, validation of the results in two independent, largely different populations from South and Northern/Center Italy supports a general involvement of GCKR rs780094 C>T polymorphisms in NAFLD progression.

In conclusion, this study on a large cohort of patients with histological diagnosis of NAFLD, showed an independent link between GCKR SNPs and significant hepatic fibrosis. Further studies are needed to explore the pathogenic mechanisms underlying this association.

Author Contributions

Conceived and designed the experiments: SP. Performed the experiments: CR DC SB SG RMP. Analyzed the data: SP. Wrote the paper: SP. Had full control of the study design, data analysis and interpretation, and preparation of article: LM EB CC VD AG GM AC.

References

1. Petta S, Muratore C, Craxì A (2009) Non-alcoholic fatty liver disease pathogenesis: the present and the future. Dig Liver Dis 41:615–25.
2. Marchesini G, Bugianesi E, Forlani G, Cerrelli F, Lenzi M, et al. (2003) Nonalcoholic fatty liver, steatohepatitis, and the metabolic syndrome. Hepatology 37:917–23.
3. Bedogni G, Miglioli L, Masutti F, Tiribelli C, Marchesini G, et al. (2005) Prevalence of and risk factors for nonalcoholic fatty liver disease: the Dionysos nutrition and liver study. Hepatology 42:44–52.
4. Petta S, Craxì A (2010) Hepatocellular carcinoma and non-alcoholic fatty liver disease: from a clinical to a molecular association. Curr Pharm Des 16:741–52.
5. Targher G, Marra F, Marchesini G (2008) Increased risk of cardiovascular disease in non-alcoholic fatty liver disease: causal effect or epiphenomenon? Diabetologia 51:1947–53.
6. Petta S, Tripodo C, Grimaudo S, Cabibi D, Cammà C, et al. (2011) High liver RBP4 protein content is associated with histological features in patients with genotype 1 chronic hepatitis C and with nonalcoholic steatohepatitis. Dig Liver Dis 43:404–10.
7. van der Poorten D, Milner KL, Hui J, Hodge A, Trenell MI, et al. (2008) Visceral fat: a key mediator of steatohepatitis in metabolic liver disease. Hepatology 48:449–57.
8. Bugianesi E, Marchesini G, Gentilcore E, Cua IH, Vanni E, et al. (2006) Fibrosis in genotype 3 chronic hepatitis C and nonalcoholic fatty liver disease: Role of insulin resistance and hepatic steatosis. Hepatology 44:1648–55.
9. Argo CK, Northup PG, Al-Osaimi AM, Caldwell SH (2009) Systematic review of risk factors for fibrosis progression in non-alcoholic steatohepatitis. J Hepatol 51:371–9.
10. Tilg H, Moschen A (2010) Update on nonalcoholic fatty liver disease: genes involved in nonalcoholic fatty liver disease and associated inflammation. Curr Opin Clin Nutr Metab Care 13:391–6.
11. Sookoian S, Castano GO, Burgueno AL, Fernandez GT, Rosselli MS, et al. (2009) A nonsynonymous gene variant in adiponutrin gene is associated with nonalcoholic fatty liver disease severity. J Lipid Res 50:2111–2116.
12. Rotman Y, Koh C, Zmuda JM, Kleiner DE, Liang TJ (2010) The association of genetic variability in patatin-like phospholipase domain-containing protein 3

(PNPLA3) with histological severity of nonalcoholic fatty liver disease. Hepatology 52:894–903.

13. Speliotes EK, Butler JL, Palmer CD, Voight BF, Hirschhorn JN (2010) PNPLA3 variants specifically confer increased risk for histologic nonalcoholic fatty liver disease but not metabolic disease. HEPATOLOGY 52:904–912.
14. Valenti L, Al-Serri A, Daly AK, Galmozzi E, Rametta R, et al. (2010) Homozygosity for the patatin-like phospholipase-3/adiponutrin I148M polymorphism influences liver fibrosis in patients with nonalcoholic fatty liver disease. Hepatology 51:1209–1217.
15. Sookoian S, Pirola CJ (2011) Meta-analysis of the influence of I148M variant of patatin-like phospholipase domain containing 3 gene (PNPLA3) on the susceptibility and histological severity of nonalcoholic fatty liver disease. Hepatology 53:1883–94.
16. Petta S, Grimaudo S, Cammà C, Cabibi D, Di Marco V, et al. (2012) IL28B and PNPLA3 polumorphisms affect histological liver damage in patients with nonalcoholic fatty liver disease. J Hepatol 56:1356–62.
17. Petta S, Ferraro D, Cammà C, Cabibi D, Di Cristina A, et al. (2012) Vitamin D levels and IL28B polymorphisms are related to rapid virological response to standard of care in genotype 1 chronic hepatitis C. Antiviral Therapy 17;823–31.
18. Ge D, Fellay J, Thompson AJ, Simon JS, Shianna KV, et al. (2009) Genetic variation in IL28B predicts hepatitis C treatment-induced viral clearance. Nature 461:399–401.
19. Speliotes EK, Yerges-Armstrong LM, Kim LJ, Palmer CD, Gudnason V, et al. (2011) Genome-wide association analysis identifies variants associated with nonalcoholic fatty liver disease that have distinct effects on metabolic traits. PLoS Genet 7: e1001324.
20. Santoro N, Zhang CK, Zhao H, Pakstis AJ, Kim G, et al. (2012) Variant in the Glucokinase Regulatory Protein (GCKR) Gene is Associated With Fatty Liver in Obese Children and Adolescents. Hepatology 55:781–789.
21. Palmer ND, Musani SK, Yerges-Armstrong LM, Feitosa MF, Bielak LF, et al. (2013) Characterization of European-ancestry NAFLD-associated Variants in individuals of African and Hispanic descent. Hepatology 2013 Apr 8. doi: 10.1002/hep.26440 [Epub ahead of print] PubMed PMID: 23564467.
22. Hernaez R, McLean J, Lazo M, Brancati FL, Hirschhorn JN, et al. (2013) Association Between Variants in or Near PNPLA3, GCKR, and PPP1R3B With Ultrasound-Defined Steatosis Based on Data From the Third National Health and Nutrition Examination Survey. Clin Gastroenterol Hepatol. 2013 Feb 13. doi:pii: S1542-3565(13)00188-2. 10.1016/j.cgh.2013.02.011 [Epub ahead of print] PubMed PMID: 23416328.
23. American Diabetes Association (2000) Report of the Expert Committee on the diagnosis and classification of diabetes mellitus. American Diabetes Association: Clinical Practice Recommendations 2000 Committee Report, Diabetes Care 23:S4–19.
24. Matthews DR, Hosker JP, Rudenski AS, Naylor BA, Treacher DF, et al. (1985) Homeostasis model assessment: insulin resistance and beta-cell function from fasting plasma glucose and insulin concentrations in man. Diabetologia 28:412–419.
25. Ikeda Y, Suehiro T, Nakamura T, Kumon Y, Hashimoto K (2001) Clinical significance of the insulin resistance index as assessed by homeostasis model assessment. Endocr J 48:81–86.
26. University of Oxford website. Available at: Diabetes Trials Unit,University of Oxfor, at http://www.dtu.ox.ac.uk/homa. Accessed 2013 December 4.
27. Colloredo G, Guido M, Sonzogni A, Leandro G (2003) Impact of liver biopsy size on histological evaluation of chronic viral hepatitis: the smaller the sample, the milder the disease. J Hepatol 39:239–244.
28. Kleiner DE, Brunt EM, Van Natta M, Behling C, Contos MJ, et al. (2005) Nonalcoholic Steatohepatitis Clinical Research Network, Design and validation of a histological scoring system for nonalcoholic fatty liver disease. Hepatology 411:313–321.
29. SAS Technical Report (1992) SAS/STAT software: changes and enhancement, Release 6.07. Cary, NC: SAS Institute, Inc.
30. Anstee Q, Darlay R, Leathart J, Liu Y, Tordjman J, et al. (2013) A CANDIDATE-GENE APPROACH TO VALIDATION OF GENETIC MODIFIER ASSOCIATIONS USING A LARGE COHORT WITH HISTOLOGICALLY CHARACTERISED NON-ALCOHOLIC FATTY LIVER DISEASE. Journal of Hepatology vol. 58,S46, 104
31. Tan HL, Zain SM, Mohamed R, Rampal S, Chin KF, et al. (2013) Association of glucokinase regulatory gene polymorphisms with risk and severity of non-alcoholic fatty liver disease: an interaction study with adiponutrin gene. J Gastroenterol 2013 Jun 26. [Epub ahead of print] PubMed PMID: 23800943.
32. Peter A, Stefan N, Cegan A, Walenta M, Wagner S, et al. (2011) Hepatic glucokinase expression is associated with lipogenesis and fatty liver in humans. JCEM 96:e1126–30.
33. Bechmann LP, Gastaldelli A, Vetter D, Patman GL, Pascoe L, et al. (2012) Glucokinase links Krüppel-like factor 6 to the regulation of hepatic insulin sensitivity in nonalcoholic fatty liver disease. Hepatology 55:1083–93.
34. Beer NL, Tribble ND, McCulloch LJ, Roos C, Johnson PR, et al. (2011) The P446L variant in GCKR associated with fasting plasma glucose and triglyceride levels exerts its effect through increased glucokinase activity in liver. Hum Mol Gene 18:4081–4088.
35. Yang Z, Wen J, Tao X, Lu B, Du Y, et al. (2011) Genetic variation in the GCKR gene is associated with nonalcoholic fatty liver disease in Chinese people. Mol Biol Rep 38:1145–1150.

NIKEI: A New Inexpensive and Non-Invasive Scoring System to Exclude Advanced Fibrosis in Patients with NAFLD

Münevver Demir[1*], Sonja Lang[1], Martin Schlattjan[2], Uta Drebber[3], Inga Wedemeyer[3], Dirk Nierhoff[1], Ingrid Kaul[4], Jan Sowa[2], Ali Canbay[2], Ulrich Töx[1], Hans-Michael Steffen[1]

1 Clinic for Gastroenterology and Hepatology, University Hospital of Cologne, Cologne, Germany, 2 Clinic for Gastroenterology and Hepatology, University Hospital of Essen, Essen, Germany, 3 Institute for Pathology, University Hospital of Cologne, Cologne, Germany, 4 Institute of Medical Statistics, Informatics and Epidemiology, University Hospital of Cologne, Cologne, Germany

Abstract

Aims: To develop, validate and compare a non-invasive fibrosis scoring system for non-alcoholic fatty liver disease (NAFLD) derived from routinely obtained clinical and biochemical parameters.

Methods: 267 consecutive patients with biopsy proven fatty liver or non-alcoholic steatohepatitis were randomly assigned to the estimation (2/3) or validation (1/3) group to develop a model for the prediction of advanced fibrosis. Univariate statistics were performed to compare patients with and without advanced fibrosis, and following a multivariate logistic regression analysis a new scoring system was constructed. This non-invasive Koeln-Essen-index (NIKEI) was validated and compared to the FIB-4 index by calculating the area under the receiver operating characteristic curve (AUC). We evaluated a stepwise combination of both scoring systems for the precise prediction of advanced fibrosis. To set in contrast, we additionally tested the diagnostic accuracy of the AST/ALT ratio, BARD score and the NAFLD fibrosis score in our cohort.

Results: Age, AST, AST/ALT ratio, and total bilirubin were identified as significant predictors of advanced fibrosis and used to construct the NIKEI with an AUC of 0.968 [0.937; 0.998] compared to 0.929 [0.869; 0.989] for the FIB-4 index. The absence of advanced fibrosis could be confirmed with excellent accuracy (99–100%). The positive predictive value of the FIB-4 index was higher (100% vs. 60%), however, the false negative rate was also high (33%). With a stepwise combination of both indices 82%–84% of biopsies would have been avoidable without a single misclassification. The AUROC for AST/ALT ratio, the NAFLD fibrosis score, and the BARD score were 0.81 (95% CI, 0.72–0.90), 0.96 (95% CI 0.92–0.99), and 0.67 (95% CI 0.55–0.78), respectively.

Conclusion: The NIKEI can reliably exclude advanced fibrosis in subjects with NAFLD. In combination with the FIB-4 index misclassification with inadequate clinical management can be avoided while the need for liver biopsies can be reduced.

Editor: Wing-Kin Syn, Institute of Hepatology, Foundation for Liver Research, United Kingdom

Funding: The authors have no support or funding to report.

Competing Interests: The authors have declared that no competing interests exist.

* E-mail: muenevver.demir@uk-koeln.de

These authors contributed equally to this work.

Introduction

Non-alcoholic fatty liver disease (NAFLD) has become the leading cause of chronic liver disease with prevalence rates ranging from 6% to 35% worldwide [1]. It is typically associated with type 2 diabetes mellitus (T2DM), hypertension, obesity, or dyslipidemia and can be considered as the hepatic manifestation of the metabolic syndrome [2]. NAFLD encompasses a histological spectrum ranging from simple steatosis (NAFL) to non-alcoholic steatohepatitis (NASH) with subsequent cirrhosis. Recent findings even suggest progression of NASH to hepatocellular carcinoma, in the absence of cirrhosis. While simple steatosis carries a relatively benign prognosis, the risk of cardiovascular as well as liver-related events is increased in individuals with NASH [3], and in a recently published study advanced fibrosis demonstrated the best independent association with long-term liver-related mortality in patients with NAFLD [4].

Currently, percutaneous liver biopsy is considered as the gold standard for the assessment of hepatic fibrosis and inflammation in chronic liver disease. However, liver biopsy is an invasive procedure with associated costs, complications, and inherent inaccuracy due to sampling error and inter- and intraobserver variability in histopathological interpretation [5,6]. Therefore, it has been attempted to establish non-invasive methods for the detection of liver fibrosis. Various biochemical markers reflecting inflammatory activity [7–11], activity of apoptosis [12], and oxidative stress [13] have been evaluated. None of these markers has proven sufficient diagnostic accuracy and numbers of cases were rather low [14]. Furthermore, several scoring systems and specialized biomarkers for the prediction of fibrosis in NAFLD have been developed by combining various serologic and clinical parameters [15–22]. However, even with the best non-invasive simple scoring systems, 11% to 26% of patients with advanced fibrosis will be misclassified as no or mild fibrosis leading to an inappropriate clinical management [23]. Additionally, some of the parameters used in these scoring systems are not available on a routine basis.

As long as there are no approved therapeutic modalities it seems reasonable to target the clinical management at those patients most in need for surveillance and monitoring of complications. Thus, the aim of this study was (*i*) to define independent predictors of advanced fibrosis in a large cohort of patients with biopsy-proven NAFLD from two separate tertiary care medical centers in Germany (University hospitals of Cologne and Essen), (*ii*) to develop and validate a simple noninvasive fibrosis scoring system for NAFLD derived from routinely obtained and easily available clinical and biochemical parameters, and (*iii*) to compare the diagnostic accuracy and clinical utility of this noninvasive Koeln-Essen-index (NIKEI) alone or in combination with the FIB-4 index, a validated scoring system for the prediction of advanced fibrosis in NAFLD [19]. To set in contrast to these results, we aimed to analyze the diagnostic performance and clinical utility of the AST/ALT ratio, BARD score [22] and the NAFLD fibrosis score [17] in our study population.

Patients and Methods

Study population

Data from 408 consecutive patients with suspected NAFL/NASH who presented to the Clinic for Gastroenterology and Hepatology, University Hospital of Cologne (n = 323) or to the Clinic for Gastroenterology and Hepatology, University Hospital of Essen (n = 85) between July 1998 and November 2009, were analyzed retrospectively. Written informed consent from the participants and a votum of the local ethics committee were not obtained. In accordance with German law, a votum of a local ethics committee is not required to conduct strictly retrospective studies (paragraph 15, sentence 1, Nordrhein Medical Association's professional code of conduct from 14 November 1998 as amended on 19 November 2011). There is also no need to get written informed consent from the participants if the considered data was collected and analysed retrospectively (paragraph 6, sentence 1, Health Data Protection Act of Nordrhein-Westfalen).

While almost all patients in Cologne had been referred to the outpatient department for further work-up after abnormal liver function tests had been detected by their treating primary care physicians, patients in Essen had been recruited at the Department II of Surgery, Alfred-Krupp Hospital Essen or the Clinic for Surgery, Visceral and Vascular Surgery, Protestant Hospital Dinslaken. Patient charts were reviewed for the following parameters: age, gender, body height, body weight, arterial blood pressure, pulse rate, concomitant diseases and medication, alcohol consumption, serology for chronic viral infections (HBV, HCV, HIV), and autoimmune liver disease (ANA, AMA, Anti-SMA, Anti-LKM1, Anti-SLA, p-ANCA). In addition, laboratory parameters (hemoglobin, WBC, platelet count, aspartate aminotransferase (AST), alanine aminotransferase (ALT), gamma glutamyl transferase (GGT), alkaline phosphatase, total bilirubin, cholinesterase, creatinine, urea, glomerular filtration rate according to the MDRD formula, albumin, quantitative immunoglobulins, ferritin, urinary copper excretion, coeruloplasmin, triglycerides, total blood cholesterol, high-density lipoprotein cholesterol, low-density lipoprotein cholesterol, prothrombin time, INR, prothrombin time, fasting glucose, and alpha-fetoprotein (AFP)), histological data of liver biopsies, and results of abdominal ultrasonography as well as number and date of follow-up visits were documented. All laboratory parameters were taken under fasting conditions.

Arterial hypertension was defined as a blood pressure ≥140/90 mmHg in the medical record or a history of taking antihypertensive drugs. The diagnosis of concomitant diseases such as diabetes mellitus, arterial hypertension or dyslipidemia was based on findings from patient charts.

A diagnosis of NAFLD was made if the following conditions were met: elevated aminotransferase levels for at least six months, fatty liver degeneration >5% and if applicable additional inflammation, after exclusion of other chronic liver diseases, e.g. viral hepatitis, autoimmune hepatitis, toxic liver injury, alcoholic steatohepatitis, cholestatic liver disease, hemochromatosis. Patients were excluded if they suffered from a malignancy, had decompensated liver cirrhosis or received drugs with well-known effects on steatosis, e.g. methotrexate or glucocorticoids. They were also excluded if the time interval between liver biopsy and date of laboratory examination exceeded 120 days or if data to definitely exclude other chronic liver diseases were missing. Patients were included if alcohol consumption was less than 30 g/d in men and 20 g/d in women. According to these criteria, 141 patients had to be excluded from our study leaving 267 patients for further analyses.

Liver histology

All liver specimens were taken under local anesthesia (17G Hepafix® Menghini type needle, Fa. Braun, Melsungen, Germany) at the Clinic for Gastroenterology and Hepatology, University of Cologne, or during surgery at the Department II of Surgery, Alfred-Krupp Hospital Essen or the Clinic for Surgery, Visceral and Vascular Surgery, Protestant Hospital Dinslaken and were assessed at the Institute for Pathology, University of Cologne. Liver biopsies were read twice by two experienced liver pathologists (D.U., W.I.), who were blinded for all clinical and laboratory patient data. Discordant ratings between these two were solved by majority decision. The stage of fibrosis was scored based on the 5-point scale proposed by Brunt et al. [24] and modified by Kleiner et al. [25].

Statistical analysis and model building

The aim of the study was the development of a prediction model for advanced fibrosis (F3–F4) by applying routinely measured clinical and laboratory parameters. Patients from both centers were pooled, and 2/3 were then randomly assigned to the estimation group (n = 170) for model building and the remaining to the validation group (n = 97). The Kolmogorov-Smirnov test was used to test for normal distribution and means ± SD were calculated for continuous variables, frequencies for categorical variables. Univariate statistics were performed to look for differences between the estimation and validation groups and to compare patients with (F3–F4) and without (F0–F2) advanced fibrosis using the Student's t-test or the X^2-test. All variables with significant differences between the two fibrosis groups (p-value <0.05) were included in a multivariate logistic regression analysis to identify variables predicting the presence or absence of advanced fibrosis. Variables with p-values <0.05 in the regression analysis were then used to construct a new scoring system to predict advanced fibrosis. The overall diagnostic accuracy of this noninvasive Koeln-Essen-index (NIKEI) was determined by calculating the area under the receiver operating characteristic curve (AUROC) with its 95% confidence intervals. Validation was performed in the subset of patients with complete data (n = 92) from the validation group. From the ROC curve of the final model, two cutoff points were selected, with sensitivity and specificity for advanced fibrosis of at least 90%. The diagnostic accuracy of the two cutoff points was determined by calculating sensitivity, specificity, PPV, NPV, and likelihood ratios. Finally, AUROC with 95% confidence intervals (95% CI) was employed to compare performance of the NIKEI, the FIB-4 index the NAFLD fibrosis score, the AST/ALT ratio and the BARD score using previously published cut-off levels [17;22;26]. All analyses were performed with SPSS Statistics 19.0.0 (Release 19.0 SPSS Inc. Chicago, USA).

Results

Characteristics of study cohort

The demographic and laboratory characteristics of all included patients (n = 267) are shown in table 1. There were no statistically significant differences between the estimation and validation groups. 218 patients (82%) were overweight or obese, and 245 patients (92%) had no or mild fibrosis stages (F0–F2). As the identification of patients with advanced fibrosis is of clinical importance, the clinical and laboratory features of subjects with no/mild fibrosis (F0–F2) were compared to those with advanced fibrosis (F3–F4). The univariate analysis in the estimation group showed that patients with advanced fibrosis were significantly older, had lower platelet counts and albumin levels ($p<0.001$ in all cases), while values for AST ($p<0.001$), the AST/ALT ratio ($p = 0.001$), GGT ($p<0.001$), total bilirubin ($p = 0.016$), INR ($p = 0.041$), glucose ($p<0.001$, and AFP ($p = 0.020$) were all significantly increased.

Generation of the NIKEI

By multivariate analysis, four variables remained significant including age, AST, AST/ALT ratio, and total bilirubin. No statistically significant interactions were identified. Using these four variables, we constructed an index to calculate the probability P of advanced fibrosis:

$$\text{LogitP} = \ln(P/1\text{-}P) = -24.214 + 0.225 * \text{age} + 0.056 * \text{ASTU/I} + 5.044 * \text{AST/ALTratio} + 3.631 * \text{totalbilirubinmg/dl}$$

The area under the ROC curve (AUROC) for this NIKEI was 0.968±0.016 (95% CI: 0.937, 0.998) that compared favorable to the well-established FIB-4 index: 0.929 (0.869, 0.989; see figure 1a). From this ROC curve two cutoff points were selected for the regression function to identify the presence (≥0.2294) or absence (≤0.0535) of advanced fibrosis.

Comparison of NIKEI and FIB-4 demonstrates superior NPV for NIKEI

By applying the lower cutoff point (≤0.0535), 128 (85%) of the 150 patients without advanced fibrosis were correctly identified. However, the absence of advanced fibrosis could be confirmed with excellent accuracy (NPV of 100%). In contrast, although the positive predictive value of the FIB-4 index for the prediction of advanced fibrosis was higher (100%), the false negative rate was 4 out of 12 patients.

Evaluation of the NIKEI in separate patient cohort supports high NPV

The diagnostic accuracy of the NIKEI was then cross-validated in a separate set of 92 patients from the validation group. Results were similar to those of the estimation group. The AUROC was 0.961±0.023 (95% CI: 0.916, 1.000), again comparing favorably to the well-established FIB-4 index (see figure 1b). By applying the lower cutoff point (≤0.0535), 74 (89%) of the 83 patient without advanced fibrosis were correctly staged, whereas 3 (3%) were misclassified as having advanced fibrosis. 6 of 9 patients (67%) with values above the higher cutoff point (≥0.2294) were correctly identified as having advanced fibrosis. However, one patient (11%) with advanced fibrosis was misclassified (table 2). As in the estimation group, the positive predictive value of the FIB-4 index for the prediction of advanced fibrosis was higher (100%).

Stepwise scoring with FIB-4 and NIKEI enhances overall performance

We then evaluated a stepwise combination of both scoring systems in a subgroup of 154 patients with complete data for calculating both indices, i.e. the FIB-4 index first, followed by the NIKEI only for patients with indeterminate or negative prediction of advanced fibrosis. Assuming that a liver biopsy reasonably could have been avoided in patients with test results above (presence of advanced fibrosis) or below (absence of advanced fibrosis) the respective cut-offs, 82% of biopsies could have been omitted without missing a single case of advanced fibrosis (figure 2). Also, combining both scoring systems in the same stepwise fashion in the validation group would have allowed avoiding liver biopsy in 84% of cases without a single misclassification (not shown).

Evaluation of the NAFLD fibrosis score in our study population

Additionally we calculated the NAFLD fibrosis score in our cohort and then compared to the NIKEI index (see table 3). Although AUROC and NPV showed similar results compared to the NIKEI index, the false negative rate was 25% for the NAFLD fibrosis score. However, only 120 patients were included to test the NAFLD fibrosis score because of incomplete data.

Evaluation of the AST/ALT ratio and the BARD score in our study population

We also evaluated the AST/ALT ratio and the BARD score in our cohort. The AUROC were as follows: AST/ALT ratio 0.81 (95% CI, 0.72–0.90), and BARD score 0.67 (95% CI 0.55–0.78) with negative predictive values for advanced fibrosis of 96% and 95%, respectively (see table S1 and figure S1).

Discussion

Liver fibrosis results from chronic injury [3], and in the absence of approved treatment modalities for NAFLD most attention has to be focused on the detection of advanced fibrosis (F3–F4) indicating the need for specific monitoring of complications such as portal hypertension and surveillance for hepatocellular carcinoma. The majority of our patients have been recruited from primary care physician practices. In this regard, our patient population is comparable to a recently published prospective study where advanced fibrosis was found in 9 of 134 liver biopsies (7%) performed in a middle-aged cohort of male and female US army personnel recruited from a primary care clinic [27]. An algorithm starting with the calculation of the FIB-4 index followed by calculating NIKEI only for patients with negative or indeterminate

Table 1. Characteristics of the study population.

Variable	All patients (n = 267)	Estimation G. (n = 170)	Validation (n = 97)	Koeln (n = 183)	Essen (n = 84)
Age (years)	43.8±12.1	43.9±11.9	43.7±12.6	44.8±12.6	41.8±10.8
Female n, (%)	141 (52.8)	89 (52.4)	52 (53.6)	70 (38.3)	71 (84.5)
BMI (kg/m^2)	37.0±12.7	37.2±13.0	36.6±12.9	29.0±6.1	52.4±7.6
BMI normal/overweight/obese, n	25/79/139	13/53/91	12/26/48	25/79/56	0/0/82
Stage of fibrosis 0/1/2/3/4, n	8/107/130/18/4	7/68/82/11/2	1/39/48/7/2	8/91/63/17/4	0/16/67/1/0
Hypertension n, (%)	112 (41.9)	74 (43.5)	38 (39.6)	73 (39.9)	39 (46.4)
Diabetes n, (%)	53 (19.9)	33 (19.4)	20 (20.6)	19 (10.4)	34 (40.5)
Platelet (1.000/μl)	265.0±80.0	265.4±80.9	264.3±78.7	247.8±71.5	299.0±85.2
AST (IU/ml)	36.8±32.4	34.9±22.8	40.2±44.7	40.9±37.5	27.9±13.5
ALT (IU/ml)	56.6±55.2	54.8±44.4	59.8±70.5	66.4±62.6	35.5±22.8
AST/ALT ratio	0.8±0.3	0.8±0.4	0.7±0.3	0.7±0.3	0.9±0.3
<1,0 n, (%)	214 (80.5)	135 (79.4)	79 (82.3)	154 (84.2)	60 (71.4)
≥1,0 n, (%)	52 (19.5)	35 (20.6)	17 (17.7)	28 (15.4)	24 (28.6)
GGT (IU/ml)	111.4±186.1	128.8±222.7	80.5±82.8	136.8±201.2	56.2±133.4
Total bilirubin (mg/dl)	0.7±0.7	0.7±0.9	0.6±0.4	0.8±0.9	0.5±0.3
Prothrombin time %	101.5±14.6	100.3±15.8	103.8±11.9	103.7±13.5	97.0±15.8
INR	1.0±0.10	1.0±0.1	1.0±0.1	1.0±0.1	0.97±0.1
Creatinine (mg/dl)	0.9±0.7	0.9±0.8	0.8±0.2	0.9±0.8	0.8±0.5
Albumin (g/l)	44.6±3.4	44.8±3.5	44.4±3.3	44.6±3.4	no data
Glucose (mg/dl)	102.8±30.6	103.1±32.6	102.3±26.8	102.8±30.6	110.9±48.7
Alkaline phosphatase (IU/ml)	111.9±52.9	114.1±57.5	108.1±43.8	111.9±52.9	no data
AFP (kU/l)	3.0±1.8	3.1±2.0	2.7±1.4	3.0±1.8	no data

Data are shown as mean ± SD. Percentages (%) are given in brackets and refer to patients inside of respective subset. Abbreviations: BMI = body mass index; AST = aspartate aminotransferase; ALT = alanine aminotransferase; GGT = gamma glutamyl transferase; INR = International normalized ratio; AFP = alpha-fetoprotein.

test results proved to be clinically very useful, since 82–84% of liver biopsies could have been avoided without missing a single case of advanced fibrosis in this low prevalence study population.

Several diagnostic panels have been developed to facilitate the noninvasive assessment of NAFLD and differentiation between different stages of disease. One approach utilizes the testing of biochemical markers of liver fibrosis: hyaluronic acid [8,28], adiponectin [11], high-sensitivity CRP [9], type IV collagen [8], serum IL-6 [10], leptin [28], laminin [8,28], c-peptide [7], and cytokeratin-18 [29,19]. Using only a single biochemical marker to predict significant fibrosis has been evaluated in a few studies with inadequate diagnostic accuracy [14,30]. In order to achieve a higher diagnostic accuracy in predicting fibrosis, scoring systems have been developed which combine multiple clinical and laboratory parameters, e.g. the FibroTest-FibroSURE® by Ratziu et al. [21], the OELF (**O**riginal **E**uropean **L**iver **F**ibrosis) score by

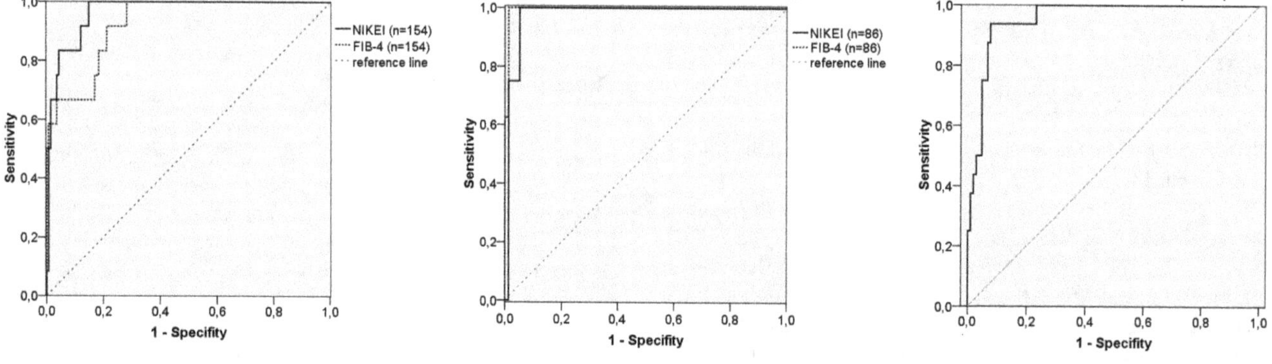

Figure 1. ROC-curve analysis for the prediction of advanced fibrosis with NIKEI, FIB-4 index and NAFLD fibrosis score. a) estimation group (n = 154 with complete data for calculating both indices); b) validation group (n = 86 with complete data for calculating both indices). c) NAFLD fibrosis score (n = 120).

Table 2. NIKEI test performance in estimation group (EG) and validation group (VG).

	≤0.0535		0.0536–0.2293		≥0.2294		All patients	
	EG	VG	EG	VG	EG	VG	EG	VG
All patients n	128	75	19	8	15	9	162	92
F0–F2 n	128	74	16	6	6	3	150	83
F3–F4 n	0	1	3	2	9	6	12	9
Sensitivity %	100	88.9			75.0	66.7		
Specifity %	85.3	89.2			96.0	96.4		
PPV %	35.3	47.1			60.0	66.7		
NPV %	100	98.7			98.0	96.4		
Likelihood Ratio (+)	6.8	8.2			18.8	18.5		
Likelihood-Ratio (−)	0.0	0.1			0.3	0.3		
AUC (95% CI) EG: 0.968±0.016 (0.937; 0.998) VG: 0.961±0.023 (0.916; 1.000)								

Cut-off levels and the classification of patients on the basis of the individual scores within the estimation (EG) and validation group (VG). A patient with a value below the lower cut-off level was classified as healthy (no advanced fibrosis), with a value above the upper cut-off level as morbid (advanced fibrosis). Patients with values between the cut-off levels are intermediate/not classifiable.

Rosenberg et al. [15] and its modification, the ELF (**E**nhanced **L**iver **F**ibrosis) score by Ghua et al. [16]. However, the unavailability of the above mentioned serum markers in most centers prevent application of the proposed scoring systems on a day-to-day basis.

We developed and validated a simple noninvasive scoring system composed of routinely measured clinical and laboratory parameters to predict the presence or absence of advanced fibrosis in patients with NAFLD and BMI ranging from 18.8 to 71.8 kg/m^2. This NIKEI consists of four variables (age, AST, AST/ALT ratio, and total bilirubin) and was highly accurate in predicting the absence of advanced fibrosis reaching negative predictive values of 99–100%.

The prevalence of NAFLD and NAFLD-related fibrosis increases with age. In addition to this association, older patients with NAFLD have a higher likelihood of disease progression or

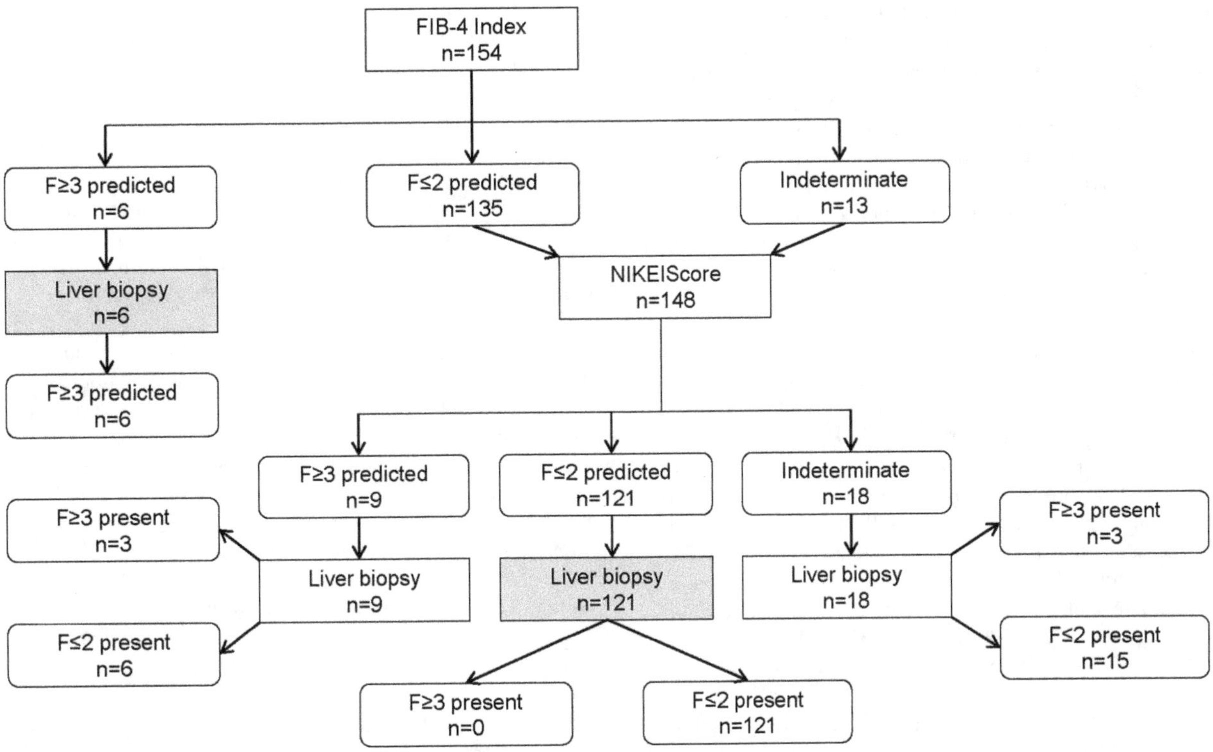

Figure 2. Stepwise combination of FIB-4 index and NIKEI. Algorithm for the prediction of advanced fibrosis in NAFLD patients (estimation group, n = 154 with complete data for calculating both indices). Algorithm starts with the calculation of the FIB4 index followed by calculating NIKEI only for patients with negative or indeterminate test results. Shaded rectangles: liver biopsies which could have been avoided.

Table 3. Diagnostic performance of the NAFLD score.

NAFLD score	≤−1.455	−1.454 −0.675	≥0.676	All patients
All patients, *n (%)*	101 (84)	16 (13)	3 (3)	120
F0–F2, *n (%)*	97 (93)	7 (7)	0	104
F3–F4, *n (%)*	4 (25)	9 (56)	3 (19)	16
Sensitivity, %	75		19	
Specifity, %	93		100	
PPV, %	63		100	
NPV, %	96		89	
Likelihood-Ratio (+)	11.2		∞	
Likelihood-Ratio (−)	0.27		0.81	
Diagnostic accuracy 0.83				
AUC (95% CI) 0.96 (0.92; 0.99)				

Cut-off values and the classification of patients on the basis of the NAFLD fibrosis score (n = 120). A patient with a value below the lower cut-off level was classified as healthy (no advanced fibrosis), with a value above the upper cut-off level as morbid (advanced fibrosis). Patients with values between the cut-off levels are intermediate/not classifiable.

mortality [31,32]. Our study results confirm this observation. An older age was highly significant associated with the presence of advanced fibrosis ($p<0.001$). It has previously been described, that NAFLD is more prevalent in cohorts of patients with pre-existing metabolic conditions than in the general population [1]. Our results confirm this observation as many patients of the study population were overweight/obese with further features of the metabolic syndrome. However, none of these conditions showed a statistically significant association with advanced fibrosis. Bilirubin levels were within the normal range. However we found bilirubin to be an independent predictor for advanced fibrosis in patients with NAFLD. These results are in line with findings from other studies [17;21;33;34]. Although bilirubin is not included in the NAFLD fibrosis score, it showed to be an independent predictor in univariate analysis [17]. Ratziu et al. and Stepanova et al. found bilirubin to be an independent predictor of significant fibrosis in patients with NAFLD in univariate and multivariate analysis [21,34].

Among several algorithms, the NAFLD fibrosis score and the FIB-4 index have been validated most widely [19,23]. Angulo et al. developed the "NAFLD fibrosis score", a panel comprising six variables of age, glycaemia, BMI, platelet count, albumin and AST/ALT ratio. In the original study, the score had a NPV of 93% and 88% for advanced fibrosis in the estimation and validation groups, respectively. The AUROC was 0.84, and application of this model to the study population would have avoided liver biopsy in 75% of patients, with a correct prediction in 90% [17]. The evaluation in our study population showed an AUROC of 0.96, PPV of 100% and NPV of 96% (table 3). However the false negative rate was 25%, too high to be clinically useful.

The FIB-4 index, developed by Sterling et al. [26] from a database of 832 HIV/HCV coinfected patients, combines age, AST, ALT and platelet count and has been validated in NASH patients for the detection of fibrosis stages F3 and F4 with an AUROC of 0.802, and NPV and PPV of 90% and 80%, respectively [19].

Compared to the NAFLD fibrosis score and the FIB-4 index we achieved a better NPV with almost 100% and a better test performance with an AUROC of 0.96. Previously reported PPVs from the NAFLD fibrosis score and the validation of FIB-4 in NAFLD patients (86% and 80% respectively) were higher than in our study (60% in the estimation and 67% in the validation group), which may be due to differences in the prevalence of advanced fibrosis. However, if the clinical decision for closer follow-up and surveillance were based only on test results from these two scoring systems without liver biopsy, 8–23% of patients with advanced fibrosis would have been missed [17,19,23]. We achieved a lower misclassification rate by combining the FIB-4 and NIKEI indices in a stepwise fashion, which could possibly avoid inappropriate clinical management despite a large number of dispensable liver biopsies.

The AST/ALT ratio and the BARD score achieved worse results in our collective. Only 66% (AST/ALT ratio) and 56% (BARD score) would have been correctly classified, 27% (AST/ALT ratio) and 30% (BARD score) of the patients with advanced fibrosis would have been missed (see table S1 and figure S1).

However, the low prevalence of advanced fibrosis (8%) in our study population has to be taken into account when comparing our test results with other large series (prevalences of 26% [19] and 27% [17], respectively). This could have affected the high false negative rate of the tested scoring systems in our patient population.

In order to achieve a homogeneous study population truly consisting of patients only with NAFLD we had to exclude a large number of patients with preexisting diseases or accompanying medications, which may have introduced a selection bias. Due to the retrospective design of our study, clinical and laboratory data were incomplete in several cases, leaving only a limited number of patients to develop our scoring system as well as for the direct comparison with the well-established FIB-4 index. Furthermore, in order to increase the range of obesity and the number of patients with NASH in our study cohort we included cases from two tertiary liver centers in Germany with clearly different populations. While almost all patients recruited in Cologne were metabolic patients who had been referred to the outpatient department for further work-up after abnormal liver function tests had been detected by their treating primary care physicians, patients recruited in Essen, showed relatively normal liver enzymes, were severe obese and scheduled for bariatric surgery. Although the comparison of this two populations showed no statistically significant differences in laboratory or clinical parameters, especially concerning the prevalence of advanced fibrosis (see table 1), we can not exclude a potential impact on the score and its accuracy due to differences in pathogenic mechanisms among this two patient groups. This makes it necessary to confirm our results in further studies with a more homogeneous study population. Liver biopsy specimens were assessed by two experienced hepatopathologists who followed established histopathological criteria for the diagnosis and staging of NAFLD [24;25]. Histological slides were reexamined at a different time point by the same pathologists, who were blinded to all clinical and laboratory data. Inter and intra variability could have caused a bias.

Recently an algorithm for the work-up of patients with NAFLD has been proposed that incorporates FibroScan® for patients with indeterminate or high risk according to the NAFLD fibrosis score [35]. Although measuring liver stiffness with FibroScan® has been shown to produce reliable results in diagnosing advanced fibrosis in patients with various chronic liver diseases including NAFLD, this method reaches its limits in overweight and obese patients where as much as 20% of measurements are uninterpretable [36].

In summary, we developed and validated a simple noninvasive scoring system, the NAFLD-NIKEI, which relies on only four routinely measured laboratory parameters and as such has the potential to be used in every day practice. Our results suggest, that this index can reliably exclude advanced fibrosis in a large proportion of subjects with NAFLD. In combination with the FIB-4 index, misclassification with inadequate clinical management can be avoided while the need for liver biopsies can be reduced by more than 80%. Therefore, if our results can be confirmed in independent study samples from community dwelling patient populations with obesity and/or elevated liver enzymes and comparably low prevalence of advanced fibrosis, the proposed algorithm could play an important role in targeting the most appropriate candidate for liver biopsy.

Supporting Information

Figure S1 a. ROC-curve analysis for the prediction of advanced fibrosis with *AST/ALT ratio >0.8 (n = 266)* in our study population. **b.** ROC-curve analysis for the prediction of advanced fibrosis with *BARD score (n = 242)* in our study population.

Table S1 a. Cut-off values and the classification of patients on the basis of the *AST/ALT ratio >0.8 (n = 266)*. A patient with a value below the lower cut-off level was classified as healthy (no advanced fibrosis), with a value above the upper cut-off level as morbid (advanced fibrosis). Patients with values between the cut-off levels are intermediate/not classifiable. **b.** Cut-off values and the classification of patients on the basis of the *BARD score (n = 242)*. A patient with a value below the lower cut-off level was classified as healthy (no advanced fibrosis), with a value above the upper cut-off level as morbid (advanced fibrosis). Patients with values between the cut-off levels are intermediate/not classifiable.

Author Contributions

Conceived and designed the experiments: MD SL HMS. Performed the experiments: MD SL UD IW AC JS MS HMS. Analyzed the data: MD SL IK DN UT HMS. Contributed reagents/materials/analysis tools: MD SL IK UD IW AC JS MS HMS. Wrote the paper: MD SL DN HMS JS AC.

References

1. Vernon G, Baranova A, Younossi ZM (2011) Systematic review: the epidemiology and natural history of non-alcoholic fatty liver disease and non-alcoholic steatohepatitis in adults. Aliment Pharmacol Ther 34: 274–285.
2. Kim CH, Younossi ZM (2008) Nonalcoholic fatty liver disease: a manifestation of the metabolic syndrome. Cleve Clin J Med 75: 721–8.
3. Ekstedt M, Franzén LE, Mathiesen UL, Thorelius L, Holmqvist M, et al. (2006) Long-term follow-up of patients with NAFLD and elevated liver enzymes. Hepatology 44: 865–873.
4. Younossi ZM, Stepanova M, Rafiq N, Makhlouf H, Younoszai Z, et al. (2011) Pathologic criteria for nonalcoholic steatohepatitis: interprotocol agreement and ability to predict liver-related mortality. Hepatology 53: 1874–1882.
5. Myers RP, Fong A, Shaheen AA (2008) Utilization rates, complications and costs of percutaneous liver biopsy: a population-based study including 4275 biopsies. Liver Int 28: 705–12.
6. Ratziu V, Charlotte F, Heurtier A (2005) Sampling variability of liver biopsy in nonalcoholic fatty liver disease. Gastroenterology 128(7): 1898–906.
7. Dixon JB, Bhathal PS, O'Brien PE (2001) Nonalcoholic fatty liver disease: predictors of nonalcoholic steatohepatitis and liver fibrosis in the severely obese. Gastroenterology 121: 91–100.
8. Santos VN, Leite-Mór MMB, Kondo M, Martins JR, Nader H, et al. (2005) Serum laminin, type IV collagen and hyaluronan as fibrosis markers in non-alcoholic fatty liver disease. Brazilian Journal of Medical and Biological Research 38: 747–753.
9. Yoneda M, Mawatari H, Fujita K, Lida H, Yonemitsu K, et al. (2007) High-sensitivity C-reactive protein is an independent clinical feature of nonalcoholic steatohepatitis (NASH) and also of the severity of fibrosis in NASH. J Gastroenterol 42: 573–582.
10. Wieckowska A, Papouchado BG, Li Z, Lopez R, Zein NN, et al. (2008) Increased hepatic and circulating Interleukin-6 levels in human nonalcoholic steatohepatitis. Am J Gastroenterol 103: 1372–1379.
11. Nazal L, Riquelme A, Solís N, Pizarro M, Escalona A, et al. (2010) Hypoadiponectinemia and its association with liver fibrosis in morbidly obese patients. Obes Surg 20(10): 1400–7.
12. Feldstein AE, Canbay A, Angulo P, Taniai M, Burgart LJ, et al. (2003) Hepatocyte apoptosis and fas expression are prominent features of human nonalcoholic steatohepatitis. Gastroenterology 125(2): 437–43.
13. Horoz M, Bolukbas C, Bolukbas FF, Sabuncu T, Aslan M, et al. (2005) Measurement of the total antioxidant response using a novel automated method in subjects with nonalcoholic steatohepatitis. BMC Gastroenterology 5: 35.
14. Lewis JR, Mohanty SR (2010) Nonalcoholic fatty liver disease: a review and update. Dig Dis Sci 55: 560–578.
15. Rosenberg WM, Voelker M, Thiel R, Becka M, Burt A, et al. (2004) Serum markers detect the presence of liver fibrosis: a cohort study. Gastroenterology 127(6): 1704–13.
16. Guha IN, Parkes J, Roderick P, Chattopadhyay D, Cross R, et al. (2008) Noninvasive markers of fibrosis in nonalcoholic fatty liver disease: validating the European Liver Fibrosis Panel and exploring simple markers. Hepatology 47: 455–460.
17. Angulo P, Hui JM, Marchesini G, Bugianesi E, George J, et al. (2007) The NAFLD Fibrosis Score: a noninvasive system that identifies liver fibrosis in patients with NAFLD. Hepatology 45: 846–854.
18. Musso G, Gambino R, Cassader M, Pagano G (2010) Meta-analysis: Natural history of non-alcoholic fatty liver disease (NAFLD) and diagnostic accuracy of non-invasive tests for liver disease severity. Ann Med Nov 2. [Epub ahead of print].
19. Shah AG, Lydecker A, Murray K, Tetri BN, Contos MJ, et al. (2009) Comparison of noninvasive markers of fibrosis in patients with nonalcoholic fatty liver disease. Clin Gastroenterol Hepatol 7: 1104–1112.
20. Miller MH, Ferguson MA, Dillon JF (2011) Systematic review of performance of non-invasive biomarkers in the evaluation of non-alcoholic fatty liver disease. Liver Int 31: 461–473.
21. Ratziu V, Massard J, Charlotte F, Messous D, Imbert-Bismut F, et al. (2006) Diagnostic value of biochemical markers (FibroTest-FibroSURE) for the prediction of liver fibrosis in patients with non-alcoholic fatty liver disease. BMC Gastroenterology 6: 6.
22. Harrison SA, Oliver D, Arnold HL, Gogia S, Neuschwander-Tetri BA (2008) Development and validation of a simple NAFLD clinical scoring system for identifying patients without advanced disease. Gut 57: 1441–7.
23. McPherson S, Stewart SF, Henderson E, Burt AD, Day CP (2010) Simple non-invasive fibrosis scoring systems can reliably exclude advanced fibrosis in patients with non-alcoholic fatty liver disease. Gut 59: 1265–9.
24. Brunt EM, Janney CG, Di Bisceglie AM, Neuschwander-Tetri BA, Bacon BR (1999) Nonalcoholic steatohepatitis: a proposal for grading and staging the histological lesions. Am J Gastroenterol 94: 2467–2474.
25. Kleiner DE, Brunt EM, Van Natta M, Behling C, Contos MJ, et al. (2005) for the Nonalcoholic Steatohepatitis Clinical Research Network. Design and validation of a histological scoring system for nonalcoholic fatty liver disease. Hepatology 41: 1313–1321.
26. Sterling RK, Lissen E, Clumeck N, Sola R, Correa MC, et al. (2006) for the APRICOT Clinical Investigators. Development of a simple noninvasive index to predict significant fibrosis in patients with HIV/HCV coinfection. Hepatology 43: 1317–1325.
27. Williams CD, Stengel J, Aike MI, Torres DM, Shaw J, et al. (2011) Prevalence of nonanlcoholic fatty liver disease and nonalcoholic steatohepatitis among a largely middle-aged population utilizing ultrasouind and liver biopsy: a prospective study. Gastroenterology 140: 124–31.
28. Lydatakis H, Hager I-P, Kostadelou E, Mpousmpoulas S, Pappas S, et al. (2006) Non-invasive markers to predict the liver fibrosis in non-alcoholic fatty liver disease. Liver International 26: 864–871.
29. Feldstein AE, Wieckowska A, Lopez AR, Liu YC, Zein NN, et al. (2009) Cytokeratin-18 fragment levels as noninvasive biomarkers for nonalcoholic steatohepatitis: a multicenter validation study. Hepatology 50: 1072–8.
30. Torres DM, Harrison SA (2008) Diagnosis and therapy of nonalcoholic steatohepatitis. Gastroenterology 134(6): 1682–98.
31. Ong JP, Pitts A, Younossi ZM (2008) Increased overall mortality and liver-related mortality in non-alcoholic fatty liver disease. J Hepatol 49: 608–12.
32. Ascha MS, Hanouneh IA, Lopez R, Tamimi TA, Feldstein AF, et al. (2010) The incidence and risk factors of hepatocellular carcinoma in patients with nonalcoholic steatohepatitis. Hepatology 51: 1972–8.
33. Francque SM, Verrijken A, Mertens I, Hubens G, Van Marck E, et al. (2012) Noninvasive assessment of nafld in obese or overweight patients. Clin Gastroenterol Hepatol. 10: 1162–8.

PRO-C3-Levels in Patients with HIV/HCV-Co-Infection Reflect Fibrosis Stage and Degree of Portal Hypertension

Christian Jansen[1☯], Diana J. Leeming[2☯], Mattias Mandorfer[3], Inger Byrjalsen[2], Robert Schierwagen[1], Philipp Schwabl[3], Morten A. Karsdal[2], Evrim Anadol[1], Christian P. Strassburg[1], Jürgen Rockstroh[1,4], Markus Peck-Radosavljevic[3], Søren Møller[5], Flemming Bendtsen[6], Aleksander Krag[7], Thomas Reiberger[3¶], Jonel Trebicka[1*¶]

1 Department of Internal Medicine I, University of Bonn, Bonn, Germany, **2** Nordic Bioscience, Fibrosis Biology and Biomarkers, Herlev, Denmark, **3** Division of Gastroenterology and Hepatology, Department of Internal Medicine III, Medical University of Vienna, Vienna, Austria, **4** German Centre for Infection Research (DZIF), partner site Bonn-Cologne, Bonn, Germany, **5** Center of Functional and Diagnostic Imaging and Research, Department of Clinical Physiology, Hvidovre Hospital, University of Copenhagen, Copenhagen, Denmark, **6** Gastro Unit, Medical Division, Hvidovre Hospital, Faculty of Health Sciences, University of Copenhagen, Copenhagen, Denmark, **7** Department of Medical Gastroenterology, Odense University Hospital, Odense, Denmark

Abstract

Background: Liver-related deaths represent the leading cause of mortality among patients with HIV/HCV-co-infection, and are mainly related to complications of fibrosis and portal hypertension. In this study, we aimed to evaluate the structural changes by the assessment of extracellular matrix (ECM) derived degradation fragments in peripheral blood as biomarkers for fibrosis and portal hypertension in patients with HIV/HCV co-infection.

Methods: Fifty-eight patients (67% male, mean age: 36.5 years) with HIV/HCV-co-infection were included in the study. Hepatic venous pressure gradient (HVPG) was measured in forty-three patients. The fibrosis stage was determined using FIB4 -Score. ECM degraded products in peripheral blood were measured using specific ELISAs (C4M, MMP-2/9 degraded type IV collagen; C5M, MMP-2/9 degraded type V collagen; PRO-C3, MMP degraded n-terminal propeptide of type III collagen).

Results: As expected, HVPG showed strong and significant correlations with FIB4-index ($r_s = 0.628$; $p = 7*10^{-7}$). Interestingly, PRO-C3 significantly correlated with HVPG ($r_s = 0.354$; $p = 0.02$), alanine aminotransferase ($r_s = 0.30$; $p = 0.038$), as well as with FIB4-index ($r_s = 0.3230$; $p = 0.035$). C4M and C5M levels were higher in patients with portal hypertension (HVPG>5 mmHg).

Conclusion: PRO-C3 levels reflect liver injury, stage of liver fibrosis and degree of portal hypertension in HIV/HCV-co-infected patients. Furthermore, C4M and C5M were associated with increased portal pressure. Circulating markers of hepatic ECM remodeling might be helpful in the diagnosis and management of liver disease and portal hypertension in patients with HIV/HCV coinfection.

Editor: Matias A. Avila, University of Navarra School of Medicine and Center for Applied Medical Research (CIMA), Spain

Funding: This work was supported by: 1. Deutsche Forschungsgemeinschaft (SFB TRR57 P18 to Jonel Trebicka); 2. J. & W. Hector-Foundation (to Jonel Trebicka); 3. unrestricted research grants from Roche Austria (to Markus Peck-Radosavljevic); 4. MSD Austria (to Markus Peck-Radosavljevic); 5. DZIF TTU HIV Project 05.803; 6. German Center for Infection Research (DZIF); 7. Danish Science Foundation; and 8. Danish Ministry of Science and Technology. The funders had no role in study design, data collection and analysis, decision to publish, or preparation of the manuscript.

Competing Interests: Diana J. Leeming, Morten A. Karsdal, and Inger Byrjalsen are employees of Nordic Bioscience, a company engaged in the development of biochemical markers. Morten A. Karsdal is a stockholder of Nordic Bioscience. The other authors have no conflict of interest.

* Email: jonel.trebicka@ukb.uni-bonn.de

☯ These authors contributed equally to this work.

¶ These authors also contributed equally to this work

Introduction

Combined antiretroviral treatment (cART) is able to control the HIV replication in the majority of HIV patients, and thereby reduce mortality [1,2]. While a decrease of AIDS-related deaths are noted, mortality related to chronic liver diseases is steadily increasing in HIV patients [3–5]. Nearly 24% of non-AIDS related deaths in HIV-infected patients are due to end-stage liver disease (ESLD), with 66% being attributed to HCV co-infection and 17% to HBV co-infection [5]. This represents an important socioeconomic problem, given the fact that more than 30% of HIV-patients in Europe and USA are co-infected [4]. HCV replication is increased in HIV coinfection [6], whereas HCV-specific immune responses are attenuated [7–10], which may be the cousal factors to the progression of liver fibrosis and accelerated development of ESLD in patients with HCV/HIV co-infection as compared to HCV mono-infected patients [11,12]. ESLD is associated with complications and mortality mainly due to portal hypertension. Measurement of hepatic venous pressure gradient (HVPG) is the best available tool to directly assess portal hypertension[13–16]. Thus, the early detection of fibrosis and portal hypertension especially in HIV/HCV co-infected patients represents an unmet clinical need.

During progression of liver fibrosis both, the synthesis and degradation of extracellular matrix (ECM) are increased – referred to as ECM remodeling [17–19]. Endopeptidases, such as matrix metalloproteinases (MMPs) MMP-2 and MMP-9 are enhanced during ECM remodeling, especially in HIV-positive patients [20–22]. During the synthesis and degradation of collagen by MMPs small fragments are released into the circulation, and their levels mirror the extent of liver dysfunction and portal hypertension in patients with alcoholic cirrhosis [17].

The aims of the present study were to evaluate circulating collagen fragments as biomarkers for (i) liver fibrosis stage and (ii) portal hypertension in patients with HIV/HCV coinfection.

Materials and Methods

Study design

We retrospectively included fifty-eight (67% male) patients with HIV/HCV coinfection. The median age was 36.5 years (range 19 to 63). HVPG was measured in forty-three patients. The fibrosis stage was determined using Fibroscan and FIB4-Score (Table 1). Circulating collagen fragments in peripheral serum were measured in all patients during routine blood sampling as previously described (Table S1). Furthermore, biochemical parameters were analyzed using standard methods (Table 2). The patients gave their written consent for the procedures and the local ethics committee of the University of Bonn (Nr. 069/10) as well as the local ethics committee of the University of Vienna (EK 005/2005) approved the study [23] in accordance with the Declaration of Helsinki.

Measurement of HVPG, liver stiffness by transient elastography and calculation of FIB-4 Index

HVPG measurements were performed as previously described [13,24,25]. Under local anesthesia and ultrasound guidance, the right internal jugular was canulated by usage of the Seldinger technique. A balloon catheter was placed under continuous radiological control in a major hepatic vein. To calculate HVPG, three repeated measurements of free and wedged hepatic venous pressure were performed. Pressure curves were continuously recorded using a licensed software (S5 Collect, Vienna, Austria).

Transient elastography (Fibroscan, Echosens, France) was used for measurement liver stiffness as previously described [25–27].

FIB4-index was calculated in 43 patients, as previously described [28]. FIB4-index is based on AST, ALT, platelet count, and age: FIB4 = (age [years] $\times$ AST [IU L^{-1}])/(platelet count [10^9 L^{-1}] $\times \sqrt{ALT}$ [IU L^{-1}]).

Enzyme-linked immunosorbentassay

Specific enzyme-linked immunosorbentassay (ELISA) were assessed in the described patient group following a protocol as previously described [17] to detect degradation of ECM fragments. In detail: PRO-C3 (true collagen type III formation) [29] C4M (MMP-2/9 degraded type IV collagen) [30] and C5M (MMP-2/9 degraded type V collagen) [31] were quantified (Table S1).

Statistical analysis

Mann-Whitney-U test was used for unpaired comparisons. The correlations were analyzed by the use of Spearman correlation coefficient. Significant differences in levels of circulating biomarkers in peripheral blood between more than two groups were analyzed using Kruskal-Wallis-Test. $p<0.05$ was considered as statistically significant. Statistical analyses were performed with SPSS 22 (SPSS Inc. Chicago, IL, USA).

Results

Clinical, biochemical, and haemodynamic characteristics of patients

The clinical characteristics of the study population are shown in Table 1. The biochemical parameters including the levels of ECM markers are shown in Table 2. All patients were treated with cART and HIV viral load was under detection level.

FIB-4 index was calculated in forty-three patients as previously described [28]. Seven patients showed no or F1 fibrosis, 30 patients showed stage F2 or F3 and six patients showed fibrosis F4 (Table 1; Figure 1C). Using transient elastography with a median of 7 kPa (range 3–22 kPa), more patients showed a mild fibrosis (F0/1 n = 23; F2/3 n = 18; F4 n = 5) (Table 1). HVPG was measured in forty-three patients. The median pressure was 3 mmHg (range: 2–13 mmHg). HVPG correlated with FIB-4 index ($r_s = 0.628$; $p = 7*10^{-7}$), liver stiffness ($r_s = 0.621$; $p = 9*10^{-5}$), and inversely with platelet counts ($r_s = -0.366$; $p = 0.016$) (Figure S1). The strong correlation of HVPG with liver stiffness serves as internal quality control of the data raised in the patients.

Table 1. Clinical parameters of patients.

Parameters	n	value
Gender (female/male, % male)	58	19/39 (67%)
Age	58	36.5 (19–63)
Weight (kg)	58	69 (45–103)
HVPG (mmHg)	43	3 (2–13)
Liver Stiffness (kPa)	46	7 (3–22)
FIB-4 Index	43	2 (0–4)

HVPG: hepatic venous pressure gradient; FIB-4 Index: Fibrosis 4 Score.
Data are shown as median (range) and n numbers of patients per group.

Table 2. Biochemical parameters of included patients.

Parameters	n	value
ALT (U/L)	48	71 (13–348)
PLT (10^9/L)	48	184 (55–330)
HCV-RNA (IU/mL)	48	1,052,500 (5,590–36,700,000)
CD4 (U/μL)	48	515 (134–1,222)
PRO-C3 (ng/mL)	58	22 (10–50)
C4M (ng/mL)	58	141 (54–411)
C5M (ng/mL)	58	375 (182–727)

ALT, alanine aminotransferase; PLT, platelets; HCV-RNA, hepatitis C virus ribonucleic acid; CD4, CD4+ T helper cells; PRO-C3, degraded n-terminal propeptide of type III collagen; C4M, degraded type IV collagen; C5M, degraded type V collagen. Data are shown as median (range).

Relationship between PRO-C3 levels and parameters of liver injury

Interestingly, serum PRO-C3 levels significantly correlated with HVPG ($r_s = 0.354$; $p = 0.020$; Figure-1A; Table 3). Furthermore, PRO-C3 levels significantly correlated with ALT as a marker of liver injury ($r_s = 0.30$; $p = 0.038$; Figure 1B; Table 3).

Moreover, serum PRO-C3 correlated with FIB-4 index ($r_s = 0.323$; $p = 0.035$; Table 3) and was significantly higher in patients with advanced fibrosis as indicated either by FIB-4 index or transient elastography (Figure 1C, 1D).

Relationship between serum C4M and C5M levels and parameters of liver injury

Levels of serum C5M significantly correlated with FIB-4 index ($r_s = 0.314$; $p = 0.04$; Figure 2B) and were higher in patients with portal hypertension defined as HVPG above 5 mmHg (Figure 2C). Interestingly, serum levels of C4M were significant higher ($p = 0.014$) in patients with portal hypertension (Figure 2A).

Discussion

This study demonstrated that serum PRO-C3 levels may serve as biomarkers for the extent of liver fibrosis, liver injury, and portal hypertension in HIV/HCV-co-infected patients. Additional markers of ECM remodeling such as serum C4M and C5M levels might be useful in these patients to non-invasively diagnose the presence of portal hypertension.

ECM remodelling occurs as an attempt to repair damaged tissue response to liver injury [14,32–34], while ongoing hepatic injury leads to a non-regenerative wound healing characterized by high turnover of ECM and ultimately, a net accumulation of fibrotic scar tissue in the liver. The deposition of fibrotic material continuously increases intrahepatic vascular resistance to portal blood flow and thereby causing portal hypertension [35,36]. Therefore, the progression of fibrosis and development of portal hypertension are closely associated [37]. Especially in patients with HIV/HCV co-infection the evaluation of fibrosis and portal hypertension represents a major issue, since disease progression is accelerated [38] and liver-related mortality is increasing [3–5]. These patients might be asymptomatic until clinical decompensation occurs, but at this stage preventing morbidity and mortality represents a major clinical challenge. Therefore, non-invasive biomarkers are needed for early detection of liver fibrosis and portal hypertension - before clinically significant complications and decompensation occur.

The present study showed that the collagen type III formation marker PRO-C3 correlated with liver injury, fibrosis, and portal hypertension in HIV/HCV co-infected patients. This marker was previously described to derive from the diseased liver and reflects fibrosis and portal hypertension in animal models of fibrosis [18] and in humans with alcoholic cirrhosis [17]. The PRO-C3 ELISA is different and may be superior to other commercial available assays since other commercial PIIINP assays available utilize either a monoclonal- or polyclonal antibody, from which the precise epitope is not known. The Pro-C3 ELISA utilized a monoclonal antibody specific for the PIIINP cleavage site resulting in a stronger surrogate for collagen III formation. This has been described in Nielsen et al. [29]. In the present work we confirmed that PRO-C3 reflects ECM remodelling and liver fibrogenesis in HIV/HCV coinfected patients. Most importantly, PRO-C3 seems to be a valuable biomarker for liver fibrosis stage and portal hypertension in HIV/HCV coinfection.

Furthermore, systemically assessed type IV (C4M) and V collagen (C5M) fragments were significantly higher in HIV/HCV-co-infected patients with portal hypertension. Interestingly, the level of C4M and C5M reflects not only the release of ECM-fragments, but also the turnover of ECM [18], and thereby may mirror the extent and activity of fibrotic processes. In contrast to PRO-C3, C4M is a marker of basement membrane degradation [30]. But similarly to the formation marker PRO-C3, C4M levels were also shown to be elevated in BDL and CCl4-treated rats [18]. In addition, we showed recently that C4M together with PRO-C3 has the highest diagnostic power as single marker to identify clinically relevant HVPG in patients with alcoholic cirrhosis [17]. Thus the present data are in alignment. Moreover, in a rat model of liver fibrosis C4M was correlated with the effect of antifibrotic treatment, which has still not deep validated in human studies [18]. All these studies have demonstrated that collagen degradation occurs in fibrotic processes and is may act as a mirror of the synthesis of collagen at a similar extent as the synthesis of collagen. Once again this study reinforces the strong causal association between ECM remodeling and portal hypertension. The present study confirms the importance of PRO-C3 and C4M as predictor of portal hypertension also in patients with HIV/HCV coinfection.

Interestingly, this study underlines a potential role of collagen type V degradation marker in the HIV/HCV patients. Fibrosis of lymphoid tissue has been described as a milestone of disease progression in HIV, and besides spleen, gut and lymph nodes, the liver is a major organ involved in the immune response towards pathogens [39]. In the presence of additional HCV infection, the liver disease may be the major couse of morbidity and mortality

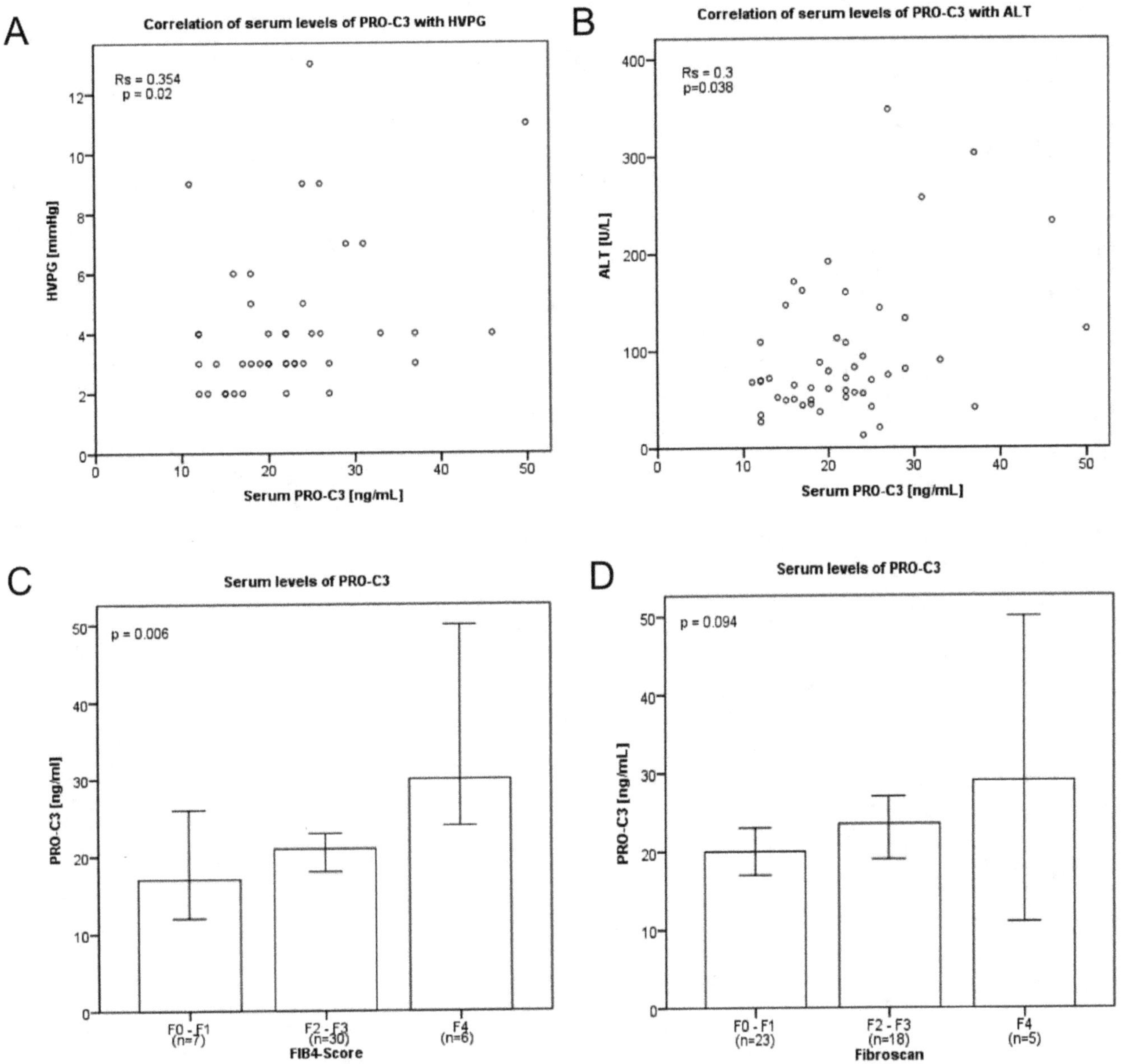

Figure 1. Levels of PRO-C3 measured in blood of patients with HIV/HCV co-infection correlated with hemodynamic and liver function parameters as well with FIB4-Score. The levels of PRO-C3 (A) correlated with HVPG ($r_s = 0.354$; $p = 0.02$) as well as the levels of ALT ($r_s = 0.3$; $p = 0.038$) (B). Furthermore significant higher levels of PRO-C3 could be observed in patients with advanced fibrosis stratified using FIB4-Score ($p = 0.006$) (C). Instead using fibroscan to stratify patient in the same way only a tendency could be seen ($p = 0.094$) (D).

and this study is the first to highlight the potential pathogenetic role of collagen type V degradation in the progression of fibrosis and development of portal hypertension. Thus, our previous results in patients with alcoholic cirrhosis [18] also apply in

Table 3. Correlations of PRO-C3 with fibrosis, portal hypertension and liver function.

PRO-C3	n	Rs	p-value
FIB4-Score	43	0.323	0.035
HVPG (mmHg)	43	0.354	0.020
ALT (U/L)	48	0.300	0.038

ALT, alanine aminotransferase; HVPG hepatic venous pressure gradient.

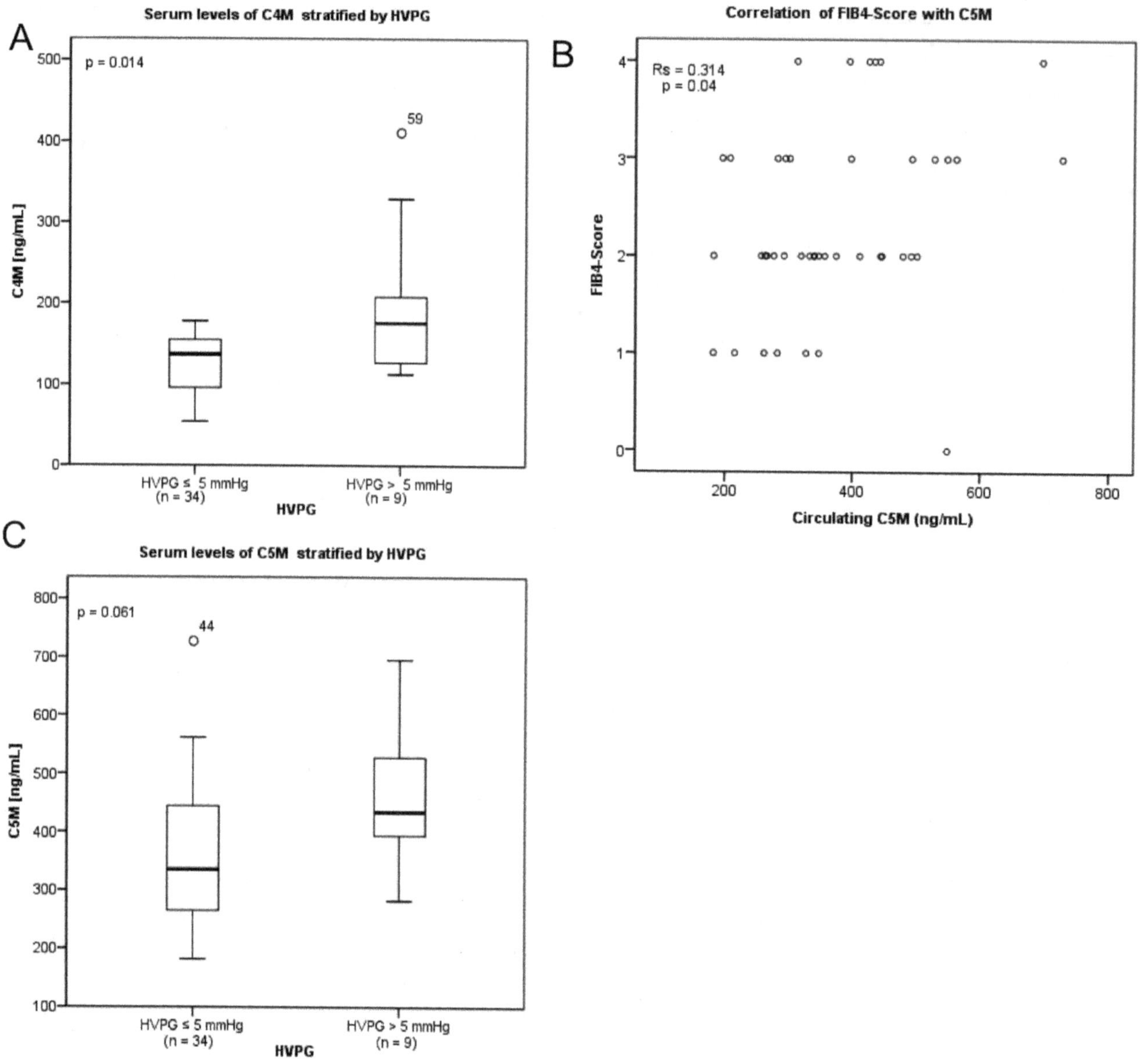

Figure 2. FIB4 score correlated significant with C5M (B). Serum levels of C5M (C) and C4M (A) stratified between patients with higher and lower or equal hepatic venous pressure gradient than 5 mmHg differ. Levels of serum C5M (B) correlated significantly with FIB4-score ($r_s = 0.314$; $p = 0.04$). Stratified patients between higher and lower hepatic venous pressure gradient than 5 mmHg showed significant differ in levels of serum C4M ($p = 0.014$) (A). Levels of C5M ($p = 0.061$) (C) only showed a tendency. Data are shown by using box-plots and were analyzed with the Wilcoxon test.

patients with HIV/HCV-co-infection. As previously described type V collagen is a key player in formation and assembly of other collagens. Therefore it is not surprising that also increased levels of C5M has been described in diseases with abnormally high collagen remodeling such as chronic obstructive pulmonary disease [40] and idiopathic pulmonary fibrosis [40] and ankylosing spondylitis [31].

Limitations

Although these patients were well characterized the present study has several limitations. We examined in this study a very selective small group of patients, which might be a bias of the study. Besides that, the validity of the results is strengthened, since they are well in line with previously published findings of correlation of HVPG with FIB-4 score, transient elastography assessed by Fibroscan, platelet count and aminotransferases levels [41–44]. Therefore, our identified markers may serve as early marker of liver injury, fibrosis and portal hypertension.

In conclusion, this study demonstrates that liver fibrosis and liver injury might be reflected by PRO-C3-levels in HIV/HCV-co-infected patients. PRO-C3 correlated with HVPG and parameters of hepatic dysfunction. Furthermore higher levels of C4M and C5M were associated with degree of portal hypertension.

Supporting Information

Figure S1 Correlation of HVPG with FIB4-Score (A), fibroscan (B) and PLT (C). HVPG correlates with FIB4-Score ($r_s = 0.628$; $p = 7*10^{-7}$) (A) as well with fibrosacan ($r_s = 0.621$; $p = 9*10^{-5}$) (B) and inversely with PLT ($r_s = -0.366$; $p = 0.016$) (C). Data are presented using Spearman coefficient r_s and p-values.

Table S1 Overview of technical specification of the novel ECM assays presented in this study.

Acknowledgments

We thank Gudrun Hack, Lise Larsen and Silke Bellinghausen for their excellent technical assistance.

Author Contributions

Conceived and designed the experiments: DJL MAK TR JT. Performed the experiments: CJ MM RS PS EA. Analyzed the data: CJ IB DJL TR JT. Contributed reagents/materials/analysis tools: DJL MAK CPS JR MPR SM FB AK TR JT. Contributed to the writing of the manuscript: CJ DJL MAK MM RS PS EA CPS JR MPR SM FB AK TR JT.

References

1. Lee LM, Karon JM, Selik R, Neal JJ, Fleming PL (2001) Survival after AIDS diagnosis in adolescents and adults during the treatment era, United States, 1984–1997. JAMA 285: 1308–1315.
2. Mocroft A, Ledergerber B, Katlama C, Kirk O, Reiss P, et al. (2003) Decline in the AIDS and death rates in the EuroSIDA study: an observational study. Lancet 362: 22–29.
3. Mocroft A, Soriano V, Rockstroh J, Reiss P, Kirk O, et al. (2005) Is there evidence for an increase in the death rate from liver-related disease in patients with HIV? AIDS 19: 2117–2125.
4. Rosenthal E, Pialoux G, Bernard N, Pradier C, Rey D, et al. (2007) Liver-related mortality in human-immunodeficiency-virus-infected patients between 1995 and 2003 in the French GERMIVIC Joint Study Group Network (MORTAVIC 2003 Study). J Viral Hepat 14: 183–188.
5. Joshi D, O'Grady J, Dieterich D, Gazzard B, Agarwal K (2011) Increasing burden of liver disease in patients with HIV infection. Lancet 377: 1198–1209.
6. Deng A, Chen C, Ishizaka Y, Chen X, Sun B, et al. (2014) Human immunodeficiency virus type 1 Vpr increases hepatitis C virus RNA replication in cell culture. Virus Res 184C: 93–102.
7. Vali B, Jones RB, Sakhdari A, Sheth PM, Clayton K, et al. (2010) HCV-specific T cells in HCV/HIV co-infection show elevated frequencies of dual Tim-3/PD-1 expression that correlate with liver disease progression. Eur J Immunol 40: 2493–2505.
8. Bowen DG, Walker CM (2005) Adaptive immune responses in acute and chronic hepatitis C virus infection. Nature 436: 946–952.
9. Cooper S, Erickson AL, Adams EJ, Kansopon J, Weiner AJ, et al. (1999) Analysis of a successful immune response against hepatitis C virus. Immunity 10: 439–449.
10. Gerlach JT, Diepolder HM, Jung MC, Gruener NH, Schraut WW, et al. (1999) Recurrence of hepatitis C virus after loss of virus-specific CD4(+) T-cell response in acute hepatitis C. Gastroenterology 117: 933–941.
11. Rotman Y, Liang TJ (2009) Coinfection with hepatitis C virus and human immunodeficiency virus: virological, immunological, and clinical outcomes. J Virol 83: 7366–7374.
12. Pineda JA, Romero-Gomez M, Diaz-Garcia F, Giron-Gonzalez JA, Montero JL, et al. (2005) HIV coinfection shortens the survival of patients with hepatitis C virus-related decompensated cirrhosis. Hepatology 41: 779–789.
13. Bosch J, Abraldes JG, Berzigotti A, Garcia-Pagan JC (2009) The clinical use of HVPG measurements in chronic liver disease. Nat Rev Gastroenterol Hepatol 6: 573–582.
14. Tsochatzis EA, Bosch J, Burroughs AK (2014) Liver cirrhosis. Lancet.
15. Garcia-Pagan JC, Di Pascoli M, Caca K, Laleman W, Bureau C, et al. (2013) Use of early-TIPS for high-risk variceal bleeding: results of a post-RCT surveillance study. J Hepatol 58: 45–50.
16. Garcia-Pagan JC, Reverter E, Abraldes JG, Bosch J (2012) Acute variceal bleeding. Semin Respir Crit Care Med 33: 46–54.
17. Leeming DJ, Karsdal MA, Byrjalsen I, Bendtsen F, Trebicka J, et al. (2013) Novel serological neo-epitope markers of extracellular matrix proteins for the detection of portal hypertension. Aliment Pharmacol Ther 38: 1086–1096.
18. Schierwagen R, Leeming DJ, Klein S, Granzow M, Nielsen MJ, et al. (2013) Serum markers of the extracellular matrix remodeling reflect antifibrotic therapy in bile-duct ligated rats. Front Physiol 4: 195.
19. Leeming D, He Y, Veidal S, Nguyen Q, Larsen D, et al. (2011) A novel marker for assessment of liver matrix remodeling: an enzyme-linked immunosorbent assay (ELISA) detecting a MMP generated type I collagen neo-epitope (C1M). Biomarkers 16: 616–628.
20. Karsdal MA, Nielsen MJ, Sand JM, Henriksen K, Genovese F, et al. (2013) Extracellular matrix remodeling: the common denominator in connective tissue diseases. Possibilities for evaluation and current understanding of the matrix as more than a passive architecture, but a key player in tissue failure. Assay Drug Dev Technol 11: 70–92.
21. Larrousse M, Laguno M, Segarra M, De Lazzari E, Martinez E, et al. (2007) Noninvasive diagnosis of hepatic fibrosis in HIV/HCV-coinfected patients. J Acquir Immune Defic Syndr 46: 304–311.
22. Schaefer L, Babelova A, Kiss E, Hausser HJ, Baliova M, et al. (2005) The matrix component biglycan is proinflammatory and signals through Toll-like receptors 4 and 2 in macrophages. J Clin Invest 115: 2223–2233.
23. Reiberger T, Payer BA, Ferlitsch A, Sieghart W, Breitenecker F, et al. (2012) A prospective evaluation of pulmonary, systemic and hepatic haemodynamics in HIV-HCV-coinfected patients before and after antiviral therapy with pegylated interferon and ribavirin. Antivir Ther 17: 1327–1334.
24. Reiberger T, Rutter K, Ferlitsch A, Payer BA, Hofer H, et al. (2011) Portal pressure predicts outcome and safety of antiviral therapy in cirrhotic patients with hepatitis C virus infection. Clin Gastroenterol Hepatol 9: 602–608 e601.
25. Reiberger T, Ulbrich G, Ferlitsch A, Payer BA, Schwabl P, et al. (2013) Carvedilol for primary prophylaxis of variceal bleeding in cirrhotic patients with haemodynamic non-response to propranolol. Gut 62: 1634–1641.
26. Reiberger T, Ferlitsch A, Payer BA, Pinter M, Schwabl P, et al. (2012) Noninvasive screening for liver fibrosis and portal hypertension by transient elastography–a large single center experience. Wien Klin Wochenschr 124: 395–402.
27. Schwabl P, Bota S, Salzl P, Mandorfer M, Payer B, et al. (2014) New reliability criteria for transient elastography increase the number of accurate measurements for screening of cirrhosis and portal hypertension. Liver Int.
28. Vallet-Pichard A, Mallet V, Nalpas B, Verkarre V, Nalpas A, et al. (2007) FIB-4: an inexpensive and accurate marker of fibrosis in HCV infection. comparison with liver biopsy and fibrotest. Hepatology 46: 32–36.
29. Nielsen MJ, Nedergaard AF, Sun S, Veidal SS, Larsen L, et al. (2013) The neo-epitope specific PRO-C3 ELISA measures true formation of type III collagen associated with liver and muscle parameters. Am J Transl Res 5: 303–315.
30. Veidal SS, Karsdal MA, Nawrocki A, Larsen MR, Dai Y, et al. (2011) Assessment of proteolytic degradation of the basement membrane: a fragment of type IV collagen as a biochemical marker for liver fibrosis. Fibrogenesis Tissue Repair 4: 22.
31. Veidal SS, Larsen DV, Chen X, Sun S, Zheng Q, et al. (2012) MMP mediated type V collagen degradation (C5M) is elevated in ankylosing spondylitis. Clin Biochem 45: 541–546.
32. Liedtke C, Luedde T, Sauerbruch T, Scholten D, Streetz K, et al. (2013) Experimental liver fibrosis research: update on animal models, legal issues and translational aspects. Fibrogenesis Tissue Repair 6: 19.
33. Trebicka J, Anadol E, Elfimova N, Strack I, Roggendorf M, et al. (2013) Hepatic and serum levels of miR-122 after chronic HCV-induced fibrosis. J Hepatol 58: 234–239.
34. Buck M, Garcia-Tsao G, Groszmann RJ, Stalling C, Grace ND, et al. (2014) Novel inflammatory biomarkers of portal pressure in compensated cirrhosis patients. Hepatology 59: 1052–1059.
35. Bosch J, Garcia-Tsao G (2009) Pharmacological versus endoscopic therapy in the prevention of variceal hemorrhage: and the winner is. Hepatology 50: 674–677.
36. Bosch J (2000) Prevention of variceal rebleeding: endoscopes, drugs, and more. Hepatology 32: 660–662.
37. Mandorfer M, Payer BA, Schwabl P, Steiner S, Ferlitsch A, et al. (2014) Revisiting liver disease progression in HIV/HCV-coinfected patients: the influence of vitamin D, insulin resistance, immune status, IL28B and PNPLA3. Liver Int.
38. Alesiani M, Pellegrini Giampietro DE, Cherici G, Galli A, Moroni F (1990) The guinea pig myenteric plexus as a tool to characterize drugs active at the glycine recognition site of the NMDA receptors. Pharmacol Res 22 Suppl 1: 15–16.
39. Estes JD (2013) Pathobiology of HIV/SIV-associated changes in secondary lymphoid tissues. Immunol Rev 254: 65–77.
40. Leeming DJ, Sand JM, Nielsen MJ, Genovese F, Martinez FJ, et al. (2012) Serological investigation of the collagen degradation profile of patients with chronic obstructive pulmonary disease or idiopathic pulmonary fibrosis. Biomark Insights 7: 119–126.
41. Sanchez-Conde M, Miralles P, Bellon JM, Rincon D, Ramirez M, et al. (2011) Use of transient elastography (FibroScan(R)) for the noninvasive assessment of portal hypertension in HIV/HCV-coinfected patients. J Viral Hepat 18: 685–691.

24

Rapamycin Ameliorates Inflammation and Fibrosis in the Early Phase of Cirrhotic Portal Hypertension in Rats through Inhibition of mTORC1 but not mTORC2

Weijie Wang[1,2], Jiqi Yan[1,2]*, Huakai Wang[1,2], Minmin Shi[2], Mingjun Zhang[2], Weiping Yang[1], Chenghong Peng[1], Hongwei Li[1]

1 Department of Surgery, Ruijin Hospital, Shanghai Jiaotong University School of Medicine, Shanghai, China, **2** Key Laboratory of Systems Biomedicine verified by Ministry of Education, Shanghai Institute of Digestive Surgery, Ruijin Hospital, Shanghai Jiaotong University School of Medicine, Shanghai, China

Abstract

Objective: Hepatic stellate cells (HSCs) transdifferentiation and subsequent inflammation are important pathological processes involved in the formation of cirrhotic portal hypertension. This study characterizes the pathogenetic mechanisms leading to cholestatic liver fibrosis and portal hypertension, and focuses on mammalian target of rapamycin (mTOR) pathway as a potential modulator in the early phase of cirrhotic portal hypertension.

Methods: Early cirrhotic portal hypertension was induced by bile duct ligation (BDL) for three weeks. One week after operation, sham-operated (SHAM) and BDL rats received rapamycin (2 mg/kg/day) by intraperitoneal injection for fourteen days. Vehicle-treated SHAM and BDL rats served as controls. Fibrosis, inflammation, and portal pressure were evaluated by histology, morphometry, and hemodynamics. Expressions of pro-fibrogenic and pro-inflammatory genes in liver were measured by RT-PCR; alpha smooth muscle actin (α-SMA) and antigen Ki67 were detected by immunohistochemistry; expressions of AKT/mTOR signaling molecules, extracellular-signal-regulated kinase 1/2 (ERK1/2), p-ERK1/2, and interleukin-1 beta (IL-1β) were assessed by western blot.

Results: The AKT/mTOR signaling pathway was markedly activated in the early phase of cirrhotic portal hypertension induced by BDL in rats. mTOR blockade by rapamycin profoundly improved liver function by limiting inflammation, fibrosis and portal pressure. Rapamycin significantly inhibited the expressions of phosphorylated 70KD ribosomal protein S6 kinase (p-P70S6K) and phosphorylated ribosomal protein S6 (p-S6) but not p-AKT Ser473 relative to their total proteins in BDL-Ra rats. Those results suggested that mTOR Complex 1 (mTORC1) rather than mTORC2 was inhibited by rapamycin. Interestingly, we also found that the level of p-ERK1/2 to ERK1/2 was significantly increased in BDL rats, which was little affected by rapamycin.

Conclusions: The AKT/mTOR signaling pathway played an important role in the early phase of cirrhotic portal hypertension in rats, which could be a potential target for therapeutic intervention in the early phase of such pathophysiological progress.

Editor: Matias A. Avila, University of Navarra School of Medicine and Center for Applied Medical Research (CIMA), Spain

Funding: This study was jointly supported by the Foundation of Shanghai Natural Science (09ZR1418600) and the National Natural Science (81070358) of China. The funders had no role in study design, data collection and analysis, decision to publish, or preparation of the manuscript.

Competing Interests: The authors are grateful to Pfizer Inc (USA) for their kindly donation of rapamycin.

* E-mail: jiqiyan@yahoo.com

Introduction

Liver cirrhosis is a very complex disease in which multiple pathological processes are closely involved, including inflammatory infiltration and fibrogenesis [1,2]. In fact, liver fibrosis represents a wound-healing process in response to a variety of chronic stimuli, which is characterized by an excessive deposition of extracellular matrix proteins (ECM) [3,4]. Induction of secondary biliary cirrhosis by bile duct ligation is a widely used model to investigate the pathophysiological changes that take place during the development of hepatic fibrogenesis and portal hypertension [5–8]. Along with cholangiocytes proliferation, quiescent HSCs transform into proliferative, fibrogenic, and contractile myofibroblasts, and then produce bulk of ECM, predominated by type I collagen [6,8]. They are both key players in the development of cholestatic liver fibrosis and portal hypertension [5,8].

To date, there is still limited specific medical therapy for hepatic fibrosis and portal hypertension. The precise pathogenetic mechanisms of cirrhotic portal hypertension have not yet been made entirely clear. Mammalian target of rapamycin (mTOR) and AKT, also called protein kinase B (PKB), are serine/threonine protein kinases akin to the phosphatidylinositol 3-kinase-related kinase (PI3K) protein family [9–11]. One of the functions of AKT

Table 1. Nucleotide sequences of RT-PCR primers.

Target mRNA	Direction Sequence (Forward/Reverse)	Accession Number
GAPDH	GAGGACCAGGTTGTCTCCTG	NM 017008.4
	GGATGGAATTGTGAGGGAGA	
mTOR	GACAACAGCCAGGGCCGCAT	NM 019906.1
	ACGCTGCCTTTCTCGACGGC	
P70S6K	CGGGGAAGCTTCAGCGCCAC	NM 031985.1
	TACGCAGGTGCTCTGGCCGT	
4EBP1	CTGCACAGCAGCCCGGAAGA	NM 053857.2
	TGCCGGGTACAAGGCCTGACT	
PCα1	TCCGGCTCCTGCTCCTCTTA	NM 053304.1
	GTATGCAGCTGACTTCAGGGATGT	
α-SMA	GCTGACAGGATGCAGAAGGA	NM 031004.2
	GCCGATCCAGACAGAATATTTG	
PDGF	CCGCTCCTTTGATGACCTTC	NM 031524.1
	GCTCAGCCCCATCTTCGTC	
PDGFRβ	TGGCCAATGGCATGGAAT	NM 031525.1
	CCAACTTGCCCTCACAGATGA	
TGF β1	AGAAGTCACCCGCGTGCTAA	NM 021578.2
	TCCCGAATGTCTGACGTATTGA	
TIMP 1	TCCTCTTGTTGCTATCATTGATAGCTT	NM 053819.1
	CGCTGGTATAAGGTGGTCTCGAT	
TNF-α	GACCAGGCTGTCGCTACATCA	NM 012675.3
	GTAGGGCGATTACAGTCACGG	
iNOS	AGCGGCTCCATGACTCTCA	NM 012611.3
	AAATGCTTTCTCCGCTCTGA	

is activation and phosphorylation of mTOR [9,11,12]. AKT/mTOR signaling pathway, the major downstream effector of PI3K, regulates a wide array of cellular processes such as cell growth, proliferation, motility, survival, apoptosis, protein synthesis and transcription [9,12–14]. Emerging experimental data showed that AKT/mTOR signaling pathway positioned itself at the center in the activation of hepatic stellate cells (HSCs) [3,15,16], and the pathway blockade by rapamycin could reduce fibrogenesis, improve liver function, and lower portal pressure in established cirrhotic animal models [5–7]. Therefore, we became especially interested in its conceivable mechanisms during portal hypertension's early pathophysiologic progress.

mTOR is the catalytic subunit of two molecular complexes: mTOR Complex 1 (mTORC1) and Complex 2 (mTORC2). They have distinct substrate specificities and are differentially sensitive to rapamycin, therefore differentially regulated [14,17]. mTORC1 integrates signals from growth factor receptors, then activates the 40S ribosomal protein S6 kinase (P70S6K) and inhibits the eukaryotic initiation factor (eIF) 4E-binding protein-1 (4E-BP1) by phosphorylation, forming two parallel signaling pathways regulating mRNA translation to control protein synthesis [14,18]. mTORC2 appears to possess the activity to phosphorylate the serine/threonine protein kinase AKT/PKB at a serine residue Ser473 [2]. Phosphorylation of the serine residue stimulates AKT phosphorylation at a threonine Thr308 residue by phosphoinositide-dependent kinase-1 (PDK1) and leads to full AKT activation [2,17].

Rapamycin as a bacterial macrolide with antifungal and immunosuppressive properties forms a complex with the FK binding protein (FKBP-12) that binds with high affinity to mTOR [19]. Several documents showed that rapamycin could inhibit the activation and proliferation of HSCs in vitro [15,20,21]. Mejias and Fernandez also confirmed that rapamycin had the inhibitory effect on lymphocyte proliferation, neovascularization and fibrogenesis in splenomegaly, as well as on the development of pathological angiogenesis in mesenteric tissues [22,23]. However, there is still little known about the specific role of the AKT/mTOR signaling pathway in the early pathophysiologic progress of cirrhotic portal hypertension. Comprehensive and in-depth researches on the pathway in cirrhotic portal hypertension have rarely been reported. We hypothesized that AKT/mTOR signaling pathway was activated in the pathophysiological onset of early cirrhotic portal hypertension, and rapamycin treatment would have multiple mechanisms of action against hepatic fibrosis and portal hypertension progression. Thereafter, we explored its potential therapeutic mechanisms in an animal model of early cirrhotic portal hypertension.

Materials and Methods

Ethics Statement

All animal care and experimental procedures complied with the guidelines for the Care and Use of Laboratory Animals, formulated by the Ministry of Science and Technology of the People's Republic of China, were approved by the Ethical

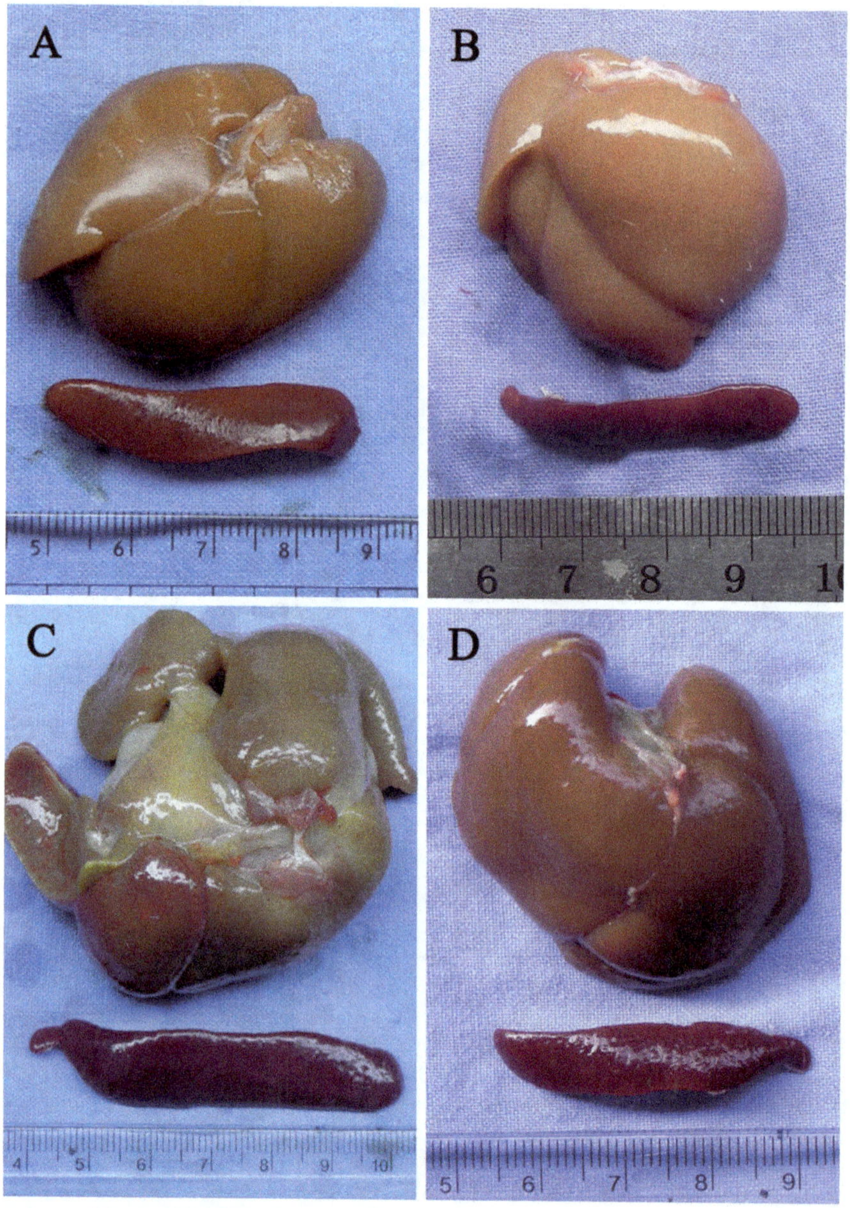

Figure 1. Rapamycin treatment ameliorates liver size and splenomegaly in BDL-Ra rats. Representative photographs of liver and spleen from (A) SHAM, (B) SHAM-Ra, (C) BDL, (D) BDL-Ra rats.

Committee on Animal Experiments at Ruijin Hospital (protocol approval number SYXK 2011-0113).

Materials

Antibody against α-smooth muscle actin (α-SMA) was from Doka (Denmark). Antibody against interleukin 1 beta (IL1-β) and Ki67 were bought from Santa Cruz Biotechnology (USA). Antibody against p-ERK1/2 was purchased from R&D (USA). Antibodies against AKT, mTOR, P70S6K, ribosomal protein S6 and their phosphorylated forms, including total protein ERK1/2, as well as peroxidase-conjugated secondary antibodies, were from Cell Signaling Technology (USA). Antibody against β-Actin was from Sigma (USA). Rapamycin was kindly donated by Pfizer Inc (USA).

Animals and Rapamycin Treatment Schedule

Liver cirrhotic portal hypertension was induced in male Sprague-Dawley rats (230–250 g body weight) by bile duct ligation (BDL). Sham-operated (SHAM) rats underwent the same surgical procedure, with the bile duct being isolated and manipulated, but not ligated. Rapamycin (5% DMSO solution with rapamycin; 2 $mgkg^{-1}$ day^{-1}; BDL-Ra: $n = 12$; SHAM-Ra: $n = 10$) or vehicle (5% DMSO solution; BDL: $n = 12$; SHAM: $n = 10$) was administered intraperitoneally for a 2-week period, starting one week after ligation, when it was still at an early stage of cirrhotic portal hypertension.

Table 2. Animal characteristic and hemodynamic parameters.

Indicators	SHAM (n = 10)	SHAM-Ra (n = 10)	BDL (n = 12)	BDL-Ra (n = 12)	P
BW (g)	340.90±24.00***	263.60±15.47###	289.30±35.56	247.70±25.93***	<0.0001
LW (LW/BW%)	4.05±0.46***	4.18±0.34	8.33±1.45	5.73±0.69***	<0.0001
SW (SW/BW%)	0.26±0.06***	0.18±0.02###	0.68±0.16	0.30±0.06***	<0.0001
HR (bpm)	376.20±26.24**	438.50±41.3	393.50±29.19	405.00±26.24**	<0.0001
MBP (mmHg)	104.30±10.96***	130.30±10.17	117.30±13.49	119.70±12.24	<0.0001
PP (mmHg)	8.71±0.93***	9.07±1.39	15.78±1.97	11.58±2.10***	<0.0001

Abbreviations: BW, body weight; LW, relative liver weight; SW, relative spleen weight; HR, heart rate; MBP, mean arterial blood pressure; PP, portal pressure.
*p<0.05;
**p<0.01;
***p<0.005 vs. BDL;
###p<0.005 vs. SHAM (mean±SD; Pairwise comparison with Mann Whitney U Test; P, non-parametrical one-way ANOVA, Kruskal-Wallis Test).

Haemodynamic Measurements, Liver Function and Tissue Conservation

At the end of the respective treatment phases, haemodynamic measurements - heart rate (HR) and mean arterial blood pressure (MBP) - were monitored by Tail-cuff method (BP-98A, Softron, Japan) in awake rats, and portal vein pressure (PP) was performed under pentobarbital anaesthesia. To maintain stable anesthesia, the measurement was started 20 min after the injection of pentobarbital. A segment of the mesenteric branch vein was cannulated with a 24-g cannula needle, and the tip of the cannula was advanced just into the trunk of the superior mesenteric vein. The PP was measured via a pressure transducer and recorded by a multichannel computer-based recorder (PowerLab, ADInstruments, Australia). Pressure measurement lasted for 1 min, and the average value was regarded as the portal pressure (PP). Rats were killed by exsanguination while taking blood samples for analyzing the serum levels of aspartate aminotransferase (AST), alanine aminotransferase (ALT), alkaline phosphatase (ALP), total bilirubin (TB), bile acids (BA), creatinine (CREA) and albumin (ALB). All of which were measured in the Department of Clinical Chemistry of Ruijin Hospital, Shanghai Jiaotong University School of Medicine. Liver and spleen were removed and weighed. Liver tissue samples were either fixed in 10% formalin, 4% glutaraldehyde or stored at −80°C.

Histology and Immunohistochemistry

Glutaraldehyde-fixed liver tissue was used for transmission electron microscope examination to observe the microscopic changes in the intrahepatic cells. Formalin-fixed and paraffin-embedded liver tissue was used for evaluation of liver pathological changes after HE, Masson and immunohistochemistry staining.

For immunohistochemistry, antigen retrieval was performed with citrate buffer (pH 6.0; 15 min at 95°C), followed by blocking with 0.6% H_2O_2 and 2% goat serum. Antibodies against α-SMA (1:400) and Ki67 (1:200) were applied 37°C for 1–2 hours, followed by biotinylated the corresponding secondary antibodies (DAKO, Denmark) at 1:350 for 45 min at room temperature (RT), streptavidin-HRP for 30 min at RT, and diaminobenzidine (DAB) detection. HE-, Masson- and DAB-stained liver tissue slides were analysed by morphometry. Morphometry was performed from three random fields of every slide using the Image-Pro plus software (Media Cybernetics Inc, USA). For each microscopic field, the positive area was calculated automatically by the software, and this positive area was in turn divided by the total area of the microscopic field. Morphometric results were then expressed as volume fractions (percentage of specific positive area in relation to the total counted area) and given as means ±SEM.

RNA Isolation and Quantitative Real-time PCR

Total RNA was isolated from about 30 mg of liver tissue with Trizol Reagent (Invitrogen, USA) according to the manufacturer's instructions. Then reverse transcription was done using Reverse Transcription Kit (Promega, USA). Quantitative real-time PCR was carried out on a 7900HT Fast Real-Time PCR System (Applied Biosystems, USA). The rat nucleotide sequences and accession numbers of primers were summarized in Table 1. Data were normalized to the housekeeping gene glycerinaldehyd-3-phosphatdehydrogenase (GAPDH).

The results were expressed as the number of cycles (CT value) at which the fluorescence signal exceeded a defined threshold. The difference in CT values of the target cDNA and GAPDH was expressed as ΔCT values. Therefore, lower ΔCT values denoted higher mRNA levels. The $2^{-\Delta CT}$ method was used for quantification of the results.

Western Blot Analysis

Tissue samples were put in ice-cold Tissue Protein Extraction Reagent (Pierce, USA) containing a mixture of proteinase inhibitors cocktails (Sigma, USA) and phosphatase inhibitors (Roche, Switzerland) to be homogenated by the tissue homogenizer. Samples were then centrifuged for 30 minutes at 10,000 g. The supernatant was collected, and the protein concentration was measured using the BCA Protein Assay Kit (Pierce, USA). Proteins (80~120 μg) were separated by SDS–PAGE and subsequently transferred to polyvinylidenefluoride membranes. The membranes were blocked with 5% bovine serum albumin (BSA) in incubation buffer for 2 h at room temperature. Afterwards, they were incubated with the corresponding primary antibodies at 4°C overnight and then with the peroxidase-conjugated secondary antibody at room temperature for 2 h. Finally, the signal was detected by enhanced chemiluminescence. Loading accuracy was evaluated by membrane rehybridization with anti-β-Actin antibodies. ImageJ software was used to quantify western blot signals.

Statistics

Comparison between multiple groups was performed with the one-way ANOVA Kruskal–Wallis test, and pairwise comparison with Mann Whitney U Test using the Graph Pad statistics software (Graph Pad Software Inc, USA). Results were considered statistically significant with a p-value <0.05. Results in the Tables

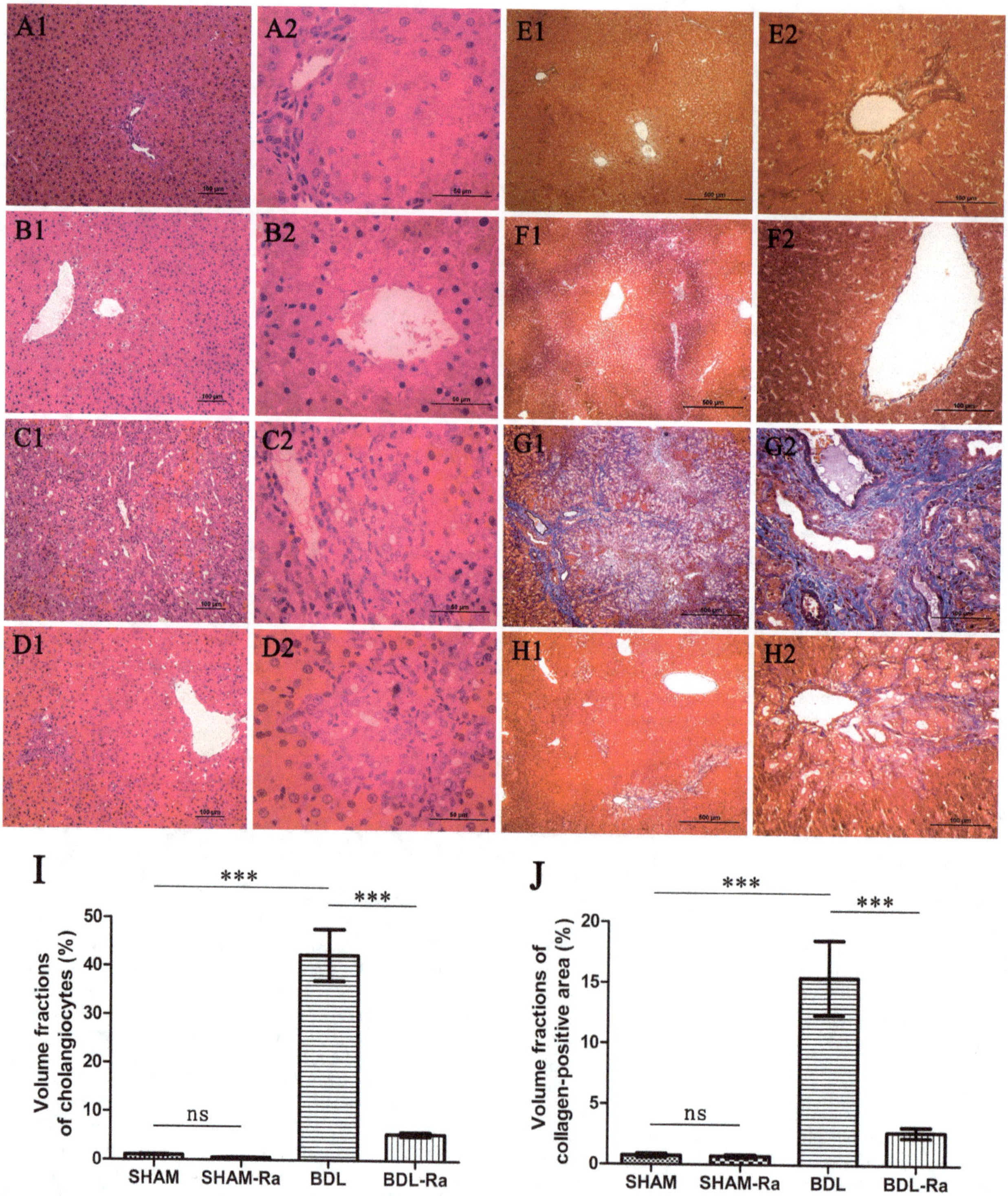

Figure 2. Rapamycin treatment reduces cholangiocytes proliferation and ECM deposition in BDL-Ra rats. Representative liver sections of (A) SHAM, (B) SHAM-Ra, (C) BDL, and (D) BDL-Ra rats, following HE-staining (magnification 100× and 400×, respectively). Representative microphotographs of Masson-stained liver sections from (E) SHAM, (F) SHAM-Ra, (G) BDL, and (H) BDL-Ra rats (magnification 40× and 200×, respectively). Graphs (I) and (J): Quantitative analysis of HE and Masson staining in representative liver sections respectively (mean±SEM; *$p<0.05$; **$p<0.01$; ***$p<0.005$; ns - nonsignificant).

were given as means ± standard deviation (SD). The columnar diagram results indicated means ± standard error of the mean (SEM).

Table 3. Serum enzymes.

	SHAM (n = 8)	SHAM-Ra (n = 8)	BDL (n = 12)	BDL-Ra (n = 12)	P
ALT	52.58±6.25***	57.80±19.28	200.40±123.70	78.00±13.73***	<0.0001
AST	160.80±23.19***	191.40±68.38	759.50±271.10	323.80±163.10***	<0.0001
ALP	324.60±65.49*	245.20±63.86#	420.60±79.80	316.00±86.17**	0.0011
TB	5.75±1.18***	9.12±3.59	158.00±27.64	122.90±49.39*	<0.0001
BA	13.46±7.46***	23.26±9.03#	109.70±14.71	73.37±33.79**	0.0007
CREA	17.22±3.12**	22.27±5.67	46.44±29.22	27.75±18.43	<0.0001
ALB	14.79±0.98**	11.20±2.14	10.13±1.99	9.00±1.91	0.0322

Abbreviations: ALT, alanine aminotransferase (IU/L); ALP, alkaline phosphatase (IU/L); AST, aspartate aminotransferase (IU/L); BA, bile acids (μmol/L); TB, total bilirubin (μmol/L); CREA, creatinine (μmol/L); ALB, albumin (g/L). (mean±SD; *p<0.05; **p<0.01; ***p<0.005 vs. BDL; #P<0.05 vs. SHAM; Pairwise comparison with Mann Whitney U Test; P, non-parametrical one-way ANOVA, Kruskal-Wallis Test).

Results

Rapamycin Ameliorates Liver Size, Splenomegaly and Portal Pressure

BDL for three weeks markedly impaired body weight gain by 15.2% (p<0.005) and significantly resulted in increased liver (p<0.005) and spleen (p<0.005) size compared with SHAM rats (Figure 1). The ratio of spleen weight to body weight, which is a measure of organ size, markedly increased by 1.6-fold (p<0.005) in BDL compared with SHAM rats, indicating the formation of portal hypertension. However, treatment with rapamycin for fourteen days obviously altered not only the growth of the body, but also the organ weights in the BDL-Ra animals (Table 2). Compared with SHAM and BDL animals, SHAM-Ra and BDL-Ra groups reduced body weight gain by 22.5% (p<0.005) and 14.7% (p<0.005) respectively. No significant differences were obtained comparing SHAM rats with SHAM-Ra animals in relative liver weight. However, liver size of BDL rats was clearly higher than that of SHAM (p<0.005) and BDL-Ra (p<0.005) groups. Rapamycin also profoundly ameliorated splenomegaly in BDL-Ra rats (p<0.005). These results demonstrated that rapamycin treatment attenuated the increase in liver and spleen size that typically succeeded BDL.

As the Table 2 showed the hemodynamic parameters were favorably influenced by the rapamycin treatment. MBP was higher in the BDL (P<0.005) than that in SHAM animals but not significantly different between BDL and BDL-Ra groups, which was highest in the SHAM-Ra group. Consistent with splenomegaly, portal pressure was markedly elevated in BDL rats compared with SHAM controls (P<0.005). However, it was decreased by 26.6% (P<0.005) with rapamycin treatment, with no significant difference between SHAM and SHAM-Ra rats. Detailed values were given in Table 2.

Rapamycin Reduces Cholangiocytes Proliferation and ECM Deposition, as Well as Improves Liver Function

The histological detection demonstrated that rapamycin treatment did not affect morphometry in SHAM and SHAM-Ra rats, but significantly attenuated cholangiocytes proliferation as well as the ECM deposition in BDL-Ra rats (Figure 2). Statistics of HE and Masson staining under the same conditions showed that volume fractions of bile ducts and ECM correspondingly decreased by 87.0% (P<0.005) and 82.5% (P<0.005) in BDL-Ra group compared with BDL rats.

Paralleled by an inhibition of the histological changes succeeding BDL, rapamycin also improved liver function greatly (Table 3). We could easily observe a poor liver function in BDL rats. However, treatment with rapamycin distinctly decreased ALT (P<0.005), AST (P<0.005), ALP (P<0.01), TB (P<0.05), and BA (P<0.01) in BDL-Ra group compared with BDL rats, but had little influence on ALB, and CREA, indicating the therapeutic effect of rapamycin on liver function. The data also showed no significant differences in ALP, AST, TB, ALB, and CREA between SHAM and SHAM-Ra animals. But the ALP of SHAM-Ra was higher (P<0.05) and the BA was lower (P<0.05) than those in SHAM.

Rapamycin Reveals Inverse Effects on Fibrosis- and Inflammatory-related mRNA

Multiple pathological processes such as inflammatory infiltration and fibrogenesis are closely involved in the development of hepatic fibrosis. Since AKT/mTOR signaling pathway plays a central role in immunological processes and fibrogenesis [22], we next assessed mTOR signaling molecules, intrahepatic inflammation and fibrosis at transcription level.

RT-PCR results showed that mRNA expressions of the mTOR, P70S6K and 4EBP1 were not significantly different among the four groups and not obviously affected by rapamycin. Our findings however showed that profibrogenic genes such as α-SMA, procollagen α1(I) (PC α1), transforming growth factor beta 1 (TGF β1), platelet-derived growth factor (PDGF), PDGF-receptor beta (PDGFRβ), and tissue inhibitor of metalloproteinase 1 (TIMP-1), as well as the proinflammatory genes tumor necrosis factor alpha (TNF-α) and inducible nitric oxide synthase (iNOS) were significantly upregulated approximately 6.1-, 16.0-, 2.4-, 5.5-, 2.8-, 15.5-, 5.7- and 22.2-fold in the BDL rats respectively compared with the SHAM group (Figure 3). Treatment with rapamycin reduced mRNA expressions of the α-SMA, PC α1, PDGFRβ, TIMP-1, and iNOS by 69.6% (P<0.005), 83.9% (P<0.005), 32.5% (P<0.05), 56.3% (P<0.05) and 73.1% (P<0.05) in the BDL-Ra rats. While genes of PDGF, TGF β1, and TNF-α were not significantly different between BDL and BDL-Ra groups, rapamycin showed a beneficial tendency for downregulating the genes of PDGF and TGF β1 with the exception of TNF-α. In addition, no striking difference was acquired between SHAM and SHAM-Ra groups. Primer sequences information detailed in Table 1.

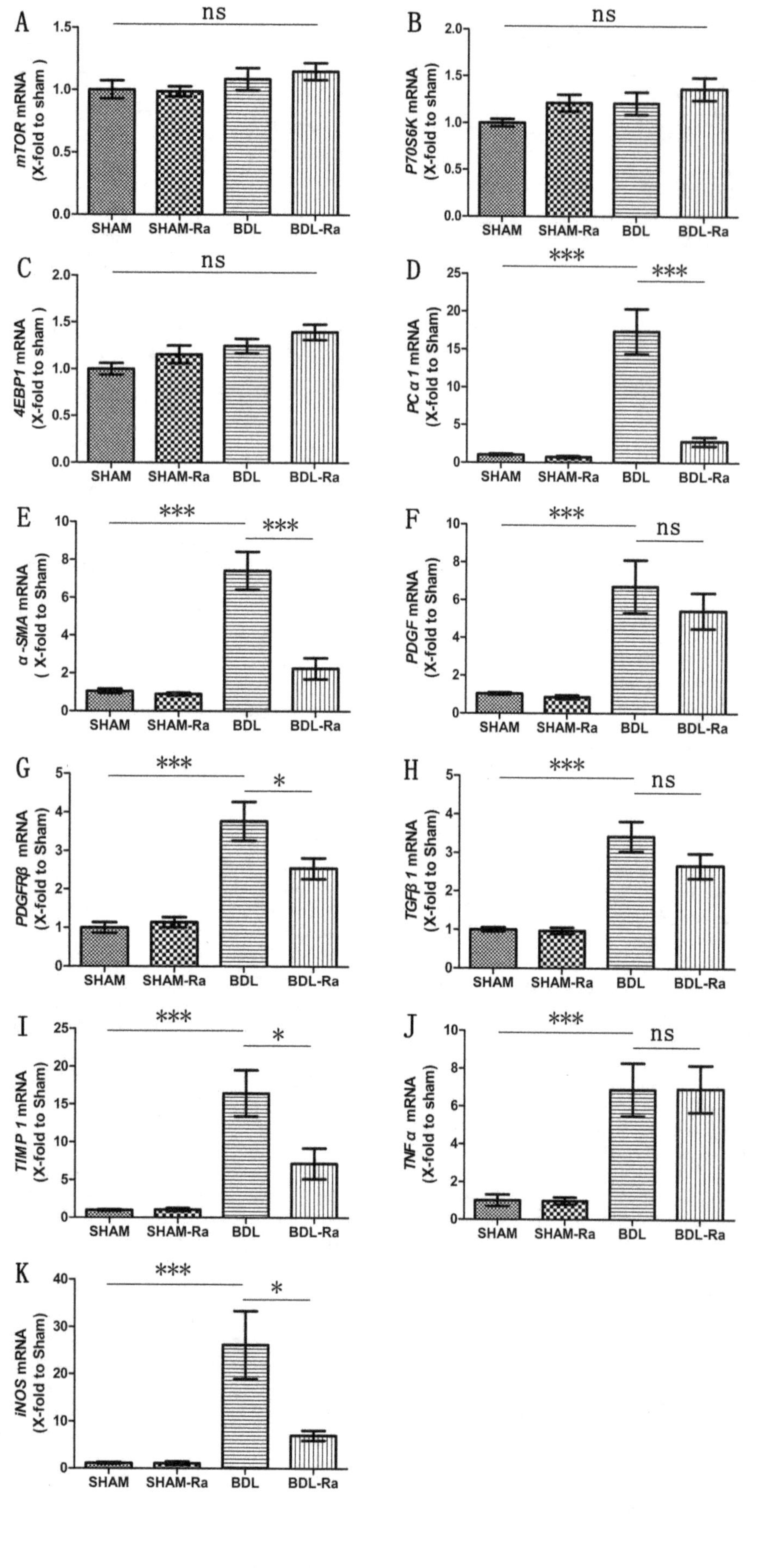
A
mTOR mRNA (X-fold to sham)
B
P70S6K mRNA (X-fold to sham)
C
4EBP1 mRNA (X-fold to sham)
D
PCα1 mRNA (X-fold to Sham)
E
α-SMA mRNA (X-fold to Sham)
F
PDGF mRNA (X-fold to Sham)
G
PDGFRβ mRNA (X-fold to Sham)
H
TGFβ1 mRNA (X-fold to Sham)
I
TIMP1 mRNA (X-fold to Sham)
J
TNFα mRNA (X-fold to sham)
K
iNOS mRNA (X-fold to Sham)
SHAM
SHAM-Ra
BDL
BDL-Ra
ns
***
*

Figure 3. Rapamycin treatment downregulates liver fibrosis- and inflammatory-related genes in BDL-Ra rats. (A) mTOR, (B) P70S6K, (C) 4EBP1, (D) Procollagen (PC) α1(I), (E) α-SMA, (F) PDGF, (G) PDGFRβ, (H) TGF β1, (I) TIMP-1, (J) TNF-α, and (K) iNOS mRNA, measured by fluorescence quantitative PCR and normalized to GAPDH (mean±SEM; *p<0.05; **p<0.01; ***p<0.005; ns - nonsignificant).

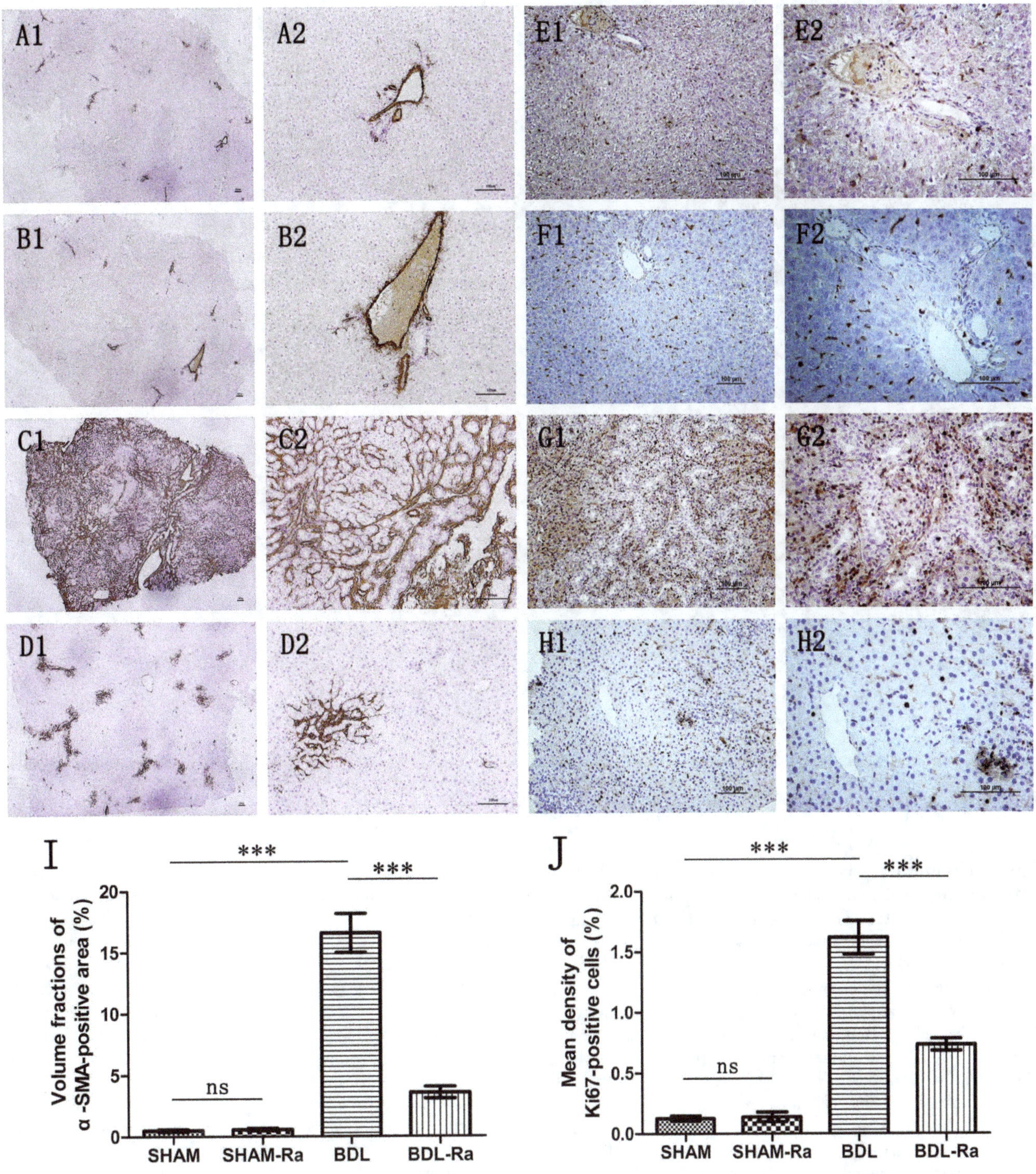

Figure 4. Rapamycin treatment decreases α-SMA and Ki67 expression in livers of BDL-Ra rats. Representative liver microphotographs of (A) SHAM, (B) SHAM-Ra, (C) BDL, and (D) BDL-Ra, following immunohistochemistry staining of α-SMA (magnification 40× and 100×, respectively). Representative liver sections of (E) SHAM, (F) SHAM-Ra, (G) BDL, and (H) BDL-Ra, using anti-ki67 for immunohistochemistry (magnification 100× and 200×, respectively). Graphs (I) and (J): Quantitative analysis of α-SMA- and Ki67-positive cells in representative liver sections respectively (mean±SEM; *p<0.05; **p<0.01; ***p<0.005; ns - nonsignificant).

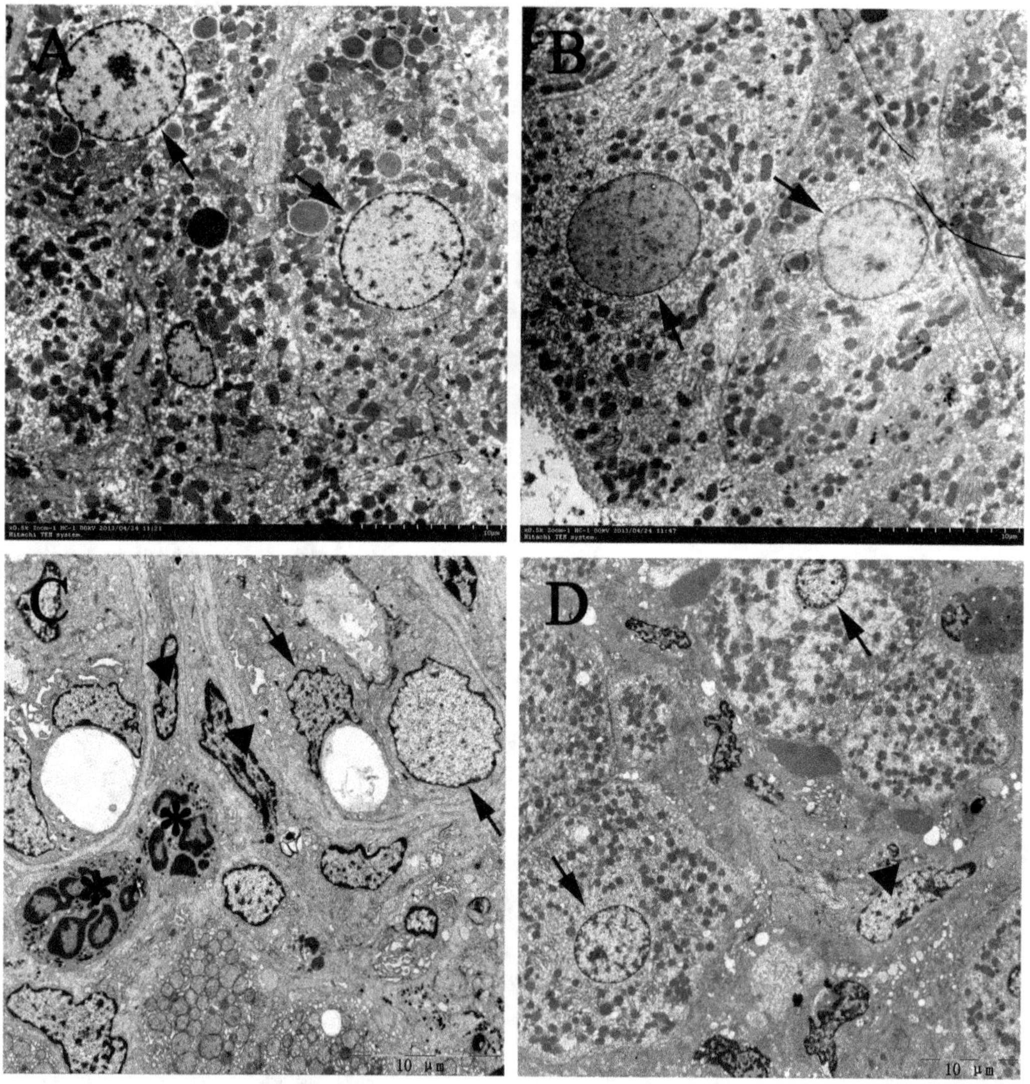

Figure 5. Rapamycin treatment improves the intrahepatic microstructure in BDL-Ra rats, evaluated by transmission electron microscopy (TEM). Representative liver TEM micrographs of (A) SHAM, (B) SHAM-Ra, (C) BDL, (D) BDL-Ra (magnification A, B: 5000×; C, D: 3000×, respectively). Arrow heads point to liver nuclei, triangles represent fibroblasts and asterisks denote neutrophils.

Rapamycin Improves Liver Fibrosis and Inflammation

Along with the biliary ducts hyperplasia, the transdifferentiation and proliferation of HSCs mainly contributed to the development of hepatic fibrosis in cholestatic liver diseases.

Our results showed the expression of Ki67, a nuclear protein expressed only in proliferating cells, was makedly increased in BDL rat livers. Treatment with rapamycin evidently reduced the Ki67-positive cells in BDL-Ra rats, indicating the suppression of intrahepatic cell proliferation by rapamycin (Figure 4). α-SMA is commonly used as a marker of activated HSCs [3,6–8]. We next found that α-SMA-positive cells appeared around the proliferative bile ducts, which increased significantly in livers of BDL compared with those of SHAM groups. More importantly, bile ducts proliferation as well as numbers of periductular α-SMA-positive cells were significantly reduced by rapamycin (Figure 4), which was consistent with our Masson staining.

Moreover, enhanced inflammation plays an important role in early stage of cholestatic liver injury and always aggravates the fibrogenesis processes [1,24]. Our electron microscopy results showed no significant differences between SHAM and SHAM-Ra. The hepatocytes had intact structure, and seemed nearly normal in cytoplasm and interstitial. In contrast, the shape of the hepatocyte nuclei became irregular, and some even appeared pyknotic in the BDL group. The mitochondria partly disappeared in damaged hepatic cytoplasm, with vacuolar degeneration visible occasionally. Furthermore, the structure of hepatic interstitial was disordered, where bile duct endothelial cells, fibroblasts, macrophages, lymphocytes and neutrophils obviously increased. The normal structure of sinusoidal endothelial fenestrae also disappeared. However, treatment with rapamycin reduced the amount of intrahepatic neutrophils, lymphocytes, fibroblasts and ECM, as well as hepatocellular injury (Figure 5).

IL-1β is one of proinflammatory cytokines thought to be involved in many acute and chronic diseases [25,26]. It is produced by a variety of cells, including macrophages, monocytes, and keratinocytes [27]. IL-1β activity is tightly controlled and requires the conversion of the primary transcript, the inactive IL-1β precursor, to the active mature IL-1β by limited proteolysis.

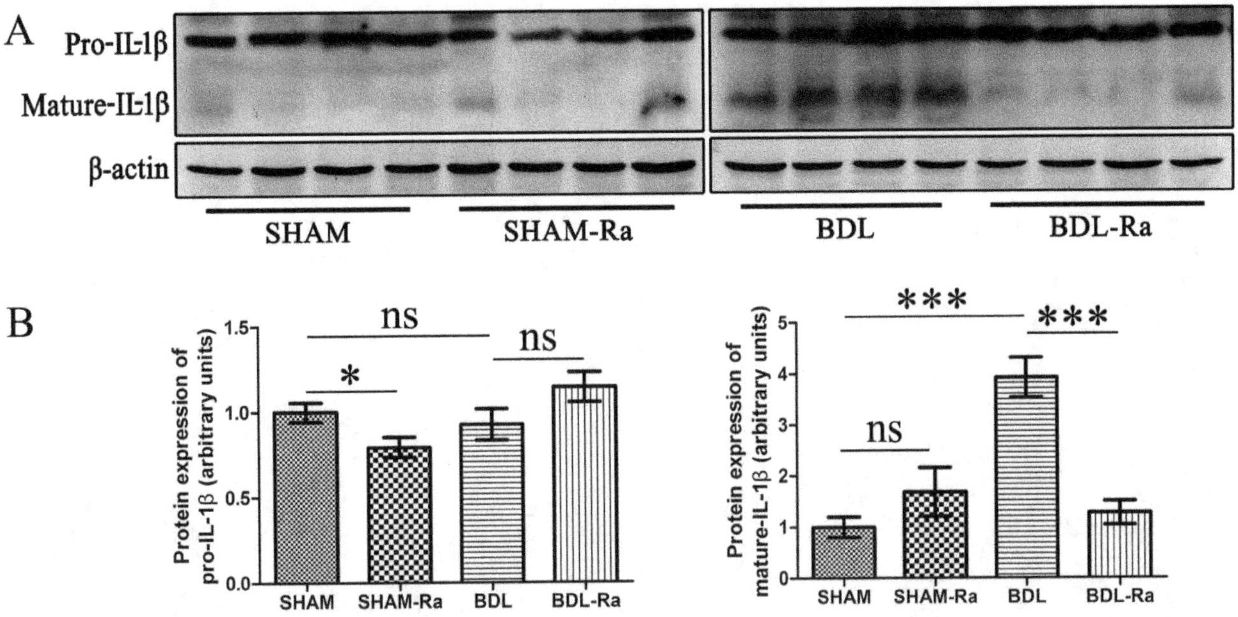

Figure 6. Rapamycin treatment attenuates intrahepatic inflammation in BDL-Ra rats. Representative western blot (A) and densitometric analyses (B) for precursor- and mature-IL-1β expressions in rat livers respectively (mean±SEM; *$p<0.05$; **$p<0.01$; ***$p<0.005$; ns - nonsignificant).

Our western blot result suggested that while the IL-1β precursor expression was not significantly different between BDL and BDL-Ra groups, the mature IL-1β evidently increased in BDL livers, indicating inflammation was involved in the pathophysiological onset and being consistent with the neutrophil infiltration showed by electron microscopy. Rapamycin might suppress the tranformation from IL-1β precursor to mature IL-1β and then markedly decreased mature IL-1β (Figure 6).

Taken together, these results indicated that the molecular basis for the rapamycin induced improvement in BDL-Ra rats involved reduction of HSCs and cholangiocytes proliferation, as well as the blockade of inflammatory process at least in part.

The Role of AKT/mTOR Signaling Pathway in the Early Phase of Cirrhotic Portal Hypertension

AKT is an important upstream mediator of mTOR and also regulated by mTORC2 [2]. We detected, using the western blot technique, a significant upregulation of the p-AKT Ser473 and Thr308 to total protein in the livers of BDL rats compared with SHAM animals (Figure 7A). The levels of the immediate downstream target proteins p-mTOR, p-P70S6K and p-S6 to their total proteins were also higher in the livers from BDL rats than those from SHAM animals (Figure 7BCD). Moreover, our results suggested that the expressions of AKT and mTOR were also increased, with the exception of P70S6K and S6. Taken these results together, we firstly demonstrated that AKT/mTOR signaling pathway was significantly overactivated and might be involved in the early pathogenesis of cirrhotic portal hypertensive rats.

To gauge the impact of targeting mTOR pathway on liver fibrosis and portal hypertension induced by BDL, we treated BDL rats with the mTOR inhibitor rapamycin for two weeks. Chronic rapamycin treatment efficiently downregulated the mTOR signaling pathway in the livers of BDL-Ra rats, as showed by the downward trend of p-mTOR and the significant reduction of p-P70S6K and p-S6 to their total proteins compared with BDL rats (Figure 7BCD). Similarly, the mTOR signaling pathway in SHAM-Ra rats was also evidently inhibited by rapamycin compared with SHAM group (Figure 7CD). In addition, we found no significant differences in the relative expressions of p-AKT (Ser473) and p-AKT (Thr308) between SHAM and SHAM-Ra group. However, the relative expression of p-AKT Thr308 in BDL-Ra rats was decreased compared with BDL group (Figure 7A). In contrast, the expression of p-AKT (Ser473) to AKT in BDL-Ra was much higher than that in BDL groups. Besides, rapamycin had little effects on the expressions of mTOR, P70S6K, and S6 compared with SHAM and BDL groups respectively, as well as on the expression of AKT between SHAM and SHAM-Ra groups. While rapamycin significantly reduced the expression of AKT compared with BDL group, the level of AKT in BDL-Ra rats was still much higher than that in SHAM group.

Rapamycin has no Evident Effect on the Level of p-ERK1/2 to ERK1/2

Many investigations suggested that there existed a cross talk between mitogen-activated protein kinase (MAPK)/extracellular signal-regulated kinase (ERK) and PI3K/mTOR pathways to co-regulate the proliferation and survival of the hepatocytes [20,28–31], cholangiocytes [20,32,33] and HSCs [11,15,20,34]. We also detected the expressions of p-ERK1/2 and ERK1/2 by western blot technique. We found that both the expressions of p-ERK1/2 and ERK1/2 increased in BDL rats, and rapamycin markedly decreased the expression of ERK1/2 in BDL-Ra rats, with the exception of p-ERK1/2.

Moreover, the level of p-ERK1/2 to ERK1/2 in BDL rats was significantly higher than in SHAM animals (Figure 8), indicating that MAPK/ERK cascade was manifestly overactivated. However, treatment with rapamycin had no obvious effect on the expression of p-ERK1/2 to ERK1/2 compared with their controls respectively. Based on the therapeutic action of rapamycin, these data implied that AKT/mTOR singnaling did play a vital role in the formation of hepatic fibrosis and portal hypertension induced by BDL from another perspective.

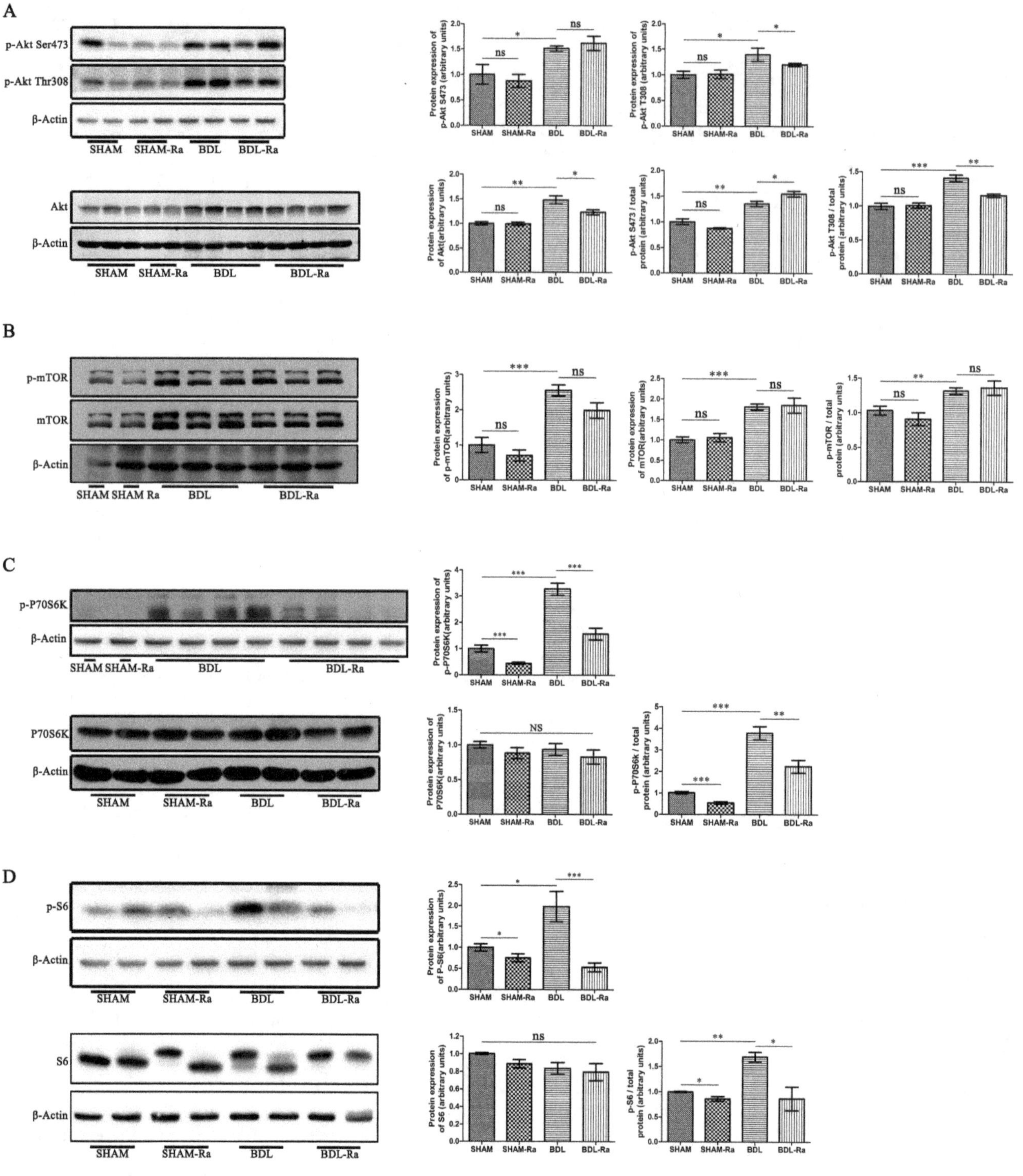

Figure 7. Rapamycin treatment blocks mTORC1 but not mTORC2 in rat livers. Representative immunoblot and densitometric analyses of hepatic (A) p-AKT and AKT, (B) p-mTOR and mTOR, (C) p-P70S6K and P70S6K, and (D) p-S6 and S6 in rat livers respectively (mean±SEM; $^{*}p<0.05$; $^{**}p<0.01$; $^{***}p<0.005$; ns - nonsignificant).

Discussion

Liver cirrhosis is the endpoint of the fibrogenic process in which inflammation and fibrogenesis are closely integrated [1]. Several studies have established a role for mTOR as an attractive target for portal hypertension and antifibrotic therapy [5–7,19,22,35]. However, comprehensive and in-depth researches on the AKT/mTOR signaling pathway in cirrhotic portal hypertension have rarely been reported, especially ones on the early phase of this disease. In this study an early cirrhotic portal hypertensive rat model was successfully established at three weeks after BDL, when portal vein pressure and spleen size were significantly increased

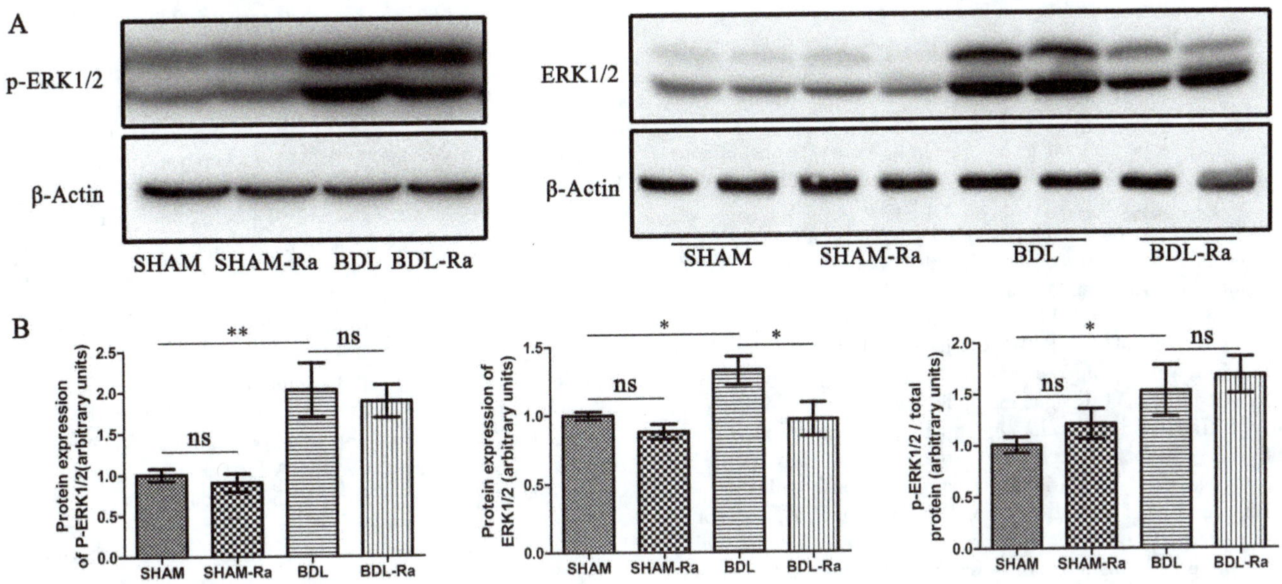

Figure 8. Rapamycin treatment has no evident effect on p-ERK1/2 expression in rat livers. Representative western blot (A) and densitometric analyses (B) of p-ERK1/2 and ERK1/2 in rat livers respectively (mean±SEM; $^*p<0.05$; $^{**}p<0.01$; $^{***}p<0.005$; ns - nonsignificant).

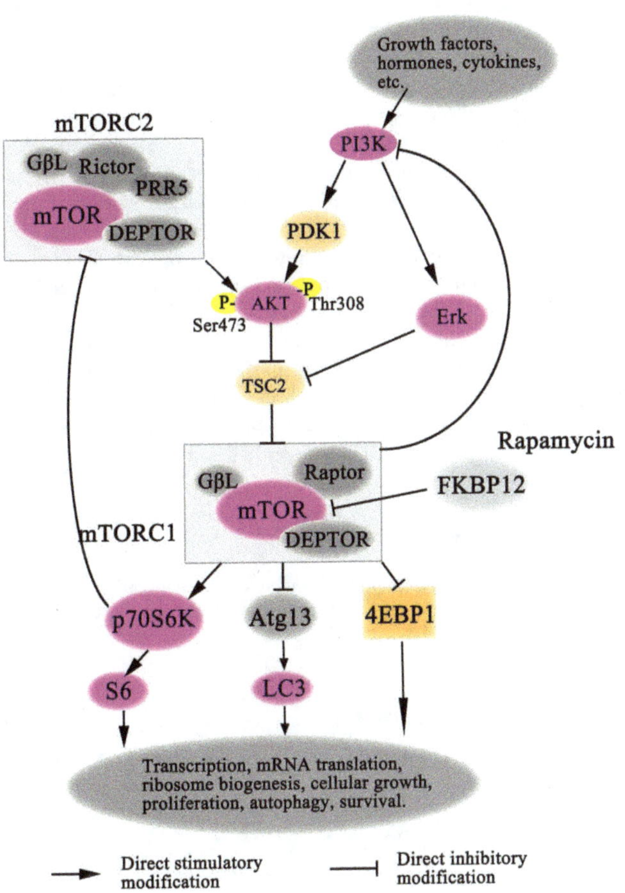

Figure 9. PI3K/AKT/mTOR signaling pathway. Rapamycin bound to FKBP12 mainly blocked the activity of mTORC1.

but intrahepatic nodules and fiber spacing had not yet formed (Figure 2). We extensively evaluated the early pathological processes and systematically explored AKT/mTOR signaling pathway in the early phase of cirrhotic portal hypertension.

The present study suggested that HSCs transdifferentiation, cholangiocytes proliferation and inflammatory infiltration mainly contributed to the development of hepatic fibrosis and portal hypertension in cholestatic liver fibrosis. HSCs play a crucial role in the process of hepatic fibrosis, as they are responsible for excessive deposition of ECM proteins [11,15], amplification of inflammatory response by inducing infiltration of mono- and polymorphonuclear leukocytes [4], as well as increase in intrahepatic resistance [36], which is consistent with our Masson-staining result and the elevated portal pressure in BDL rats. Morphological change with HSCs activation is evident in appearance of the cytoskeletal protein α-SMA [3,6–8]. Our RT-PCR and immunohistochemical detections consistently demonstrated a high expression of α-SMA in BDL rats, indicating the activation and proliferation of HSCs. In this regard, we even intuitively witnessed the fibroblasts transformed from HSCs and collagen fiber structure in the liver interstitial using electron microscopy. HE-staining and electron microscopy also showed a large number of proliferative cholangiocytes and infiltration of neutrophils in BDL rats.

PDGF and TGFβ1 are the most potent mitogen and stimulus for HSCs to produce ECM proteins respectively [5,37]. The former is not only secreted in an autocrine fashion by HSCs but also synthesized by cholangiocytes during cholestasis. The latter is derived from both paracrine and autocrine sources of HSCs [5]. TIMP1, a tissue inhibitor of metalloproteinases, is a natural inhibitor of the matrix metalloproteinases (MMPs), a group of peptidases involved in degradation of the extracellular matrix. We demonstrated a significant up-regulation of the powerful profibrogenesis genes PDGF, PDGFRβ, TGF-β1, PC-α1 and TIMP1, as well as pro-inflammatory genes TNF-α and iNOS in the liver of cirrhotic portal hypertensive rats. Moreover, the western blot result of IL-1β further suggested an enhanced inflammation during the development of hepatic fibrosis. Treatment with rapamycin effectively ameliorated these pathological processes as well as improved liver function and portal pressure, implying that AKT/mTOR signaling pathway contributed to the early pathology of cirrhotic portal hypertension, consistent with the studies conducted by Reif on HSCs culture and by Neef on the established cirrhotic rat models [3,6].

In order to better explain our research, we based on previous studies to draw a schematic diagram of AKT/mTOR signaling pathway in Figure 9 [9,12–14]. To our knowledge, we for the first time demonstrated that the AKT/mTOR signaling pathway was significantly overactivated and mTORC1 rather than mTORC2 was inhibited by rapamycin in the early phase of cirrhotic portal hypertension in rats (Figure 9). We evaluated the mRNA expressions of mTOR, P70S6K and 4EBP1, but no significant differences were obtained from all of the four groups. These results suggestted that mTOR signaling molecules had no obvious change at the transcription level, and rapamycin showed no evident influence on their mRNA expressions in the early phase of cirrhotic portal hypertension. Afterwards, we consistently detected the expressions of p-AKT (Ser473/Thr308), p-mTOR, p-P70S6K and p-S6 relative to their total proteins in BDL rats, all of which were profoundly higher than those in SHAM rats, indicating the activation of AKT/mTOR signaling pathway. However, treatment with rapamycin significantly inhibited the expressions of p-P70S6K and p-S6 but not p-AKT (Ser473) to their total proteins in BDL-Ra rats. Since p-P70S6K and p-AKT (Ser473) are the direct downstream effectors of mTORC1 and mTORC2 respectively (Figure 9), it indirectly proved that rapamycin blocked mTORC1 but not mTORC2, which was consistent with the researches of Sarbassov and Feldman [2,17]. Whereas, investigations in vitro suggested rapamycin treatment for more than 24 h might also inhibit mTORC2 assembly to suppress AKT/PKB (Ser473) phosphorylation in certain cell lines [38]. In our study, however, the relative expressions of p-mTOR and p-AKT (Ser473) were still much higher in BDL-Ra livers than those in SHAM. These results suggested treatment with rapamycin (2 mg/kg/day) for two weeks did not block mTORC2 assembly, nor did it reduce the levels of mTORC2 below those needed to maintain AKT/PKB signaling in this pathophysiologic progress of cirrhotic portal hypertension.

While mTOR activation is a downstream effector of AKT, mTORC1 reciprocally regulates the growth-factor responsiveness of PI3K and AKT through feedback inhibition (Figure 9) [39,40]. As is known, AKT/PKB activation requires the phosphorylation of Thr308 and Ser473 [2]. Our data showed that the relative expressions of p-AKT (Thr308) and p-AKT (Ser473) were still much higher in BDL-Ra rats than those in SHAM group. Thus it was possible that inhibition of mTOR and P70S6K by rapamycin partly induced AKT Ser473 and Thr308 phosphorylation in BDL-Ra rats by feedback (Figure 9).

On the other hand, the MAPK/ERK signaling cascade, which belongs to the mitogen activated protein kinases (MAPKs) family, is another major player in the mitogenic and antiapoptotic response in many cells [16,20,41]. Existing researches show that MAPK/ERK and AKT/mTOR signaling pathways are colsely related in cholestatic liver injury [20,41]. They are two parallel regulatory pathways to control cell survival, differentiation, proliferation, metabolism, and motility in response to extracellular cues [42]. However there also exists an important cross-talk, in which ERK modulated mTOR signaling through phosphorylation and inactivation of tuberous sclerosis complex 2 (TSC2) (Figure 9) [43].

Our study clearly showed that both AKT/mTOR (Figure 7) and ERK1/2 (Figure 8) signaling cascade were profoundly overactivated in livers of early cholestatic fibrosis, indicating both of them were closely involved in the formation of this disease. However, we found that treatment with rapamycin had no obvious influence on the expression of p-ERK1/2 to ERK1/2, but distinctly inhibited the expressions of p-P70S6K and p-S6 to their total proteins. The expression of p-mTOR to mTOR in BDL-Ra rats was still significantly higher than that in SHAM animals (Figure 9). Therefore, it was also possible that the high expression of p-ERK1/2 to ERK1/2 might stimulate the activation of mTOR to partly antagonize the inhibitory effect of rapamycin in this disease. Collectively, these data indicated that MAPK/ERK and AKT/mTOR signaling pathways might participate in the disease in a collaborative manner. A further investigation with a single or joint specific inhibition of the two pathways is needed to explore the exact mechanisms.

Another finding of the present study was that rapamycin markedly decreased the body weight in both SHAM-Ra and BDL-Ra rats compared with their controls. mTOR pathway mainly regulates protein synthesis, transcription, cell growth, cell proliferation, cell motility, and cell survival in almost all the cells [9,12–14]. Thus mTOR blockade by rapamycin may slow down the normal growth of rats. Other study also described weight loss of rats caused by rapamycin at a low dosage 0.2 mg/kg/d [44]. Therefore, it was not surprising to find the similar phenomenon in our study. Despite the loss in body weight, all the rats in SHAM-Ra group seemed healthy. Moreover, rapamycin is a FDA–approved immunosuppressive drug to inhibit transplant rejection in clinical application. Therefore, rapamycin should be a safe and stable drug in this study.

In conclusion, this study demonstrated that the activation of AKT/mTOR signaling pathway was clearly involved in the pathophysiological onset of early cirrhotic portal hypertension in rats. Early treatment with rapamycin did effectively ameliorate intrahepatic inflammation and fibrosis, improve liver function, decrease splenomegaly and portal pressure, as well as reduce the expressions of p-AKT T308, p-P70S6K and p-S6 relative to their total proteins. These evidences indicated the essential role of AKT/mTOR signaling pathway in the early pathophysiologic progress. The supression of p-P70S6K and p-S6 but not p-AKT S473 to their total proteins by rapamycin indirectly confirmed that it mainly inhibited mTORC1 rather than mTORC2 in the early phase of cirrhotic portal hypertension.

Acknowledgments

We are grateful to Pfizer Inc (USA) for their kindly donation of rapamycin. We thank Dr. Gele Li for the technical guidance in the animal experiments. We also thank Dr. Yaofei Pei and Xiqiang Liu for friendly help in molecular biology experiments.

Author Contributions

Conceived and designed the experiments: JY WW. Performed the experiments: WW HW MS. Analyzed the data: JY WW. Contributed reagents/materials/analysis tools: JY MZ. Wrote the paper: JY WW. Revised the manuscript: WY CP HL.

References

1. Tugues S, Fernandez-Varo G, Muñoz-Luque J, Ros J, Arroyo V, et al. (2007) Antiangiogenic treatment with sunitinib ameliorates inflammatory infiltrate, fibrosis, and portal pressure in cirrhotic rats. Hepatology 46: 1919–1926.
2. Sarbassov DD, Guertin DA, Ali SM, Sabatini DM (2005) Phosphorylation and regulation of Akt/PKB by the rictor-mTOR complex. Sci Signal 307: 1098–1101.

3. Reif S (2002) The role of focal adhesion kinase-phosphatidylinositol 3-kinase-Akt signaling in hepatic stellate cell proliferation and type I collagen expression. J Biol Chem 278: 8083–8090.
4. Mehal WZ, Friedman SL (2007) The role of inflammation and immunity in the pathogenesis of liver fibrosis. Liver Immunology: Principles and Practice 9: 111–121.
5. Biecker E (2005) Long-term treatment of bile duct-ligated rats with rapamycin (sirolimus) significantly attenuates liver fibrosis: analysis of the underlying mechanisms. J Pharmacol Exp Ther 313: 952–961.
6. Neef M, Ledermann M, Saegesser H, Schneider V, Reichen J (2006) Low-dose oral rapamycin treatment reduces fibrogenesis, improves liver function, and prolongs survival in rats with established liver cirrhosis. J Hepatol 45: 786–796.
7. Patsenker E, Schneider V, Ledermann M, Saegesser H, Dorn C, et al. (2011) Potent antifibrotic activity of mTOR inhibitors sirolimus and everolimus but not of cyclosporine A and tacrolimus in experimental liver fibrosis. J Hepatol 55: 388–398.
8. Bridle KR, Popa C, Morgan ML, Sobbe AL, Clouston AD, et al. (2009) Rapamycin inhibits hepatic fibrosis in rats by attenuating multiple profibrogenic pathways. Liver Transplant 15: 1315–1324.
9. Hay N, Sonenberg N (2004) Upstream and downstream of mTOR. Gene Dev 18: 1926–1945.
10. Inoki K, Guan K-L (2006) Complexity of the TOR signaling network. Trends Cell Biol 16: 206–212.
11. Shegogue D, Trojanowska M (2004) Mammalian target of rapamycin positively regulates collagen type I production via a phosphatidylinositol 3-kinase-independent pathway. J Biol Chem 279: 23166–23175.
12. Yang Q, Guan KL (2007) Expanding mTOR signaling. Cell Res 17: 666–681.
13. Schmelzle T, Hall MN (2000) TOR, a central controller of cell growth. Cell 103: 253–262.
14. Sarbassov DD, Ali SM, Sabatini DM (2005) Growing roles for the mTOR pathway. Curr Opin Cell Biol 17: 596–603.
15. Gabele E (2005) The role of P70S6K in hepatic stellate cell collagen gene expression and cell proliferation. J Biol Chem 280: 13374–13382.
16. Gabele E, Brenner DA, Rippe RA (2003) Liver fibrosis: signals leading to the amplification of the fibrogenic hepatic stellate cell. Front Biosci 8: d69–d77.
17. Feldman ME, Apsel B, Uotila A, Loewith R, Knight ZA, et al. (2009) Active-site inhibitors of mTOR target rapamycin-resistant outputs of mTORC1 and mTORC2. PloS Biol 7: 0371–0383.
18. Choo AY, Yoon SO, Kim SG, Roux PP, Blenis J (2008) Rapamycin differentially inhibits S6Ks and 4E-BP1 to mediate cell-type-specific repression of mRNA translation. P Natl Acad Sci USA 105: 17414–17419.
19. Geerts AM, Vanheule E, Van Vlierberghe H, Leybaert L, Van Steenkiste C, et al. (2008) Rapamycin prevents mesenteric neo-angiogenesis and reduces splanchnic blood flow in portal hypertensive mice. Hepatol Res 38: 1130–1139.
20. Svegliati-Baroni G, Ridolfi F, Caradonna Z, Alvaro D, Marzioni M, et al. (2003) Regulation of ERK/JNK/P70S6K in two rat models of liver injury and fibrosis. J Hepatol 39: 528–537.
21. Wang Y, Jiang XY, Liu L, Jiang HQ (2008) Phosphatidylinositol 3-kinase/Akt pathway regulates hepatic stellate cell apoptosis. World J Gastroentero 14: 5186–5191.
22. Mejias M, Garcia-Pras E, Gallego J, Mendez R, Bosch J, et al. (2010) Relevance of the mTOR signaling pathway in the pathophysiology of splenomegaly in rats with chronic portal hypertension. J Hepatol 52: 529–539.
23. Fernandez M, Mejias M, Garcia-Pras E, Mendez R, Garcia-Pagan JC, et al. (2007) Reversal of portal hypertension and hyperdynamic splanchnic circulation by combined vascular endothelial growth factor and platelet-derived growth factor blockade in rats. Hepatology 46: 1208–1217.
24. Gujral JS, Farhood A, Bajt ML, Jaeschke H (2003) Neutrophils aggravate acute liver injury during obstructive cholestasis in bile duct-ligated mice. Hepatology 38: 355–363.
25. Kolb M, Margetts PJ, Anthony DC, Pitossi F, Gauldie J (2001) Transient expression of IL-1β induces acute lung injury and chronic repair leading to pulmonary fibrosis. J Clin Invest 107: 1529–1536.
26. Girón-González JA, Martínez-Sierra C, Rodriguez-Ramos C, Macias MA, Rendon P, et al. (2004) Implication of inflammation-related cytokines in the natural history of liver cirrhosis. Liver Int 24: 437–445.
27. Lee DF, Hung MC (2007) All roads lead to mTOR: integrating inflammation and tumor angiogenesis. Cell Cycle 6: 3011–3014.
28. Rao YP, Studer EJ, Stravitz RT, Gupta S, Qiao L, et al. (2003) Activation of the Raf-1/MEK/ERK cascade by bile acids occurs via the epidermal growth factor receptor in primary rat hepatocytes. Hepatology 35: 307–314.
29. Qiao L, Yacoub A, Studer E, Gupta S, Pei XY, et al. (2003) Inhibition of the MAPK and PI3K pathways enhances UDCA-induced apoptosis in primary rodent hepatocytes. Hepatology 35: 779–789.
30. Schoemaker MH, Conde de la Rosa L, Buist-Homan M, Vrenken TE, Havinga R, et al. (2004) Tauroursodeoxycholic acid protects rat hepatocytes from bile acid-induced apoptosis via activation of survival pathways. Hepatology 39: 1563–1573.
31. Dixon M, Agius L, Yeaman SJ, Day CP (2003) Inhibition of rat hepatocyte proliferation by transforming growth factor β and glucagon is associated with inhibition of ERK2 and p70S6 kinase. Hepatology 29: 1418–1424.
32. Alvaro D, Onori P, Metalli VD, Svegliati-Baroni G, Folli F, et al. (2003) Intracellular pathways mediating estrogen-induced cholangiocyte proliferation in the rat. Hepatology 36: 297–304.
33. Werneburg NW, Yoon JH, Higuchi H, Gores GJ (2003) Bile acids activate EGF receptor via a TGF-α-dependent mechanism in human cholangiocyte cell lines. Am J Physiol-Gastr L 285: G31-G36.
34. Svegliati-Baroni G, Ridolfi F, Hannivoort R, Saccomanno S, Homan M, et al. (2005) Bile acids induce hepatic stellate cell proliferation via activation of the epidermal growth factor receptor. Gastroenterology 128: 1042–1055.
35. Chen G, Chen H, Wang C, Peng Y, Sun L, et al. (2012) Rapamycin ameliorates kidney fibrosis by inhibiting the activation of mTOR signaling in interstitial macrophages and myofibroblasts. PloS One 7: 1–14.
36. Cichoż-lach H, Celiński K, Słomka M, Kasztelan-Szczerbińska B (2008) Pathophysiology of portal hypertension. J Physiol Pharmacol 59: 231–238.
37. Friedman SL (2008) Hepatic fibrosis-overview. Toxicology 254: 120–129.
38. Sarbassov DD, Ali SM, Sengupta S, Sheen JH, Hsu PP, et al. (2006) Prolonged rapamycin treatment inhibits mTORC2 assembly and Akt/PKB. Mol cell 22: 159–168.
39. O'Reilly KE, Rojo F, She Q-B, Solit D, Mills GB, et al. (2006) mTOR inhibition induces upstream receptor tyrosine kinase signaling and activates Akt. Cancer Res 66: 1500–1508.
40. Zhang HH, Lipovsky AI, Dibble CC, Sahin M, Manning BD (2006) S6K1 regulates GSK3 under conditions of mTOR-dependent feedback inhibition of Akt. Mol cell 24: 185–197.
41. Coutant A, Rescan C, Gilot D, Loyer P, Guguen-Guillouzo C, et al. (2003) PI3K-FRAP/mTOR pathway is critical for hepatocyte proliferation whereas MEK/ERK supports both proliferation and survival. Hepatology 36: 1079–1088.
42. Mendoza MC, Er EE, Blenis J (2011) The Ras-ERK and PI3K-mTOR pathways: cross-talk and compensation. Trends Biochem Sci 36: 320–328.
43. Ma L, Chen Z, Erdjument-Bromage H, Tempst P, Pandolfi PP (2005) Phosphorylation and functional inactivation of TSC2 by Erk: implications for tuberous sclerosisand cancer pathogenesis. Cell 121: 179–193.
44. Tao Y, Kim J, Schrier RW, Edelstein CL (2005) Rapamycin markedly slows disease progression in a rat model of polycystic kidney disease. J Am Soc Nephrol 16: 46–51.

Permissions

All chapters in this book were first published in PLOS ONE, by The Public Library of Science; hereby published with permission under the Creative Commons Attribution License or equivalent. Every chapter published in this book has been scrutinized by our experts. Their significance has been extensively debated. The topics covered herein carry significant findings which will fuel the growth of the discipline. They may even be implemented as practical applications or may be referred to as a beginning point for another development.

The contributors of this book come from diverse backgrounds, making this book a truly international effort. This book will bring forth new frontiers with its revolutionizing research information and detailed analysis of the nascent developments around the world.

We would like to thank all the contributing authors for lending their expertise to make the book truly unique. They have played a crucial role in the development of this book. Without their invaluable contributions this book wouldn't have been possible. They have made vital efforts to compile up to date information on the varied aspects of this subject to make this book a valuable addition to the collection of many professionals and students.

This book was conceptualized with the vision of imparting up-to-date information and advanced data in this field. To ensure the same, a matchless editorial board was set up. Every individual on the board went through rigorous rounds of assessment to prove their worth. After which they invested a large part of their time researching and compiling the most relevant data for our readers.

The editorial board has been involved in producing this book since its inception. They have spent rigorous hours researching and exploring the diverse topics which have resulted in the successful publishing of this book. They have passed on their knowledge of decades through this book. To expedite this challenging task, the publisher supported the team at every step. A small team of assistant editors was also appointed to further simplify the editing procedure and attain best results for the readers.

Apart from the editorial board, the designing team has also invested a significant amount of their time in understanding the subject and creating the most relevant covers. They scrutinized every image to scout for the most suitable representation of the subject and create an appropriate cover for the book.

The publishing team has been an ardent support to the editorial, designing and production team. Their endless efforts to recruit the best for this project, has resulted in the accomplishment of this book. They are a veteran in the field of academics and their pool of knowledge is as vast as their experience in printing. Their expertise and guidance has proved useful at every step. Their uncompromising quality standards have made this book an exceptional effort. Their encouragement from time to time has been an inspiration for everyone.

The publisher and the editorial board hope that this book will prove to be a valuable piece of knowledge for researchers, students, practitioners and scholars across the globe.

List of Contributors

Kyu Sik Jung, Ji Hong Kim and Do Chang Moon and In Ji Song
Department of Internal Medicine, Yonsei University College of Medicine, Seoul, Korea

Seung Up Kim, Beom Kyung Kim, Jun Yong Park, Do Young Kim, Sang Hoon Ahn and Kwang-Hyub Han
Department of Internal Medicine, Yonsei University College of Medicine, Seoul, Korea
Institute of Gastroenterology, Yonsei University College of Medicine, Seoul, Korea
Liver Cancer Special Clinic, Yonsei University College of Medicine, Seoul, Korea
Liver Cirrhosis Clinical Research Center, Seoul, Korea

Kijun Song
Department of Biostatistics, Yonsei University College of Medicine, Seoul, Korea

Gi Hong Choi
Department of Surgery, Yonsei University College of Medicine, Seoul, Korea

Young Nyun Park
Department of Pathology, Yonsei University College of Medicine, Seoul, Korea

Stéphanie Bonnafous
INSERM, U1065, Equipe 8 Complications hépatiques de l'obésité, Nice, France
Centre Hospitalier Universitaire de Nice, Hôpital de l'Archet, Département Digestif, Nice, France

Stéphanie Patouraux and Marie-Christine Saint-Paul
INSERM, U1065, Equipe 8 Complications hépatiques de l'obésité, Nice, France
Université de Nice-Sophia Antipolis, Faculté de Médecine, Nice, France
Centre Hospitalier Universitaire de Nice, Hôpital de l'Archet, Département de Biologie, Nice, France

Rodolphe Anty, Yannick Le Marchand-Brustel, Albert Tran and Philippe Gual
INSERM, U1065, Equipe 8 Complications hépatiques de l'obésité, Nice, France
Université de Nice-Sophia Antipolis, Faculté de Médecine, Nice, France
Centre Hospitalier Universitaire de Nice, Hôpital de l'Archet, Département Digestif, Nice, France

Cosmin S. Voican
INSERM, U996, IPSIT, Clamart, France
Univ. Paris-Sud, Faculté de Médecine Paris-Sud, Kremlin-Bicêtre, France
Universitatea de Medicina si Farmacie Craiova, Craiova, Romania

Micheline Njike, Nadége Barri-Ova, Gabriel Perlemuter, Hélène Agostini and Sylvie Naveau
INSERM, U996, IPSIT, Clamart, France
Univ. Paris-Sud, Faculté de Médecine Paris-Sud, Kremlin-Bicêtre, France
AP-HP, Hôpital Antoine Béclère, Service d'hépato-gastroentérologie, Clamart, France

Maria-Alessandra Rosenthal-Allieri
Centre Hospitalier Universitaire de Nice, Hôpital de l'Archet, Département d'Immunologie, Nice, France

Pascal Veillon and Paul Calès
Centre Hospitalier Universitaire d'Angers, Service d'Hépatologie, Angers, France

Yue-Jin Liang, Jie Luo, Quan Yuan, Dan Zheng, Ya-Ping Liu, Lei Shi, Ying Zhou, Ai-Ling Chen, Yan Sun, Yong Wang and Zhao-Song Zhang
Department of Pathogen Biology, Key Laboratory of Pathogen Biology of Jiangsu Province, Nanjing Medical University, Nanjing, Jiangsu, China

Yong-Ya Ren
Department of Pathology, Nanjing Medical University, Nanjing, Jiangsu, China

Ke-Yi Sun
Department of Microbiology and Immunology, Nanjing Medical University, Nanjing, Jiangsu, China

Jia-bo Wang, Yan-ling Zhao, Cheng Jin, Dao-jian Liu, Hong-juan Wang and Xiao-he Xiao
Integrative Medicine Center, 302 Military Hospital, Beijing, People's Republic of China

Hai-ping Zhao
Integrative Medicine Center, 302 Military Hospital, Beijing, People's Republic of China
Key Laboratory of Modern Preparation of Traditional Chinese Medicine, Ministry of Education, Jiangxi University of Traditional Chinese Medicine, Nanchang, People's Republic of China

Wei-jun Kong, Fang, Fang and Lin Zhang
Integrative Medicine Center, 302 Military Hospital, Beijing, People's Republic of China
Chengdu University of Traditional Chinese Medicine, Chengdu, People's Republic of China'

Shuji Sumie, Ryoko Kuromatsu, Akio Takata, Masahito Nakano, Manabu Satani, Shingo Yamada and Takashi Niizeki
Division of Gastroenterology, Department of Medicine, Kurume University School of Medicine, Kurume, Japan

Takumi Kawaguchi and Michio Sata
Division of Gastroenterology, Department of Medicine, Kurume University School of Medicine, Kurume, Japan
Department of Digestive Disease Information and Research, Kurume University School of Medicine, Kurume, Japan

Takuji Torimura
Liver Cancer Research Division, Research Center for Innovative Cancer Therapy, Kurume University, Kurume, Japan

Susan S. Baker, Robert D. Baker, Wensheng Liu and Lixin Zhu
Digestive Diseases and Nutrition Center, Department of Pediatrics, The State University of New York, Buffalo, New York, United States of America

Norma J. Nowak
Department of Biochemistry and the New York State Center of Excellence in Bioinformatics and Life Sciences, The State University of New York at Buffalo, Buffalo, New York, United States of America
Microarray and Genomics Facility, Roswell Park Cancer Institute, Buffalo, New York, United States of America

Andreas Nellen, Daniel Heinrichs, Marie-Luise Berres, Hacer Sahin, Petra Schmitz, Christian Trautwein and Hermann E. Wasmuth
Medical Department III, University Hospital Aachen, Aachen, Germany

Amanda E. Proudfoot
Merck Serono, Geneva Research Centre, Geneva, Switzerland

Hanno Ehlken, Vangelis Kondylis, Jan Heinrichsdorff, Laura Ochoa-Callejero and Manolis Pasparakis
Institute for Genetics, Centre for Molecular Medicine (CMMC), Cologne Excellence Cluster on Cellular Stress Responses in Aging-Associated Diseases (CECAD), University of Cologne, Cologne, Germany

Tania Roskams
Department of Pathology, Catholic University of Leuven, Leuven, Belgium

Prince Kwaku Awuah, Byung Han Rhieu, Sucha Singh and Amalea Misse
Department of Pathology, University of Pittsburgh, Pittsburgh, Pennsylvania, United States of America

Satdarshan P. S. Monga
Department of Pathology, University of Pittsburgh, Pittsburgh, Pennsylvania, United States of America
Department of Medicine, University of Pittsburgh, Pittsburgh, Pennsylvania, United States of America

Henning W. Zimmermann, Sebastian Seidler, Tom Luedde, Christian Trautwein and Frank Tacke
Department of Medicine III, University Hospital, Aachen, Germany

Nikolaus Gassler
Institute of Pathology, University Hospital, Aachen, Germany,

Jacob Nattermann
Department of Medicine I, University of Bonn, Bonn, Germany

Yuxia Zhang
Department of Microbiology and Parasitology, Anhui Medical University, Hefei, Anhui, People's Republic of China

Miao Liu, Qingsi Wu, Dake Huang, Cuiping Ren, Xin Hou and Jijia Shen
Department of Microbiology and Parasitology, Anhui Medical University, Hefei, Anhui, People's Republic of China
Anhui Provincial Laboratory of Microbiology and Parasitology, Anhui Medical University, Hefei, Anhui, People's Republic of China

Peng Chen
College of Clinical Medical Sciences, Anhui Medical University, Hefei, Anhui, People's Republic of China

Berthold Büchele and Thomas Simmet
Institute of Pharmacology of Natural Products & Clinical Pharmacology, Ulm University, Ulm, Germany

Maohong Bian
Department of Blood Transfusion, The First Affiliated Hospital, Anhui Medical University, Hefei, Anhui, People's Republic of China

Shengjian Dong
Department of Clinical Laboratory, Hefei Second People's Hospital, Hefei, Anhui, People's Republic of China

Liang Peng and Geng-lin Zhang
Department of Infectious Diseases, the Third Affiliated Hospital of Sun Yat-Sen University, Guangzhou, Guangdong Province, China

Pei-pei Wang, Dong-ying Xie, Chan Xie and Zhi-liang Gao
Department of Infectious Diseases, the Third Affiliated Hospital of Sun Yat-Sen University, Guangzhou, Guangdong Province, China
Key Laboratory of Tropical Disease Control, Ministry of Education, Sun Yat-sen University, Guangzhou, Guangdong Province, China

Xu-Jing Liang
Department of Infectious Disease, the First Affiliated Hospital, Jinan University, Guangzhou, Guangdong, China

Yi-nong Ye
Department of Infectious Diseases, the First Peoples Hospital of Foshan City, Foshan, Guangdong Province, China

George M. Philips, Marzena Swiderska, Gamze F. Karaca, Cynthia Moylan, Wing-Kin Syn, Rafal P. Witek, Steve Choi, Gregory A. Michelotti and Anna Mae Diehl
Division of Gastroenterology, Department of Medicine, Duke University Medical Center, Durham, North Carolina, United States of America

Isaac S. Chan
Division of Gastroenterology, Department of Medicine, Duke University Medical Center, Durham, North Carolina, United States of America
Department of Genetics, The University of North Carolina School of Medicine, Chapel Hill, North Carolina, United States of America

Youngmi Jung
Division of Gastroenterology, Department of Medicine, Duke University Medical Center, Durham, North Carolina, United States of America
Department of Biological Science, Pusan National University, Pusan, Korea

Vanessa T. Schroder
Department of Surgery, Duke University Medical Center, Durham, North Carolina, United States of America

Cynthia Guy
Department of Pathology, Duke University Medical Center, Durham, North Carolina, United States of America

Talaignair Venkatraman, Sebastian Feuerlein, Elmar Merkle and Christopher Lascola
Department of Radiology, Duke University, Durham, North Carolina, United States of America

Fatima Rangwala
Divisions of Cell Therapy, Hematology and Medical Oncology, Duke University Medical Center, Durham, North Carolina, United States of America

M. Ujue Latasa, Raquel Urtasun, Saioa Goñi, Miriam Méndez, Nerea Juanarena, Carmen Berasain, Fernando J. Corrales and Matías A. Ávila
Division of Hepatology and Gene Therapy, CIMA, University of Navarra, Pamplona, Spain

Carmen Gil-Puig and Jon Lecanda
Division of Hepatology and Gene Therapy, CIMA, University of Navarra, Pamplona, Spain
Digna Biotech, Madrid, Spain

Maite G. Fernández-Barrena, Carlos M. Rodríguez-Ortigosa, Jesús M. Banales and Jesús Prieto
Division of Hepatology and Gene Therapy, CIMA, University of Navarra, Pamplona, Spain
CIBERehd, University Clinic, University of Navarra, Pamplona, Spain

Sara Arcelus
CIBERehd, University Clinic, University of Navarra, Pamplona, Spain

Juan A. Recio
Vall d'Hebron Research Institute, Institute of Oncology and Hospital, Barcelona, Spain

Sophie Lotersztajn
Inserm, U955, Créteil, France
Université Paris-Est, Faculté de Médecine, UMR-S955, Créteil, France

Pavel Strnad, Ozlem Kucukoglu, Mariia Lunova and Nurdan Guldiken
Department of Internal Medicine I, University Medical Center Ulm, Ulm, Germany

Tim C. Lienau
Medizinische Klinik mit Schwerpunkt Hepatologie und Gastroenterologie, Charite, Universitätsmedizin Berlin, Berlin, Germany

Felix Stickel
Department of Medicine I, University of Erlangen-Nuremberg, Erlangen, Germany

M. Bishr Omary
Department of Molecular and Integrative Physiology, University of Michigan Medical School, Ann Arbor, Michigan, United States of America

Lu Zhu, Lingdi Wang, Xiao Wang, Xiaolin Luo, Ling Yang, Rui Zhang, Hongkun Yin, Dong Xie, Yi Pan and Yan Chen
Key Laboratory of Nutrition and Metabolism, Institute for Nutritional Sciences, Shanghai Institutes for Biological Sciences, Graduate School of the Chinese Academy of Sciences, Chinese Academy of Sciences, Shanghai, China

Yoshiki Murakami
Department of Hepatology, Graduate School of Medicine, Osaka City University, Osaka, Japan

Hidenori Toyoda and Takashi Kumada
Department of Gastroenterology, Ogaki Municipal Hospital, Ogaki, Japan

Toshihito Tanahashi
Department of Medical Pharmaceutics, Kobe Pharmaceutical University, Kobe, Japan

Junko Tanaka
Department of Epidemiology, Infectious Disease Control and Prevention, Hiroshima University Graduate School of Biomedical Sciences, Hiroshima, Japan

Yusuke Yoshioka, Nobuyoshi Kosaka and Takahiro Ochiya
Division of Molecular and Cellular Medicine, National Cancer Center Research Institute, Tokyo, Japan

Y-h Taguchi
Department of Physics, Chuo University, Tokyo, Japan

Giorgio Sesti, Teresa Vanessa Fiorentino, Franco Arturi, Maria Perticone, Angela Sciacqua and Francesco Perticone
Department of Medical and Surgical Sciences, University "Magna Graecia" of Catanzaro, Catanzaro, Italy

Andrea De Gottardi, Ranka Vukotic and Sith Siramolpiwat
Hepatic Hemodynamic Laboratory, Liver Unit, Hospital Clinic, Institut d'Investigacions Biomediques August Pi i Sunyer (IDIBAPS), Barcelona, Spain

Annalisa Berzigotti, Juan G. Abraldes, Juan Carlos García-Pagan and Jaime Bosch
Hepatic Hemodynamic Laboratory, Liver Unit, Hospital Clinic, Institut d'Investigacions Biomediques August Pi i Sunyer (IDIBAPS), Barcelona, Spain
Centro de Investigación Biomédica en Red de Enfermedades Hepáticas y Digestivas (CIBERehd), University of Barcelona, Barcelona, Spain

Thijs Feuth, Joop E. Arends and Andy I. M. Hoepelman
Department of Internal Medicine and Infectious Diseases, University Medical Center Utrecht (UMCU), Utrecht, The Netherlands

Justin H. Fransen and Debbie van Baarle
Department of Internal Medicine and Infectious Diseases, University Medical Center Utrecht (UMCU), Utrecht, The Netherlands
Department of Immunology, University Medical Center Utrecht (UMCU), Utrecht, The Netherlands

Nening M. Nanlohy
Department of Immunology, University Medical Center Utrecht (UMCU), Utrecht, The Netherlands

Karel J. van Erpecum and Peter D. Siersema
Department of Gastroenterology and Hepatology, University Medical Center Utrecht (UMCU), Utrecht, The Netherlands

Salvatore Petta, Calogero Cammà, Vito Di Marco, Stefania Grimaudo, Rosaria Maria Pipitone and Antonio Craxì
Sezione di Gastroenterologia, Dipartimento Biomedico di Medicina Interna e Specialistica, University of Palermo, Palermo, Italy

Luca Miele, Stefania Boccia and Antonio Grieco
Institute of Internal Medicine, School of Medicine, Catholic University of the Sacred Heart, Rome, Italy

Elisabetta Bugianesi and Chiara Rosso
Division of Gastroenterology, Dept. of Medical Sciences, University of Turin, Turin, Italy

Daniela Cabibi
Cattedra di Anatomia Patologica, University of Palermo, Palermo, Italy

Giulio Marchesini
Dipartimento di Medicina e Gastroenterologia, "Alma Mater Studiorum," Università di Bologna, Bologna, Italy

Münevver Demir, Sonja Lang, Dirk Nierhoff, Ulrich Töx and Hans-Michael Steffen
Clinic for Gastroenterology and Hepatology, University Hospital of Cologne, Cologne, Germany

Martin Schlattjan, Jan Sowa and Ali Canbay
Clinic for Gastroenterology and Hepatology, University Hospital of Essen, Essen, Germany

Uta Drebber and Inga Wedemeyer
Institute for Pathology, University Hospital of Cologne, Cologne, Germany

Ingrid Kaul
Institute of Medical Statistics, Informatics and Epidemiology, University Hospital of Cologne, Cologne, Germany

Weijie Wang, Jiqi Yan and Huakai Wang
Department of Surgery, Ruijin Hospital, Shanghai Jiaotong University School of Medicine, Shanghai, China
Key Laboratory of Systems Biomedicine verified by Ministry of Education, Shanghai Institute of Digestive Surgery, Ruijin Hospital, Shanghai Jiaotong University School of Medicine, Shanghai, China

Weiping Yang, Chenghong Peng and Hongwei Li
Department of Surgery, Ruijin Hospital, Shanghai Jiaotong University School of Medicine, Shanghai, China

Index

www.ingramcontent.com/pod-product-compliance
Lightning Source LLC
LaVergne TN
LVHW081028210926
848485LV00004B/970